FOURTH EDITION

Group Dynamics
in Occupational Therapy

The Theoretical Basis and Practice Application of Group Intervention

FOURTH EDITION

Group Dynamics
in Occupational Therapy

The Theoretical Basis and Practice Application of Group Intervention

Marilyn B. Cole, MS, OTR/L, FAOTA

Professor Emerita of Occupational Therapy
Quinnipiac University
Hamden, Connecticut

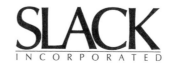

www.slackbooks.com

ISBN: 978-1-61711-011-5

Marilyn B. Cole has no financial or proprietary interest in the materials presented herein.

Group Dynamics in Occupational Therapy: The Theoretical Basis and Practice Application of Group Intervention, Fourth Edition includes ancillary materials specifically available for faculty use. Included are assignments and PowerPoint slides. Please visit www.efacultylounge.com to obtain access.

The procedures and practices described in this publication should be implemented in a manner consistent with the professional standards set for the circumstances that apply in each specific situation. Every effort has been made to confirm the accuracy of the information presented and to correctly relate generally accepted practices. The authors, editors, and publisher cannot accept responsibility for errors or exclusions or for the outcome of the material presented herein. There is no expressed or implied warranty of this book or information imparted by it. Care has been taken to ensure that drug selection and dosages are in accordance with currently accepted/recommended practice. Off-label uses of drugs may be discussed. Due to continuing research, changes in government policy and regulations, and various effects of drug reactions and interactions, it is recommended that the reader carefully review all materials and literature provided for each drug, especially those that are new or not frequently used. Some drugs or devices in this publication have clearance for use in a restricted research setting by the Food and Drug and Administration or FDA. Each professional should determine the FDA status of any drug or device prior to use in their practice.

Any review or mention of specific companies or products is not intended as an endorsement by the author or publisher.

SLACK Incorporated uses a review process to evaluate submitted material. Prior to publication, educators or clinicians provide important feedback on the content that we publish. We welcome feedback on this work.

Published by: SLACK Incorporated
                  6900 Grove Road
                  Thorofare, NJ 08086 USA
                  Telephone: 856-848-1000
                  Fax: 856-848-6091
                  www.slackbooks.com

Contact SLACK Incorporated for more information about other books in this field or about the availability of our books from distributors outside the United States.

Library of Congress Cataloging-in-Publication Data

Cole, Marilyn B.,
  Group dynamics in occupational therapy : the theoretical basis and practice application of group intervention / Marilyn B. Cole. -- 4th ed.
      p. ; cm.
  Includes bibliographical references and index.
  ISBN 978-1-61711-011-5 (alk. paper)
  1. Occupational therapy. 2. Group psychotherapy. 3. Social groups. I. Title.
  [DNLM: 1. Occupational Therapy--methods. 2. Psychotherapy, Group--methods. WM 450.5.O2]
  RC487.C65 2011
  616.89'165--dc23
                              2011025318

Printed in the United States of America.

Last digit is print number: 10   9   8   7   6   5   4   3   2

Contents

Group Dynamics in Occupational Therapy: The Theoretical Basis and Practice Application of Group Intervention, Fourth Edition includes ancillary materials specifically available for faculty use. Included are assignments and PowerPoint slides. Please visit www.efacultylounge.com to obtain access.

ACKNOWLEDGMENTS

For the *Fourth Edition*, I'd like to thank Mary Donohue, Anne Scott, Valnere McLean, Jennifer Creek, Mary Law, Mildred Ross, Ann Burkhart, Anne Golensky, and Roseanna Tufano for their feedback, contributions, editing, and helpful suggestions. A special thanks also goes to my husband, Marty, for his support and encouragement as I worked overtime to complete this project while recovering from an injury of the lumbar spine.

About the Author

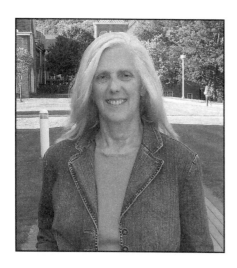

Marilyn B. (Marli) Cole, MS, OTR/L, FAOTA, is a Professor Emeritus of Occupational Therapy at Quinnipiac University, Hamden, Connecticut, and an Occupational Therapy Consultant. After 25 years of teaching, she has now become a full-time writer. She holds a bachelor's degree in English from the University of Connecticut, a graduate certificate in occupational therapy from the University of Pennsylvania, and a Master's degree in Clinical Psychology from the University of Bridgeport. Also, she is licensed by the state of Connecticut to practice occupational therapy and is certified by the Center for Study of Sensory Integrative Dysfunction to administer the Southern California Sensory Integration Tests. She has more than 24 years of practice experience in mental health, pediatrics, and geriatrics. Places of employment include Eastern Pennsylvania Psychiatric Institute in Philadelphia, and Middlesex Memorial Hospital, Lawrence and Memorial Hospitals, and Newington Children's Hospital, all in Connecticut. While teaching, courses included psychiatric clinical media, group leadership, group dynamics, frames of reference, fieldwork I and II, psychopathology, sensorimotor integration, computer technology lab, evaluation, intervention, problem-based learning, research, and geriatrics. She has also served as a consultant for the West Haven VA Medical Center, the Portland Public Schools, Fairfield Hills Hospital, the Institute of Living, St. Joseph's Manor, and Baldwin Senior Center, all in Connecticut. In conjunction with Quinnipiac University, she escorted groups of fieldwork students to clinical and community practice sites in England, Costa Rica, and Australia.

In addition to three prior editions of *Group Dynamics* (1993, 1998, 2005), she has coauthored two books within the past 3 years: *Applied Theories in OT* (2008), with coauthor Roseanna Tufano of Quinnipiac University, and *Social Participation in Occupational Contexts* (2010), with coauthor Mary Donohue, retired professor from NYU. Her chapters for other texts include "A Preference for Activity" (1988), "Client Centered Groups" (2008), "Retirement, Volunteering, and End of Life Issues" in Meriano and Latella (2007) *OT Interventions*, "Theories of Aging" (2008), and "Occupational Theory Development and Organization" in Jacobs and Sladyk (2010) *Occupational Therapy Essentials for Clinical Competence.*

Marli has presented papers and workshops at professional conferences on many different topics. She has delivered professional presentations to Yale psychiatric residents, the Connecticut Occupational Therapy Association, the New York State Occupational Therapy Association, the Centers for Disease Control and Prevention (CDC), the American Occupational Therapy Association (AOTA), the American Psychology Association (APA), the International Positive Psychology Association (IPPA), and the World Federation of Occupational Therapy (WFOT).

Recently, Marli has edited a special edition of the *Occupational Therapy International Journal* on OT in the Third Age, focusing on the transition to retirement and productive occupations of older adults worldwide. She and husband Marty are at home in Stratford, Connecticut, and Freeport, Bahamas.

INTRODUCTION

As the health-care paradigm continues to shift away from a reductionistic medical model and toward a holistic community model, occupational therapy (OT) has expanded its practice into many new community areas. The American Occupational Therapy Association (AOTA) Practice Framework-II increases the range of OT practice for clients as individuals, caregivers, organizations, and populations and incorporates wellness, prevention, advocacy, and occupational justice as potential outcomes (AOTA, 2008). OT generally embraces a positive view of health, defined in the *International Classification of Function, Disability, and Health* (ICF) as not only the absence of disease, but also life satisfaction and a sense of well-being (World Health Organization [WHO], 2001). Additionally, ICF views participation restrictions as emanating from both people and environments. In the fourth edition of *Group Dynamics in Occupational Therapy*, our use of groups for evaluation and intervention reflects elements of this evolving new OT paradigm, which is holistic, client-centered, and systems-oriented (Cole & Tufano, 2008).

In the first decade of the 21st century, OTs have become increasingly aware of environments because of the important role they play in occupational choice and engagement (Dunn, 2007; Law & Dunbar, 2007). It has long been known that participation in groups provides feedback (environment) that increases self-awareness and the experience of emotional states (Henry, Nelson, & Duncombe, 1984). Additionally, when clients make choices in group activities, this fosters a sense of competency and self-efficacy (Bandura, 1999). A sense of self-efficacy results from the complex interaction of "cognitive, affective, and biological events, behavioral patterns, and environmental events, all operating as interactive determinants that influence one another bidirectionally...self-theory encompasses self-organizing, proactive, self-reflective and self-regulative mechanisms" (Bandura, 1999, p. 21). As evidenced by this writing, complexity theory replaces the systems theory as a backdrop to our understanding of group dynamics. A sense of self-efficacy, now a central concept of many OT frames of reference and occupation-based models, is essential for a person to act with self-determination and autonomy, also recently called personal agency. If independent occupational functioning is an OT goal, then OTs need to understand the complex environmental interactions that affect the development of self-efficacy. Bandura continues: "Human agency can be exercised through direct personal agency, through agency operating through shared beliefs of efficacy, pooled understandings, group aspirations and incentive systems, and collective action...personal agency operates within a broad network of sociostructural influences. In these agentic transactions, people are producers as well as products of social systems" (1999, p. 21). In other words, a client's participation in groups helps to build self-efficacy while simultaneously influencing others and helping to shape the entire social environment.

In Section One, Acquiring Group Skills, Chapter 1 retains the original seven steps, with added sections expanding the application of leadership skills to professional leadership, focus group leadership, and team leadership. Chapter 2 adds new evidence and examples from current literature. In the new Chapter 3, Client-Centered Groups, complexity theory (Whitford et al., 2007), professional reasoning (Schell & Schell, 2008), and the role of culture (Wells & Black, 2007) are discussed, in addition to the basic principles of client-centered practice. Added to this chapter is the Canadian Model of Occupational Performance and Engagement (CMOP-E) (Townsend & Polatajko, 2007) as well as new developments in therapeutic use of self (Taylor, 2007). Activity examples in Chapter 3 focus on increasing self-awareness and self-expression. Chapter 4, renamed Groups and the OT Practice Framework-II, is newly organized around the different parts of OT's domain and process, with group examples from the recent OT literature. A six-session protocol for families with dementia, based on Schaber's (2002) application of the family FIRO model, provides an example of how Cole's seven-step format could be adapted for a home-care setting.

Section Two of the fourth edition, renamed Group Guidelines From Six Frames of Reference, is substantially updated. Using frames of reference and occupation-based models is essential to the reasoning process occupational therapists use to evaluate clients and design interventions. These chapters illustrate how Cole's seven-step format for groups can adapt to different theoretical perspectives in meeting the needs of a wide range of client populations. While these adaptations take into account different goals and levels of client ability, they do not deviate from the original client-centered focus. Evidence, new theory developments, and group examples have been added to Chapters 5 through 10. This section now includes five OT frames of reference and five occupation-based models. Chapter 10, renamed A Model of Human Occupation Approach, also includes brief descriptions of the Ecology of Human Performance (Dunn, 2007), Occupational Adaptation (OA) (Schkade & Schultz, 1994), Person-Environment-Occupation (PEO) Model (Law & Dunbar, 2007), and the Kawa Model (Iwama, 2006). Examples of groups using each of these new models have been added. It is now acceptable to incorporate one or more frames of reference within an occupation-based model. The models take a broad view of occupation, while frames of reference zero in on specific areas of disability, retaining the overall goal of participation in life through occupational engagement.

In Section Three, Planning an Occupational Therapy Group, Chapter 11 has been updated to include a wider variety of practice areas, such as wellness, prevention, and community-based settings. In this chapter, there is a greater emphasis on the process of theory application in groups. The outcomes defined by the Framework-II are occupational performance, adaptation, health and wellness, participation, quality of life, prevention, self-advocacy, and occupational justice (AOTA, 2008). The fourth edition includes the discussion of outcomes throughout the group sessions, rather than only at the end. Outcome measures have always addressed the therapeutic goals, but the new process requires that goals be derived from those verbalized by clients during the member selection process. These additions take into account a greater emphasis on collaboration with clients in every aspect of client-therapist interaction.

Chapter 12, A Group Laboratory Experience, remains unchanged, as it serves as a venue for learning about group dynamics and leadership. Chapter 13, an additional laboratory experience entitled A Group Experience: Developing Cultural Competence, has been updated with new developments in cultural competence (Black & Wells, 2007). This group protocol incorporates current research on culture from a variety of sources and presents six original structured group activities, based primarily on the cultural competence model (Black & Wells, 2007). A recent study shows that prior training, both formal and informal, was positively correlated with higher levels of cultural competence (Suarez-Balcazar et al., 2009). In the facilitation of client-centered groups, occupational therapists need cultural competence to create an atmosphere of nonjudgmental acceptance, to recognize and encourage the expression of cultural differences among members, and to maximize the value of diversity. Teaching students about culture prepares them to interact effectively with clients and others in the ever-changing multicultural world of the 21st century.

This section ends with a new chapter taking group intervention to the community in the form of service learning. Chapter 14 provides guidelines for creating a community profile, organizing and leading focus groups to determine occupation-related needs, and designing a group protocol for organizations or populations within the community. After learning the skills of group leadership, students are well-prepared to provide valuable services in new and innovative settings with the guidance of offsite faculty supervisors, demonstrating the value of occupational therapy interventions where they have not previously been available.

The use of group interventions continues to grow in practice, not only because groups are cost-effective, but because of their potential for providing social and emotional support, encouraging client participation, and motivating clients to make therapeutic changes in their occupational choices and performance. When therapeutic groups are skillfully planned, client participation in them parallels their participation in life. There is no better arena for occupational therapists to evaluate and build upon client self-efficacy, social participation, communication, and group interaction skills than while enabling their participation in a well-designed and facilitated therapeutic group.

A revised instructor's manual for the *Fourth Edition* is also available. Please visit at www.efacultylounge.com to obtain access.

REFERENCES

American Occupational Therapy Association. (2008). Occupational therapy practice framework: Domain and process, 2nd ed. *American Journal of Occupational Therapy, 62,* 625-683.

Bandura, A. (1999). Social cognitive theory: An agentic perspective. *Asian Journal of Social Psychology, 2,* 21.

Black, R., & Wells, S. (2007). *Culture and occupation: A model of empowerment in occupational therapy.* Bethesda, MD: American Occupational Therapy Association.

Cole, M., & Tufano, R. (2008) *Applied theories in occupational therapy.* Thorofare, NJ: SLACK Incorporated.

Dunn, W. (2007). Ecology of human performance model. In S. Dunbar (Ed.), *Occupational therapy models for intervention with children and families* (pp. 127-155). Thorofare, NJ: SLACK Incorporated.

Iwama, M. K. (2006). *The Kawa Model: Culturally relevant occupational therapy.* Toronto, Canada: Churchill Livingstone.

Law, M., & Dunbar, S. (2007). Person-environment-occupation model. In S. Dunbar (Ed.), *Occupational therapy models for intervention with children and families* (pp. 27-50). Thorofare, NJ: SLACK Incorporated.

Schaber, P. (2002). FIRO model: A framework for family-centered care. *Physical & Occupational Therapy in Geriatrics, 20*(4), 1-18.

Schkade, J., & Schultz, S. (1994). Occupational adaptation: Toward a holistic approach to contemporary practice, Part 2. American *Journal of Occupational Therapy, 46,* 917-926.

Schultz, S. (2010). Theory of occupational adaptation. In E. Crepeau, E. Cohn, & B. Schell (Eds.), *Willard and Spackman's Occupational Therapy* (11th ed., pp. 462-475). Philadelphia, PA: Lippincott, Williams & Wilkins.

Schell, B. B., & Schell, J. W. (2008). *Clinical and professional reasoning in occupational therapy.* Philadelphia, PA: Wolters Kluwer, Lippincott, Williams & Wilkins.

Suarez-Balcazar, Y., Rodawoski, J., Balcazar, F., Taylor-Ritzler, T., Portillo, N., Barwacz, D., & Willis, C. (2009). Perceived levels of cultural competence among occupational therapists. *American Journal of Occupational Therapy, 63,* 498-505.

Taylor, R. (2007). *The intentional relationship.* Philadelphia, PA: Lippincott, Williams & Wilkins.

Townsend, E. A., & Polatajko, H. J. (2007). *Enabling occupation II: Advancing an occupational therapy vision for health, well-being, & justice through occupation.* Ottawa, ON: Canadian Association of Occupational Therapy.

Wells, S., & Black, R. (2007). *Cultural competency for health professionals.* Bethesda, MD: American Occupational Therapy Association.

Whiteford, G., Klomp, N., & St. Clair, V. W. (2005). Complexity theory: Understanding occupation, practice and context. In G. Whiteford & V. W. St. Clair (Eds.), *Occupation & practice in context* (pp. 3-15). London, UK: Elsevier, Churchill Livingstone.

World Health Organization. (2001). *International classification of functioning, disability, and health.* Geneva, Switzerland: Author.

ACQUIRING GROUP SKILLS

INTRODUCTION

This section begins with experiential learning. Chapter 1, Group Leadership: Cole's Seven Steps, shows the beginning occupational therapy student how to lead an occupational therapy group. This format reflects a client-centered approach that facilitates client participation at every level of the process. The chapter includes many examples, learning activities, and opportunities for practice. A review of current theories of leadership paves the way for three occupational therapy leadership styles—director, facilitator, and adviser. Students can practice the seven steps by leading groups of their peers using the practice group plan at the end of the chapter. Students often work in pairs when leading groups during fieldwork experiences. Therefore, guidelines for co-leadership of groups, a more complex process, are included. In this fourth edition, a section on focus group leadership is added as an additional application of group leadership abilities. Focus groups, traditionally used in social science and marketing research, appear in recent OT literature as a useful way to assess the needs, concerns, and preferences of community groups, organizations, and populations (Fazio, 2008; Jacobs, 2010).

Chapter 2, Understanding Group Dynamics, selects from the vast body of knowledge about group dynamics those elements of groups that have the most impact for occupational therapy. An understanding of the process of groups, group development, and group norms and roles plays an integral part in the design and leadership of group activities. Guidelines on how to approach common member problem behaviors are also helpful to the beginning therapist. Learning exercises in this chapter are intended to increase awareness of the more abstract aspects of group process. This is best accomplished concurrently with experience, such as the series of six group sessions described in Chapter 12, A Group Laboratory Experience. In this way, as students absorb the content of Chapter 2, they can apply the principles directly to their own experience.

Chapter 3, Client-Centered Groups, begins with new sections on complexity theory (Whiteford, Klomp, & St. Clair, 2005), clinical/professional reasoning (Schell & Schell, 2008), and the Canadian Model of Occupational Performance (Townsend & Polatajko, 2007). It then summarizes the basic concepts of client-centered practice as they apply to occupational therapy group leadership. Concepts such as respect, genuineness, and non-judgmental acceptance form a central core for group facilitation using Cole's seven-step format. Many of the basic assumptions are similar to the humanistic approach described in previous editions. This chapter includes skill-building exercises for the therapeutic use of self during group leadership. An outline of Cole's seven steps discusses ways in which each step applies client-centered principles.

Chapter 4, Groups and the OT Practice Framework-II, reflects the expanded use of group interventions implied in the domain and process of OT practice (American Occupational Therapy Association, 2008). Its content discusses the design and leadership of occupational therapy groups in family, work, school, social, and community group contexts. Several theoretical sections, such as role theory, culture change, social support, and teams, provide evidence of the expanded role of occupational therapy groups in community and nontraditional settings. A series of six family group interventions is given as an example. Donohue's Social Profile (Cole & Donohue, 2010; Donohue, 2003) provides an evaluation tool for Mosey's five levels of group interaction skills (Mosey, 1986; see Appendix C). This tool can apply to individual members or collectively to both therapeutic groups and naturally occurring groups in the community.

Professional leadership, promoted in the OT Centennial Vision (Moyers, 2007), implies application of OT group leadership skills in team leadership, advocacy, and community interventions to promote social change and facilitate occupational justice, all new directions implied in the Framework-II.

REFERENCES

American Occupational Therapy Association. (2008). *Occupational therapy practice framework: Domain and process, 2nd ed.* American Journal of Occupational Therapy, 62, 625-683.

Cole, M. B., & Donohue, M. (2010). *Social participation in occupational contexts: In clinics, schools, and communities.* Thorofare, NJ: SLACK Incorporated.

Donohue, M. (2003). Group profile: Studies with children: Validity measures and item analysis. *Occupational Therapy in Mental Health, 19,* 1-23.

Fazio, L. (2010). Health promotion program development. In M. Scaffa, S. M. Reita, & M. Pizzi (Eds.), *Occupational therapy in the promotion of health and wellness* (pp. 195-207). New York, NY: F. A. Davis.

Jacobs, K. (2010). Systems to organize and market occupational therapy. In K. Sladyk, K. Jacobs, & N. MacRae (Eds.), *Occupational therapy essentials for clinical competence* (pp. 389-395). Thorofare, NJ: SLACK Incorporated.

Mosey, A. C. (1986) Psychosocial components of occupational therapy. New York, NY: Press.

Moyers, P. (2007). A legacy of leadership: Achieving our centennial vision. *American Journal of Occupational Therapy, 61,* 622-628.

Schell, B. B., & Schell, J. W. (2008). *Clinical and professional reasoning in occupational therapy.* Philadelphia, PA: Wolters Kluwer, Lippincott, Williams & Wilkins.

Townsend, E. A., & Polatajko, H. J. (2007). *Enabling occupation II: Advancing an occupational therapy vision for health, well-being & justice through occupation.* Ottawa, ON: Canadian Association of Occupational Therapy.

Whiteford, G., Klomp, N., & St. Clair, V. W. (2005). Complexity theory: Understanding occupation, practice and context. In G. Whiteford & V. W. St. Clair (Eds.), *Occupation & practice in context* (pp. 3-15). London, UK: Elsevier, Churchill Livingstone.

Chapter 1

GROUP LEADERSHIP
COLE'S SEVEN STEPS

Initially, students often learn best by experience. They are anxious to know how to "do" occupational therapy. They are both eager and afraid to begin working with clients. To the beginning student, occupational therapy is just a label. Only when students are put in the role of a professional do they become aware of what needs to be learned.

Acting like a professional is often difficult for students, whose only experience in group leadership is often with groups of their peers. Part of making the transition to a professional role is learning that it is different from a social role. Professionalism carries with it an authority and a directness of purpose that will need to be practiced by students before they begin interacting with clients.

This book begins with a technique that is a concrete form of group leadership training. This allows students to practice the role of a professional. It is as generic as any technique can be and is intended as a beginning experience for students entering the profession. As the educational process continues, it is expected that the technique will be modified many times over to match the needs of each unique group. It is changed in content to meet new goals and address different age groups and health conditions. It is changed in process and structure to align with different professional models and frames of reference.

Depending on the goals and contexts, these seven steps may occur in different sequence from the one presented here. Aside from introduction, activity, and summary, the experienced leader allows the group to flow naturally and self-organize, making sure the necessary elements of processing, sharing, generalization, and application are appropriately addressed. The seven-step model is holistic and incorporates the basic "dynamic occupation and client-centered process of the American Occupational Therapy Association (AOTA) Framework-II, promoting health and participation of people, organizations, and populations through engagement in occupation" (AOTA, 2008, p. 626). All seven-step group interventions described in this text are client centered. The primary purpose for which this method of group facilitation was designed is to enable the participation of members in doing a shared task or activity and to reflect upon its meaning for each of them. Every step in the process calls for the group leader's therapeutic use of self to enact the principles of client-centered practice. While the seven steps can be adapted for use with different frames of reference and occupation-based models, their basic approach remains client centered. Chapter 3 reviews some basic principles of client-centered occupational therapy practice as they relate to group interventions.

But, learning has to begin somewhere. Therefore, it is recommended that students practice the seven steps in their original sequence, even though it may seem somewhat stilted. Just as motor development precedes cognitive awareness in the infant, a concrete experience in group leadership becomes the forerunner of the knowledge and understanding of its purpose and application in practice.

Leading therapy groups represents only one of many applications for the leadership skills inherent in the seven steps. Professional leadership includes participation in professional organizations and promoting the OT profession with others and with the public. Focus group

Cole M.B. *Group Dynamics in Occupational Therapy:*
The Theoretical Basis and Practice Application
of Group Intervention (pp 3-28).
© 2012 SLACK Incorporated.

leadership has been added because of its usefulness in assessing the needs of community groups and populations and its role in marketing OT programs (in addition to its use in qualitative research). Some more advanced leadership skills apply in professional leadership, such as group decision-making strategies and conflict resolution. These leader roles supplement the basic skills in therapeutic use of self, which are covered in Chapter 3.

SEVEN-STEP FORMAT FOR GROUP LEADERSHIP (COLE'S SEVEN-STEP GROUPS)

These seven steps can meet the needs of the highest level groups and so are very appropriate for student groups. They are chosen for maximum integration of learning by the members. Clearly, this format will not fit every need, goal, or client population. However, the format is easily adapted to meet the goals of any group. How and why it will be modified will be described later. The steps in group leadership are as follows:

1. Introduction
2. Activity
3. Sharing
4. Processing
5. Generalizing
6. Application
7. Summary

The original idea for this format comes from Pfeiffer and Jones' *Reference Guide to Handbooks and Annuals* (1977), which presents a five-step format that is expanded and adapted for occupational therapy here.

Step 1: Introduction

Let us assume the occupational therapist is leading the initial session of a group. The therapist does not know the members well, although it is presumed he or she knows who they are and something about their disability and the reasons they have been assigned to the group. (In many settings, the occupational therapist would select the members himself or herself.) The members may not know one another. Once the group is gathered, the occupational therapist introduces himself or herself to the group. This introduction includes the therapist's name and title and the name of the group that is about to begin. Then, even if people know one another, the therapist asks the members to greet the group by saying their names in turn. This procedure does more than just help the members learn one another's names; it acknowledges their membership in the group and invites them to be a part of it. In subsequent groups, it

may not be necessary to say names around the room, but each member's presence should still be acknowledged. A friendly "hello" or "welcome back" from the therapist may accomplish this.

Warm-Up

The next thing the leader should be concerned with is the receptivity of the members. How alert are they? How preoccupied are they? How are they feeling? Are members ready to begin a new experience, or do they need to be "warmed up"? A warm-up is an exercise that captures the group's attention, relaxes them, and prepares them for the experience to follow. Warm-ups can be structured or casual and impromptu. An example of a structured warm-up is, "Grandma's Trunk" (Rider & Rider, 2000). Each member says, "Grandma has an old trunk up in the attic and in it I found _____." Members fill in the blank by saying the name of something that begins with each letter of the alphabet in order. All items must be repeated each time. For example, the first person says she found an acorn, the second found an acorn and a bonnet, etc. If there are eight members of the group, the eighth one must remember the seven items preceding his or her contribution.

This warm-up obviously requires members to have a good short-term memory. The occupational therapist should choose a warm-up that challenges members enough to hold their interest but is not beyond their capabilities. Warm-up activities accomplish several important goals. The game creates an atmosphere of spontaneity and fun. It also refocuses members' thoughts from whatever they came to the group thinking about to this group right here, right now. If a warm-up works properly, it gets the members listening for what will come next and encourages their cooperation in the group experience to follow.

All groups do not need a formal warm-up. Sometimes, the best warm-up is a casual conversation about how members are feeling today. If the group is to engage in a discussion, just getting the members talking may prepare them adequately. If the agenda is more creative in nature, an imaginative warm-up may be in order. Remembering what happened last week may be an appropriate warm-up to an activity that will be the next step in a sequence. It is important to make the warm-up relevant to the activity to follow. One does not set a mood of fun and games when the agenda for the group is a serious issue like coping with loss or finding new employment.

Setting the Mood

Setting an appropriate mood is an important objective in choosing the most appropriate warm-up. However, setting the mood for a group is not only accomplished with a warm-up. The environment, the therapist's facial expression and manner of speaking, and the media used all contribute to the mood. Care should be taken before the group begins to set up the environment accordingly; this includes proper lighting, getting rid of clutter, setting out equipment, supplies, and the correct number of chairs, and avoiding distractions as much as possible.

Expectation of the Group

The therapist's manner and expression should generally reflect his or her expectation of the group. A therapist cannot expect group members to take an activity seriously if the therapist does not appear to do so. The therapist will always be a role model to members, whether or not it is his or her intention. If the therapist begins by saying, "Okay you guys, listen up!" the members will be expecting a pep talk before a football game, rather than a serious discussion about managing their time. A direct and authoritative presentation of the group is one of those skills students must learn that make up the role of the professional.

Explaining the Purpose Clearly

Clearly explaining the purpose of the group is a primary task in the introduction phase. How this is done depends on the type of group and the clients' level of understanding. This is a step that should never be left out. The intent of the group and why he or she was assigned to this particular group has undoubtedly been explained individually to each member. But it should not be taken for granted that the clients remember, or even fully understand, the purpose of a group from a previous explanation. The purpose should be reiterated by the occupational therapist in a way clients are likely to understand. A higher-level group of clients will want to know why they are being asked to perform a particular activity. If they are asked to do calisthenics, it will be helpful to tell them that physical exercise has been known to change brain chemistry, to relieve stress, to elevate their mood, and to energize their muscles. Clients who understand and believe this will be much more motivated to participate.

Clients with mild to moderate cognitive disability are unlikely to understand such abstract explanations of purpose. For them, a modified explanation, such as, "These exercises will make you feel better so you can do more for yourself," may suffice. For clients with severe cognitive disability, a friendly expression and a gentle touch that says, "Trust me, this will help you," may be all it takes to engage them in the group activity (Allen, 1999; Allen, Earhart, & Blue, 1992).

We started out assuming that the occupational therapist is introducing a new group experience to a new set of clients. In an initial session, more time is taken in explaining the purpose than in subsequent sessions. In describing the purpose of the group, the goals of the whole series of group sessions should be outlined in the initial session. If possible, the goals should be spelled out in concrete terms. For example, money management is an activity of daily living that occupational therapists often help clients work on improving. In a money management group, members may be expected to plan and carry out a realistic budget for 1 month and keep accurate records in a notebook. Therapists often use behavior change as a measure of progress in their clients. When clients are informed about the behavior that is expected to change, they can keep track of their own progress. This becomes motivating when clients in groups start measuring each other's behavior change (or lack thereof). Peer pressure is a powerful motivator of change in human behavior.

Describing the purpose of each session will not take as much time as the initial explanation. However, the goals for each activity should always be stated clearly at the beginning of each session. Clients need to be reminded of how the group is expected to help them. As the therapist gets to know the members better, explanations can be more individualized and related to the problems each member presents. For example, in introducing a stress-management session, the therapist might mention that, "In the previous sessions, you've been complaining about how difficult it is to carry out daily activities when you're feeling so much stress. Today's activity will give you some new strategies for reducing the stress in your lives." Generally, when clients understand exactly how an activity will help them, they are much more interested in doing it.

Brief Outline of the Session

Finally, the introduction ends with a brief outline of the session to immediately follow. The time frame, the media, and the procedures are included. For example, if the activity for a 1-hour session is "draw yourself," the therapist might say, "We will be using the paper and markers provided to do a drawing for the next 20 minutes. After we are finished, I will ask each of you to explain your drawing to the group, and we will discuss the activity for the last half of the session." This explanation serves several purposes. It tells the client how long he or she has to complete the activity. A complex artistic drawing cannot be done in 20 minutes, so if he or she is to finish, he or she knows he or she must keep it simple. The explanation also warns him or her that he or she probably should not draw anything he or she does not wish to discuss. Although this may be seen as inhibiting the client's creativity, it also allows him or her to control the image of himself or herself that he or she projects to the group. How the therapist handles this will depend on the goal of the activity. If self-awareness is more important than social awareness, the clients may be given the option not to explain everything about their drawing. They need only say as much as they are comfortable sharing.

As well as understanding the purpose of the drawing activity, clients will want to know what is to be done with it afterward. When they know they will be expected to talk about their work, their drawing may be more focused, and they will be more prepared to speak when it is their turn. It may be helpful to tell clients ahead of time whether their drawings will be kept by the therapist or if they can keep them. The disposition of drawings produced will differ depending on the goals and the frame of reference used. However, stating the procedures ahead of time is most respectful to the client and may also prevent difficulties later in the session.

The brief outline of the session also gives members a clue to the session's focus. The example given tells clients that the activity portion is relatively short (20 minutes) compared with the discussion portion (at least 30 minutes). Members will see that the focus is on the discussion rather than the drawing and on learning and interaction rather than artistic talent. The outline helps clients and therapists get the whole session in perspective.

The introduction is one of the steps that is consistently kept in every frame of reference and every type of group. The structure may become less formal, with practice, but the essential elements must remain. An introduction can make or break a group, and each element plays a part in the effectiveness of group outcome.

Step 2: Activity

Many factors should be considered when planning the activity. In a professional setting, this is, in fact, a tremendously complex process. It incorporates all we know about clients, health conditions, and their corresponding dysfunctions, assessment, intervention planning, activity analysis and synthesis, and group dynamics. Selecting a therapeutic activity involves the entire process of clinical reasoning that occupational therapists take 2 or 3 years of academic training to learn. One of the problems in learning group technique before the theory is that the process will seem oversimplified and incomplete. However, students should have a positive experience in trying out the role of an occupational therapist, even though there is much more to be learned before they can adequately do it in the clinic or community.

Designing the group experience is a very complex process, and many issues should be considered. All of them cannot be addressed here. For the purposes of simplification, the following issues will be presented for consideration in selecting a therapeutic activity: timing, therapeutic goals, physical and mental capacities of the members, knowledge and skill of the leader, and adaptation of an activity. When leading client-centered groups, clients will participate in the activity selection whenever possible, according to their occupational needs and priorities.

Timing

With five more steps to go (sharing, processing, generalizing, application, and summary), it should be evident that the activity to be experienced should be kept fairly simple and short. This will vary, of course, but for our purposes in learning to plan and lead groups, the activity portion should last no longer than one-third of the total session. For example, in this seven-step process, for a 1-hour group, the activity used must be adapted to fit a time frame of 15 to 20 minutes and to meet a preset therapeutic goal.

Therapeutic Goals

It is impossible to plan an activity without first planning and structuring the goals. Goals are desired outcomes, something clients and therapists strive together to accomplish. Setting therapeutic goals for clients involves assessing their needs and applying our knowledge of their abilities and disabilities. The referral source, such as the hospital treatment team, the doctor, or the nursing home staff, may have already defined the problem (e.g., "This client needs to develop adequate social skills" or "Help client to learn joint protection and energy conservation techniques"). In planning our practice groups for peers, the student might first think about what goals might be useful for himself or herself. Perhaps coping with stress, setting priorities, clarifying values, managing money, managing time, and asserting oneself in social situations may be troublesome areas for students. The group goals should be chosen to meet the needs of most of the members. Once the goal is defined, an activity is designed or selected to help members achieve that goal. For example, when goals have to do with personal growth, for example, creative activities such as drawing, sculpture, dramatics, and storytelling can be helpful. Through the creative process, many parts of the self can be revealed and explored. If goals are more socially oriented, structured group tasks involving interaction of the members are appropriate (e.g., communication exercises or group decision-making and problem-solving).

Physical and Mental Capacities of the Members

Selection of the activity or experience is further determined by the physical and mental capacities of the members. If members are college students around age 20, without physical or mental disabilities, the possibilities are almost unlimited. The challenge would be to find an activity that holds their interest and from which they can learn something new and meaningful. When members of the group are geriatric clients, the physical and fine motor components of the activity may be limited. A game of balloon volleyball or a lively discussion about a topic of interest might be suitable. When cognitive limitations must be taken into account, the activity will need to be more physical and concrete (not abstract) in nature. Cooking, simple crafts, and games are often useful activities with adult clients who have developmental

Table 1-1

Activity Analysis Example—Playing a Game of Bingo

Activity Components	Skills Needed
A number and letter are called	Client must hear the call and associate it with written letters and numbers
The bingo card is scanned	Client must read and understand written letters and numbers
A marker is placed on the number called	Client must have hand-eye coordination, fine motor skills, grasp and release
When a row of five is marked, calls out "Bingo" loudly	Client must have good visual perception and must be able to speak

delays or cognitive limitations. Assessment of the physical and mental functioning of an individual client is the subject of other textbooks in occupational therapy, and so will not be covered here. In the clinical setting, assessment would be done on each member prior to starting the group.

Knowledge and Skill of the Leader

Another factor in the activity selection process is the knowledge and skill of the leader. What activities that are familiar to the leader can be adapted to this group experience? Student leaders usually choose activities for the group that they themselves are comfortable with or have done before. A student who has had dance lessons may feel very comfortable introducing a movement activity; a leader with artistic talent may choose a drawing activity. Crafts, games, and educational or social experiences may be sources of familiar activities to be adapted. There are a wealth of resource books available offering ideas for structured experiences in human relations. An example is Rider and Rider's *The Activity Card Book for Mental Health* (2000), which is updated every few years. When using these references, it should be kept in mind that most of the exercises cannot be done as written but will have to be adapted to the specific goals set by the occupational therapist.

Adaptation of an Activity

Adaptation of an activity requires some knowledge of activity analysis and synthesis. Activity analysis is the "process of examining an activity to distinguish its component parts. Activity synthesis is the process of combining component parts of the human and non-human environment so as to design an activity suitable for evaluation or intervention relative to performance" (Mosey, 1981, p. 114). The analysis of activities is the subject of other textbooks and will not be fully described here. This is yet another example of the complex process of clinical reasoning in occupational therapy, in bringing together concepts from many bodies of knowledge to influence our intervention choices.

Activity analysis is the breaking down of an activity into its component parts and matching each part with the human functions required to accomplish it. Playing bingo, for example, may be analyzed as shown in Table 1-1.

In this oversimplified illustration, the therapist must know 1) how to play bingo and 2) what physical and mental skills are required to play. Knowing this, the client's skill is matched with what is required to do the activity. Modifications can then be made in the activity to suit the client's abilities. This is activity synthesis. For example, a group of clients with poor vision may need bingo cards with larger letters and numbers and bright-colored markers. A hearing-impaired group will need to have the calls written on a blackboard or flashed on a screen. Clients with poor motor control may need a bingo card with magnetic markers that will stay in place even if the card is moved. Higher-functioning groups may need more challenging requirements to win, such as markers all around the edge or in the shape of an "H" or an "S." Additional motivation may be built in by offering appealing prizes.

Once selected, the therapeutic activity should be presented in a systematic way. First, the activity should be explained as directly and simply as possible. Procedures and instructions are given in language appropriate to the level and background of the group.

The therapist should get feedback from the group as to whether they understood the directions and should answer any questions before proceeding. Materials and supplies, if needed, should be hidden from view until they are actually needed. As the activity is in progress, the therapist may choose to participate in order to avoid making members feel self-conscious or watched. However, a leader should not allow his or her participation to detract from making relevant observations of the group to be discussed later.

When the activity portion of the group is finished, any materials used, such as pencils or paints, should be collected and placed out of sight before moving to the discussion stages. This will avoid having some members continue working after time is up or be distracted by the extraneous items. It may be necessary to stop some individuals before they are finished in order to keep the group moving along. The leader needs to be prepared to continually adapt and structure the group.

Step 3: Sharing

After completing the activity, each member is invited to share his or her own work or experience with the group. The structure and process for sharing will vary with each activity. If the activity involves drawing or writing something individually, members will show the drawing and explain it to the group or read to the group what was written. In activities involving interaction, members share what the experience was like for them or what it meant to them. In either case, the therapist is responsible for making sure each member has a chance to do this.

Another important responsibility in this phase is to make sure each member's contribution is acknowledged. Acknowledgment may be done verbally or nonverbally. Sometimes, just a smile and a nod may be all that is necessary. Members often want to respond to one another's sharing, but the therapist may need to model this to be sure the responses show caring and concern. Empathy is an important factor here. This means the therapist responds to the client in a way that communicates understanding of how the client feels. Empathy will be discussed in more depth in a later chapter.

Some members may be reluctant to share for various reasons. The therapist may need to support and encourage clients to share or to reassure them that they can do it without negative consequence. However, if a client refuses to share, this must be accepted; clients should not be unduly pressured to disclose anything about themselves that they do not feel comfortable sharing.

It does not matter in what order the members share, but often it is easier to keep track if members go in order around the circle. It is usually best to ask for a volunteer to start the process, so that clients feel some control over the group. However, the therapist can start to role model for the group what is expected to be shared. For example, in the "Best Friend" exercise from Pfeiffer and Jones (1973), the therapist might begin by getting up and standing behind a chair and saying, "This is my best friend Beth (indicating an invisible self in the empty chair). She's a person who likes cooking healthy food, doing creative projects, and helping other people. Her pet peeve is people who smoke. She has always wanted to write a book... etc." The therapist models the format the members will use in sharing (Worksheet 1-1).

There are a few activities for which sharing is not a separate step but is incorporated into a discussion activity. For example, "The Doctor's Dilemma" is a group decision-making task that involves extensive discussion as part of the activity. Expressing one's opinion on a given issue is built into the actual task. In this case, the therapist may be more involved during the activity to make sure all of the members participate and express their views and that their responses to one another are respectful and courteous.

Step 4: Processing

This is the most difficult step for students to learn. Inexperienced group leaders often skip this step entirely. Processing involves members expressing how they feel about the experience, the leader, and each other. Feelings guide our behavior more than we know, and they certainly influence clients' behavior in occupational therapy groups. If these emotions remain unexpressed, the outcome of the group can never be fully understood. Expressing feelings is not so difficult when the experience has been positive. But if there are negative feelings, people often wish to avoid expressing them, and this includes both the group members and the leader.

Done correctly, processing can reveal some important and relevant information. If members felt anxious, embarrassed, or belittled while doing an activity, this will help to explain some of their responses when sharing and discussing it. Perhaps they felt intimidated by the leader or angry with some of the other members. Feelings like this can override any possible benefit the activity may have, if they are not expressed before the group ends. When they are expressed, the therapist has the opportunity to incorporate them into the subsequent discussion and to help the clients understand the significance of the feelings related to the group experience. From the OT Framework-II perspective, this process helps to identify issues that encourage or discourage "engagement in occupation" or emotions that facilitate or present "barriers to participation" (AOTA, 2008).

Processing also includes a discussion of the nonverbal aspects of group. Underlying issues, such as struggles for power and control, subgrouping, scapegoating, conflict, attraction, and avoidance, are dynamics that may never be verbalized but will have a powerful influence on the group. These issues are highly complex for the beginning student; however, they should be well-understood by the beginning therapist. Underlying dynamics such as those mentioned can and do occur naturally in all groups. They will strongly influence the outcome of our occupational therapy groups, both positively and negatively, and must be handled openly and skillfully. More will be discussed about the underlying process of groups in a later chapter.

Step 5: Generalizing

This step addresses the cognitive learning aspects of the group. Here, the therapist mentally reviews the group's responses to the activity and tries to sum them up with a few general principles. If the activity has gone as expected, some of the general principles derived

Worksheet 1-1
Best Friend Introduction Sheet

Directions: Answer the questions as you would expect your best friend to describe you.

This is my best friend _____ (your name).

He or she is the kind of person who likes:

1.

2.

3.

He or she greatly appreciates and values:

1.

2.

3.

Some of his or her dislikes or pet peeves are:

1.

2.

3.

Someday, he or she would like to:

1.

2.

3.

from the group should closely resemble the original goals. However, few groups go exactly as planned. The general principles discussed in the group should not be preplanned but should come directly from the response of the members.

For example, an occupational therapist did an activity called "Incomplete Sentences" with a group of emotionally disturbed adolescents. The goal of the group was to clarify their values, and, in fact, the group did accomplish this. However, some additional principles were brought up during the processing phase, which are important to note. Principles of the "Incomplete Sentences" group are the following:

- The members generally value making decisions independent of their parents.

- The most valued activities were those the members chose to do themselves, such as sleeping late on Saturdays or buying their own clothes.

- Although wishing to be independent, members generally needed and wanted to be accepted by their parents as autonomous adults.

The third principle is the one not planned. During the processing phase, a member pointed out how good it was to be able to ask the leader to complete the sentences, too. The group felt positive toward this leader, who, unlike their parents, seemed to accept them as equals. The comment brought forth many spontaneous stories of parental nonacceptance, and it was evident that this was the important issue for the group.

General principles may be arrived at in several ways. The leader can look at the patterns of response among members. What opinions do they have in common? What were the common elements of their drawings or stories? For example, people with alcohol abuse may see their drinking as the obstacle to reaching their vocational ambitions; bottles or glasses may appear in their drawings, or they may talk about highly unrealistic vocational ambitions. These common elements are easily seen as general principles.

Another way to distinguish general principles is to look at areas of disagreement. What are the conflicted areas in the group? Some members, for example, may see stress as a motivator to get moving, while others may find it overwhelming and the cause of their inaction.

A third important clue to the general principles is the group's energy. The therapist should follow up on issues that seem to energize the group and stimulate spontaneous conversation. An example is the third principle in the "Incomplete Sentences" activity mentioned earlier. This is one of those unpredictable aspects of groups that makes them continually exciting and interesting.

Step 6: Application

The application phase closely follows the generalizing phase, but takes it one step further. The therapist helps the group to understand how the principles learned during the group can be applied to everyday life. The goal is for each member to understand how he or she will apply the results of this group experience to help make his or her own life more functional outside the group.

To begin this process, the therapist should attempt to verbalize the meaning or significance of the experience—"Now that we know how important it is to have our parents' respect and acceptance, each of us needs to find a way to communicate this need to our parents." Application answers the question, "Now that you know how things are, what are you going to do about it?"

The answer to this question will be different for each individual. Knowledge of the client's background is helpful. The therapist discusses with each member how the principles learned in the group relate to problems or issues each has expressed earlier. For example, Sue will have a hard time explaining to her father, who thinks of her as a child, that she needs for him to trust her judgment about whom she dates and where she goes on Saturday nights. Laura, whose mother travels extensively on business, will have difficulty just getting her mom's attention long enough to talk about it. She sometimes wonders if her mother cares about her enough to take the time. Both girls will have difficulty in communicating with their parents, but in very different ways. Application may sometimes resemble a kind of group problem solving as members help each other find ways to apply the newly learned information. In client-centered terms, this part of the group's session encourages collaboration. In the OT Framework-II (AOTA, 2008), application addresses how the group learning will facilitate "participation in life."

One way the therapist can help the group with application is through limited self-disclosure. The therapist can role-model application by saying, "When I need to discuss something with my mother and there never seems to be a good time, sometimes I suggest we make a date to go out to dinner together. She has to eat anyway and so do I, so that plan works well for both of us. How do you see that?" The self-disclosure is not so personal as to be distracting, but offers a possible method of getting parents' attention for the group to consider. It gives group members a concrete example and opens the door for them to make their own suggestions.

Step 7: Summary *(Group Closure)*

The final phase of the seven-step group is the summary. The purpose of the summary is to verbally emphasize the most important aspects of the group so that they will be understood correctly and remembered. Like generalizing, there is really no way to preplan a summary. The points to emphasize should come directly from the group's responses. A good summary may take 4 or 5 minutes. It reviews the goals, the content, and the process of the group. Sometimes, the therapist asks the group members to help summarize by remembering the activity and giving their ideas about what was learned. The general principles are almost always included in the summary. Having members explain their own views of the group and how it can be applied often reinforces the learning that took place.

The emotional content of the group is also important to summarize. Especially when the group feels positive or the mood has changed for the better, verbal recognition of the good feelings by the therapist will help members remember the group as a positive experience.

One way for the therapist to acknowledge feelings is to thank the members for their participation in the group. While this is not a formula, addressing and thanking individuals for their openness, honesty, and willingness to share or trust in the group is always welcomed.

A final responsibility of the therapist is to end the group on time. If the group is well-planned and well-led, this will mark the completion of all seven steps. If, for some reason, all the steps have not been completed by the end of the session, the missing parts and the reasons for this can also be dealt with in the summary.

Before leaving the "how to" section, two more functions of group leadership will be addressed: group motivation and setting limits. OT leaders should apply these important skills throughout the seven steps as they are needed.

Group Motivation

Ideally, the therapist will have a group that comes to meetings with enthusiasm and interest to participate. Such a group will be eager to listen to the therapist and take direction. A group that is motivated will interact freely with one another, will share with one another easily, and will spontaneously seek to know the meaning of the group activity and how it can be applied. Such a group is probably too healthy to need therapy. Therefore, the leader needs to develop skills in how to motivate groups that may not be so eager.

Confidence in the Leader

An important factor in the group's motivation is its confidence in the leader. If the leader takes charge of the group with some authority and sounds like he or she knows what to do, the leader will inspire the group's confidence and trust. This confidence is further enhanced by the support and encouragement offered to the members. If clients feel that the therapist empathizes with them and understands their situation, they will tend to be more cooperative in accepting leadership. Trust is the important issue here. Clients need to feel that the leader is sensitive to them and that he or she can and will respond to their needs. They also need to know the leader is in control in order to feel safe.

Encouraging Enthusiasm

A leader also motivates the group members by encouraging their enthusiasm. This can be done in a number of ways. First, the leader can show enthusiasm for the group both verbally and nonverbally. A leader who smiles and speaks in a lively tone, makes frequent eye contact, and demonstrates energetic movements often passes on enthusiasm to the group. Talking to members individually and encouraging them to participate may be effective. The approach to clients has to be adapted to the cognitive level of the clients. An explanation of how the group will make a difference in their lives will work for higher-level clients. A more immediate benefit may need to be offered to lower-functioning clients (e.g., "Doing this activity will make you feel more relaxed"). Activities such as games or creative efforts chosen for the group may stimulate enthusiasm. Some activities will have built-in rewards (e.g., cooking groups and craft groups).

Encouraging Interaction

A final motivating factor is encouraging group interaction. It has been said that people get as much out of a group activity as they put into it. When group members are interacting with one another, they are not only participating, but also taking over some of the responsibility for the group. Interaction should be encouraged, especially in the sharing, processing, generalizing, and application phases of the group. A good leader allows the group members to share the leadership to the extent that they are capable. If they can support one another during sharing, express how they feel about one another during processing, notice similarities and differences during generalizing, and offer ideas to each other about application, they will then learn a lot more than if the leader does all these things for them. The leader can get the group to interact by indirectly encouraging them or by asking them to do so directly; the leader might ask, "Susan, what do you think of Peter's drawing?" or "Peter, what do you think the group had in common?" Often, the leader only needs to ask questions a few times in order for the group to understand what is expected.

A leader who does all the talking in the seven-step group is working too hard. It benefits both the leader and the group by getting the group to talk more. Members who interact, respond, and ask questions are showing their enthusiasm and helping others to become enthusiastic also. With the leader's guidance, the group can help accomplish many of its goals through interaction.

Setting Limits

This has to do with how the leader exerts authority over the group. The goal is to achieve a balance between control and leniency. Some of the ways to set limits in OT groups are assuming appropriate authority, giving members equal time to participate, limiting inappropriate behaviors, and respectful limit setting.

Assuming Appropriate Authority

The leader should assume appropriate authority, guiding the group through all of its stages, while giving members the freedom to express their thoughts, feelings, and opinions. A good leader will guide the group assuredly but will not dominate or intimidate its members. Neither does a good leader allow himself or herself to be dominated by the group. If the group goes its own way unguided, the members will not learn and make therapeutic change, and the group may never reach its goals.

Equal Time

Another part of setting limits is allowing sufficient time for each member to contribute. There are always a few members of a group who seem to take up more time and attention than the others. It is up to the therapist to see that all the members have a chance to participate. The leader controls the pace of the group and lets members know when they are taking more than their share of the time available. In this way, the group can be guided through each stage and can end on time.

Limiting Inappropriate Behavior

Limiting inappropriate behavior is perhaps the most difficult for students to learn. It generally requires that the leader interrupt the process going on in order to request that it be changed. If Joe has embarked on a lengthy discussion about a staff member who has treated him unfairly, but the issue has nothing to do with the goals of the group, it may be necessary for the leader to stop him and redirect the group back to the task at hand.

Respectful Limit Setting

Limits are best set with respect, and without anger, so that the group members will not become defensive. The therapist should develop skill in empathizing with the offending client. When the leader asks Joe to stop his tirade about the staff member, it is more likely to be heard if he or she first acknowledges his anger: "Joe, it sounds like you're very angry at _____, and I'd be happy to listen to you tell me about it after the group. But for now, I'd like to hear what all the members have to say about leisure planning." Other types of inappropriate behavior might be members showing disrespect for or disinterest in one another or physical expressions of emotion.

One important principle to keep in mind is always put the good of the group first. When individuals behave in ways that distract the group from benefiting in an occupational therapy activity, the leader is obligated to intervene on behalf of the group. Techniques for dealing with specific client behaviors that are difficult will be discussed in the next chapter.

THEORIES OF GROUP LEADERSHIP

The leadership style a therapist uses will profoundly affect the outcome of the group. Furthermore, different frames of reference require very different leadership approaches. Knowing the characteristics of several approaches and their likely effects on the group allows us to be flexible and use our skills more effectively to achieve desired outcomes. This section will review several theories from social psychology and will propose three basic leadership approaches for OT groups: directive, facilitative, and advisory.

General Theories of Group Leadership

Lewin

According to Lewin and colleagues (Lewin & Lippitt, 1938; Lewin, Lippitt, & White, 1939), there are three fundamental leadership styles: autocratic, democratic, and laissez-faire. Autocratic leadership implies complete control of the group with little or no input from the members. Democratic leadership allows members to make choices and to have a say in what the group does and becomes. Laissez-faire is a French expression meaning literally "to let do" or to let the people do as they choose. Laissez-faire leadership implies a minimum of control and a deliberate noninterference in the natural forces of a group or the freedom of individuals within it. Lewin studied the effects of these three styles of leadership at a boys' summer camp. He found that autocratic leadership resulted in the greatest productivity, but created hostility and resentment, poor quality of work, and dependency on the leader. Laissez-faire leadership produced independence in the members, but morale was not very high. It was democratic leadership that resulted in the highest morale and the most group cohesiveness. However, Lewin's study should be understood in the context of the boys' camp. The democratic style that worked best for campers may not work for other populations, and other styles may be more appropriate.

Situational Leadership

Situational leadership, developed from studies of work-management practices (Hersey & Blanchard, 1969; Hersey, Blanchard, & Johnson, 1996), outlines four leader styles based on the abilities and motivation of the workers.

1. *Telling:* Leader focuses on workers getting the job done with very little interaction or input from them.
2. *Selling:* Leader focuses on the task, but also encourages relationship building and worker development.

3. *Participating:* Leader focuses on building relationships and supporting worker initiatives.

4. *Delegating:* Leader gives workers independence in how they do their jobs, with minimal direction.

In management of an OT department, the supervisor may change his or her leadership style according to the situation, as well as the traits and performance of each individual employee. New graduates need first to be told what is expected, while more experienced therapists benefit from more interactive and supportive approaches. Likewise, in OT client groups, the style of leadership changes according to the needs of group members.

Transformational Leadership

Transformational leaders (Bass & Avolio, 1996; Burns, 1978) create a vision and give followers the encouragement and resources needed to achieve that vision. Four behaviors comprise transformational leadership: idealized influence, inspirational motivation, intellectual stimulation, and individualized consideration. Such leaders often lead by role-modeling or by example and inspire followers to perform exceptionally through encouraging them personally to use their creativity, innovation, and autonomy in pursuing shared values and beliefs. Transformational leaders go beyond requiring workers to meet certain standards and expectations; rather, they seek to help workers fulfill their own potential. Reiss (2000) compared transformational (inspirational) with transactional (setting goals and expectations) styles among the leadership of OT clinical administrators and OT program directors. He found a negative correlation between transactional leadership and overall organizational effectiveness. In other words, truly effective OT leaders need to go beyond a task focus; they need to also inspire students and therapists to reach higher to achieve their potential.

Path-Goal Theory of Leadership

Path-Goal theory (Evans, 1970; House, 1971) calls for leaders to motivate workers to perform well and to achieve job satisfaction. This leader also adapts the style of leadership to individual needs, but in addition adapts the task and the environment so that the worker more easily achieves the goal. A part of the leader's role is to provide appropriate incentives for workers to meet their goals. Four behaviors of the leader are incorporated into this theory:

1. *Directive:* Involves telling workers what they need to do, in as much detail as needed. Incentives might be built into this approach. OT educators might give out a syllabus that establishes the criteria for receiving a good grade.

2. *Supportive:* This style of leadership emphasizes creating a friendly climate, showing concern for the well-being and concerns of members, and remaining open and approachable, treating members as equals (Pennington, 2002). A supportive approach includes many aspects of OT's therapeutic use of self (see Chapter 3). In OT, groups mainly concerned with building social support, such as facilitating groups of family caregivers or people adjusting to being recently widowed, might require this type of leadership. Stewart, Shamdasani, and Rook (2007) suggest that supportive leadership is often used for focus groups, described later in this chapter.

3. *Participative:* Leadership in teams of one's peers often follows this approach, in which the leader consults with group members about topics, schedules, and activities; often asks for opinions and suggestions; and generally shares the leadership roles with mature group members. Participative leadership encourages all the team members to take equal responsibility for creating and working toward the stated group goals and solving problems along the way. This type of leadership is similar to facilitative leadership in that member interaction is encouraged and members' ideas and views are taken into account (Pennington, 2002; Stewart et al., 2007).

4. *Achievement-oriented:* Leaders motivate members through high-level challenges and by setting high expectations. A sports team coach might use this approach to motivate players to win a championship game.

These theories of leadership, borrowed from the field of business management and social psychology, have many useful applications for OT group leaders (Dunbar, 2009).

Occupational Therapy Group Leadership Styles

How might these theories of leadership be applied in OT groups? Posthuma (2002) suggests that characteristics from all the above styles become a part of each leader's repertoire. Mosey (1986) identified different roles for leaders at each of five levels of group development: parallel, project, egocentric-cooperative, cooperative, and mature. Donohue's social profile assessment tool builds on Mosey's original concepts, showing member leadership roles increasing at each of five levels of group maturity: parallel, associative, basic cooperative, supportive-cooperative, and mature (Donohue, 2010).

Three types of occupational therapy group leadership are presented in this text: directive, facilitative, and advisory. All may be defined as democratic in spirit, but with varying amounts of member input. Each is appropriate in different situations and for different levels of client functioning.

Directive Leadership

In politics, an autocratic leader rules a dictatorship; he or she fashions the nation according to his or her own vision, setting up the structures of government and making all the decisions. In therapy, it would not be ethical nor desirable to hold this much control over a group of clients. However, as a director, the occupational therapist defines a group, selects activities, and structures the group in ways that he or she knows to be therapeutically appropriate for a specific group of clients. The director uses authority sparingly, only as necessary to make the group therapeutic for its members. Used inappropriately, too much direction can cause members to feel infantilized, treated like children who cannot think for themselves; it can stunt the growth and development of a group by crushing attempts to question or challenge the leader.

However, directive leadership is absolutely necessary for lower-functioning clients who do not have the cognitive capabilities to make decisions or solve problems. These clients do not feel safe when the therapist is not in control. In a sense, the therapist is always in control, even in the more democratic approaches. The leader sets the goals, the level of structure, the media used, and the extent to which leadership responsibilities are shared with the group. The therapist's decisions about how to lead are, hopefully, based not only on his or her own preference or style, but on the therapist's expert assessment of the needs of the group. For example, Allen suggests that the therapist structure the environment and the task demand, but, within that context, allow clients to do as much as they can for themselves (Allen et al., 1992). If the therapist is knowledgeable about Allen's theory, he or she will be able to predict fairly accurately how much assistance the clients will need to accomplish a task and will plan the structure of the group accordingly.

Frames of reference for which a directive leadership style is most appropriate are cognitive-behavioral, sensorimotor, and cognitive disabilities. (Note: The term *directive* as used here does not relate to Kaplan's "Directive Group," which is discussed in Chapter 10.)

Facilitative Leadership

The next style of leadership on the control versus freedom continuum is democratic. Just as the democratic leader is voted into power by the citizens, a facilitator gathers support from constituents. The facilitative leader must convince the members of the group that he or she is on their side and represents their best interests. The facilitator earns the support of the members by allowing them to make choices and showing care and concern. Decisions are made by the group with the facilitator's guidance. The therapist is a resource person, providing the group with needed information, needed structure, and needed equipment and supplies. The occupational therapist facilitator openly discusses the purpose and goals of the group. Just as a democratic government presumes and requires a certain level of education in its citizens in order to work effectively, democratic leadership in therapy requires that the members have a certain level of knowledge and skill. Without the required knowledge, members cannot make good decisions or share the leadership effectively. So, the role of a facilitator is also that of an educator. The therapist explains the therapeutic aspects of activity so that the group can choose tasks that are likely to be of benefit to them.

Lewin said that democratic leadership is the most likely to lead to group cohesiveness. This is confirmed in reviewing the group developmental process (further described in Chapter 2). As a group reaches the "control" phase, members must challenge the leadership, the structure, and/or the group task. A facilitator can allow himself or herself to be challenged, use reason and logic to explain the way things have been, and give the group choices about changing them in ways that are not destructive to the group's integrity.

Group facilitation also has its limitations. It is not suitable for clients functioning at a low cognitive level. It presumes a certain level of self-awareness, intelligence, insight, and self-understanding. It is most useful in frames of reference that make personal direction and choice a priority. The developmental, psychodynamic, and model of human occupation approaches depend on a facilitative leadership style to promote a certain level of independent functioning and decision making in client group members. However, when the goals of intervention are to develop specific skills and abilities or to promote neurophysiological or cognitive development, a democratic approach may not be appropriate.

Facilitation is very useful in motivating clients and getting them involved and, as such, is most compatible with a client-centered approach. It is a widely recognized phenomenon that people tend to be more committed to pursuing goals that they have a part in choosing. The more cognitively aware they are, the more they resent goals that are imposed on them. Therefore, discussions that precede a group may use a facilitative approach as a motivator, even when the group itself is more directive.

Group Leader as Advisor

The advisor is the most passive of leadership styles. Occupational therapy consultants use advisory leadership when working with groups of professionals or community groups. Its use in therapy is limited to the most highly functioning groups working on goals like problem solving or attitude change. An occupational therapy consultant/advisor may be appropriate in emerging practice areas like prevention or health maintenance. Clients who seek assistance with specific problems may need an occupational therapist to advise them on issues such as coping with stress on the job, conserving energy in the home, or eliminating architectural and social barriers.

Table 1-2

Leadership Style Guidelines

Member Characteristics	Directive Leadership	Facilitative Leadership	Advisory Leadership
Cognitive level	Low	Medium-high	High
Insight capacity	Minimal	Fair-good	Very good
Group maturity	Immature	Medium-high	Mature
Verbal skills	Poor	Average	High
Motivation	Low	Medium	High

Activity Characteristics	Directive Leadership	Facilitative Leadership	Advisory Leadership
Structure	Therapists selects activity	Therapist and members select activity	Members select activity
Goals	Accomplish task	Learn skill from experience	Understand process
Instruction	Therapist demonstrates/ teaches	Therapist and members teach process	Members seek advice as needed
Group maintenance roles	Mostly done by therapist	Members share in leadership	Members lead themselves
Feedback	Given mostly by therapist	Members encouraged to give to each other	Natural consequences from environment

The advisor offers expertise as needed or requested, but does not provide structure or goals. Motivation comes from the group itself, and change is produced intrinsically as a result of the internal processes of each member or extrinsically as a result of social action. This type of leadership is most appropriate when working with families, caregivers, self-help groups, or community organizations.

GENERAL PRINCIPLES OF GROUP LEADERSHIP

Leaders of therapy groups, whatever their particular style, have certain obligations to the group. Designing the group is the most obvious of these. This planning phase involves choosing the members, setting or acknowledging the goals, setting the time and place, organizing the environment, and choosing the activity or media (sometimes with help from members). The group protocol described in Chapter 11 serves as a guide for how to design a therapy group. Decisions about the best leadership style to use within a given client setting are often complex. Table 1-2 may be helpful in choosing the best leadership style for certain member and activity characteristics.

The ongoing functions of the leader are to help the group achieve its goals (task function) and to maintain the group's integrity (maintenance function). The therapist may need to focus the group on the task to prevent it from getting sidetracked. He or she may have to adapt the activity or task along the way. Maintaining the group can involve the use of many leader skills. Setting group norms, like confidentiality and mutual respect, can be important. Modeling behaviors to be learned or effective interaction skills can help the group communicate and resolve its conflicts. The counseling skills that Egan (1986) writes about are all useful in leading a therapeutic group; accurate empathy, concreteness, genuineness, confrontation, and self-disclosure are examples. These are elaborated in Chapter 3. Giving members feedback and helping members to give and receive feedback is an important function of the leader. Keeping the communication channels open is vital to the survival and growth of groups. These norms and roles are elaborated in Chapter 2.

Co-Leadership

While leadership skills are best learned individually for practice purposes, students may feel more comfortable facing client groups in the company of a co-leader. Having a co-leader in an occupational therapy group with six to eight clients has a number of advantages. Some of these are mutual support, increased objectivity, collective knowledge, modeling for each other, and taking different roles.

Advantages of Co-Leadership

- *Mutual support.* Even if your co-leader is an inexperienced peer, you will be able to encourage one another and cover for each other's weaknesses. One of you is bound to remember what the other one forgets. Overcoming one's fear of coping with difficult clients and situations in the group will be easier when you have a partner to fall back on.

- *Increased objectivity.* Much more can be learned by the group when there are two leaders who can compare observations and give each other feedback. An objective understanding of the process of the group will be easier to achieve using both leaders' points of view. This is especially advantageous during supervision.

- *Collective knowledge.* Two leaders means twice as much knowledge and experience available for the group. Both leaders will be able to contribute ideas in the planning stage, as well as provide skilled interventions and leadership during the group itself. A discussion between co-leaders after the group is over is an important learning tool for novice leaders. Yalom and Leszcz (2005) writes that discussion is an "essential ingredient" of a good co-therapy team. He suggests at least 5 minutes before each meeting and 15 to 20 minutes after each meeting be reserved for planning strategy and sharing reflections about each other's behavior during the group. If there are differences of opinion about how to handle difficult clients or interactional problems, this post-group discussion would be the time to work them out. Co-leaders who cannot come to terms with their differences would be well-advised to seek out supervision before they re-enter the group arena for another session.

- *Models for each other.* Peer co-leaders have much to learn from each other. Every leader has different strengths and weaknesses, as well as different styles of intervention. Co-leader teams can help each other best by taking turns being active or directive and being attentive listeners and observers. In the clinic, students may have practicing therapist as co-leaders; beginning therapists may have experienced co-leaders as models. Each has its obvious advantages. However, ongoing co-leadership teams should eventually equalize their roles so that both are contributing and sharing the responsibility.

- *Different roles.* Good co-leadership teams learn to take advantage of each other's strengths by taking on different leadership roles. Some leaders are especially effective in setting limits when group members lose control. Other leaders are better at giving empathetic support. Co-leaders should take turns doing the confronting and rescuing so that no one has to play the "bad guy" all the time.

A much discussed issue in co-leadership is whether or not the group leaders should air their disagreements openly during the group or save them for the post-group discussion. Yalom (2005) points out that timing is the deciding factor here. Newly formed groups should not be exposed to disagreement among the leadership. However, more stable and cohesive groups have much to learn from observing two mature leaders model the open discussion and respectful consideration of their differences of opinion.

Male/female co-leadership can be particularly enlightening to group members when they model different roles. Their interaction during the group generally brings up issues relating to the primary family. They are also prone to the stereotyping of gender roles. That is, typically, the female leader is expected to take on supportive and nurturing roles, while the male leader is perceived as critical and judgmental. Male/female co-therapy teams are well-advised to share a variety of confrontational and harmonizing roles, so that both are perceived as capable leaders with mutual respect for one another's professional strengths.

Occupational therapists in the clinic may be asked to co-lead groups with professionals from other disciplines. Physicians, psychologists, social workers, nurses, recreation therapists, and dietitians are some of the many possibilities. An occupational therapist and a registered nurse may co-lead a medication education group. An occupational therapy assistant may co-lead a sensory awareness group with a recreation therapist. Each profession brings a different knowledge base and a different point of view. Teams such as these require careful planning to be sure the goals and leadership roles are clear and that their attitudes are compatible. Interdisciplinary collaboration has many potential advantages, but also pitfalls for the inexperienced occupational therapist. A well-established professional identity should be in place before attempting to co-lead a group with a person from another discipline. It is not recommended for students.

Disadvantages of Co-Leadership

Although there are many advantages to co-leading groups, there are a few common difficulties to be wary of. These difficulties must be overcome if the co-leadership is to be effective.

- Splitting. When there are two leaders, group members have a tendency to favor one over the other. Clients often put pressure on one co-leader to take sides against the other. Like children who, when they are criticized by one parent, turn to the other for refuge, so clients in groups will try to get the co-leaders to disagree or to form alliances with subgroups. Co-leaders should be watchful for such attempts and openly discuss them in the group. Not doing so can divide the group and create power struggles, which usually have nontherapeutic consequences.

- Competition. A certain amount of competition in co-leading a group is normal. Leaders seek to establish themselves as competent therapists, and the approval of others does much to enhance their self-esteem. Student leaders or beginning therapists may be looking for high marks from a supervisor as well. While competition is not a bad thing, open communication about the feelings it evokes between co-leaders is necessary in order to avoid destructive consequences.

- Unequal contribution. This disadvantage occurs when one leader does most of the work, while the other sits back and watches. Resentment is bound to develop on both sides. Students have often complained of this problem during supervision of fieldwork experiences. In resolving this dilemma, it must first be acknowledged that both parties are to blame. Once again, the problem must be openly discussed, and supervision sought as needed. The partner who is more active may not see the situation as problematic. It is usually the silent partner who feels uncomfortable and increasingly afraid to speak up. Often, the passive leader feels dominated by his or her partner, prevented from doing his or her part in leading the group, and deprived of the opportunity for needed experience. This problem does not resolve itself and only grows worse as time goes on. Considerable effort and determination on both sides must be given, to set aside the blame and to equalize the balance of leadership, in fairness to the group members.

Stages of Co-Leadership

Lessler, Dick, and Whiteside (1979) studied the development of the co-therapy relationship. They identified four developmental stages, that parallel the group's development (described in Chapter 2).

1. Formative stage. In this stage, co-leaders are preoccupied with their feelings of self-worth as a leader and are plagued by fears of inadequacy. These feelings naturally lead co-leaders to compete with one another. By trying too hard to be "good" leaders, they could end up in a power struggle with one another or a popularity contest with the group members.

2. Development stage. This stage requires much interpersonal discussion and the recognition of differences. This stage must be resolved if the co-therapy team is to work effectively together.

3. Stabilization. After having their fights and talking it out, co-therapists view each other as individuals and recognize each other's strengths and weaknesses as well as their own. They are able to capitalize on their differences by taking on different leadership roles and discussing their perceptions openly during the group as well as afterwards.

4. Refreshment. From the process of the first three stages, a relationship between co-leaders forms that allows each to grow in his or her role as leader. Their interaction results in renewed enthusiasm for the group experience and its potential to help others. They may experiment with new ideas, do research together, or present their group experiences at professional meetings. They take pride and enjoyment from working with each other, and this energizes the group members with a sense of hope and anticipation.

The lesson from this classic research outcome is that competition in co-leadership can lead to a positive outcome when it is openly discussed and dealt with constructively. However, some leaders may find that, after a few sessions, they are incompatible as partners. If mutual respect cannot be achieved through discussion of differences, it is best to find another co-leader. The focus of the group should be therapy for its members, not training for the co-leaders.

Recently, three students from Tufts University developed a tri-leadership model while on assignment leading a Nintendo Wii (Nintendo of America Inc., Redmond, WA) sports/fitness group at an adult day care center in Medford, MA. (Bresnahan, 2010). They shared group facilitation roles of task accomplishment, group support, and standby assistance to group members as they moved from sitting to standing while engaged in Wii sports games. They felt the third leader added to their resources in planning groups and increased their ability to provide each other feedback and analyze group process. They provided each other with opportunities to exchange roles in game play, safety, and moral support to members, deciding ahead of time who would play each role during the group.

Co-leadership has many advantages in practice. However, co-leaders should be chosen carefully and matched for compatibility. Students are advised to master individual leadership first before attempting co-leadership of groups. Those who take on co-leadership should be prepared to work hard, be open to feedback, and take time to discuss the issues of working together on a regular basis.

PROFESSIONAL GROUP LEADERSHIP

Several years ago, leaders of our profession created a "Centennial Vision" of what they hope occupational therapy will become by the 100th anniversary of occupational therapy's founding in 1917 (Moyers, 2007). Goals include making our profession more visible, advocating for OT roles in public policy, and establishing nontraditional OT programs in the community, among many others. Hine and Toth-Cohen (2010) write, "leadership is essential for developing a partnership to achieve the Centennial Vision and will be pivotal in achieving success" (p. 13). These authors describe an innovative leadership development program called "Building OT Leaders for Today (BOTLT)" for the large OT staff at Thomas Jefferson University Hospital in Philadelphia. Transformational leadership provides the structure and inspiration for this grassroots program, which included education regarding leader skills of collaboration, communication, negation techniques, and assertiveness training; and topics chosen based on a needs assessment of their large rehabilitation staff, including OTs, physical therapists, speech-language pathologists, therapy aides, and management staff. Additionally, the AOTA has conducted ongoing workshops in leadership development for state association presidents, OT assistants, and others as a strategy for facilitation of the Centennial Vision.

In education, team teaching and leading student problem-based learning groups are examples of applications of group leadership in professional education. Part of leadership is leading by example, thus inspiring others "to dream more, do more, and become more" (Hine & Toth-Cohen, 2010, quoting John Quincy Adams). Fieldwork directors may have opportunities to model leadership within the clinic, school, or community setting. Those who wish to use OT skills in community service might join existing organizations, such as the Industrial Areas Foundation (www.industrialareasfoundation.org), which specializes in organizing collective grassroots actions not connected with corporations or political parties. There is ample evidence of the need for OT leadership in the nonprofit sector.

Leadership always implies that there are followers, members of groups who look for guidance from a person with a vision, the right connections, and/or the ability to organize and mentor them. If OTs wish to take on leadership roles within the profession, the workplace, or the community, some more advanced skills will be needed, such as group decision-making strategies, conflict resolution, collaborative partnership building, focus group leadership, and team building.

Group Decision-Making Strategies

Group leaders beginning a new group will already have made some decisions concerning membership criteria, goals, purpose, and initial activity for the members to begin to form relationships with one another and establish a culture of caring and support. However, as groups move toward cohesive maturity, they will become more capable of participating in the decisions that affect the group's activities, goals, and outcomes. Groups in the community might be expected to function at a mature level from the outset. Therefore, leaders need to be aware of the typical ways that groups make decisions (Tomlinson & Moore, 2009). Johnson and Johnson (2009) list seven ways for group decision making:

1. Decision by authority without discussion.

2. Decision by authority after discussion.
3. Identification of an expert member who leads the group decision.
4. Identification of an average of the members' opinions.
5. Decision by a minority of the group.
6. Democratic decision—a majority of the group by vote (51% or 2/3 majority).
7. Consensus.

As a group leader, the OT will control to what extent a group becomes involved in making decisions about the content, procedures, structure, and other aspects of the group's activities. It is well-known that group involvement in decisions that affect the members helps motivate engagement in the work and commitment to the group members. While simple democratic majority may seem the most fair, research tells us that repeated majority votes tend to disenfranchise members with minority positions and may be based on criteria other than doing what is right or best for all the members. As such, decisions by majority vote may have a negative impact on group cohesion (Tomlinson & Moore, 2009).

In work settings, group decisions are believed to be superior to those made individually because of the collective knowledge and diversity of the group members. However, some work groups may prefer to identify the member who is most knowledgeable about the issue at hand to lead a discussion, collect relevant information, and make the final decision for the group. Likewise, some senior managers may prefer to have the final say on certain issues because of an unwillingness to share authority with the more junior members.

Depending on the task, the goal, and the culture of the organization or system within which the group is involved, different strategies for group decisions will be favored. In large community groups, elected officials have the power to make decisions for the group or to represent their interests within a larger decision-making group. For example, a politician might wish to have input from voters on a particular issue before deciding how to vote on a bill before local, state, or national legislature. A group might discuss the issue and argue different points of view, but the elected politician will make the final decision (decision by authority after discussion).

Decisions by consensus require that everyone in the group agree. This has been recognized by some as the best strategy because it requires the members to carefully explore all aspects of a problem on which they disagree and to deliberate, collaborate, compromise, and, in some cases, negotiate differences and resolve conflicts between members or subgroups. The group leader must consider the importance of the issue and reserve this strategy for only the most critical issues because it is often quite time consuming and difficult for the group to accomplish. A next best strategy might be for the leader to summarize opinions of members and try to find a way to accommodate more than one decision, such as combining two or more activities or adopting more than one group goal to address. When decision making skills are a part of the group's goal, such as when members wish to increase their social or communication skills, and to be able to find meaningful roles within their communities, the OT leader can focus the group more on process than outcome. A good example of this type of group is the task-oriented group described by Fidler (Appendix B) and further developed in Chapter 5 as a student learning activity.

Groups that have experienced a great deal of conflict or have members with compromised cognitive abilities or communication difficulties may not be capable of the higher-level reasoning, compromise, and collaboration involved in making group decisions, and in such cases, the OT leader limits the decisions to be made by the group. While group members should be allowed to participate in the leadership roles of groups, including group decision-making, to the best of their ability, leaders must continually evaluate the benefits and costs to the entire group experience. While too much authority makes groups dependent, too much leniency makes them feel emotionally unsafe and detracts from the meaning of the group experience. OT leaders sometimes need to make decisions for the group in order to provide them with the structure and means to reach an occupational goal and to experience a sense of accomplishment and group pride.

Conflict Resolution

Conflict resolution is defined as a "process by which people from opposing positions on issues arrive at mutually acceptable solutions through collaborative problem solving" (Murray, 2010, p. 499). When OT professionals are faced with conflicts in the work environment, they might react in a number of ways.

Arguing

This involves defending one's position in a nonconciliatory way, which is geared to winning through power and dominance.

Avoiding

People who do not like conflict often hope it will just go away. They may be concerned with creating animosity or damaging relationships. It seems like a "do no harm" approach, but unresolved conflicts tend to build resentment and can resurface in moments of weakness, often inappropriately. Avoiding is temporary, and the conflict must be addressed at some point.

Compromise

This is a positive solution used when neither party is willing to fully concede his or her position. Each side conceded some portion of his or her argument. The goal of compromise is to work together as a team to arrive at the best solution.

- Step 1—Agree to engage in a dialogue.
- Step 2—Each side acknowledges some validity to the opponent's argument.
- Step 3—Communicate the most important point on each side, and acknowledge concessions being made by each side.

The benefits of compromising are to build consensus and teamwork, promoting an understanding of other perspectives on an issue, and each party is viewed as open and willing to listen to others. No one wins or loses in a compromise resolution.

Collaborative Partnership Building

Both sides hold different views but put them aside in favor of trying to work out the best solution for the situation and organization involved. Opposing parties enter a partnership that is mutually beneficial for themselves and the organization. Neither party tries to persuade the other that he or she is right. A true dialog is entered by both sides, reframed as doing what is best for all in a particular situation. This is considered the best solution because no one compromises his or her own position.

Arbitration

When the power for resolution is conveyed to another person or persons, both parties give up their right to engage in collaboration, making them dependent on a higher authority. This might be a last resort, but it hurts both sides by reducing the need for collaboration or compromise.

OTs working with others to resolve conflicts should first create a culture of openness and collaboration. Before a resolution can be reached, mutual trust and a willingness to listen to contrary views must be established. The focus is uncovering basic issues and beliefs and mutual understanding through dialogue. Murray (2010) suggests that OTs be proactive in planning how potential conflicts can be addressed. A worker can often avoid conflicts with the company by fully understanding its culture, both the written and the unwritten rules. He suggests the following strategies to address a potential or emerging conflict:

- Identify the desired outcome of the conflict, the end goal you wish to achieve.
- Create a tactical plan. What are the steps to achieve the goal?

- Affirm the relationship, and focus on the positive aspects first (empathy statements).

- Prepare to ask questions and gather facts about the situation. Try putting self in the other person's place.

- Listen to answers to the questions and engage in active listening, including body language.

- Clearly explain one's own viewpoint.

The process of setting the stage for collaborative conflict resolution may take time and patience. It requires that one first fully understand all aspects of the conflict. Complex conflicts that involve several individuals may take time to work out, and collaboration can be an ongoing process, with sequential meeting allowing time for reflection in between. Some conflicts may require an outside mediator, such as a manager, human resources in work settings, and professional networks.

When working with groups to resolve conflicts, OTs need to be aware that clients fear open hostility and often process it poorly, with the expected end result being a winner and a loser (Kottler & Englar-Carlson, 2010). If a conflict in the group emerges unexpectedly, the OT leader should model calmness under fire and protect group members from becoming victims. The group leader reframes the conflict and uses it as a positive learning experience by doing the following:

- Bringing attention to underlying issues of power.

- Using group energy to prevent stagnation.

- Regulating the distance between people, by becoming aware of what is comfortable.

- Using emotional expression to ease tension.

- Promoting reflection and growth through open discussion.

- Realizing that resolution of conflict, done without hostility, can lead to greater intimacy.

- Providing a model of resolution without injuring those involved.

As a group leader, OTs in the conflict environment can model compassion, respect, empathy, warmth, and nonjudgmental acceptance. No technique can substitute for a kind and supportive therapeutic leader. Groups, as systems, tend to seek equilibrium. After an outbreak of conflict, they tend to self-correct based on feedback. The peaceful resolution of conflict can be the most important lesson derived from groups (Kottler & Englar-Carlson, 2010).

Johnson and Johnson (2009) suggest the following steps for group conflict resolution:

- Identify and define the problem

- Gather relevant information

- Consider alternative actions

- Examine barriers to decision making

- Decide

- Take action

- Evaluate the outcome

When individuals within the group present problems, the OT can follow this sequence with the individual and invite group members to participate in the process as a learning experience for the whole group.

Focus Group Leadership

Most students and professionals recognize focus groups as a data-gathering method in connection with qualitative research. However, these structured group interviews have recently emerged in the OT literature as a clinical tool as well. OT practitioners can use focus groups to evaluate the occupational features and issues of a community group, to construct a group or organizational profile, or to establish a need for and/or further define OT programs within any specific setting. For example, in implementing the University of Southern California (USC) well-elderly study, Mandel, Jackson, Zemke, Nelson, and Clark (1999) used focus groups in the exploratory stages of their lifestyle re-design program These authors found that focus groups could "gather valuable information about a particular topic through input generated by a group of persons with the guidance of a moderator" (p. 21).

There are many advantages of using focus groups as part of a needs assessment before implementing a group intervention. Some include the following:

- They validate participants by recognizing their unique cultural dimensions.

- Participants feel privileged to provide input to the initial program design.

- Program leaders show respectful appreciation of client's perspective.

- The dynamic process of the group interaction allows clients to stimulate and build upon one another's ideas.

- The flexible structure of the focus groups allows for unanticipated ideas and questions to be explored. (adapted from Mandel et al., 1999, p. 22).

Jacobs (2010) recommends that OT practitioners use focus groups as a marketing strategy when establishing new community or organizational programs. Groups of six to 10 participants meet for a few hours with a skilled interviewer, usually called a "moderator," who asks the group questions related to a specific topic or "focus." The participants might be referral sources, funding sources, or potential clients. Jacobs (2010) suggests their use in exploring the feasibility of specific OT programs in schools, organizations, or the workplace. When planning programs for community health, Brownson (2001) suggests conducting focus groups as part of an overall needs assessment. She highlights the advantages of focus groups in establishing rapport with community leaders and others who may add support for OT programming in later stages of development. Likewise, Fazio (2010) suggests using focus groups with both providers (physicians, educators) and the potential recipients of service when establishing health maintenance or wellness programs for specific populations within the community. When OTs need to measure the outcomes of an OT group intervention, focus groups are a good way to determine the benefits and pitfalls from the clients' perspective and to gain insight about the group process as well as overall client satisfaction.

How are focus groups different from other OT group interventions? As a research tool, focus groups have more structure because they are generally used to gather information about a specific topic. The leader of a focus group is called a "moderator." This person introduces the topic and goal of the group and asks primary and follow-up questions around a specified issue. Stewart and colleagues (2007) define the moderator's role as mainly facilitative, although this may change according to the needs and responses of the group. A good moderator:

...gently draws consumers into the process; deftly encourages them to interact with one another for optimum synergy; lets the intercourse flow naturally with a minimum of intervention; listens openly and deeply; uses silence well; plays back consumer statements in a distilling way, which brings out more refined thoughts and explanations; and remains completely non-authoritarian and non-judgmental. Yet the facilitator will subtly guide the proceeding when necessary and intervene to cope with various kinds of troublesome participants who may impair the productive group process (Karger, 1987, p. 54 in Stewart et al., 2007, p. 69).

In other words, for both therapy groups and focus groups, many of the same leadership skills apply, such as facilitating group interaction and setting norms for mutual respect and cultural sensitivity. Focus groups generally last for only one or two sessions. The open questions provided by the leader become the group task, rather than a concrete activity. The steps in designing focus groups as outlined by Stewart and colleagues (2007) are as follows:

1. Clearly define the issue or problem, for example, assessing the need for an after-school bicycle safety program for preteens.

2. Identify a sampling frame, consisting of groups or organizations that include people who can provide insight about the identified issue or problem, such as Parent Teacher Association members, local police, and students who ride bicycles, to continue the above example.

3. Identify a moderator, in this case, the OT practitioner.

4. Generate an interview guide, consisting of open and closed questions related to the specific issue. The OT practitioner specifies what information might determine the need for a bicycle safety program, such as traffic safety issues around neighborhoods and schools, parent attitudes and concerns, and student input about their use of bicycles for transportation and recreation.

5. Recruit the group participants from the groups specified in the sampling frame. Stewart and colleagues (2007) recommend that the focus groups be homogeneous. In other words, groups of parents, police, and students should meet in separate groups, not mixed together.

6. Conduct the group, taking notes or otherwise recording the data collected.

7. Analyze the data or, for nonresearch purposes, a narrative summary of the issues discussed. For example, the pros and cons of a bicycle safety program and its feasibility within a specific school system (for research purposes, more formal analysis methods would apply).

8. Applying what was learned in program planning: designing the OT program itself.

For practice, students can choose a population in the community for which to design an OT wellness intervention and then plan a focus group to determine its feasibility using the above steps.

For OT practitioners, the focus group format might best be used in the planning stages, before designing a client-centered therapeutic group intervention. In this way, potential group members can identify the occupational issues most important for them, and the OT can gain needed insights from their perspective. Such discussions with potential clients take advantage of the benefits outlined earlier, such as conveying respect for their input, gathering information about their background, and incorporating ideas generated through focus group interaction into the group design (see group protocols, Chapter 11).

Focus group leaders might apply the seven-step leadership structure as a guide to ensure that all members participate, substituting the preplanned questions about a specific topic or issue for Step 2: Activity. The introduction would be the same for any group, ensuring that all members are included by name and explaining the purpose and goals of the session. Sharing takes the form of making sure all members have equal time to respond, and processing gives the group an opportunity to express emotional reactions. Generalizing might take the form of summarizing member thoughts and ideas, for example, topics they might want included in a program design, to ensure that the moderator has correctly understood member issues. Continuing the example of the program design, the application step asks each member how the resulting topics listed might be relevant and meaningful for them. Ending with a summary, particularly with member input, leaves members with a sense of accomplishment that the objectives of the group have been met. Beginning a new program with potential client focus groups is consistent with the client-centered approach discussed in Chapter 3.

Team Building

The concept of teams in business management dates back to the 1930's when organizational behavior researchers found that grouping employees into effective work teams produced more effective outcomes for America's corporations (Dyer, 1984). Today's team building strategies are commonly directed to businesses, schools, sports teams, and religious or non-profit organizations. Team building activities have the goal of helping team members work better together to solve problems, make decisions, design new products, and generally produce more effective outcomes.

The original sports team metaphor, once synonymous with any autonomous work group, has broadened in the 21st century. In a well-managed organization, multiple teams also need to work in synergy with the organization as a whole. The role of a manager or leader in this environment includes the design of a well-constructed team which can engage in mutual assessment and can accept collective responsibility for what they achieve (Belbin, 2002). The team leader tasks most predictive of positive outcomes are: 1) involving employees in decision making, 2) coaching team members, and 3) promoting effective communication (Gilley, McConnel, & Veliquette, 2010). In a meta-analytic study of four specific team building strategies: goal setting, interpersonal relations, problem solving, and role clarification, results suggest that team building does have a "moderate positive effect across all team outcomes" but more strongly relates to "affective and process outcomes" such as group cohesiveness (Klein et al., 2009, p.181). Interestingly, team building efforts become less effective as the size of the team increases (Salas, Nichols, & Driskell, 2007)

Business managers must evaluate team members not only by their individual abilities and expertise, but by how well they work with the team as a whole. When clients in OT have a goal of returning to work or re-integrating with communities, they can often benefit from participating in group team building activities that help them become better team players. Also known as team bonding, an abundance of specific team building activities and exercises may be found on the internet, many of which OT group leaders can adapt for therapeutic groups for a variety of populations. This example, intended for team bonding with high school cheerleaders, builds group decision making, peer coaching, and communication among members:

- Cheerleader Tic-Tac-Toe: "You need nine chairs set up in three rows. Divide the squad into Xs and Os. Just like in regular tic-tac-toe, the Xs and Os alternate, except they sit in the chairs instead of drawing it out on paper. Ask questions about the rules of football, basketball, or any sport. If she is right, then she sits in one of the chairs. The first team to get three in a row, diagonally, vertically, or horizontally, wins." (Headridge, 2011).

A LEADERSHIP EXPERIENCE FOR STUDENTS

To practice the seven-step group leadership, students may be divided into groups of eight members. Each student should plan and lead a group of his or her peers for 45 minutes, followed by a 15-minute feedback session from the instructor (and members). Students who are beginning their professional training should not attempt to play the roles of clients. There are plenty of goals students will find useful to work on for themselves in these groups.

To help the student plan a group, the Practice Group Plan (Worksheet 1-2) is suggested. The student's leadership skills may be evaluated by using Worksheets 1-3 and 1-4.

SUMMARY

Section 2 will review some occupation-based models and frames of reference that occupational therapists have used to guide them in planning and leading groups. However, students often understand theory best when it relates to their experience. Therefore, it is suggested that students learn to lead groups first. They can practice their skills by leading groups of their peers.

Although the seven steps of group leadership are described without reference to theory, it should be noted that no approach is entirely nontheoretical. The theoretical basis for this approach is client centered and has some elements of the cognitive-behavioral frame of reference as well. It has a sequence of steps that may be seen as developmental in their hierarchical order. These approaches and their application to occupational therapy groups will be discussed in later chapters. Cole's seven-step approach is not intended to meet all needs for all clients. It can be adapted in many ways to reflect differing clients, goals, models, and frames of reference.

Worksheet 1-2
Practice Group Plan

1. Title of group:

2. Purpose of group:

3. Brief description of activity:

4. Supplies and equipment needed:

5. Goals of the group:

6. Questions for discussion in:

    □ Processing

    □ Generalizing

    □ Application

7. Points of Summary:

From Cole, M. B. *Group dynamics in occupational therapy: The theoretical basis and practice application of group intervention* (4th ed.). Thorofare, NJ: SLACK Incorporated. © 2012 SLACK Incorporated.

Worksheet 1-3
Leadership Evaluation

Student Name: _____ Date: _____ Time: _____

Group Title: _____

,_____ Written Group Plan (10 points)

_____ Introduction (10 points)
- Explains purpose clearly
- Uses warm-up to relax/prepare group
- Communicates expectations
- Outlines timeframe/structure of group

_____ Activity (10 points)
- Adequately prepared
- Asks for feedback from the group
- Directions clearly given
- Timing appropriate
- Materials appropriate
- Environment appropriate

_____ Sharing (10 points)
- Invites each member to share
- Uses appropriate verbal and nonverbal communication
- Empathizes and acknowledges feelings of members

_____ Processing (10 points)
- Elicits members' feelings about the experience
- Elicits members' feelings about each other
- Elicits members' feelings about the leader (when appropriate)
- Helps group understand its own processes

_____ Generalizing (10 points)
- Points out like and similar responses
- Points out contrasts of differences
- Develops one or two principles learned

_____ Group Motivation (10 points)
- Inspires confidence of group
- Encourages enthusiasm
- Encourages group interaction

From Cole, M. B. *Group dynamics in occupational therapy: The theoretical basis and practice application of group intervention* (4th ed.). Thorofare, NJ: SLACK Incorporated. © 2012 SLACK Incorporated.

Leadership Evaluation (Continued)

_____ Limit Setting (10 points)
- Allows sufficient time to each member
- Limits inappropriate behavior
- Assumes appropriate authority (but not too controlling)

_____ Application (10 points)
- Verbalizes meaning of this experience (significance)
- Shows how this experience can relate to everyday life
- Relates this experience to issues/problems of members
- Uses concrete examples and/or self-disclosure

_____ Summary (10 points)
- Chooses most important points to emphasize
- Verbally reinforces group learning
- Acknowledges contributions of members
- Ends group on time

_____ Total Leadership Score

Member Evaluation Summary (from Worksheet 1-4)

Average leadership score: _____

Summary of strengths:

Summary of suggestions for improvement:

Worksheet 1-4
Member Evaluation of Leader

Directions: This form may be used to obtain reactions of student members prior to discussion of student leader's performance in practice groups. The forms are then collected by the instructor and are considered when rating the student leader. Member evaluations are anonymous.

Date and Time: _____ Title of Activity: _____

How satisfied were you with the way the group was planned and led? (Please check one of the following.)
- ☐ 1 Not at all satisfied
- ☐ 2 Somewhat satisfied
- ☐ 3 Satisfied
- ☐ 4 Very satisfied
- ☐ 5 Extremely satisfied

Please comment on how you found this group experience.

What did you see as the leader's strengths?

What did you see as the leader's weaknesses? (Must state at least one.)

From Cole, M. B. *Group dynamics in occupational therapy: The theoretical basis and practice application of group intervention* (4th ed.). Thorofare, NJ: SLACK Incorporated. © 2012 SLACK Incorporated.

REFERENCES

Allen, C. (1999). *Structures of the cognitive performance modes.* Ormond Beach, FL: Allen Conferences, Inc.

Allen, C., Earhart, C., & Blue, T. (1992). *Occupational therapy treatment goals for the physically and cognitively disabled.* Bethesda, MD: American Occupational Therapy Association.

American Occupational Therapy Association. (2008). Occupational therapy practice framework: Domain and process, 2nd ed. *American Journal of Occupational Therapy, 62,* 625-683.

Bass, B. M., & Avolio, B. J. (1996). *Transformational leadership development. Manual for the multifactor leadership questionnaire.* Palo Alto, CA: Consulting Psychologists Press.

Belbin, M. (2002). Building teams in the 21st century: How do we define their role? *The Team Building Directory.* Retrieved from http://www.innovativeteambilding.co.uk/pages/articles/21stcentury.htm

Bresnahan, J. (2010). Tri-leadership: Learning as a group within a group. *OT Practice, Nov. 8,* 17-19.

Brownson, C. (2001). Program development for community health: Planning, implementation, and evaluation strategies (pp. 95-118). In M. Scaffa (Ed.), *Occupational therapy in community-based practice settings.* Philadelphia, PA: F. A. Davis.

Burns, J. M. (1978). *Leadership.* New York, NY: Harper & Rowe.

Donohue, M. (2010). The social profile. Retrieved from http://www.socialprofile.com

Dunbar, S. B. (2009). Leadership theories. In S. B. Dunbar (Ed.), *An occupational perspective on leadership: Theoretical and practical dimensions* (pp. 1-10). Thorofare, NJ: SLACK Incorporated.

Dyer, J. L. (1984). Team research and team training: A state of the art review. *Human Factors Review,* 285-319. Retrieved from http://www.innovativeteambilding.co.uk/pages/history.htm

Egan, G. (1986). *The skilled helper* (3rd ed.). Monterey, CA: Brooks/Cole.

Evans, M. G. (1970). The effects of supervisory behavior on the path-goal relationship. *Organizational Behavior and Human Performance, 5,* 277-298.

Fazio, L. (2010). Health promotion program development. In M. Scaffa, S. M. Reita, & M. Pizzi (Eds.), *Occupational therapy in the promotion of health and wellness* (pp. 195-207). New York, NY: F. A. Davis.

Gilley, J. W., McConnell, C. W., & Veliquette, A. (2010). Competencies used by effective managers to build teams: An empirical study. *Advances in Developing Human Resources, 12,* 29-45.

Headridge, P. (2011). Team building games. *Oak Harbor Cheer.* Retrieved from http://www.oakharborcheer.com/TeamBuildingGames.html

Hersey, P., & Blanchard, K. (1969). *Management of organizational behavior: Utilizing human resources.* Englewood Cliffs, NJ: Prentice Hall.

Hersey, P., Blanchard, K., & Johnson, D. (1996). *Management of organizational behavior: Utilizing human resources* (7th ed.). Upper Saddle River, NJ: Prentice Hall.

Hine, T. E., & Toth-Cohen, S. (2010). Facilitating OT leaders: A grassroots approach. *OT Practice. 15,* 12-15.

House, R. J. (1971). A path-goal theory of leader effectiveness. *Administrative Science Quarterly, 16,* 321-338.

Jacobs, K. (2010). Systems to organize and market occupational therapy. In K. Sladyk, K. Jacobs, & N. MacRae (Eds.), *Occupational therapy essentials for clinical competence* (pp. 389-395). Thorofare, NJ: SLACK Incorporated.

Johnson, D. W., & Johnson, F. P. (2009). *Joining together: Group theory and group skills* (10th ed.). Upper Saddle River, NJ: Pearson Education.

Karger, T. (1987). Focus groups are for focusing, and for little else. *Marketing News, Aug,* 52-55.

Klein, C., DiazGranados, D., Salas, E., Huy, L., Burke, C. S., Lyons, R., & Goodwin, G. F. (2009). Does team building work? *Small Group Research, 40,* 181-222.

Kottler, J. A., & Englar-Carlson, M. (2010). *Learning group leadership: An experiential approach* (2nd ed.). Los Angeles, CA: Sage Publications.

Lessler, K., Dick, R., & Whiteside, J. (1979). Stages of cooperation: Co-therapy viewed developmentally. *Transactional Analysis Journal, 9*(1), 67-73.

Lewin, K., & Lippitt, R. (1938). An experimental approach to the study of autocracy and democracy: A preliminary note. *Sociometry, I,* 292-300.

Lewin, K., Lippitt, R., & White, R. (1939). Patterns of aggressive behavior in experimentally created social climates. *Journal of Social Psychology, 10,* 271-299.

Mandel, D. R., Jackson, J. M., Zemke, R., Nelson, L., & Clark, F. *Lifestyle redesign: Implementing the Well Elderly Program.* Bethesda, MD: AOTA.

Mosey, A. C. (1986). *Psychosocial components of occupational therapy.* New York, NY: Raven Press.

Moyers, P. (2007). A legacy of leadership: Achieving our Centennial Vision. *American Journal of Occupational Therapy, 61,* 622-628.

Murray, J. (2010). Conflict resolution. In J. Jacobs & J. Sladyk (Eds.), *Occupational therapy essentials for clinical competence* (pp. 497-505). Thorofare, NJ: SLACK Incorporated.

Pennington, D. C. (2002). *The social psychology of behavior in small groups.* New York, NY: Taylor & Francis.

Pfeiffer, J., & Jones, J. (1977). *Reference guide to handbooks and annuals* (2nd ed.). La Jolla, CA: University Associates.

Posthuma, B. (2002). *Small groups in therapy settings: Process and leadership.* Toronto: Little, Brown & Co.

Reiss, R. (2000). Leadership theories and their implications for occupational therapy practice and education. *OT Practice Continuing Education, 5,* 12, CE1-CE8.

Rider, B., & Rider, J. (2000). *The activity card book for mental health.* Kalamazoo, MI: Author.

Salas, E., Nichols, D., & Driskell, J. E. (2007). The effect of team building on performance: An integration. *Small Group Research, 38,* 471-488. Sage Journals Online. Retrieved from http://sgr.sagepub.com/content/30/3/309.abstract

Stewart, D. W., Shamdasani, P. N., & Rook, D. W. (2007). *Focus groups: Theory and practice* (2nd ed.). Thousand Oaks, CA: Sage Publications.

Tomlinson, J., & Moore, O. (2009). Occupation and activity in groups. In J. Hinojosa & M. L. Blount (Eds.), *The texture of life* (3rd ed., pp. 253-283). Bethesda, MD: AOTA.

Yalom, I., & Leszcz, M. (2005). *Theory and practice of group psychotherapy* (5th ed.). New York, NY: Basic Books.

Chapter 2

UNDERSTANDING GROUP DYNAMICS

The large body of knowledge regarding group dynamics developed by behavioral scientists over the past 60 years offers a great deal of help in our understanding of how groups work. This body of knowledge comes from a variety of theoretical bases: psychoanalytic, existential, behavioral, cognitive behavioral, and, more recently, systems theory. Around the mid-1970s, a paradigm shift occurred in group dynamics research. Older theories were challenged, and new theories and models have come into focus since then. This chapter retains the best of traditional research while presenting an overview of representative updated theories.

Because of the verbal nature of the groups being researched, some assumptions have been made about the populations upon which these theories are based. Although even the most dysfunctional groups achieve some level of social organization, members of a group who have verbal skills and are capable of interaction can more easily demonstrate the dynamics described. Another assumption is that when there is enough freedom within the group structure for members to initiate and make choices, the dynamics will be more obvious. A third assumption is that the members are intrinsically motivated to self-improve through self-understanding and by increasing their interaction skills. All of these assumptions are consistent with the client-centered approach described in Chapter 3.

Group dynamics may be defined as the forces that influence the interrelationships of members and ultimately affect group outcome. It is important for occupational therapists to understand these forces when planning and implementing group interventions. Groups have predictable stages of development and will respond best to different activities at different stages. As leaders, our recognition of our group's stage of development should influence our selection of activities. How we design and lead groups also depends on our recognition and understanding of the various dynamics. Some of the dynamics that will be included in this chapter are group process, group development, group culture, norms and roles, client problem behaviors, and termination of groups. A section on evidence for therapy group effectiveness concludes this chapter, along with examples of occupational therapy groups recently reported in the literature.

Group membership experiences are emphasized in this chapter so that students can gain an appreciation for what clients might be experiencing under different group conditions. It is hoped that membership experiences will help occupational therapy students to be more observant and empathetic group leaders.

GROUP PROCESS

We have already discussed processing as one step in group leadership. An awareness of the underlying process of groups is essential to our approach as therapists. It gives us many clues as to the feelings and motives of members and helps the therapist to make clients aware of these and their impact on wellness and on group function. Yalom and Leszcz (2005) have written a great deal about the process of psychotherapy groups. Process is often first understood by what it is not. It is not content. The content of a group is what is done and what is said.

Cole M.B. *Group Dynamics in Occupational Therapy: The Theoretical Basis and Practice Application of Group Intervention (pp 29-58).* © 2012 SLACK Incorporated.

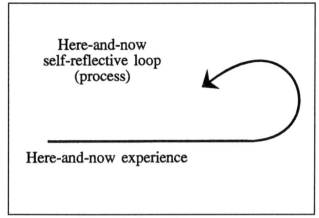

Figure 2-1. Yalom's self-reflective loop.

For example, the group did pencil drawings, and topics discussed were the jobs members had and how they liked them. Bob said he likes being a carpenter, but Sarah hates being a teacher. Process does not include past history or even recent history of the members. Its thrust is what is happening in the group, between and among members, right now. Process concerns the interpersonal relationships among the participants.

There are two parts to process in groups, according to Yalom: "If the powerful therapeutic factor of interpersonal learning is to be set into motion, the group must recognize, examine, and understand process. It must study itself; it must study its own transactions; it must transcend pure experience and apply itself to the integration of that experience" (Yalom & Leszcz, 2005, p. 142). So the process is experienced first, and then it "performs a self-reflective loop," examining what just occurred. The "processing" step in the preceding chapter represents a simplified self-reflective loop (Figure 2-1). Members are asked to reveal how they felt about the activity they just experienced, as well as how they felt about the leader and each other. So the process commentary begins. Its emphasis is often on emotion, and its purpose is to establish a cognitive framework that permits members to retain the group experience so that it can be generalized and applied.

The process comments are largely the responsibility of the therapist. The leader can and should request member participation, but he or she chooses the direction of intervention according to the needs of the group.

Example

In a task-oriented group, the occupational therapist had taken considerable time in helping the group plan their next activity. They were going to construct kites. The plan for Monday was to walk to a craft store (about four blocks from the hospital) to buy paper, string, sticks, and paint. The kites would be constructed during the next two sessions. The seven members of the group assembled, wearing jackets and sneakers and ready for the walk. Hannah, age 63, the eldest member of the group, was not feeling well and refused to go. Dave, a 23-year-old member, bluntly asked the therapist if Hannah was too sick to walk. The reply was that she was fine medically. So, Dave proceeded to call Hannah a "lazy, do-nothing complainer." The other members verbally attacked Dave for his rudeness and insensitivity to the elder member, and a heated argument ensued until it was too late to carry out the plan.

Content

As an occupational therapy leader, how would you process this group? First, it is helpful to identify content. What was the overt experience? The group came prepared to walk to the craft store as planned. The plan was not carried out because Hannah refused to go. What was verbalized? Dave was verbally abusive to Hannah. The other members verbally attacked Dave for being abusive, and he defended himself with counter attacks, shouting loudly at the group. The virtue of courtesy to one's elders was discussed.

Process

The process involves what is implied by the content. The therapist might consider the following possibilities:

- Hannah wanted some attention and chose to pursue it by her passivity. Perhaps her refusal was her way of exerting control over the group, or perhaps illness is her usual way of getting attention.

- The other group members were frustrated at not being able to carry out their plan and were looking for someone to blame.

- Hannah was to blame, but she seemed too frail and vulnerable to be verbally accused.

- Dave was impatient and expressed his frustration aggressively. Perhaps aggressiveness is his usual way of coping with frustration, a habit that often gets him into trouble, or perhaps he feels guilt and is looking for a way to be punished.

- The group's frustration, diverted from Hannah by her vulnerability, was vented onto Dave instead. Dave was made the scapegoat of the group. A scapegoat is something that symbolizes all the badness of the group or someone who is blamed for its problems. The scapegoat generally serves the purpose of allowing the group to avoid its own responsibility for what has occurred.

- Perhaps the group wanted to avoid either the walk or the activity. Dave and Hannah gave them an excuse to avoid doing any task-oriented problem-solving.

Needs to Be Addressed

Which hypothesis is correct? Any or all of them could be true. How, then, should the therapist intervene to help the group understand its process? The first thing a leader should ask himself or herself is, "What does this group really need?" Here are some possible needs to be addressed:

- The foremost need is to get Dave off the "hot seat." He may have been rude and aggressive, making him an easy target for the group, but he is certainly not the direct cause of their frustration. If Dave is not rescued, he will probably be forced out of the group and will be left feeling angry and hurt. Being scapegoated is not a therapeutic experience. For Dave, the therapist might point out how his behavior tends to elicit this kind of response from others, and how he set himself up to be the scapegoat. For the members of the group, the therapist might discuss their feelings about Hannah. They need to understand why they avoided blaming her, how they ended up in a struggle with Dave, and what they themselves were avoiding by pursuing the argument.

- The therapist might then want to examine the issue of Hannah's control. What are her real needs (attention, respect), and how might they be pursued more appropriately? An awareness of her pattern of controlling others with her illness, real or otherwise, might be very helpful as a beginning step toward therapeutic change. The group's collusion with her in achieving her goal to keep the group from acting is another important issue. Why did they allow her to exert such control? What purpose did it serve for them? Why did they not exclude her instead of Dave?

- The final issue of importance is the group's relationship to the task. How did they feel about the activity they chose? Were they really that invested? Or were they looking for an excuse not to pursue it? What were the group's choices? Could they have found an alternative way to get their supplies? Could they have reorganized their roles so that Hannah would not have to go on the walk, without excluding her from the group as a whole? If walking is important to them in getting out of the hospital to enjoy the spring weather, perhaps Hannah could have been wheeled in a wheelchair, or she could have walked part of the way and then waited with another member.

If the group is to learn from this rather frustrating and upsetting experience, it is evident that they need the OT's guidance in problem solving. Finding alternative solutions and compromising are essential if the group is to accomplish its task. Learning depends on the effectiveness of the group's reflection about the reasons for the unfortunate outcome. The occupational therapist guides the group to discover what steps should be taken before the end of this group to avoid a reoccurrence of frustration in the next session.

Discovering the Process of Groups

The best way for students to learn about group process is to experience it. Therefore, a real example taken from a student group experience is best used for this exercise. However, if that is not available, the student may use the following case example. Use Worksheet 2-1 to evaluate the experience.

Case Example

The group was engaged in doing an assertiveness exercise. All the members had anonymously written down situations on a card and put them in a basket in the center of the table. Members had to draw a card, read it, and tell what they would do to assertively handle the situation described on the card. Mary drew a card and read it to the group. It said, "On my fieldwork experience, I was working with two clients and one of them started to cry. I didn't know why she was crying so I ran down the hall to find a nurse, leaving the two clients alone in the clinic. I couldn't believe that my supervisor, Miss Hunt, failed me for leaving the clients alone." Mary looked bewildered. "How could the supervisor expect you to know what to do? You're just a student." Maureen, another member said, "How could the student be so stupid? If she doesn't know what to do, she shouldn't be in occupational therapy." Susan added, "But I had Miss Hunt, too. She's really a hard nose." Several others commented on Miss Hunt's inadequacy as a supervisor. Laurie agreed with Maureen, "Yes, but the student should have known better." Roberta listened silently to this debate, looking more and more distressed as the end of the session approached.

YALOM'S THERAPEUTIC FACTORS— A BRIEF REVIEW

These well-known therapeutic factors, originally conceived to explain what makes group therapy work, represent an attempt to simplify a highly complex system of group interactions. Once understood, their presence within the process of group can easily be recognized and commented upon by group leaders as a way to help build a therapeutic culture within the group. Yalom's classic therapeutic factors have recently been researched and updated and can serve here to explain how the process of group interaction becomes the incentive for therapeutic change. Yalom and Leszcz (2005) and others have conducted studies with multiple therapeutic groups on the original 11 therapeutic factors using a Q-sort format in order to better understand the way client group members perceive their relative importance in promoting positive

Worksheet 2-1
Content-Process Reaction

Directions: Write the answers to these questions after you have participated in the group session.

I. Content

    A. Give a brief description of the activity.

    B. Identify three major participants and what topics they discussed. If there were more than three, choose the three you think were most important.

        1. Person:

          Topic:

          Others offering feedback:

          Approximate length of time:

        2. Person:

          Topic:

          Others offering feedback:

          Approximate length of time:

        3. Person:

          Topic:

          Others offering feedback:

          Approximate length of time:

II. Process

    A. Name three feelings you personally experienced during the group. To whom or what were the feelings directed?

        1.

        2.

        3.

    B. Based on your observations of verbal and nonverbal behavior, what are some hypotheses (possible explanations or interpretations) about the process of the group?

        1.

        2.

        3.

        4.

        5.

    C. Based on the above hypotheses, what therapeutic intervention(s) would you make as a leader and why?

From Cole, M. B. *Group dynamics in occupational therapy: The theoretical basis and practice application of group intervention* (4th ed.). Thorofare, NJ: SLACK Incorporated. © 2012 SLACK Incorporated.

change. The resulting rank order follows, with one new addition, that of "self-understanding" as a twelfth factor. Interpersonal has also been split into input and output components.

1. *Interpersonal learning (input):* Through participation and feedback from the group, members learn how they are viewed by others, can reflect upon how this compares with their own self-concept, and can become aware of negative social behaviors or habits that could be undermining their real-life relationships. Many OT structured group activities are designed to facilitate this process through group interaction in the context of a group activity.

2. *Catharsis:* Best known as an emotional unburdening, the therapeutic value of this factor lies in its connection with some form of cognitive learning and reflection on its meaning. When a member expresses strong emotions in an OT group, the leader may guide the focus of the group to facilitate member reactions to the event before the group ends. Interpretation of the emotional discharge by the leader and members can be critical to the promotion of positive change.

3. *Group cohesiveness:* The sum total of complex interactions and interrelationships that engage and connect therapist and members with one another, forming a positive bond. Cohesive groups represent the end stage of group development. There is general consensus among researchers that this high sense of group solidarity correlated with a higher rate of attendance, participation, and mutual support. Cohesiveness is a powerful force of attraction for group members that is also a precondition for the other therapeutic factors to function optimally.

4. *Self-understanding:* Described as the intellectual component denoting "insight," self-understanding clarifies the continuity of past and present in one's life. A complex category containing more than one element, Yalom and Leszcz (2005) describe self-understanding as "discovering and accepting previously unknown or unaccepted parts of the self" (p. 92). This self-discovery has both positive and negative elements, accepting one's previous shameful thoughts or behavior as part of an imperfect self, and also discovering new strengths and abilities that can enrich one's life. "Clients want to be liberated from pathogenic beliefs; they seek personal growth and control over their lives. As they gain fuller access to themselves, they become emboldened and increase their sense of ownership of their personhood" (Yalom & Leszcz, 2005, p. 92). For occupational therapists, demonstrating occupational talents and performance might contribute highly to this process.

5. *Interpersonal learning (output):* Members learn to better express their thoughts and feelings, practice resolving differences, and build skills in getting along better with others. Many occupational therapy group activities can be designed to help members build social skills.

6. *Existential factors:* Factors relating to the human condition, such as acceptance of pain and death as realities of life, and realizing that life is not always fair. The concepts of freedom and responsibility from existential philosophy can help group members to discover their own role in choosing the path their life has taken and accepting responsibility for their life choices, rather than blaming others.

7. *Universality:* The feeling that one is not alone is most often expressed by members in the early stages of groups, when members seek to identify similarities between themselves and other members. In groups, this provides members a powerful sense of relief.

8. *Instillation of hope:* Coming to the group with high expectations that one will receive needed help can become a self-fulfilling prophecy. Therapists' guidance is key to sustaining the initial hope over time.

9. *Altruism:* In helping others, members can raise their status in the group and feel a greater sense of well-being. Groups are unique in offering often very disabled individuals a way to be of benefit to others (rather than a burden). OTs encourage this when they ask members to help one another with group tasks.

10. *Family re-enactment (corrective emotional experiences):* Although not highly valued by clients, this factor may operate at an unconscious level. Clients who have varying degrees of problematic family backgrounds often express their distortions through the roles they choose to play in the group, as well as their response to the group leader. With guidance from the leader, members have the opportunity to break free from rigid family role scripts in which they have "unknowing been long locked" (Yalom & Leszcz, 2005, p. 97).

11. *Imparting information (guidance):* Includes didactic educational information or instruction as well as direct guidance and suggestions from others. However, advice-giving among members in the early stages of groups may be a sign of group immaturity. This can be counter-therapeutic, when members reject initial advice, or when they feel others do not fully understand their situations or viewpoints.

12. *Imitative behaviors (identification):* The factor least valued by clients may be due to their misinterpretation that copying behaviors of others negates one's individuality. At an unconscious level, much social learning occurs through observing others and modeling the successful social behaviors of one's peers. This factor is basic to the role-playing

Table 2-1

Comparison of Various Theories of Group Development

Theorist	Year*	Beginning of Group				End of Group
Bion	1961	Flight		Flight		Unite
Schutz	1958	Inclusion		Control		Affection
Tuckman	1977	Forming	Norming	Storming	Performing	Reforming
Yalom	1985	Orientation		Conflict	Cohesiveness	Maturity
Poole	1983	Multiple sequences, cycles, and breakpoints; multiple activity tracks				
Gersick	1984	First meeting	Phase 1	Midpoint transition	Phase 2	Conclusion

*Years represent earliest introduction of group development theory.

exercises used by OT group facilitators, relative to the context of a variety of social situations.

Although each factor represents a separate concept, all are interdependent, and in keeping with complex systems theory, the whole group experience cannot be fully appreciated by separation into component parts.

GROUP DEVELOPMENT

Group development refers to the stages that groups go through as they progress from initiation to termination. Several theorists have contributed to this aspect of groups, including Tuckman (1965), Bion (1961), Schutz (1958), Yalom, Poole (2003), and Gersick (2003) (Table 2-1). Knowing the characteristics of each stage helps the therapist to anticipate problems. It helps him or her predict how the group will respond to certain activities and, therefore, plan appropriately.

Traditional researchers (Bion, Schutz, Tuckman, Yalom, and many others) suggest that all groups progress through a series of predictable stages. Many theories have been suggested as to what these stages are, and, in fact, all seem to have similar characteristics. There is an initial stage of orientation, with its search for structure, goals, and dependency on the leader. Next, there is a stage of conflict with its struggle for dominance and rebellion against the leader. Following resolution of conflicts, interpersonal harmony and intimacy emerge, sometimes called cohesiveness.

Newer theorists (Poole, Gersick) challenge traditional phase theories and tend to use systems theory to study the process of small group communication, behaviors, and decision making. Our knowledge of group development comes from a collection of studies including observations of therapy groups, training groups (educational), natural groups, laboratory groups, and work teams. The final outcome of development is a mature working group characterized by high cohesiveness and commitment

to the goals of the group. This outcome is agreed upon by older and newer theorists. Cohesiveness is the ideal to which we will aspire as occupational therapy group leaders.

Tuckman

Tuckman (1965) published the first major review of these studies from which he abstracted a theory of five-stages of group development:

1. Forming
2. Storming
3. Norming
4. Performing
5. Reforming

Tuckman believed that all the stages occur in some way regardless of the duration of the group (e.g., shorter length groups impose the requirement of the problem-solving stages to be reached quickly); therefore, the rate of development tends to adjust to the time available.

Tuckman's initial stage, forming, involves orientation and testing regarding the group task and a dependence on the leader for guidance. Storming involves conflict among group members as they challenge the task, the rules, and the leader. In the norming stage, harmony prevails, and members accept and trust one another while conflicts are avoided. The fourth stage, performing, goes beyond cohesiveness to a point where conflict can be openly discussed and resolved. A performing group can effectively work together in a supportive emotional environment that encourages growth and therapeutic change.

In 1977, Tuckman and Jenson revisited the stages of groups adding the fifth stage "reforming" whose task it is to review an evaluate past performance, learn from both the positive and negative experiences, and re-organize itself accordingly for the future. Tuckman's stages have recently been redefined as stage of team development (Ryan, 2010).

Bion

Bion's work is also frequently quoted, especially with the easy-to-remember titles of the three stages:

1. Flight
2. Fight
3. Unite

Bion (1961) looked at the behavior of groups at conferences, having a task rather than a therapeutic focus. Flight represents an avoidance of some problem or threat. Members tend to turn to each other in pairs for more intimate emotional response in this stage. The fight stage represents the challenge of the leader (and possibly scapegoating a rival member-leader). Uniting follows these two emotional states; it settles down the members to a stable working group with relatively little emotionality. Bion's work, although emerging from the corporate and industrial arena, has many parallels in the therapeutic group. This may be especially applicable to the occupational therapy group, which, although therapeutic in its goal, tends to be more task-focused.

Schutz

Schutz's (1958) theory, while similar to those previously described, tends to have the clearest interpersonal focus. He says that every individual has three interpersonal needs:

1. Inclusion
2. Control
3. Affection

These needs parallel those of a child in the family and are generalized to any interpersonal relationship among two or more individuals. In other words, groups follow the same sequence of interpersonal concerns as individuals do. Schutz's stages are shown to have both individual and group characteristics.

Inclusion Stage

In the inclusion stage, the individual is concerned with being accepted: "Where do I fit in? Will I be important, respected? Can I be myself? How will the leader respond to me?" The group behaviors observed are over-talking, attention-seeking, territoriality, and individual self-centeredness. Members listen but do not really hear what others say. They tend to look to the leader when they speak rather than each other. In this initial phase, the rational approach is dominant; emotions do not flow freely. The group explores the goals, rationale, and structure. The leader is looked to for the answers. There are multiple attempts at sizing each other up. Members look for similarities and tend to downplay differences. There is concern over those who have not made a contribution, and rightly so. If members are continually passive, they can become blockers to the progress of the group as a whole.

Control Stage

Schutz's control stage also has individual and group concerns. The individual now questions the following: "Where do I stand in relation to power and authority? How much influence do I have? Will I have too much responsibility?" The group is generally, at some point, engaged in a leadership struggle. The once all-powerful and all-knowing leader (therapist) is now viewed with skepticism and mistrust.

If the leader abdicates (i.e., gives up the leadership), a struggle among members ensues to fill the void. Scapegoating of a would-be leader is common, and attempts to lead are often met with severe criticism or are ignored. Members often disagree about how much structure is needed or how the group should be led, and subgroups may arise. There is ambivalence about the leader; like a 2-year-old child, the group at once wants to be autonomous but needs the leader's support and protection.

The importance of all this for occupational therapists is in knowing that rebellion and challenge among group members is normal and necessary to the healthy development of the group. Be prepared to be challenged, and do not take it as a personal affront. How then should we as occupational therapists handle the challenge? There are three choices:

1. An advisor as leader would tend to back down, to abdicate leadership. To do so invites intra-group conflict that could be more stressful than clients can handle.

2. A director would subdue the rebellion. In this case, the therapist remains the leader and encourages further dependency of the group. Such an approach has been known to stifle group development.

3. The facilitative leader would not abdicate all the control, but would encourage the group to share the leadership. This is Yalom's approach. He states that the group needs to experience the freedom and the responsibility for the group outcome. He suggests the leader not abdicate, but allow expression of dissension and acknowledge it. The therapist should "take the blows" and not allow any group members to become a scapegoat. Ideally, the therapist will make some changes in response to the group to allow the conflict to resolve while preserving the integrity of the group.

Affection Stage

If the conflict in leadership is resolved successfully, the group progresses to the affection stage. This is the stage of group cohesiveness when attention focuses on "How do others feel about me?" and then "How do we feel about each other?" The group is characterized by expression of positive feeling and emotional investment in the group. Members are able to really listen to each other, and even direct hostility may be expressed without devastating consequences.

The affection stage is the goal for any therapy group. Here is where members feel safe, cherished, and trusting in one another. This allows members to explore new behaviors and to grow. They value one another, and therefore, they value themselves. There is real altruism and real consensual validation; members want to help each other and accept feedback from each other to validate their own self-perceptions. It is part of our role, as occupational therapists, to help our groups reach this stage.

Nevertheless, there are some real barriers to achieving the affection stage. Schutz (1958) tells us that groups tend to regress easily, even after they have reached this stage. Events such as the arrival of a new member, leaving of an old member, leadership changes, and long holidays will all cause a group to regress. Furthermore, clients who are lacking in social and interpersonal skills and/or who are unable to trust others may be incapable of reaching the affection stage. Anticipation of termination of the group inevitably causes the development to reverse. A cohesive group may sink, once again, into conflict in preparation for breaking the ties and moving on.

Yalom incorporates characteristics of Schutz's theoretical group phases in his theory. He dubs Schutz's Stage 1, In or out, Stage 2, Top or bottom, and Stage 3, Near or far.

Yalom

In the most recent update of his classic textbook on group psychotherapy, Yalom synthesizes much of the previous research regarding group development. He concedes that the issues of each phase may, in fact, be revisited in later phases. That being said, the "imperfect but nonetheless useful schema of developmental phases" (p. 309) he describes are as follows:

- Orientation (hesitant participation, search for meaning, dependency)
- Conflict (dominance, rebellion)
- Cohesive maturity (Yalom & Leszcz, 2005, pp. 311-320)

Orientation

Yalom points out that the group therapist's preparation of members regarding the purpose for joining the group will affect its early development. In occupational therapy groups, pre-group interviews with potential clients might serve a dual purpose of determining collaborative goals and discussing group membership as an intervention strategy. According to Yalom, a client's hesitant participation in the initial stage of the group stems from his or her need to understand how group membership will help meet individual goals. Socialization is also inherent in the process of a therapeutic group. Accordingly, members size each other up in order to determine whether or not they belong as they search for acceptance and approval.

Dependency, another characteristic of the initial stage, stems from the members' wish to be rescued from the dilemma that brings them to therapy in the first place. Yalom suggests that group leaders take advantage of this early need for structure and answers to shape therapeutic norms in the orientation stage.

Conflict

In the second stage, members are preoccupied with issues of power and control. As social conventions are abandoned, members feel free to make personal comments and criticism. Yalom states that "the struggle for control is a part of the infrastructure in every group" (Yalom & Leszcz, 2005, p. 314). However, the urge to rebel might not be a conscious process. For example, latent conflict may create group stagnation or boredom. Or, rebellion might take the form of complaining about the structure, such as the time or place of group meetings, or some other aspect of group content. In this case, the leader's role will be to promote awareness of the conflict through processing. Hostility toward the leader, as mentioned earlier, might be the most overt expression of conflict. How the therapist handles the hostility or criticism has a powerful effect upon group development.

Cohesive Maturity

In their 2005 update, Yalom and Leszcz have combined the final two phases of group development. The earliest phase of cohesiveness occurs when the group successfully resolves the conflicts of the previous stage. It is characterized by the emergence of a group spirit, high morale, and heightened mutual support. Competition among members is replaced by intimacy and trust, and an emotional atmosphere of nonjudgmental acceptance is created. As members feel free to self-disclose, "long past transgressions are shared" (Yalom & Leszcz, 2005, p. 319), and previously unexpressed emotions from past sessions may surface. However, the early stage does not represent true cohesiveness because negative affect remains suppressed.

Not until both negative and positive can be freely expressed does the group reach true cohesiveness or maturity. The mature working group will demonstrate "true teamwork in which tension emerges not out of a struggle for dominance but out of each member's struggle with his or her own resistances" (Yalom & Leszcz, 2005, p. 320). This is the more advanced stage of group cohesiveness.

Yalom, in his review of criticisms of group development theory, states that the boundaries between phases are not clearly demarcated. As such, the above stages may be more accurately named developmental tasks, not phases. Research shows that the same themes are repeatedly revisited and that some group events have an unpredictable effect on group development.

Poole's Multiple Sequence Model

This model is included as representative of an updated approach that challenges the validity of previous group development phase theory. Poole (2003) focused on decision making in work groups for his research. He suggests that group decision making generates multiple clusters of associated behaviors along at least three activity tracks:

1. Task process activities, which the group enacts to manage its task

2. Relational activities, which reflect or manage relationships among the members (process)

3. Topical focus, which includes issues and arguments of concern to the group (discussion, conflict resolution)

Central to Poole's developmental theory is the concept of breakpoints. Breakpoints are points of change or transition, and Poole (2003) acknowledges three types:

1. Normal (changes in discussion topic, different parts of the task)

2. Delays (setbacks due to emerging problems, group problem solving)

3. Disruptions (major conflicts, major changes required for the group to proceed)

Poole suggests that no distinct phases occur in all groups, but that different tasks, goals, and group member characteristics produce unique patterns of content and process.

Gersick's Time and Transition Model of Group Development

Gersick (2003) studied eight diverse work teams to discover how their function changed over time. Her findings also contradict prior stage theories, but she replaces them with an alternate structure. Gersick points out that most organizations consist of permanent and temporary groups, which function as teams to carry out the work of the organization. She changes the focus of group development from one of typical behaviors to one that attempts to explain the mechanisms of change and considers environmental contingencies. In a broad-based research study, Gersick observed that while groups use a wide variety of behaviors, "the way they worked was highly congruent" (p. 62). Her model consists of a first meeting, phase 1, midpoint transition, phase 2, and completion. The theory Gersick identifies is called "punctuated equilibrium" (Eldridge & Gould, 1972), which theorizes that systems progress through an alternation of stasis (inertia) "punctuated by concentrated revolutionary periods of quantum change" (Gersick, 2003, p. 62).

Phase 1

The first half of the group's calendar time is an inertial movement whose direction is set by the end of the group's first meeting. This places great importance on the first meeting as a time that the group's process and content may be easily shaped. During the first meeting, Gersick speculates, member behaviors may be influenced by prior expectations, contexts relating to the sponsoring organization (social, cultural contexts), and preferred behaviors or strategies characteristic of their personalities (client factors).

Midpoint Transition

At the midpoint of the allotted calendar time, groups undergo a transition during which the direction of the group is revised for phase 2. Gersick calls this a "problemistic search and pacing," which stems from the group's awareness of problems with initial norms and the pressure exerted by external deadlines. The group transition is compared to Levinson's "midlife crisis" in which, around age 40 to 45, an adult reappraises his or her life so far and redefines his or her remaining life as "time left to live" (see Chapter 8). At the midpoint transition, the group faces the reality of limited time left to complete its task and picks up the pace accordingly. The ideal outcome gives way to a more realistic one, and both content and process change to accommodate this altered goal.

Phase 2

The second period of inertia focuses on carrying out the plan formulated during the transition. Progress may spurt ahead in order to reach a markedly accelerated conclusion, in which the group finishes off the work generated during phase 2.

Role of Context

The environmental influences on groups, not addressed by phase theorists, play a significant role in Gersick's model. Context impacts the group's development at three critical periods:

1. Design of the group

2. The first meeting

3. The midpoint transition

Translated into occupational therapy terms, the OT's selection of members for the group, structuring of the task, and support for the group from outside sources greatly influences the initial group functions. During the group's first meeting, both content (the task and its purpose) and process (the norms for interaction and reflection) have a lasting impact on subsequent groups. During the phases of inertia, groups are less responsive to environmental influence. The next and final time the group opens itself to outside influence is the midpoint transition. At this time in the life of the group, members are familiar enough with the task to realize that outside resources, requirements, and guidance are needed as a basis for re-charting their work, and the stress of a rapidly approaching deadline motivates them to pick up the pace while there's still time to produce a reasonably successful outcome.

Relevance for Occupational Therapy

The importance of Gersick's study for occupational therapy group leaders is to acknowledge the importance of initial planning and to establish therapeutic norms aggressively during the first meeting. Secondly, occupational therapy group leaders should anticipate the midpoint transition in ongoing task groups and use it as a second chance to redirect and refine goals, correct nontherapeutic norms, and provide needed resources to increase the likelihood of a positive outcome.

How Groups Reach Cohesive Maturity

Why should occupational therapists study group development? There are several reasons. First, understanding the progression to cohesive maturity in groups gives us something to strive for; it shows us the true capacity of a mature, cohesive group. We, as therapists, should do whatever we can to help the group reach a mature, working stage. Corey, Corey, Callanan, and Russel (1988) suggest one way to speed up the process is to prepare members to get the most from a group. Corey's guidelines are helpful to students participating in a group lab and may be kept in mind as suggestions for our higher-functioning clients. Some of the suggestions are summarized as follows.

Have a Focus

Think about what you would like to get from the group, what issues you would like to explore, and what changes you would like to make. Writing down your goals prior to each group is often helpful.

Pay Attention to Feelings

Groups are an opportunity to explore personal issues that are often heavily laden with emotion. It is often the emotions that emerge that offer important insights and an opportunity for personal growth. The group is not a place to censor expression of emotions, but rather to let them flow. Feelings that are bottled up session after session will eventually "dam up the flow of the group" (Corey et al., 1988, p. 48).

Be an Active Participant

You will help yourself most if you take an active role in the group. Silent observers are not as likely to get as much from their participation in the group, and others may believe their silence means they are being judgmental (Corey et al., 1988).

Give Feedback

Whether positive or negative, your honest and direct response to others will move the group toward a deeper level of trust. Occupational therapists look forward to a long career of giving constructive feedback to clients. It is essential for occupational therapy students to develop the skill of giving honest feedback in ways that are empathetic and respectful of the other member.

Be Open to Feedback

Others in the group may not have perfected the art of giving constructive feedback. When someone responds honestly but bluntly, it is natural to get defensive in justifying your own standard and therefore to reject his or her feedback. Instead of letting defenses sabotage your work in the group, use the group as an opportunity to discover your defenses, which might include "rationalizing, withdrawing, denying, or turning a specific criticism into a global 'I'm no good'" (Corey et al., 1988, p. 51). Try to get beyond your defenses and learn to use feedback constructively.

Take Responsibility for What You Accomplish

It is easy to blame others when you are bored, annoyed, or unable to self-disclose in the group. Take a look at your own contribution to this state of affairs, and, instead of blaming the group, think about what you could do to make things better. You have a great deal of control and choice about how you interact with others in the group, and in the final analysis, what you accomplish is up to you. Corey's suggestions are some individual behaviors and beliefs that can help groups move toward cohesiveness. We as occupational therapists have many activities at our disposal that encourage the group to move in the direction of cohesiveness. An example is the structured group activity called "Giving and Receiving Feedback" (Session 3 in Chapter 12).

Second, because the stages are predictable, knowledge of group development prepares us for what is coming next. It makes us better able to plan occupational therapy activities that are appropriate at each stage of development. For example, a "Trust Circle" exercise, requiring members to intentionally fall into the arms of other group members and trust that they will be protected, may not be a good activity to introduce in the control stage of a group. Even the best laid plans might have to be changed because of changes in the stage of the group's development. For example, in a student training group, I had planned a structured exercise in setting priorities for the sixth session of the group. The group had developed beyond the control stage to a level of intimacy that made them almost cohesive. Sharing their priorities seemed too superficial, so they rejected it and modified the activity to a discussion of how to rescue

Table 2-2

Schutz's Stages of Development of Groups

I. Inclusion—behaviors	II. Control—behaviors	III. Affection—behaviors
1. Depend on leader to structure	1. Ambivalence toward leader; challenge structure/purpose; challenge leader style; challenge authority of leader; test limits/rules; need for leader protection/approval	1. Focus on feeling; express feelings about each other; express feelings about the leader; consensual validation occurs; direct hostility expressed constructively
2. Look to leader for answers	2. Disenchantment with group; subgroups struggle among selves; leader viewed with mistrust; members critical and discounting group	2. Delight in company of others; identify with group; feel one is lovable and loved; concern that one is not lovable and not loved; altruistic desire to help others; separation anxiety; new behaviors are explored
3. Rational approach dominates; discuss topics/opinions/thoughts; avoid feelings; look for purpose/goals for group	3. Sharing group responsibility; dependence-independence struggle; members share leadership functions; suggestions for change in structure and task emerge; members-leaders emerge; competition, not cooperation, predominates; leader bends toward will of group	
4. Individual behaviors predominate attention-getting or withdrawal humor/laughter, territoriality/pairing, talking but not listening, referring back to prior experiences		
5. Search for similarities; energy is in keeping harmony; find "what we agree on"; avoid conflicts		
6. Concern over belonging/approval; only say what will be accepted; eye contact, verbalize mostly with leader; seating changes frequently		

their troubled relationships. The group let me know very quickly that they needed to deal with something on a deeper level.

Another reason for studying group development is that the role of the leader changes with each stage. As occupational therapy leaders, we need to know what to expect. Imagine if you were a student leading a group, and one week the clients all decided to rebel against you. Suppose you did not know that this is a normal process for groups? How would you feel? One student leading a time-management group for substance abusers was faced with a client uprising. Quite unexpectedly, several members of the group refused to do the prescribed activity. Rather than forcing them to do it, she changed the agenda to a discussion of what they did and did not like about the group. This student did not get defensive (fortunately) but listened intently to the clients' complaints and wrote down their suggestions. Group development theory had given this student some guidelines about how to handle the conflict. She knew she could not give up her leadership role, but neither was there any way she was going to force six grown men to do an activity they did not want to do. By listening to them and taking them seriously, she allowed them to challenge her in a way that did not threaten her and did not threaten the integrity of the group, either. The following week, they were able to approach the activity (one they themselves had suggested) with renewed interest and enthusiasm.

Identifying Group Stages

A good way to learn about the stages of group development is to reflect on a group one has participated in for several sessions. If the group meets for 10 weeks, the self-reflection about the stage of development should not start until at least the fifth session. If the stages are discussed too soon, before the conflicts begin, the discussion will not be meaningful.

Furthermore, too close a scrutiny will make the group self-conscious and, therefore, inhibit its flow. The leader takes his or her cue from the group itself in the timing of a discussion of developmental stages.

As a self-learning tool, the student group member might look at the characteristics of each stage and see if these behaviors can be found in his or her group. Table 2-2 may be useful in assisting with this process. As behaviors are recognized, examples of these in one's own group may be cited. Generally, if three or four of the behaviors are present for a given stage, that one is likely to be correct. As an example, my student group lab was scheduled to do the "Giving and Receiving Feedback" exercise. Some of them questioned if they were ready for it. They claimed they did not know each other well enough to say anything critical. They asked me to allow them to modify the activity so they would not have to say anything negative. A few said, with hostility, they would just have to "make something up." A few others counterattacked with the rationale that they would soon have to give constructive feedback to clients, and this would give them some practice. I did not allow them to modify the activity but did allow them to vent their frustrations and fears and make their suggestions. Clarification and examples were given on how to give constructive feedback. The activity was carried out with a great deal of anxiety, but ended in relief when it was "not as hard as we thought."

Considering the above example, try Worksheet 2-2.

THE CULTURE OF GROUPS

Each group, whether in therapy or in life, develops its own unique culture. Both the leader and the members influence the culture of groups, which becomes more stable over time. Culture defines the way the group interacts and gets its work done. In OT groups, culture becomes evident in the norms and roles that emerge within it. Group leaders take care to set therapeutic norms from the beginning session, because once the culture becomes established, it later becomes much harder to change.

Norms

Norms are present in every group; they incorporate certain attitudes and standards of behavior that are acceptable to the group. Norms may be specified and verbalized by the leader, or they may not be verbalized but only implied by the behavior and interactions of members. The norms of a group may change as it develops or as members come and go. The therapist's awareness of the norms and their acceptance by the group helps him or her understand better the behaviors observed in the members.

The leader is responsible for establishing explicit ground rules for the group, like being on time and respecting the opinions of others. These are expectations the leader will announce at the outset and enforce as the group continues. Confidentiality has been mentioned earlier as a common explicit norm of groups. This means that what members say and do during group sessions should not be revealed or discussed with nonmembers. The agreement to keep group work confidential is an extension of the client-therapist relationship: what clients say and do is considered privileged information. Knowing this, the clients can trust one another and are more likely to open up to the group.

Nonexplicit norms are more elusive because they are seldom verbalized. These may even be beyond the group's awareness. They may be understood in terms of behaviors that are acceptable or nonacceptable in the group. For example, the avoidance of conflict may be a norm in the beginning stages of groups. Certain topics may be considered taboo, to be discouraged or avoided. Norms develop in all groups, therapeutic or otherwise. They are a part of the culture of any social or therapeutic group.

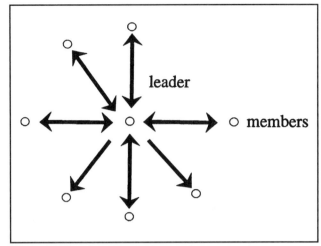

Figure 2-2. Leader-centered interaction.

Culture Building Role of the Leader

To a great extent, the leader is responsible for shaping the group into a therapeutic social system. The establishment of therapeutic norms creates a culture that is maximally conducive to effective group interaction. Yalom points out that the norms of a therapy group are radically different from the rules of etiquette in social groups. In therapy, members interact freely and also feel free to comment spontaneously on their immediate feelings about each other and the leader. Yalom describes the desirable norms of a therapy group as "active involvement in the group, non-judgmental acceptance of others, extensive self-disclosure, desire for self-understanding, dissatisfaction with present modes of behavior, and eagerness for change" (Yalom & Leszcz, 2005, p. 121). These norms do not develop automatically. The leader uses considerable influence to shape the norms of a therapy group, with necessary help from its members.

Furthermore, the leader should closely monitor the nonexplicit norms of the group. The adoption of nontherapeutic norms must be avoided at all costs because, once norms are established, they are very difficult to change. The therapist is the key influence in shaping norms. Yalom suggests that therapists do this in two ways: as a technical expert and as the model-setting participant.

As technical expert, the therapist relies on his or her experience and knowledge to introduce therapeutic norms and the reasons for them. Then, as the group goes on, the therapist may use social reinforcement to encourage the enactment of therapeutic norms, while discouraging antitherapeutic norms. For example, one pattern that should be discouraged is the group members speaking only to the leader. We have already learned that dependence on the leader is a characteristic of the early stages of groups. A typical picture of this interaction is shown in Figure 2-2.

Worksheet 2-2
Group Development Evaluation

Directions: List six different behaviors or events in the group in the first column. Then in the second column, identify the stage of development in which this behavior would best be categorized.

Group Behaviors	Stage
1.	
2.	
3.	
4.	
5.	
6.	

Stage of development for this group is _____ .

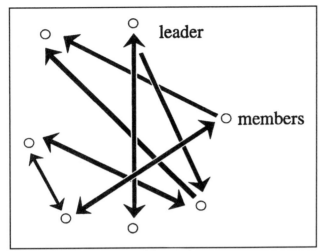

Figure 2-3. Group-centered interaction.

In the earliest stages, the leader establishes a norm of group interaction in several ways. He or she can refuse to answer the questions of members and reflect these to other members. For example, Mary asks the leader, "What are we supposed to talk about?" The leader does not answer, but responds with a question, "What might be some meaningful issues to talk about today?" As members begin to give their ideas, the therapist might ask, "Mary, what do you think about Sally's idea?" or "Sally, why don't you give Bill some feedback about his suggestion?" In this way, the leader tactfully establishes a communication pattern that looks more like Figure 2-3, above.

Members are speaking not only to the leader, but are addressing each other as well. This is an important norm to set in an interactive occupational therapy group, where members are expected to give each other feedback and learn from each other. This norm also helps the group to progress beyond the initial stage of development.

In this example, the therapist has used his or her role as both technical expert and model-setting participant. The therapist has guided the group by telling them that they should interact with one another and has demonstrated the behaviors by asking specific group members to respond to one another.

Self-disclosure might be another way to model expected behaviors. When asking members to share their feelings, the leader may begin by sharing his or her own. Referring to the situation described earlier, the therapist might say, "When Maureen criticized the student for not knowing what to do with a client who cried, I felt very concerned about how that student was feeling. Yet I was frustrated, because the situation was presented anonymously and I didn't know who wrote it. I didn't want to force this student to reveal herself, but I was afraid she would really be hurt and I wanted to protect her from the attack. I wonder if other members had some of these feelings also." This example demonstrates several expectations. The norm of free expression of emotion in the group is demonstrated by the leader's expression of both concern (fear) and frustration. The focus on "here and now" is demonstrated in the leader's encouragement of responses to one another within the group about what just occurred. The therapist's encouragement of concern for one another and not allowing members to criticize one another in a hurtful way helps establish a norm of safety and trust. Finally, this self-disclosing comment invites the group to reflect on its own process, encouraging a norm of self-reflection in the group.

The norms in this example are some of what Yalom considers to be therapeutic norms. Some therapeutic norms Yalom refers to include the following:

- Self-reflection of the group
- Encouraging self-disclosure
- Encouraging free interaction among members
- Reinforcing the importance of the group
- Regarding members as agents of change and setting an atmosphere of safety and support

Norms will necessarily change in different groups. In occupational therapy groups, norms will vary with the client populations with which we deal and our frame of reference. Norms also change as the group moves through the stages of development. A comment that is unacceptable in Stage 1 may be right on target in Stage 2 or 3. For example, the avoidance of conflict may be normal in Stage 1, but gives way to open criticism of the leader and the group structure in Stage 2. The norm of open conflict in turn gives way to a norm of acceptance of constructive feedback in Stage 3.

Taking Risks

If a group is to progress in its development, norms must, from time to time, be challenged. Members who do so are considered to be taking a risk. Risks involve revealing yourself to the group in a way that makes you vulnerable and taking the chance that you will be accepted and supported. In risks, there is always the chance that you may not get the response you are looking for. For example, after a very tense session in "Giving and Receiving Feedback," Roberta shared with the group that she was rather hurt that someone in the group considered her to be aggressive and intimidating. Another member, Jennifer, took Roberta's cue and shared that she was confused by someone's comment that she was a snob and "looked down her nose" at peers who were not as smart as she was. The comments of Roberta and Jennifer were met with silence. Shortly afterward, the group ended.

What risks did Jennifer and Roberta take? How did the group respond? How do you think the group changed (or should change) as a result of their risk-taking behaviors? What norms did these two students challenge? Use Worksheet 2-3 to evaluate a group experience.

Worksheet 2-3
Monitoring Norms

Directions: As a learning exercise, complete the following after each group experience. Your comments can address many individual and group behaviors, but here are some suggestions: seating pattern, structure and format of the group, timing, silence, topics discussed, communication pattern, expression of emotion, discussion of process, and leader intervention.

List three behaviors that were accepted by the group.

1.

2.

3.

List three behaviors that were not (or would not be) accepted by the group.

1.

2.

3.

List three expectations established by the leader.

1.

2.

3.

List three of your own expectations for this group.

1.

2.

3.

What norms have changed from the last group? Which norms would you like to see changed?

1.

2.

3.

In considering the example of Roberta and Jennifer, it is clear that neither left the group happy. They were both angry and silent during the next group session. The group, left on its own, perhaps would have continued to ignore the behavior, which in some way threatened the group's status quo. In this case, the therapist has to make some judgment calls. Are Jennifer and Roberta mature and stable enough to handle the group's response, or do they need support in continuing to take risks? Is the group ready to change its norms and open up to challenge and conflict? In the group exercise "Giving and Receiving Feedback" (Chapter 12, Session 3), the members' feedback to one another is anonymous. At what point are members ready to accept responsibility for their comments and give up the safety of anonymity? The leader's intervention should be protective of Roberta and Jennifer and supportive of their vulnerability, while being sensitive to the level of trust within the group. The best intervention, considering these factors, would be to use these members' risk-taking behaviors as a way of encouraging the silent members to take risks also. Only when the writers of the seemingly hurtful comments take the risk of revealing themselves can the issues be discussed and resolved. Members can learn a great deal from this process, not the least of which is learning to give critical feedback in a caring and helpful way and learning to accept critical feedback as an opportunity to grow and make therapeutic change.

GROUP ROLES

Roles are the result of the members dividing the work of the group among themselves. Members play roles, such as follower, initiator, energizer, and blocker, spontaneously as the group progresses, or roles may be assigned by the leader. Researchers have identified the more frequent roles played in groups and have organized these according to their functions. Some roles tend to help the group accomplish a task, while others help maintain the group's lines of communication. Still other roles tend to interfere with group function, such as an attention seeker or a monopolist. The therapist not only needs to recognize these roles, he or she also should help members take on a variety of roles and to change those roles that are detrimental to the group. It is often through taking on different roles that much of the therapeutic learning takes place in the group setting.

The concept of group roles was introduced in 1948 by two researchers, Kenneth Benne and Paul Sheats. Their idea was to look at leadership of the group not as solely present in the identified leader or therapist, but as a shared responsibility of all the members. These writers suggest that "the quality and amount of group production is the 'responsibility' of the group ...(and) the setting of goals and the marshalling of resources to move toward these goals is a group responsibility in which all members of a mature group come variously to share" (Cathcart & Samovar, 1974, p. 180). Benne and Sheats (1948) developed from their research at the National Training Lab in Group Development in 1947 their now-classic breakdown of member roles into the following:

- Group task roles
- Group building and maintenance roles
- Individual roles.

A group role is a behavior pattern or structured way of behaving within the group. Group roles tend to remain stable regardless of who is in them. Thus, a single group member can take on a variety of roles within the group, and members can change their roles as often as they wish. Because there is a relationship between personality and the roles one typically plays with others, the roles that members find themselves taking on can, in itself, be revealing. However, the roles themselves are interchangeable. Maturity has been measured by the ability to take on a variety of group roles.

Group Task Roles

These are the 12 roles that help the group to get its work done:

1. Initiator-contributor: Suggests new ideas, innovative solutions to problems, unique procedures, and new ways to organize.

2. Information seeker: Asks for clarification of suggestions, focuses on facts.

3. Opinion seeker: Seeks clarification of values and attitudes presented.

4. Information giver: Offers facts or generalizations "automatically."

5. Opinion giver: States beliefs or opinions.

6. Elaborator: Spells out suggestions and gives examples.

7. Coordinator: Clarifies relationships among various ideas.

8. Orienter: Defines position of group with respect to its goals.

9. Evaluator-critic: Subjects accomplishments of group to some standard of group functioning.

10. Energizer: Prods the group into action or decision.

11. Procedural technician: Expedites group's movement by doing things for the group such as distributing materials, arranging seating.

12. Recorder: Writes down suggestions and group decisions, acts as the "group memory."

Group Building and Maintenance Roles

These are seven supportive roles that keep the group functioning together:

1. Encourager: Praises, agrees with, and accepts the contributions of others.
2. Harmonizer: Mediates the differences between other members.
3. Compromiser: Modifies his or her own position in the interest of group harmony.
4. Gatekeeper and expediter: Keeps communication channels open by regulating its flow and facilitating participation of others.
5. Standard-setter: Expresses ideal standards for the group to aspire to.
6. Group observer and commentator: Comments on and interprets the process of the group.
7. Follower: Passively accepts ideas of others and goes along with the movement of the group.

Individual Roles

These are opposed to group roles and indicate the use of the group to serve one's individual needs. These roles tend to interfere with group functioning. Benne and Sheats (1948) suggest that a high incidence of individual behaviors is symptomatic of various group malfunctions, such as inadequate group skills of members (including the leader); low level of group maturity, discipline, and morale; or an inappropriately chosen and inadequately defined group task. There are eight individual roles defined by these authors:

1. Aggressor: Deflates the status of others; expresses disapproval of the values, acts, or feelings of others; attacks the group or group task, etc.
2. Blocker: Tends to be negativistic or stubbornly resistant, opposing beyond reason or maintaining issues the group has rejected.
3. Recognition-seeker: Calls attention to self through boasting, acting in unusual ways, or struggling to remain in the limelight.
4. Self-confessor: Uses group as an audience for expressing non-group-oriented feelings, insights, or ideologies.
5. Playboy: Displays lack of involvement through joking, cynicism, or nonchalance.
6. Dominator: Monopolizes group through manipulation, flattery, giving directions authoritatively, or interrupting the contributions of others.
7. Help-seeker: Looks for sympathy from the group through unreasonable insecurity, personal confusion, or self-deprecation.
8. Special interest pleader: Cloaks his or her own biases in the stereotypes of social causes, such as the laborer, the housewife, the homeless, or the small businessman.

Admittedly, the group roles are, in part, a function of the group's stage of development. More of the task and maintenance roles can be observed in a mature group than one that is less mature. No statements are made as to the relative value of the various roles. It can be assumed that all roles are equally valuable and necessary to the group's positive outcome. Too many opinion givers and not enough compromisers are likely to create chaos rather than productivity. A well-functioning group needs a balance of roles, and this requires members to take on a mixture of roles that are compatible.

As a learning experience, it is helpful to analyze member roles (Worksheet 2-4). This gives members some feedback about what roles they tend to take on in groups and how they are contributing to the group outcome. It is easiest to see roles in groups that require extensive interaction, problem solving, and decision making. Remember, a single member can take on several roles. After everyone has written down his or her ideas, group members should compare notes and discuss their answers and the reasons for them. See if the group can reach a consensus about who played which roles.

For further self-awareness, the questions in the Self-Role Analysis (Worksheet 2-5) can be answered concerning your own role in the group. Because flexibility in roles is considered a sign of maturity, it may be set as a goal in groups to have each member try a few new roles over the course of group meetings.

CLIENT PROBLEM BEHAVIORS

It is evident from our discussion of individual roles that certain member behaviors can interfere with or severely constrict the functioning of groups. Knowledge of group dynamics also helps the leader know how to deal with special problems. For example, if the leader understands why the monopolist needs to monopolize and how his or her behavior affects the other group members, then the type of therapeutic intervention needed can be determined. Sometimes, the problems that arise are best dealt with by the leader, while others are handled more effectively by the group itself.

Yalom and Leszcz (2005) point out that all clients are problems. Indeed, clients are often assigned to therapy groups for the purpose of attempting to change problem behaviors. The behaviors to be reviewed here are monopolizing, attention-getting, silence, and psychosis. It is very important for the occupational therapist leading groups to gain an understanding of each member's needs and develop skills in handling problem behaviors.

Worksheet 2-4
Role Analysis Exercise

Directions: After your group ends, take a few minutes to identify which members played the various identified roles. Give an example of the behavior that supports your choices.

Group Task Roles

Role	Member Name	Sample Comment or Behavior
1. Initiator-contributor		
2. Information seeker		
3. Opinion seeker		
4. Information giver		
5. Opinion giver		
6. Elaborator		
7. Coordinator		
8. Orienter		
9. Evaluator-critic		
10. Energizer		
11. Procedural technician		
12. Recorder		

From Cole, M. B. *Group dynamics in occupational therapy: The theoretical basis and practice application of group intervention* (4th ed.). Thorofare, NJ: SLACK Incorporated. © 2012 SLACK Incorporated.

Worksheet 2-4
Role Analysis Exercise (Continued)

Group Building and Maintenance Roles

Role	Member Name	Sample Comment or Behavior
1. Encourager		
2. Harmonizer		
3. Compromiser		
4. Gatekeeper/expeditor		
5. Standard-setter		
6. Group observer/ commenator		
7. Follower		

Individual Roles

Role	Member Name	Sample Comment or Behavior
1. Aggressor		
2. Blocker		
3. Recognition-seeker		
4. Self-confessor		
5. Playboy		
6. Dominator		
7. Help-seeker		
8. Special interest pleader		

Worksheet 2-5
Self-Role Analysis

1. What role(s) did you see yourself playing in the group?

2. Were these the same or different from the role(s) others saw you playing?

3. How does your role in this group compare with the one you usually play in groups?

4. What other roles would you like to try?

5. What comments or behaviors can you use to help you take on a new role?

Members who display these problem behaviors are those who play the individual roles in groups, often blocking the group's progress and frustrating its members. Dealing effectively with these clients in the group involves several challenges for the therapist. First, the therapist should develop an understanding of the individual dynamics of the client: What does this client really need? Second, the therapist needs to develop strategies for preserving the integrity and cohesiveness of the group: What does the group need? How can the leader handle this client so that the group can continue to function therapeutically? Ideally, both the client need and the group need can be satisfied. Realistically, it is not always possible for the leader to do both. If a choice is to be made, the group should be preserved first, even if that means an individual member must leave it. A good group therapist will never sacrifice the whole group for the sake of an individual member.

Unequal Participation

The two extremes of participation, dominance and passivity, each present unique challenges for the group leader. Because the group time and resources are meant to benefit all its members, setting limits for participation becomes the responsibility of the therapeutic group leader (Kottler & Englar-Carlson, 2010). Cultural influences are highly likely to influence member participation, according to recent research (DeLucia-Waack & Donigian, 2004). Unacknowledged power hierarchies within the group with respect to gender, ethnicity, race, age, or other individual diversities can create frustration and resentment within the group, especially in the conflict stage of development. For this reason, OT leaders need to facilitate constructive discussion around these issues in a culturally competent manner.

The Monopolist (Dominance)

Harry came into the group angry. He refused to listen to the purpose of the group or to participate in the activity. "I'm not going to draw like I'm in kindergarten. Excuse me, but you girls (occupational therapy student leaders) don't know anything about alcohol abuse. When I was in County Hospital, they had me doing paintings and sculptures, and what-all, and it never did anything for me...." Five other members listened to this outburst in silence. They had heard Harry's routine before.

How should the leaders handle Harry? First, let us ask two key questions. What does Harry need? Perhaps he needs to control the group, to maintain the group's (or leader's) attention, or to avoid his own hurtful issues. What do the members of the group need? Probably, they need to get Harry to "shut up." However, when a silent group allows a monopolist to control things, there is always an element of ambivalence. In some ways, Harry may be serving their needs as well, particularly if they, too, wish to avoid revealing hurtful issues or feelings.

In this example, Harry is playing the role of the aggressor, by devaluing both the task and the leaders of the group. The leaders, in this case, are more likely to stop Harry's tirade by appealing to the other group members. Ask them, "Why do you allow Harry to monopolize the group? Why are you silent?" The group might be encouraged to give Harry feedback by completing the sentence, "When you speak like that, it makes me feel _____." If the group is able to express its frustration with Harry, then Harry might be helped by learning to control the behaviors that elicit negative feelings from others.

The Silent Member (Passivity)

Silent behaviors occur frequently in occupational therapy groups. In active groups, silent members may go unnoticed for a session or two, but will eventually block the group's progress. Why? Because, as the group becomes aware of a member's silence, members begin to imagine what the silent member must be thinking. Soon, resentment develops over the silent, passive member's "not pulling his or her weight" in the group. In truth, a silent member might feel inadequate, out of tune with the others, and fearful of self-disclosure. What the group wants most is for the silent member to talk and to allay its fears about what he or she may be thinking. For example, in a group of students, Patty usually made two or three noncommittal comments in each session, just enough to keep her from being noticed. Patty's greatest fear was becoming the center of attention. But as members got to know one another through mutual participation in group activities, it soon became clear that no one was getting to know Patty. Two group members finally confronted her angrily at the beginning of a group. Once begun, she continued speaking in a very pressured way, hard to interrupt: "I've been listening to you all discussing your life in the dorms and your problems with your boyfriends. But I'm a commuter. I leave right after class and go to my evening job, and I don't get home until midnight. On weekends, I help my handicapped mother with the housework and help her shop and pay her bills. I don't have time for a boyfriend and homework, too. I can't think about having fun when I'm wondering how I'll manage to pay next semester's tuition or how I'll get the money to fix my car. I have nothing in common with this group. I'm not resentful or angry, and I learn a lot from listening, but don't ask me to join in when I have nothing say." After allowing the group to respond, the occupational therapist suggested that the group try to find things Patty and they had in common, rather than things that singled her out as being different. Patty was still quiet and had a hard time feeling like part of the group. But after this "event," the group no longer regarded her as an impediment. They empathized with her and collaborated to help involve her as much as she could tolerate.

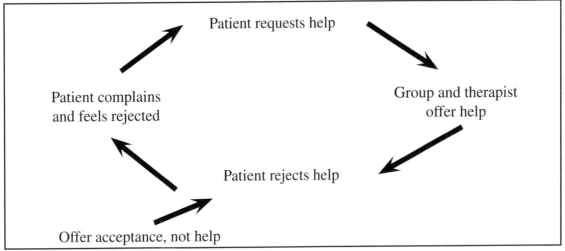

Figure 2-4. Self-defeating cycle of the help-rejecting complainer.

Attention-Getting Behaviors

There are various forms of attention-getting behavior. Most represent self-centered patterns of interaction that reflect low self-esteem and the need for external evidence of one's worth. The three types we will discuss are self-depreciation, complaining, and narcissism or self-love.

The Self-Deprecator

The self-deprecator is the client whose stories you hear over and over. He's/she's always putting himself or herself down and seems unresponsive to overtures of acceptance from others. Janice loved to do activities, so she participated willingly in occupational therapy group. But whenever she finished a project, she talked on and on about all of its flaws and imperfections. The group used to argue with her and tell her how nice her project looked. But, the routine was repeated too often, so they stopped responding to Janice at all. This "fed up" group behavior made Janice feel all the more rejected. Getting the group to help Janice to see her self-defeating behavior was a key intervention here. Through group feedback, Janice learned how she made her expectation of rejection a self-fulfilling prophecy. The leader encouraged Janice to accept the group's support and stop devaluing herself before the group gave up on her.

The Help-Rejecting Complainer

The help-rejecting complainer, referred to by Yalom as the "HRC" (1995, p. 379), chronically rejects the very help he or she asks for from the group. Yalom explains this behavior as unresolved dependency: the HRC is dependent on authoritative others, but at the same time is unable to trust others. After the fifth or sixth "yes, but..." response, the group usually becomes frustrated and angry at having all of its advice rejected. The HRC is seen as using up a lot of time and energy and getting nowhere. Marge, for example, had chronic headaches and was addicted to several medications, which, in turn,

caused a barrage of other symptoms from constipation to irrational anger. An unknowing doctor tried to help Marge by lowering her pain medication prescription. Predictably, the doctor's well-meaning action not only did not help Marge, it made him the target of all her irrational anger. She complained incessantly in group and would not be consoled. Marge had once again painted herself into a corner. Not only had the group rejected her, but she had rejected the only person (the doctor) who had the credentials to help her with her addiction problem. Why does this happen? Because the client is stuck in a self-defeating cycle (Figure 2-4).

What to do? Do not give the client the help requested. Why? Because he or she will reject the help and therefore reinforce the self-defeating cycle. The only hope for the HRC is to break the cycle. The therapist can help the group to empathize with Marge, to understand and acknowledge her feelings of defeat and frustration. As a bond with the group forms, the client might be helped to see how her own behavior invites rejection.

The Narcissistic Member (Entitled)

These attention-seekers seem to demand the constant and undivided attention of the group. Narcissistic clients have an exaggerated self-love; they feel entitled to concern, compliments, gifts, and surprises, although they give none of these to others. For example, Franklin, a small, clever, and attractive man, seemed to have a natural talent for comedy. He held the group's attention with his humor, but rarely listened to the other members. Franklin did a lot of talking about the women he had affairs with; he could not understand why these relationships never lasted. The group's need was to have Franklin contribute to the group by listening to and empathizing with others.

Groups can be very useful to clients like this, who need to alter their perception of themselves and others. It is important, however, for the therapist to protect them because of their high degree of vulnerability. The group's feedback can be accepted if it is presented in a gentle and caring way. Franklin, for all his humorous over-confidence about his sex appeal to women, had a very fragile sense of self-worth. He was highly dependent on the acceptance or rejection of others. The group, in their anger, could easily burst his bubble, and their rejection would sink him to the depths of depression. Franklin needed the group's high regard to sustain him through their feedback about how his lack of caring makes them feel. The therapist might look for an opportunity to ask the group to comment about Franklin's rejection of them in ways that are not likely to evoke defensiveness.

Psychotic Client Behavior

The client who becomes psychotic and is out of touch with reality does not benefit from group intervention, according to Yalom and Leszcz (2005). Irrational and illogical clients take up vast amounts of group energy and may bring the group process to a halt. Such clients should be removed from the group until their psychosis comes under control through medical treatment. Posthuma (2002), however, suggests that psychotic clients may benefit from occupational therapy group intervention in which the activity is the focus, rather than discussion and social interaction. People with a potential for psychosis, when stabilized with medication, have been found to benefit more from the structure of occupational therapy task groups when compared to traditional psychotherapy group treatment (Greene & Cole, 1991).

Additionally, psychosis may not always be easy to identify. Some clients continue to interact in a seemingly rational manner and may deceive the group by creating distractions or personal crises to cover their breaks with reality. Clients with borderline personality disorder (BPD) provide good examples of this problem behavior. BPD has been identified as exceedingly difficult to treat. Yalom describes these clients as having an "outward veneer of integration" that "conceals a chaotic, primitive personality structure" (1995, p. 399). Clients with BPD can thrive in occupational therapy groups because they have developed a great deal of skill. Often, they are excellent artists, craftsmen, and writers, as well as convincing talkers. In groups (as in life), they seem to go from crisis to crisis. Self-destructive acts can be an everyday occurrence, although they are often unpredictable. Group members and therapists alike are taken in by the borderline client's great potential to achieve and disappointed again and again by his or her impulsive self-destructiveness.

Group intervention can be valuable to the client with BPD because of the many opportunities to test reality. Feedback from the group can keep his or her numerous perceptual distortions and primitive needs and fears in check. However, the therapist needs to be constantly in touch with the amount of the group's time and energy taken in meeting the needs of the client with BPD.

Sometimes, these clients leave little time for the other group members. When any one member threatens the overall benefit of the group for all its members, the leader needs to take action and remove the disruptive member from the group.

TERMINATION: ENDING GROUPS THERAPEUTICALLY

For closed groups, with membership consistent over time, the number of sessions and the planned ending date have most likely been known from the beginning. Still, as the time for ending a group approaches, the leader will need to help the group through the process of termination. Some groups prepare for termination from the day they begin, while others avoid dealing with issues of termination altogether. The therapeutic learning that takes place in the group can be greatly enhanced by a good termination, or it can be destroyed by an inadequate termination. The leader should be keenly aware of the issues groups need to deal with in terminating so that he or she can help the group face them in a healthy and effective way.

This rather gruesome word *termination* is used here simply to mean the end of something. In the case of groups, it refers to the point at which groups cease to meet together as a group. Whether or not members expect to encounter one another as individuals in another context, termination of a group usually means the end of relationships as they exist within the group. The end of a group is a real loss and involves some of the same feelings associated with other losses.

Termination, when faced directly, usually involves pain and anxiety. Group members tend to avoid these feelings in a number of ways: withdrawal, devaluing the importance of the group, anger toward the leader or other members, silence and inactivity, or leaving the group prematurely. It was mentioned in the section on group development that some research shows group regression as the end approaches. A group that has reached maturity may go backwards and re-enter a state of conflict prior to termination. Some groups just ignore the impending termination by bringing up new issues as if the group would continue as usual.

A healthy ending is never easy. However, leaders can help group members to go through the process, which involves several steps:

- Review the group experience, the goals, and the learning that took place over the life of the group. Even though members may wish to devalue the group, the leader can encourage members to verbalize the goals they have accomplished or can help them recall positive learning experiences.

- Review concerns and feelings regarding separation and loss. A good therapist will encourage the expression of painful, sad, angry, or anxious feelings to prepare the members for separation. Often, the leader will experience these feelings and can share them with the group as an example.

- Use counseling skills. Empathy and confrontation (detailed in Chapter 3) are often useful in this process to help members acknowledge their feelings instead of avoiding them.

- Finish unfinished business. This seems obvious, but there may be various reasons why members wish to avoid doing it. A therapist should encourage members to bring up issues that are pending and follow-up on past conflicts to bring closure.

- Give feedback on skills learned. Group members may be engaged in giving one another feedback about changes they have made or learning what has been gained from the group's activities.

- Help generalize learning. As a way to help members accept separation, an emphasis can be placed on how what was learned in the group can be practiced and applied elsewhere. When members understand how they can apply their skills to their lives outside of the group, they can move on without diminishing the importance of their group experience.

THERAPEUTIC GROUP INTERVENTIONS: THE EVIDENCE

This subsection includes evidence from the social sciences and from occupational therapy. While reports of group interventions have appeared more frequently in the OT literature, most of the larger studies of group effectiveness come from the social sciences. In reviewing the existing empirical evidence of the effectiveness of group counseling, Kottler and Englar-Carlson (2010) conclude that ample evidence exists for overall effectiveness of groups. However, some features of therapeutic groups make them more or less effective. Burlingame and colleagues (2003) report that homogeneous groups tend to have better outcomes than heterogeneous or mixed groups. Groups with a behavioral orientation, such as knowledge acquisition or skill practice, are more effective than those with eclectic orientation (Burlingame et al., 2003). While inpatient and outpatient therapy groups have both been shown highly effective, outpatient groups are more so (Kosters, Burlingame, Nachtigall, & Strauss, 2006). Therapy groups that continue long-term report better outcomes than brief group interventions (Tschushke, Anbeh, & Kiencke, 2007).

In studying the nature of the change process of groups, Holmes and Kivlighan (2000) attributed positive change to the group interactions and relationships among group members as most influencing positive change. These

researchers identified the therapeutic factors of universality, altruism, and vicarious (interpersonal) learning as factors setting group interventions apart from individual sessions. Joyce, Piper, and Ogrodniczuk (2007) found that the quality of the therapeutic alliances or relationships of group members to the therapist and each other was most predictive of good outcomes. Shechtiman and Gluk (2005), in studying the dynamics of children's groups, likewise identified the relationship aspects of the group experience as most useful in bringing about positive outcomes.

In summarizing recent literature on group effectiveness across disciplines (business, education, and therapy), Kottler and Englar-Carlson (2010) compiled the following as most characteristic of groups with positive outcomes:

- High levels of trust and safety
- Individual and cultural differences are respected
- Clear boundaries and rules of conduct are in place
- Conflict is acknowledged and worked through (or resolved without hostility)
- Information and resources are openly shared
- Every member participates
- Unproductive behaviors are effectively managed so as not to block the group's progress
- The group accomplishes its objectives (efficiency)
- Nonverbal communications are acknowledged and verbalized
- There is continuity and follow-up from one session to the next
- A healthy group culture guides group behaviors, in which both caring behaviors and productive contributions are encouraged
- The group process results in some form of action (for members both inside and outside the group) (Adapted from Kottler & Englar-Carlson, 2010, p. 35).

The above list of group characteristics may guide occupational therapy group leaders in two ways. First, they can serve as goals around which to design group activities, thus supporting and helping to build a healthy group culture. Second, when groups function poorly, these factors might serve as a checklist when attempting to identify what might be causing the group to falter and what actions could be taken to address the problem. All of these characteristics relate in some way to the group culture and, as such, may be openly discussed as a group self-reflection at appropriate stages of group development.

Occupational Therapy Group Evidence

Probably the best-known evidence of OT group effectiveness comes from the USC Well Elderly study, a nationwide randomized controlled trial using multiple pre-post measures of health and well-being. This 9-month occupational therapy program for community-living older adults combined group and individual interventions. These researchers state, "the decision to execute the Lifestyle Redesign program mainly in groups was made primarily because of the therapeutic benefit of group process and only secondarily because of potential cost benefits" (Mandel, Jackson, Zemke, Nelson, & Clark, 1999, p. 26). In fact, the authors cite an earlier edition of this text in outlining the structure and leadership for their group interventions (p. 26). The groups met 2 hours per week, following a schedule of pre-determined modules, which included components of education about occupation and its importance in maintaining wellness, open discussion and interaction, and group activity participation. A report of this study in the *Journal of the American Medical Association* described the intervention as "an OT group, a social activity group, and a nontreatment control group," resulting in "significant benefits for the OT preventive treatment group...across various health, function, and quality of life domains" (Clark et al., 1997, p. 1321). In a replication of the American well elderly study, Craig and Mountain (2007) conducted similar groups in the United Kingdom, with equally positive results. Some of the benefits outlined in the UK study included the following:

- A sense of validation by older person's peer group
- Isolation broken down
- New skills practiced in a supportive environment
- Social support and friendships
- Generation of ideas through listening to each other and engaging in group problem solving
- Modeling, where other members acted as role models (adapted from Craig & Mountain, 2007)

A follow-up study by these authors attributes the benefits of the group program to an increase in self-efficacy that resulted from members doing activities with others and "[translating] skills developed within the safety of the group into real world experiences" (Mountain & Craig, 2011). In both studies, participants had maintained gains in occupational participation, health, and well-being in a 6-month follow-up measure after the program ended. Carlson, Clark, and Young (1998) conclude that "given their experience in the therapeutic use of occupation to foster health and life satisfaction, occupational therapists are ideally situated to play a major role in the design and administration of preventive health care for elders" (p. 115).

In other published studies, occupational therapists have reported many group interventions with positive outcomes. In an experimental study comparing inpatient mental health OT task groups with traditional psychotherapy groups, Cole and Greene (1988) found that all mental health clients preferred the OT task groups and that those with borderline personality disorders had a stronger preference for OT task groups. For people with stroke and resultant hemiparesis, Capasso, Gorman, and Blick (2010) report good results in their breakfast groups, which offered a social alternative to repetitive upper extremity exercise. The sharing of breakfast allowed participants to share experiences with, learn from, and encourage each other while improving upper extremity function. Kalina (2010) describes a "successful student group" to help people with multiple sclerosis to function successfully in an educational environment. Topics included taking notes, test-taking strategies, managing symptoms, asking for help, and staying connected with others.

What Is the Ideal Size for Groups?

Most sources quote Yalom and Leszcz as the authority on the size of therapy groups: they suggest seven to eight members as ideal, with numbers ranging from five to 10 (2005). Similarly, Kottler and Englar-Carlson suggest that six to eight members is a "manageable size" or eight to 12 with two co-leaders (2010, p. 269). The USC Lifestyle Redesign program used groups of eight to 10 members, meeting 2 hours per week for 9 months, with highly effective outcomes (Jackson, Carlson, Mandel, Zemke, & Clark, 1998). Howe and Schwartzberg (2001) define the minimum number for a group as two, although the ideal size changes according to the goals and the amount of interaction required to meet stated objectives. These authors concur with Yalom's ideal: "seven members can work together effectively in the activity of the group and participate fully in the process of the group" (2001, p. 147). As a contemporary update from business team research, Parkinson (2009), CEO of TransUnion, uses the "two pizza rule"—teams should not exceed the number one can feed with two large pizzas (six to nine members).

Summary

Because students best learn about group dynamics through experience, it is recommended that students meet in a series of six to 10 group sessions. These can be led by peers or by an instructor and can follow the format of Chapter 12 or 13.

As a way to enhance an awareness of group dynamics, it is suggested that the Personal Group Reaction Paper Outline (Worksheet 2-6) be used to record student reactions after each group session.

The Group Leadership Analysis Assignment (Worksheet 2-7) is intended for the more advanced student. Students in a group lab sign up to lead one of the groups described in Chapter 12 or 13 and videotape the group. The analysis assignment serves as a guide to more in-depth observation of group process from an occupational therapy leadership perspective.

Worksheet 2-6
Personal Group Reaction Paper Outline

Title (a few words expressing theme): _____

Date of Session: _____

Seating Pattern Diagram:

1. Draw a diagram of the seating arrangement, listing names of each member present and his or her position within the group.

2. Discuss significance of seating pattern, positions near leader, opposite leader, pairing, subgroups.

3. Note absences and impact of these.

```
┌─────────────────────────────────┐
│         Seating Diagram         │
│                                 │
│                                 │
│                                 │
│                                 │
│                                 │
│                                 │
└─────────────────────────────────┘
```

Norms: Identify "rules" of the group (confidentiality, respect, etc.).

1. Which are verbalized (explicit)?

2. What norms are not verbalized (implicit) (e.g., What behaviors are acceptable to the group? Not acceptable?)

3. Each week, note any changes in group norms from previous weeks.

Content: Identify the major discussion topics of the group.

Process:

1. Theme—Based on the topics discussed, identify the predominant theme of the session in a few words or a phrase (this becomes the "title" of your paper). The theme should have both a content and a process (or feeling) component. Then, explain how you arrived at this theme. How do the topics reflect the theme, and why were they verbalized (or not verbalized) in this manner?

From Cole, M. B. *Group dynamics in occupational therapy: The theoretical basis and practice application of group intervention* (4th ed.). Thorofare, NJ: SLACK Incorporated. © 2012 SLACK Incorporated.

Worksheet 2-6
Personal Group Reaction Paper Outline (Continued)

2. Stage—Identify the stage of development you think your group is in and why.

3. Verbal communication—What significant interpersonal interactions took place between group members? Be sure to name names. Vagueness is not helpful to the understanding of process. Interpret what was implied or hidden in the group discussion. What subjects were avoided and why?

4. Nonverbal communication—What was the general mood of the group? What was communicated by nonverbal behaviors of members, especially feelings of members? Interpret significance. How did nonverbal behaviors affect group functioning?

Personal Reaction: Identify your role and the impact you had on the group. Describe your personal feelings.
1. How did you respond to this group?

2. How do you feel about your relationship to individual group members (give names)?

3. How did you react to the leader (honesty counts)?

Self-Evaluation: What did you learn about yourself today in group (strengths, weaknesses, values, interactive style)?

Goal: What are your personal goals for the next session?

From Cole, M. B. *Group dynamics in occupational therapy: The theoretical basis and practice application of group intervention* (4th ed.). Thorofare, NJ: SLACK Incorporated. © 2012 SLACK Incorporated.

Group Leadership Analysis Assignment
(Due 2 Weeks After You Lead Group)

Video and Preparation

You must videotape your group. As a group leader, you are responsible for arranging to borrow a camera and tripod from AV for your assigned date. (Plan ahead!) Please purchase a good quality videotape as you will need to keep it for use in a graduate course next year. You are responsible for the quality of the finished video. Position the tripod so that you are facing the camera and all group members are visible and away from distracting noises (vents) so that voices may be clearly heard. No adjustment of taping should be necessary after you start your group, so that you will be able to give the group your full attention as a leader. Also, prepare copies of worksheets and written group plan.

Analysis Guidelines (four pages or more, double spaced, 1-inch margins)

1. *Steps:* Watch the videotape and summarize what occurred during each of the seven steps.
2. *Goals:* What were the therapeutic goals and how well were they achieved? Be specific.
3. *Process:* Discuss the process of the group. What was the prevailing theme? What feelings were expressed verbally/nonverbally? What was the level of self-disclosure (stage of group development)? What barriers or conflicts became evident (must name at least one)?
4. *Member Roles:* What roles did each member play? What emotional issues were expressed by each member? (Should list names individually and answer for each.)
5. *Meaningful Interactions:* Choose three significant interactions that occurred between members in this group; describe and discuss why they were significant.

Self-Analysis

1. *Leadership Role:* Discuss your leadership role in this group. Compare your own expectations with the group experience. What challenges did the group members represent for you as leader? What could you have improved or done differently and how?
2. *Highlights:* Identify three highlights of your leadership skills during this group (list videotape positions for these). These should represent group reactions or interactions that challenged you as a leader and for which you demonstrated effective group leadership. Write a short paragraph describing each, including what was stated, what interventions you used, and why.
3. *Transference/Counter Transference:* What emotional responses did members evoke for you, and what prior relationships or experiences help explain these responses (either positive or negative)?
4. *Personal Reaction:* How did you feel about leading this group? What was most personally meaningful about it and why?

**Videotapes of group sessions must be kept confidential. As a precaution, after you hand it in, your instructor will keep your videotape until the end of the semester.

REFERENCES

Benne, K., & Sheats, P. (1948). Functional roles of group members. *Journal of Social Issues, 2*(4), 123-135.

Bion, W. (1961). *Experiences in groups and other papers.* New York, NY: Basic Books.

Burlingame, G. M., Furhman, A., & Mosier, J. (2003). The differential effectiveness of group psychotherapy: A meta-analytic perspective. *Groups Dynamics Theory, Research, and Practice, 7,* 3-12.

Capasso, N., Gorman, A., & Blick, C. (2010). Breakfast group in an acute rehabilitation setting: A restorative program for incorporating client's hemiparetic upper extremities for function. *OT Practice, 15*(8), 14-18.

Carlson, M., Clark, F., & Young, B. (1998). Practical contributions of occupational science to the art of successful ageing: How to sculpt a meaningful life in older adulthood. *Journal of Occupational Science, 5*(3), 107-118.

Cathcart, R., & Samovar, L. (1974). *Small group communication: A reader* (2nd ed.). Dubuque, IA: W. C. Brown Co.

Clark, F., Azen, S., Zemke, R., Jackson, J., Carlson, M., Mandel, D., Hay, J., ... Lipson, L. (1997). Occupational therapy for independent-living older adults: A randomized controlled trial. *Journal of the American Medical Association, 278,* 1321-1326.

Cole, M., & Greene, L. (1988). A preference for activity: A comparative study of psychotherapy groups vs. occupational therapy groups for psychotic and borderline patients. In D. Gibson (Ed.), *Group process and structure in psychosocial occupational therapy.* New York, NY: Haworth Press.

Corey, G., Corey, M. S., Callanan, P., & Russel, J. (1988). *Group techniques* (Rev ed.). Pacific Grove, CA: Brooks/Cole.

Craig, C., & Mountain, G. (2007). *Lifestyle matters: An occupational approach to healthy ageing.* Milton Keynes, UK: Speechmark Publishing.

DeLucia-Waack, J. L., & Donigian, J. (2004). *The practice of multicultural groupwork.* Belmont, CA: Brooks.

Eldridge, N., & Gould, S. J. (1972). Punctuated equilibria: An alternative to phyletic gradualism. In Schopf (Ed.), *Models in paleobioloby.* San Francisco, CA: Freeman, Cooper & Co.

Gersick, C. J. (2003). Time and transition in work teams. In R. Hirokawa, R. Cathcart, L. Samovar, & L. Henman (Eds.), *Small group communication: Theory and practice: An anthology* (8th ed.). Los Angeles, CA: Roxbury Publishing.

Greene, L., & Cole, M. (1991). Level and form of psychopathology and the structure of group therapy. *International Journal of Group Psychotherapy, 41,* 499-521.

Holmes, S. E., & Kivlighan, D. M. J. (2000). Comparison of therapeutic factors in group and individual treatment processes. *Journal of Counseling Psychology, 47,* 478-484.

Howe, M. C., & Schwartzberg, S. L. (2001). *A functional approach to group work in occupational therapy* (3rd ed.). Philadelphia, PA: Lippincott, Williams & Wilkins.

Jackson, J., Carlson, M., Mandel, D., Zemke, R., & Clark, F. (1998). Occupation in lifestyle redesign: The well elderly study occupational therapy program. *American Journal of Occupational Therapy, 52,* 326-336.

Joyce, A. S., Piper, W. E., & Ogrodniczuk, J. S. (2007). Therapeutic alliance and cohesion variables as predictors of outcome in short term group psychotherapy. *International Journal of Group Psychotherapy, 57,* 269-296.

Kalina, J. T. (2009). Role of occupational therapy in a multiple sclerosis center. *OT Practice, 14,* 9-13.

Kosters, M., Burlingame, G., Nachtigall, C., & Strauss, B. (2006). A meta-analytic review of the effectiveness of inpatient group psychotherapy. Group Dynamics: *Theory, Research, & Practice, 10,* 146-163.

Kottler, J. A., & Englar-Carlson, M. (2010). *Learning group leadership: An experiential approach* (2nd ed.). Los Angeles, CA: Sage Publications.

Mandel, D., Jackson, J., Zemke, R., Nelson, L., & Clark, F. (1999). *Lifestyle redesign: Implementing the well elderly program.* Bethesda, MD: American Occupational Therapy Association.

Mountain, G., & Craig, C. (2011). The lived experience of redesigning lifestyle post retirement. *Occupational Therapy International* (in press).

Parkinson, J. (2009). IT project teams: Big vs. small. CIO Strategy. Retrieved from http://blogs.cioinsight.com/cio_strategy/content/it_architecture/it_project_teams_big_vs_small.html

Poole, M. S. (2003). A multiple sequence model of group decision development. In R. Hirokawa, R. Cathcart, L. Samovar, & L. Henman (Eds.), *Small group communication: Theory and practice: An anthology* (8th ed.). Los Angeles, CA: Roxbury Publishing.

Posthuma, B. (2002). *Small groups in counseling and therapy: Process and leadership* (4th ed.). Boston, MA: Little Brown.

Ryan, D. (2010). Tools for facilitating health care teamwork: 2. *University of Toronto center for interprofessional education.* Retrieved from http://www.ipe.utoronto.ca/std/ryan2.html

Schechtman, Z., Gluk, O. (2005). Therapeutic factors in group psychotherapy with children. *Group Dynamics Theory, Research, and Practice, 9,* 127-134.

Schutz, W. (1958). The interpersonal underworld. *Harvard Business Review, 36,* 123-135.

Tschuschke, V., Anbeh, T., & Kiencke, P. (2007). Evaluation of long term analytic outpatient group therapies. *Group Analysis, 40,* 140-159.

Tuckman, B. W. (1965). Developmental sequence in small groups. *Psychological Bulletin, 63,* 384-399.

Tuckman, B. W., & Jenson, M. A. (1977) Stages of small group development revisited. *Group and Organization Studies, 2,* 419-427.

Yalom, I., & Leszcz M. (2005). *The theory and practice of group psychotherapy* (5th ed.). New York, NY: Basic Books.

Chapter 3

CLIENT-CENTERED GROUPS

This chapter discusses OT group leadership in the context of some of the major theoretical trends in health care in the 21st century. These trends include complex systems theory, clinical and professional reasoning, client-centered practice, cultural competence, and therapeutic use of self. Earlier, we stated that the seven-step format for group leadership simplifies, for the purposes of student learning, an exceedingly complex process of group leadership. Here, we will discuss just how complex groups can be and how the unpredictable nature of group interactions can be harnessed to increase the probability of therapeutic outcomes. The focus on client centeredness, specified in the OT practice framework for all evaluations and interventions (AOTA, 2008), requires that group leaders begin with a thoughtful and empathetic understanding of every group member, respecting the values, wishes, preferences, and unique culture of each one. All of the information gained through therapist-client interactions combines with the therapist's knowledge of health conditions and therapeutic methods and techniques to become a part of the expert group leader's clinical thinking process. Clinical thinking in groups is a dynamic process, responsive to the changing directions, emotional reactions, and member conflicts and inter-relationships, that continues to guide leadership as the group unfolds. In this way, the group leader strategically applies all of the skills in therapeutic use of self, in the context of effective group leadership.

COMPLEXITY THEORY IN HEALTH CARE AND OCCUPATIONAL THERAPY

Complexity theory, also called complex systems theory (Cilliers, 1998), chaos theory (MacGill, 2007), and dynamical systems theory (Gray, Kennedy, & Zemke, 1996), represents the next generation of systems theory. Whiteford, Klomp, and St. Clair (2005) describe it as "the richness and variety of structure and behavior that arises from interactions between components of a system" (p. 5). Complexity science "studies systems that are too complex to accurately predict the future, but that nonetheless exhibit underlying patterns that can help us cope in an increasingly complex world" (MacGill, 2007). Complexity theory has been applied across a wide range of disciplines, including earthquakes, traffic patterns, the stock market, human evolution, and group dynamics. Its use has been augmented through the use of computers to calculate statistics involving very large numbers of components and inter-relationships.

Historically, complexity theory arose out of a need to understand phenomena that could not easily be studied through traditional reductionistic methodology (Geyer, 2004). Beginning with Newtonian or linear thinking, which Geyer dubs the "paradigm of order" in the time of the industrial revolution, scientists believed in the power of human reason. They relied upon the scientific method to reveal basic objective truth, a type of thinking also referred to as "modernism." By the mid-20th

Cole M.B. *Group Dynamics in Occupational Therapy:*
The Theoretical Basis and Practice Application
of Group Intervention (pp 59-102).
© 2012 SLACK Incorporated.

century, postmodernism challenged the idea of objective truth, proposing that truth is never static, but rather dynamic, changing with time, place, person, and situation. Postmodernists believe that there are, in fact, multiple truths, that can only be understood through the use of qualitative research, such as interviews, narratives, and participant observation, methods now widely used, especially in the social sciences. Postmodernism may be viewed as "disorderly" and therefore directly opposing the paradigm of order. Complexity theory challenges both of these opposites, calling them "equally flawed" but nonetheless "partly true." In fact, the world can be both orderly and disorderly, rational and irrational, predictable and unpredictable, often simultaneously. In this way, complexity theory seeks to build a bridge between the two extremes (Geyer, 2004).

In her AOTA presidential address, Florence Clark (2010) promoted the concept of "occupational therapy in high definition," a metaphor that illustrates how scientific reductionism and complex holistic views co-exist in OT practice. In a high-definition picture, we can zoom in for a better look at the detail of a person's face, the position of a tennis ball with respect to the foul line, or the number on a license plate, but then broaden the scope in order to take in the bigger picture, the whole situation, the multiple contexts within which the action takes place. In complexity theory, OTs do not have to choose between the application of biomechanics, notably reductionistic, and an occupation-based theory, such as the Model of Human Occupation. Both views of the person help us in different ways, and one does not exclude the other.

Whiteford and colleagues (2005) explore occupation and OT practice within the context of complexity theory as a way of framing the environmental influences upon practice: professional, organizational, socio-cultural, and political/economic contexts. They write, "to understand complex systems such as occupation and professional practice, understanding the components is clearly not enough" (p. 4, citing Kielhofner, 2000; Wilcock, 2001). In groups, "strange things happen when you put individuals together to form a system. They interact with their environment (context). They interact with one another. And the effects of all these interactions can be unpredictable. They can be profound. Studying these effects—learning to understand them—that is what complexity research is all about" (Whiteford et al., 2005, p. 4). Gray and colleagues (1996) propose complexity as an appropriate model for occupational science: "studies of complex, dynamic systems suggest that living systems are self-organizing and pattern forming. Human patterns of occupation may reflect this quality" (p. 298). Creek (2010) proposes complexity theory as the guiding model for a group of European OTs seeking to agree upon the basic concepts of the profession, which will subsequently be defined and translated into various languages. Creek suggests that competing epistemologies "may be resolved by abandoning the use of general systems theory as an organizing framework for the profession's knowledge base, and moving towards a fuller acknowledgment of the complexity of occupational therapy theory and practice" (2010, p. 2).

CLINICAL REASONING IN OCCUPATIONAL THERAPY GROUPS

If we accept complexity as an organizing principle, we also acknowledge that there is much we still do not, and may never, know. With multiple changing realities impacting the process of occupational therapy intervention, much of what we do cannot be accurately predicted. For students, this can be overwhelming and discouraging. Whiteford et al. (2005) suggest that the most important skill OT students and practitioners need today is "to know how to learn. This is, of course, underpinned by an ability to think" (p. 8). In addressing human problems, "an appreciation of multiple perspectives can ensure better communication," resulting in better solutions. "A systems thinker would deal adequately with the social dimension of a problem (political, economic, human) rather than just technical" (Mant, 1997, in Whiteford et al., 2005, p. 8). Recently, a systems orientation, or "broad band intelligence," has been identified as a key component of effective leadership (Mant, 1997; Rimmington, 2001). In the business world, the best team leaders would understand the "complex matrix of discipline and team role specialties...in the multi-disciplinary team" (Belbin, 1983, in Whiteford et al., 2005, p. 9).

Clinical reasoning is also called professional reasoning, a term some scholars feel is better suited to today's broad range of clinical and nonclinical practice settings. Professional reasoning provides a good example of complexity theory in action because of its simultaneous application of multiple perspectives: scientific, narrative, pragmatic, interactive, ethical, and conditional (Schell & Schell, 2008). Much has changed since Mattingly (1994) and Fleming (1994) first published their ground-breaking clinical reasoning study in 1994. The therapist with the "three track mind" (Fleming, 1994, p. 119) included the following types of reasoning:

- *Procedural:* Similar to medical problem solving, OTs seek to solve problems with everyday occupations using evaluation and intervention techniques that are evidence-based.

- *Interactive:* Connecting with the person as a social being, including establishing a therapeutic relationship, engaging the client in treatment, and communicating a sensitivity to and appreciation for the client's cultural background, life story, and experience of illness.

- *Conditional:* A complex metacognitive process, including broader social and temporal contexts, such as the meaning of illness and disability for the family and others, and envisioning how the health condition might change and be changed by the clinical encounter (Fleming, 1994).

- *Narrative:* This additional type of reasoning refers to the therapist's own everyday storytelling, identified by Mattingly as "a way to enlarge a therapists' practical knowledge through vicariously sharing other therapists' experience" (1994, p. 19). In groups, storytelling also enlarges the practical knowledge of all the members.

The application of just these three types of reasoning applied simultaneously by expert OTs illustrates the presence of complex systems thinking.

More recently, Schell and Schell (2008) have identified two more modes of reasoning and redefined the original three. Their five dimensions of reasoning include the following:

1. *Scientific:* Includes procedural reasoning, scientific knowledge, and methods and techniques associated with various health conditions.

2. *Narrative:* Refers to client's reports of subjective experience, life history, problem situations, and perspectives on occupational issues and contexts. Storytelling (narrative) serves two purposes—to understand the illness or disability as it affects the person's life and to provide an unfolding story of how disability and occupational therapy could change that life story.

3. *Pragmatic:* Practical considerations, including time and place of intervention, funding issues, and the OT's skill sets.

4. *Ethical reasoning:* Reasoning related to values, judgments, and doing what is right. Consideration for philosophical issues such as the values of autonomy, beneficence (doing good), nonmaleficence (doing no harm), occupational justice, confidentiality, and dignity factor into this type of reasoning.

5. *Interactive and conditional reasoning:* Schell synthesizes these two, referring to reasoning that guides therapist-client interactions, relationship building, power and practice cultures, and envisioning and preparing for changes in short- and long-term care (Schell & Schell, 2008).

Others have also expanded upon the original three tracks. For example, Neistadt (1998) reported five common types: narrative, procedural, interactive, pragmatic, and conditional.

Schwartzberg (2002) focused mainly on one type, interactive reasoning, which she summarized as "the thoughts and means used by an OT to get to know a person and engage the intervention process" (p. 35). Schwartzberg acknowledges, however, that all types of reasoning inter-relate and must also be applied and understood in relation to each other. Through interviews with OTs, Schwartzberg identified five themes within the interactive process: 1) active participation and collaboration, 2) engaging/connecting with the person, 3) exploring and interpreting motives as well as occupation-based meanings, 4) listening, and 5) understanding and use of narratives and symbols. Schwartzberg notes that the dimensions of interactive reasoning occur with groups as well as with individuals. Therefore, the same therapeutic skills apply, such as active listening, establishing trust, communicating hope and empathy, and the process of building mutual respect and rapport.

Ward (2003) studied the nature of clinical reasoning in groups through in-depth interviews and participant observation with an expert OT group therapist (Joan) in a mental health setting. Joan's reflections on group interventions revealed the simultaneous use of procedural and interactive reasoning, as well as pragmatic and narrative reasoning. Here are some examples: Joan observed a morning community meeting and began thinking about client behaviors and what they might mean when these same clients attended her two task-oriented groups (interpretation of behavioral cues is both procedural and interactive). Her interactions with clients served as a means of assessment (interactive and procedural), while they also conveyed empathy and encouraged positive interaction with other members to make them feel connected (both interactive and procedural). With some clients, she used humor to engage them in the task. When several clients needed her attention at the same time, she kidded them about taking a ticket at the deli counter. This use of metaphor illustrates a form of narrative reasoning. As members engaged in the activity, Joan noticed that some had more skill than others and suggested they help one another (pragmatic reasoning). She constantly monitors the members to make sure they continue to engage in the task (pragmatic). When Joan discusses the process of the group, she helps members understand the meaning of their interactions: some can feel a sense of efficacy at having finished a task or having helped someone else. Some client interactions, conveying empathy to one another, help them to practice social skills and to feel a sense of belonging. These process comments fall into the category of narrative reasoning. Also, a part of interactive reasoning is Joan's ongoing awareness of her own reactions to clients and the need to adjust her behaviors in order to best meet their needs, both individually and as a group. This study illustrates the complex reasoning process that occurs during OT group leadership.

O'Reilly's (1994) New York subway group leadership provides a now classic illustration of the value of narrative reasoning in addressing physical disability (in Mattingly, 1994, p. 261). O'Reilly was asked to take over an "upper extremity group" for which assigned members with spinal cord injury routinely did not show up. In preparation, O'Reilly interviewed each member and discovered they all came from New York City. As a strategy to get them engaged, O'Reilly used a combination of interactive and narrative reasoning, encouraging them to tell her stories of riding the New York subway. As the group evolved, she incorporated upper extremity exercises through the creation of graffiti (typically seen on subway walls). The members expressed their emotions through the graffiti, told each other their life stories, and suggested other subway-related activities: baking New York pretzels, grilling hot dogs, and creating a scrapbook of New York subway scenes. Through narrative storytelling, O'Reilly transformed this group of "body parts" into a compelling group theme that became the first episode of an ongoing saga to which each member felt connected.

Group leadership involves all of the identified types of clinical/professional reasoning at some point. Scientific or procedural reasoning may be most active in the design stages of groups, so that evaluation and/or intervention applies the field's best knowledge, theories, techniques, and evidence to the occupational problems of members. Interactive reasoning focuses on building relationships with individual group members, as well as facilitating their relationships with each other. Narrative reasoning concerns the meaning of group experiences and activities for members, and how they can use group learning in their own occupational lives. Conditional reasoning seeks to understand connections between experiences within the group and the environmental systems with which the group members interact outside the group. Ethical and pragmatic reasoning come into play when dilemmas emerge, requiring group problem solving. In real life, group leaders often apply several types of reasoning simultaneously, as needed by the members and the situation.

CLIENT-CENTERED PRACTICE AND THE CANADIAN MODEL OF OCCUPATIONAL PERFORMANCE AND ENGAGEMENT

This approach has also been called person-centered, and the basic concepts are similar to patient-centered and family-centered practice. Matheson prefers person-centered to client-centered "because being a person is more basic and encompassing than being a client" (1998, p. 108). Client-centered practice as an approach in occupational therapy was developed by the Canadian Occupational Therapy Association (1991, 1997) in the 1980s and earlier. Recently, the client-centered approach

takes a central place in the American Occupational Therapy Association's (AOTA's) core values (AOTA, 2004; Law, 1998) and OT practice framework (AOTA, 2002, 2008). Client-centered principles are based, in part, on the theories of Carl Rogers, Abraham Maslow, and Robert White. This set of compatible concepts has also been called the humanistic approach. In addition, the writings of Irvin Yalom and Rollo May enlighten us on how many of these principles can be enacted in groups. Irvin Yalom has long been recognized as an existential group psychotherapist, and Rollo May is credited with translating existential ideas from many sources for use in mainstream American psychotherapy (Corey, 1996). Many of the concepts reviewed here are also reflected in AOTA's core values, ethics, and philosophy of occupational therapy (Crepeau, Cohn, & Schell, 2003). People are seen as equally valuable, regardless of their race, religion, gender, level of intellectual ability, socioeconomic position, or state of health. The "Philosophical Base of Occupational Therapy," adopted by the AOTA in April 1979, states that "human beings are able to influence their physical and mental health and their social and physical environment through purposeful activity" and "adaptation is a change in function that promotes survival and self-actualization" (AOTA, 2004, p. 403). Client-centered groups using the seven steps outlined in Chapter 1 will bring our group interventions into harmony with the fundamental philosophy and values of our profession as well as with client-centered practice (Table 3-1).

The Canadian Model of Occupational Performance and Engagement (CMOP-E; Townsend & Polatajko, 2007) provides a fitting framework for OT practice with diverse populations, as well as revision and definition of its core concepts: occupation and enablement. These authors redefine OT as "the art and science of enabling engagement in everyday living through occupation; of enabling people to perform occupations that foster health and well-being; and of enabling a just and inclusive society so that all people may participate to their potential in the daily occupations of life" (2007, p. 89). The definition of the client has expanded to include individuals, families, groups, communities, organizations, and populations. This new version reflects a "deeper appreciation for the complexity of occupation and enablement" (p. 5).

The term *occupation* acknowledges Dunton's statements that "occupation is as necessary to life as food and drink, every human being should have both physical and mental occupations, and sick minds, sick bodies and sick souls may be healed through occupation". In the Canadian model, OTs look beyond occupational performance to occupational engagement, which encompasses not only performance but also its importance, meaning, and the satisfaction it provides the client. Table 3-2 lists the possible occupational interactions with which OTs are concerned.

Table 3-1

The Philosophical Base of Occupational Therapy

Man is an active being whose development is influenced by the use of purposeful activity. Using their capacity for intrinsic motivation, human beings are able to influence their physical and mental health and their social and physical environment through purposeful activity. Human life includes a process of continuous adaptation. Adaptation is a change in function that promotes survival and self-actualization. Biological, psychological, and environmental factors may interrupt the adaptation process at any time throughout the life cycle. Dysfunction may occur when adaptation is impaired. Purposeful activity facilitates the adaptive process.

Occupational therapy is based on the belief that purposeful activity (occupation), including its interpersonal and environmental components, may be used to prevent and mediate dysfunction and to elicit maximum adaptation. Activity as used by the OT includes both an intrinsic and a therapeutic purpose.

This statement was adopted by the April 1979 Representative Assembly of The American Occupational Therapy Association, Inc. as Resolution C #53-79. The text can be found as noted below:
American Occupational Therapy Association. (1979). The philosophical base of occupational therapy. *American Journal of Occupational Therapy, 33,* 785.
American Occupational Therapy Association. (1979). Policy 1.11. The philosophical base of occupational therapy. In: *Policy manual of The American Occupational Therapy Association, Inc.* Bethesda, MD: Author.

Copyright American Occupational Therapy Association. Reprinted with permission.

Table 3-2

Modes of Occupational Interaction

- *Capacity:* Mental and physical doing
- *Competence:* Both ability and potential for occupational performance
- *Deprivation:* Environmental influences limiting occupational choice and participation
- *Development:* Gradual changes over time, growth, and maturation
- *Engagement:* Participating, involving oneself in doing
- *Enrichment:* Deliberation manipulation of environmental contexts to support occupational engagement
- *History:* Occupational progressions, experiences, and transitions
- *Identity:* Occupations that contribute to one's internal and social self
- *Mastery:* Competence and belief in one's occupational abilities
- *Participation:* Involvement in a life situation (WHO, 2001) through occupation
- *Pattern:* Scheduling and routines of doing
- *Potential:* Predicted ability for occupational development
- *Role:* Occupations and tasks associated with social role expectations
- *Satisfaction:* Contentment with one's occupational engagement

Adapted from Townsend, E. A., & Polatajko, H. J. (2007). *Enabling occupation II: Advancing an occupational therapy vision for health, well-being, & justice through occupation* (pp. 26). Ottawa, ON: Canadian Association of Occupational Therapy.

The term *enablement*, unlike evaluation and intervention, implies empowering the client to take control and responsibility in partnership with the OT, and its language is embedded in cultural meanings. Culture is a dynamic process by which "meanings are ascribed to commonly experienced phenomena and objects" (Iwama, 2006). Diverse cultures require diverse forms of enablement. The authors envision enablement not only as OT's unique collection of methodology, but also as a theory of social change through occupation. The term comes from the Ottawa Charter for Health Promotion (WHO, 1986), which names three key strategies to improve/maintain health: 1) enable, 2) advocate, and 3) mediate. The CMOP-E describes enablement as reducing differences in current health status and ensuring equal opportunities and resources to enable all people to achieve their fullest health potential. The role of enablement includes advocating for and providing a supportive environment, access to information, development of life skills, and the "means and opportunity to participate in shaping their own lives."

Enabling is the basis for OTs' client-centered practice and a foundation for empowerment and justice. For CMOP-E, "enablement is the most appropriate form of helping when the goal is occupational performance" (Townsend & Polatajko, 2007, p. 99). The following occupation-based foundations further define enabling:

- *Choice, risk, and responsibility:* Based in part on the Ottawa Charter, this defines the existential belief in the human need and ability to exercise free will, make one's own decisions, and take responsibility for one's own choices. OTs and other professionals need to respect each person's right to self-direct.

- *Client participation:* The OT invites the client to explain his or her own perspective regarding occupational issues and needs and to select occupational goals, methods, and circumstances with the guidance of the therapist. This central feature forms the basis of the therapist-client partnership, in which both participate as equals and each shares different areas of expertise.

- *Vision of possibilities:* OTs and clients together explore possible and desired outcomes of intervention, providing hope and optimism for positive changes in occupational engagement and participation.

- *Change:* OT and client together define the process by which client goals and visions for the future might be achieved, such as developing, maintaining, and restoring occupational abilities, and/or preventing negative outcomes.

- *Justice:* Involves identifying and removing environmental barriers, as well as advocating for social change to equalize occupational opportunities and inclusion for diverse populations.

- *Power-sharing:* The enactment of the previous strategies to form a collaborative partnership with clients, involving genuine interest in one another, acknowledgment of each other's expertise, empathy, altruism, trust, and creative communication. Instead of "What can I do for you?" or "What will I tell you?" the OT asks him- or herself, "What will we learn from each other?" (2007, p. 107).

The Canadian model, which translates the more generic client-centered concepts into the language and practice of OT in Canada, has the benefit of a great deal of evidence to support it. According to multidisciplinary sources, while client-centered practice has its challenges, especially in overcoming power barriers within the health care system, studies suggest that client-centered practice generally leads to better outcomes (Black, 2005; Sumison, 2005). In 2006, Sumison and Law summarized the evidence for some of the basic concepts of the client-centered practice: power, listening and communication, partnership, choice, and hope. Their findings are summarized in Table 3-3.

CORE CONCEPTS OF CLIENT-CENTERED PRACTICE

Existential Concepts

Existential theory can be seen as the forerunner of humanism and person-centered therapy. Existentialism focuses on understanding the person's subjective view of the world. In client-centered practice, occupational therapy practitioners use interactive reasoning and therapeutic use of self in order to better understand the client's experience, situation, emotions, life roles, and occupational concerns. Central to existentialism is the idea that meaning in life is not predetermined and that each person must find meaning for him- or herself. Part of OT's role is to find out how occupations give meaning to the lives of clients. The major contributions of the existentialists lie in three key concepts:

1. Freedom and responsibility
2. Aloneness and relatedness
3. Existential anxiety and search for meaning

Freedom and Responsibility

Freedom implies that an individual has a capacity for self-awareness and awareness of his or her environment that allows him or her to make choices. An individual who is aware need not allow his or her present behavior to be determined by others, his or her situation, or his or her past experiences. He or she alone is responsible for his or her own life dilemmas. Therapy that uses this approach is aimed at getting clients to see that they have

Table 3-3

Client-Centered Concepts and Evidence

Power	• Barriers still exist for balancing the power between therapist and client. • Clients are disempowered by the health system (Corring, 1996). • Policies readily disempower those they are designed to help (Townsend, 2003). • People with disabilities generally lack power (Townsend, 2003). • Power sharing increases the likelihood of client-participation (Hall, Roter, & Katz, 1988).
Listening and communication	• Listening sometimes means being silent and making room for the client to explore (Harrison, 2001). • Listening to client worries and fears (empathizing) is a prerequisite of taking appropriate action (Maxmin, 2002). • More clients use technology/internet to access health information and want to discuss options for care; clients want to be involved in decisions (College of Health, 1999; Law & Mills, 1998). • Communication of information is a central focus of client-centered practice (Coulter & Dunn, 2002). Health information and evidence is essential for clients to make good decisions about their own health (Baum & Law, 1997). Professionals need better training in how to use information with clients to promote informed decision making (College of Health, 1999). • Client satisfaction is most accurately predicted by the amount of information clients receive from providers (Hall et al., 1988).
Partnership	• Many barriers exist to establishing true partnerships with clients, the most frequently cited is time constraints (Wilkins, Pollock, Rochon, & Law, 2001). • Time taken in enhancing the relationship with clients has long-standing benefits (Brown, McWilliam, & Weston, 1995; Delbanco, 1992; Jones et al., 2004) and saves time later on (Powers, Plank, Thomas, & Conkright, 2000). • Specific measures and effort are needed to make the shift from authoritarianism to partnership (Rosenbaum, King, Law, King, & Evans, 1998). • Effective professional partnership is required to ensure the best care (Edgman-Levitan, 1997; Ellers, 1993; Kalmanson & Seligman, 1992). • An outcome of partnership is the deep understanding that is achieved through taking in the other's experience (Banks, Crossman, Poel, & Stewart, 1997; Rogers, 1939).
Choice	• Client choice is central to the client-centered OT assessment, the Canadian Occupational Performance Measure (COPM) (Law, Baptiste, Carswell, McColl, Polatajko, & Pollock, 2005). • Choice is influenced by the stage of illness and client capabilities (Fallowfield, 2001). • For clients with cancer, therapists need to respect their right to choose (Harrison, 2001; McKinlay, 2001).
Hope	• A large multidisciplinary body of research supports the importance of hope and optimism to positive outcomes (Sumison & Law, 2006). • Hope is the expectation that something good will happen in the future (Von Guten, 2002). • Hope is not directly connected with severity or length of illness (Landeen, Pawlick, Woodside, Kirkpatrick, & Byrne, 2000). • Hope includes feeling connected to God, affirming relationships, staying positive, anticipating survival, living in the present, and fostering ongoing accomplishments (Saleh & Brockopp, 2001).

choices and have always had choices and helps them take responsibility for the choices that have made them who they are now. Adults can stop blaming their parents for their shortcomings and, instead, can take on the responsibility of correcting them. The concept of freedom to choose is what allows clients to take charge of their own lives, to leave the past behind, and to make positive changes for the future (Yalom & Leszcz, 2005).

Aloneness and Relatedness

Existentialists believe that we are social beings who depend on interpersonal relationships for our humanness. Awareness of our aloneness can be frightening. Some people attempt to hide their fears in superficial relationships or projects and activities. Existential therapists encourage individuals to find their own identity and inner direction before attempting to connect with others. Group interventions necessitate interactions among members and afford opportunities to practice forming meaningful connections. The work of groups in occupational therapy involves reflecting on the experience of interaction with other members and how that experience relates to social participation in the world outside the group. Additionally, occupational therapy group interventions are ideal for evaluating and learning socialization skills and for exploring and problem-solving barriers to social participation.

Existential Anxiety and Search for Meaning

Anxiety, in the existentialist view, is a necessary condition of living. Rollo May defines anxiety as "the threat to our existence or to values we identify with our existence" (1977, p. 205). The concept is based on the idea that our existence or "being" (May & Yalom, 1989) has no intrinsic predetermined meaning. The meaning of life is developed by each individual for him- or herself. Thus, in therapy, there is an emphasis on one's individual values and in finding or defining what activities are meaningful to the individual. While too much anxiety can immobilize a person, a certain amount of anxiety is normal and positive. Anxiety alerts us that all is not well and that a change is needed. In this case, anxiety is seen as a motivator to make necessary changes in behavior, values, or life structure in order to maintain or promote healthy functioning.

Humanistic Concepts

The humanistic approach is overwhelmingly positive and is appealing to most therapists. Carl Rogers was perhaps its major spokesman. Rogers developed what is known as nondirective counseling, based on the assumption that the client really knows what is best for him or her. Rogers viewed his clients with "unconditional positive regard" and allowed them to choose the direction of

therapy, to set their own goals, and to provide their own solutions to problems (Rogers, 1967). Abraham Maslow added significantly to humanistic thinking through his hierarchy of needs, leading to self-actualization. Robert White's (1959) theory of occupational competence helps us understand human motivation and the role of occupation. The Canadian Model has reorganized most of these concepts under the overarching term *enablement*, described earlier. The key concepts of the humanistic (client-centered) approach are as follows:

- Respect
- Genuineness
- Nonjudgmental acceptance
- Deep understanding
- Self-actualization
- Occupational competence and motivation
- Spirituality

Respect

Respect in therapy is not a technique, but an attitude toward the client. In the client-centered approach, the therapist sees the client as the only real expert on his or her own life. Therefore, the therapist makes no predetermined assumptions about the client, but seeks to learn all about him or her by asking open-ended questions and getting him or her to talk about him- or herself as much as possible. Yalom translates this idea in his approach to group intervention by encouraging group members to respect each other and to talk to each other as much as possible. Respect also includes a belief that when people are realistically aware of their problems, they are capable of creating their own solutions. Therefore, suggestions and advice giving are discouraged and are replaced by responses that show empathy. Empathy is expressed by both therapist and group members by statements that not only reflect what the client has said, but also acknowledge how the client is feeling. For example, a client presents the problem that his wife does not understand his need to grieve the death of his mother. The therapist would encourage the group to ask for appropriate details in order to gain a thorough understanding of how this client feels. Then, empathy would be expressed with a statement like, "You must be feeling abandoned when your wife cannot share your grief about the loss of your mother." Statements such as this encourage the client to trust the therapist and/or group members and to move ahead to even greater self-disclosure.

Genuineness

Genuineness is also an attitude rather than a technique. It means that the therapist expresses real emotional responses to the client. Clients are keen observers and are quick to sense any dishonesty on the part of therapists. When the therapist tries to cover up anger or frustration, the client usually senses something wrong, and the effect is often silence and withdrawal of trust. It is only by expressing negative feelings that honest communication with the client is facilitated. This is not to suggest that the therapist's anger (or other feelings) should be expressed indiscriminately. On the contrary, it takes considerable skill and self-understanding for a therapist to express feelings in a way that is therapeutic (Egan, 2001). Examples of genuineness in the therapeutic use of self lie in the empathy, immediacy, and self-disclosure skills discussed later in this chapter.

The value of genuineness has a profound effect upon groups. When the therapist encourages the members to be genuine, the responses they give to one another are much more meaningful and helpful. In the initial stages of groups, it is a natural tendency for members to hold back in their responses to one another. Clients are often reluctant to express negative feelings toward other members. Reasons for this have been discussed in the chapter on group dynamics. After members have established a certain degree of trust in one another, they feel much more inclined to share their real feelings. It is one of the therapist's roles to establish an atmosphere of safety and trust, which allows group members to be genuine in their responses to one another.

Nonjudgmental Acceptance

Nonjudgmental acceptance refers to the therapist's relationship with the client as one of caring. In the humanistic approach, the client is accepted for the human being that he or she is, regardless of his or her feelings or his or her behavior. This "unconditional positive regard" allows the client to reveal all of his or her inner feelings and secrets without fearing the therapist's rejection. According to Rogers, research indicates that "the greater the degree of caring, prizing, accepting, and valuing the client in a nonpossessive way, the greater the chance that therapy will be successful" (Corey, 1991, p. 214). The humanistic/client-centered therapist needs to be very careful not to allow his or her own values to enter into the therapeutic relationship. Judgments of bad and good feelings or bad and good behavior have no place in the humanistic approach.

Being judged by others is one of the greatest fears clients have in the group setting. For example, when a client speaks in the group, he or she is often uncomfortable with the silence of others. Clients often imagine that silent members are secretly disapproving of what is being said. It is most important for the therapist to establish the norm or expectation early in the group that members not judge one another in this way. All members have a right to have feelings, and feelings are neither good nor bad. Likewise, behavior should not be judged for itself, but looked upon in the context of the individual's perceptions of self and environment. If a client got drunk on a weekend pass, this behavior can be seen as one of several responses the client could have to a stressful situation. The object is not to condemn the behavior but to understand it and examine its effect on the client.

Deep Understanding

In the humanistic approach, behavior change is considered to be the by-product of a deep self-understanding. For this reason, considerable time and energy in therapy is devoted to uncovering hidden aspects of the self. In occupational therapy groups, structured activities are often helpful in fostering self-understanding among group members. The therapist should continue to gather information from the client until he or she can almost see the world through the client's eyes. Only then is the therapist able to assist the client in changing his or her behavior. New therapists have a tendency to push for behavior change too quickly. In their desire to be helpful, new therapists might even make a suggestion in the form of a question (e.g., "Have you tried talking to your wife instead of just getting drunk?"). Such a question reveals a lack of respect as well as understanding. Questions should focus on further defining the problem until it is thoroughly explored. When it is revealed that the client depends on his wife so much that he cannot risk disagreeing with her, then getting drunk to numb the pain is less contemptible. Furthermore, the problem is redefined not as one of drunkenness, but one of dependency. That dependency may be further explained by a lack of trust in oneself. Problems are seldom as simple as they may seem. Rogers believes that, "When therapists can grasp the present experience of the client's private world as the client sees and feels it without losing the separateness of their own identity, then constructive change is likely to occur" (Corey, 1991, p. 214).

Self-Actualization

Self-actualization is the innate tendency of all human beings to achieve their potential. This concept assumes that each of us has within us an inherent potential that we can actualize and through which we can find meaning. Maslow, the chief proponent of this concept, places self-actualization at the top of a continuum called the hierarchy of needs (Figure 3-1). Maslow sees at the core of human nature a push to satisfy the needs that ensure physical and psychological survival. The satisfaction of each need is a necessary prerequisite to the search for satisfaction of the next. Thus, in Maslow's hierarchy—1) physiological needs, 2) safety needs, 3) needs for belonging and love, and 4) esteem—needs are all prerequisites to the need for self-actualization. In his book *Toward a Psychology of Being*, Maslow (1968) elaborates the idea of self-actualization in his discussion of "peak experiences." These experiences are difficult to describe, but widely documented, according to Maslow. They are moments of ecstasy, self-discovery, and brilliant creativity or vision, moments when suddenly one's views

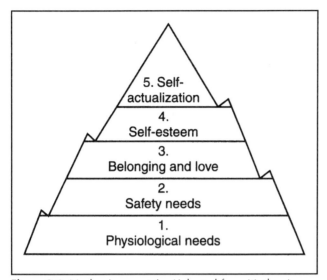

Figure 3-1. Maslow's mountain. (Adapted from Maslow.)

of him- or herself and the world change permanently forever. Peak experiences are said to cause symptoms to disappear; they can change self-perception in a healthy direction and can release the person for greater creativity, expressiveness, and growth. "The person [after such experiences] is more apt to feel that life in general is worthwhile, even if it is usually drab, pedestrian, painful, or ungratifying, since beauty, excitement, honesty, play, goodness, truth, and meaningfulness have been demonstrated to him to exist" (Maslow, 1968, p. 101). If only we, as therapists, could make our clients feel that life is worthwhile in this way!

Occupational Competence and Motivation

Robert White (1959) believed that people have an innate motivation toward competence, which translates into an innate drive to explore and master the environment. This idea is certainly compatible with the basic tenets of occupational therapy. Perhaps we would add that occupational therapy interventions improve the quality of clients' lives through engagement in meaningful occupation. Similarly, Maslow views motivation as a need for satisfaction and a kind of thrust for survival. But, this changes from physiological survival to psychological survival as it approaches the top of the needs hierarchy. Self-actualization is seen not as a search for what is missing, but an innate drive toward self-fulfillment. This differs somewhat from the existentialist view that anxiety is the major motivator and that the search for structure and meaning is largely motivated by the desire to escape the anxiety of meaninglessness and nothingness. In client-centered theory, there is an assumption that people have a natural tendency to improve the quality of their lives.

We as therapists need to find out where the dysfunction lies—where our client is stuck and the obstacles

preventing him or her from pursuing self-actualization. Perhaps the client is not aware of the freedom to make choices. Many clients I have worked with have felt so defeated by the "system," by the bureaucracy of governments and organizations or by the prejudices of society, that they no longer exercise their ability to choose. Many have had negative life experiences rather than "peak" experiences. Perhaps their more basic needs are not being satisfied; they feel unsafe, unloved, or like they do not belong. People with disabilities, both mental and physical, often feel they are misfits, controlled by others, victims of circumstance, incapacitated by anxiety, and prevented from enjoying the fulfillments of life that "normal" people enjoy. As group therapists, we sometimes facilitate the outward expression of our clients' pain before we can help them begin to find the more positive aspects of themselves.

Spirituality: The Experience of Meaning

One of the unique aspects of the CMOP-E is the place of the human spirit at the center of the person. Client-centered theory views the human spirit as the unifying force that binds the other parts (physical, psychological, social) together. Spirituality had been defined as "the experience of meaning in everyday activities" (Urbanowski & Vargo, 1994, p. 89). Its scope encompasses religious beliefs but transcends the divisiveness of organized religions. As OTs, we are concerned with the meaning of daily activities for our clients. An activity cannot be separated from its meaning. Through our various roles, it is the routines and activities of everyday life that define us. When clients' lives are disrupted by illness or injury, our first priority might be to find out how to best restore this sense of "ordinary existence," however the client might define it.

Hasselkus (2002) discusses everyday routines as rituals. Unlike other habits, rituals have a meaning not only for the individual, but also attributed by one's culture. For example, baking cookies can have meaning beyond following a recipe; it becomes a ritual when the activity symbolizes motherhood for the individual.

Dixon (1987) states that each (life) crisis has a nucleus, a nuclear problem that threatens something the person considers essential for a meaningful life (Rosenfeld, 1997). Rosenfeld suggests that OTs seek to understand this "nuclear" problem and find "nuclear tasks, that is, the things that need doing to resolve the crisis.... The functions of nuclear tasks are to express and manage feelings, sustain occupational patterns and involvements, learn vital new skills, and re-motivate by demonstrating self-reliance and symbolize recovery" (p. 26).

Using the client-centered approach, group interventions with clients might focus on some of the steps Rosenfeld defines in identifying nuclear problems and tasks. The occupational goals clients set for themselves with our help probably relate in some way to this kind of spiritual meaning.

Cultural Competence

Cultural issues are closely aligned with client-centered practice and the CMOP-E. Nonjudgmental acceptance, a core concept, implies the acceptance of diversity, and occupational justice, another core concept, implies an enduring value of equality in occupational opportunity. Inclusion refers to the social acceptance of diverse cultures within communities and adds advocacy for policy change and for removing barriers to full participation for diverse clients as one of OT's expanded roles. Black and Wells (2007) define cultural competence as a "broad term that includes cultural awareness and cultural knowledge (cognitive domain), cultural skills (behavioral domain), cultural sensitivity (affective domain), and cultural encounter (environment domain)" (Callister, 2005, p. 33). See Chapter 13 for a more thorough discussion and group laboratory activities for the development of culturally competent leadership.

APPLICATIONS

Practical application of the contributing concepts of client-centered theory will be discussed in three sections:

1. The client-centered nature of groups
2. Selecting group members using the client-centered model
3. Skills of the client-centered leader: therapeutic use of self.

The Client-Centered Nature of Groups

Ideally, clients come to us with an understanding of what occupational therapy can do for them and already knowing their goals and priorities regarding occupational participation. In reality, that level of awareness rarely exists. Care must be taken during the initial occupational therapy interview to connect with the person who is the client, to evaluate that person's status regarding self-awareness, and to facilitate further client self-understanding. Only when the OT has developed an appreciation for the client's own feelings and perceptions regarding his or her occupational status can therapist and client collaborate about what possible occupational therapy interventions might be helpful.

There are many reasons why a client may not have a good understanding of his or her own occupational issues. Psychological barriers such as denial, repression, projection, or reaction formation might prevent client insight. Cognitive disabilities often interfere with

the ability to define and communicate problems or to anticipate the consequences of impaired occupational performance. Even the most cognitively able clients may lack an understanding of the barriers to occupational engagement caused by illness or by social and cultural contexts. When the OT encounters several such clients, designing structured group activities or exercises to enable self-awareness and self-understanding may be the ideal format for initial intervention. Client-centered groups offer a structured way to facilitate client self-expression, awareness of choices, and empowerment for self-direction.

Selecting Group Members Using the Client-Centered Model

In the process of occupational therapy practice, member selection becomes a part of the initial evaluation. Within the Canadian model, OTs ask clients to identify problem areas during an informal or semi-structured interview, such as the Canadian Occupational Performance Measure (Fearing, Clark, & Stanton, 1998). While evaluation of clients is beyond the scope of this text, a general description is necessary in order to appreciate how groups can play a part.

The client-centered interview has several purposes:

- To develop a therapeutic relationship (engagement)
- To identify and prioritize problem areas in occupational functioning
- To identify potential interventions
- To discuss the effects of contexts in enabling or creating barriers to occupational performance
- To identify strengths and weaknesses
- To identify targeted outcomes and collaborative action plans

Not all clients are self-aware, and many have not given much thought to their priorities or the effects of the various contexts in which they perform occupations. Kielhofner (2004) states:

In practice, the problems that therapists and clients encounter are not immediately apparent. Rather, each client is ordinarily faced with ambiguous and complex circumstances. Converting these circumstances into a recognizable problem requires that practitioners support their clients to make sense of an uncertain and indeterminate situation. In order to identify a problem that can be addressed in therapy, the therapist and client must transform complexity and uncertainty into something that can be understood and acted upon (p. 266).

In the initial meetings with clients, OTs use therapeutic use of self to enable problem definition. In OT groups, initial sessions may be designed to assist all group members with this process. Structured group activities can

Table 3-4

The Potential Benefits of Groups

- Provide a context of social support
- Enhance communication and self-expression
- Provide an atmosphere of nonjudgmental acceptance
- Allow expression of the unique cultural values of each member
- Offer multiple opportunities to share learning and application of therapeutic strategies
- Impart information in a cost-effective way
- Facilitate client participation
- Promote all levels of client group interaction skill
- Provide ideal context for problem-solving relationships with others

help clients clarify and prioritize problem areas, explore the enabling and disabling aspects of context, identify strengths and weaknesses through group discussion and mutual feedback, and identify targeted outcomes through group problem solving.

In the client-centered evaluation and intervention process, OTs should consider the advantages of groups listed in Table 3-4. These potential group benefits should be shared with the client during the evaluation.

During the initial evaluation, clients who are good candidates for groups can be identified using an interpersonal relationships interview focus. Yalom and Leszcz (1995) suggest exploring the client's relationships with others, including spouse, family, friendships, and community groups. This can be useful in two ways. It can assist the client in identifying problems with interpersonal relationships that might be preventing meaningful social participation, and it can also help the therapist to evaluate the client's appropriateness for different types of groups.

After a client has agreed that a group intervention would be helpful, the next step is to prepare the client for group participation. The therapist should discuss the goals, benefits, and expectations of group membership. Potential members should have a clear understanding of the targeted outcomes to be worked on during the session before joining the group. When working with groups or clients, families, caregiver groups, organizations, or selected members of a population, designing a focus group as outlined in Chapter 1 may be the best way to begin the design process for a group intervention.

Therapeutic Use of Self in Occupational Therapy Group Leadership

Client-centered therapy provides guidelines that help OTs develop skills for forming and maintaining therapeutic relationships, also called therapeutic use of self. Matheson (1998) calls this therapeutic engagement. A therapeutic relationship has been defined as "a trusting connection established between therapist and client through collaboration, communication, therapist empathy, and mutual understanding" (Cole & McLean, 2003). AOTA defines therapeutic use of self as a "practitioner's planned use of his or her personality, perceptions, and judgments as part of the therapeutic process" (Punwar & Peloquin, 2000, p. 285 in AOTA, 2008, p. 653). A group therapist forms a connection with group members through the therapeutic use of self. Some of the basic communication skills outlined in the client-centered model are included in this section with worksheets for students learning to communicate empathy, understanding, concern, and guidance to clients, both as individuals and in groups.

Taylor (2007) reports that, although therapeutic use of self has appeared in the OT literature since its beginning, little is known about exactly how to use the "self" to "orchestrate the process of occupational engagement" (p. 5). In a nationwide survey of OT practitioners, a strong connection between therapeutic use of self and successful OT outcomes was reported across divergent fields of practice (Taylor, Lee, Kielhofner, & Ketkar, 2009). These researchers also report that most survey participants felt inadequately trained in the therapeutic use of self. Taylor attempts to elaborate upon the concept using a model called "the intentional relationship," which includes six "therapeutic modes for OT":

1. *Advocating:* To obtain needed services for clients, mediating and negotiating with others.

2. *Collaborating:* Forming partnership with client, communicating respect and genuineness.

3. *Empathizing:* Understanding client's views, feelings, and perspective.

4. *Encouraging:* Through giving feedback, praise, reinforcement, or positive visions for the future.

Table 3-5

Three Stages of Therapeutic Communication for Individuals and Groups

Stage	Individual Counseling	Group Development	Specific Skills Needed	OT Examples
Stage I	Problem definition	Orientation	Attending	Evaluation
			Concreteness	Setting priorities
			Primary accurate empathy	Setting therapeutic norms
			Communication of respect, genuineness, and nonjudgmental acceptance	Sharing information about each other, expressing emotions, exploring strengths
Stage II	Self-understanding	Conflict	Advanced accurate empathy	Deeper understanding of occupational complexities, supports, and barriers to occupational engagement; need for change, and occupational goal setting
			Confrontation	
			Immediacy	
			Therapist self-disclosure	
Stage III	Behavior change	Cohesive maturity	Focuses on providing support for therapeutic behavior change	OT, interventions, applying group learning, taking action to more fully participate in life

5. *Instructing:* Includes designing, planning, and sequencing interventions and interactions.

6. *Problem solving:* With client, to facilitate occupational engagement, overcome barriers (adapted from Taylor, 2008).

OTs use these modes in a flexible, dynamic way as the need arises during the process of evaluation and intervention. All of them apply when working with both individuals and groups.

The humanists say that we cannot change our clients, that they must desire to change themselves. The function of the therapist is to create an atmosphere of safety and to help the client build the kind of self-image and self-understanding that increases the likelihood of positive change. The client-centered therapist does this through the therapeutic relationship and through the facilitation of therapeutic groups. Rogers (1961, 1975) said that behavior change is really a by-product of a deep self-understanding. To change their lives in a positive way, clients must first feel and believe that they have the strength and the power to make changes. This requires feelings of self-worth and self-esteem as well as a belief that one has the needed skills and capacities required. A prerequisite for change is the belief that change is possible. All of these are appropriate issues to be addressed in occupational therapy groups.

The occupational therapy group leader focuses on skills that help develop the therapeutic relationship. These skills will be used extensively in planning and leading occupational therapy groups. The leader uses skills in therapeutic use of self to gradually transfer leadership roles, giving group members an active part in the direction and process of therapy, while allowing the leader to guide them through the establishment of therapeutic norms.

This text uses a developmental approach in organizing basic therapeutic communication skills. Knowledge of the stages of groups is important, as well as what skills are appropriate for each stage. Yalom and Leszcz's (2005) stages of group development (orientation, conflict, and cohesive maturity) parallel Egan's (2001) three stages of counseling (problem definition, self-understanding, and behavior change). These can serve as guidelines for therapeutic communication skill use within the OT group process (see Table 3-5 for a comparison of these skills and stages).

Stage I Skills

Stage I is concerned with problem definition. This stage is parallel to Yalom's orientation stage of a group, in which members get to know one another and begin to lay the ground rules for how they will interact. The communication skills Egan (2001) suggests for this stage are attending, concreteness, and primary accurate empathy (PAE). Babiss (2002) provides evidence of the need for self-awareness for people in the acute stages of mental illness. She designs expressive OT groups, using art, creative writing, music, and movement to assist clients to get in touch with their own feelings and to learn things about themselves that will later facilitate change. She writes, "it is crucial to have some awareness of what needs to be worked on before beginning the work" (p. 105). Thus, in addition to defining problems, the therapeutic goals in working with both individuals and groups in the beginning stage, is "being aware of the dynamics of the interaction in the here and now, [which will allow empathy, validation, compassion, caring, and ultimately, good treatment]" (Babiss, 2002, p. 108, paraphrasing Peloquin, 2002).

Attending

Attending is something most of us do without even thinking about it. The leader of the group needs to be especially alert and observant because he or she is attending to not one but several people at one time. Attending refers to the attentive physical presence the therapist focuses on the client. It is evident even before anyone begins to speak. Taking note of appearance, body language, posture, seating position, eye contact, and facial expression are all part of attending. The therapist gets from these factors important clues as to how members are feeling and how the group is likely to respond to various activities or interventions.

Skill Practice in Attending

To help you become aware of how powerful these first impressions really are, try sitting in a group for the first few minutes without speaking and do the following:

- Draw a diagram of where people are seated in the room.
- Write a one- or two-word phrase describing the appearance of each member. For example:
  - Glenn—Sloppy, poor hygiene
  - Mary—Dressed up, neat
  - Sue—Provocative, overly made up
  - Joe—Preppy, well-groomed
- Write one or two adjectives to describe the posture of each member. For example:
  - Glenn—Relaxed, slouching
  - Mary—Watchful, tense
  - Sue—Uncomfortable, fidgety
  - Joe—Alert, open

- Note with whom each member has eye contact. For example:
  - Glenn—Looks at no one, looks down
  - Mary—Looks at everyone
  - Sue—Looks only at Joe
  - Joe—Looks at leader primarily
- Write a word of feeling describing the emotional message given by the facial expression of each. For example:
  - Glenn—Defiant
  - Mary—Anxious, fearful
  - Sue—Distracted, blunted
  - Joe—Eager, anticipating

It is most helpful to put the descriptions of each individual together so you can begin to get a more complete picture of each (Worksheet 3-1).

Knowing these impressions before starting the group, the leader can predict some responses that can be expected from the four clients. Even if the therapist does not know anything about the clients except their names and ages, an observant leader will begin to adapt his or her approach to the group to accommodate the different expectations.

Which of these clients is most likely to be cooperative? Uncooperative? Which client is most likely to disrupt the group? Which member might be expected to leave prematurely? Attending and forming impressions of members becomes second nature to the skilled therapist, but the beginning therapist perhaps needs some practice. Worksheet 3-1 may be used to practice these observations on your own group.

Concreteness

Concreteness refers to the ability to elicit specific information about a client/problem. If the humanistic therapist's goal is to obtain a thorough understanding of the client, many clarifying questions must ultimately be asked. The most basic skill in concreteness is to ask open-ended questions. These are questions that cannot be answered with a simple "yes" or "no." Open-ended questions encourage the client to clarify his or her perceptions, elaborate on important points, and give specific personal examples. A therapist may use open-ended questions to get the client to discover concrete solutions to problems, but that often happens in a later stage of intervention.

Constructing open-ended questions is not always as easy as it seems. Some beginning therapists are in the bad habit of asking closed questions one after the other, and this kind of habit is hard to break. Consider the following opening of an occupational therapy session:

OT: Would you like to do some drawing today?
Joe: No.
OT: Are you too tired?

Worksheet 3-1
First Impressions

Directions: List names of group members in the first column. Then, use one or two descriptive words to denote appearance, posture, and facial expression. Before beginning to speak, note the person with whom each member makes eye contact. This information will make up your first impressions of group members.

Member Name	Appearance	Posture	Facial Expression	Eye Contact
1.				
2.				
3.				
4.				
5.				
6.				
7.				
8.				

From Cole, M. B. *Group dynamics in occupational therapy: The theoretical basis and practice application of group intervention* (4th ed.). Thorofare, NJ: SLACK Incorporated. © 2012 SLACK Incorporated.

Joe: Yes.

OT: Can you just talk to me for a while?

Joe: I'd rather not.

OT: Do you find it hard to talk?

Joe: Yes.

OT: Why?

Joe: I don't know.

Now consider the following alternative opening:

OT: To begin our session, I'd like to learn how well you express your feelings. What can you tell me about how you're feeling right now?

Joe: Nothing.

OT: What makes it difficult to talk about feelings with me?

Joe: It's nothing against you; I'm just in a bad mood.

OT: What put you in a bad mood?

Joe: My doctor just told me I can't go home this weekend.

In leading occupational therapy groups, open-ended questions are more effective because they encourage communication and interaction among members. Closed-ended questions tend to cut off communication. This is an important point to remember when planning questions for discussion when processing an activity group. In asking open-ended questions, it seems most useful to begin with the words "what" or "how." Using the word "why" is not advisable because it tends to elicit vague answers and because it may sound judgmental, reminding some clients of their angry parents' interrogations. Also, avoid beginning a question with "do you, can you, would you, are you, have you," because these can easily be answered with "yes" or "no," as observed in the above example. Now, try Worksheet 3-2.

Primary Accurate Empathy

PAE is discussed by several humanistic theorists, particularly Carl Rogers. The importance of its use early in therapy cannot be overemphasized. PAE is the reflection of the feeling and content expressed by the client. If composed and delivered effectively, an empathetic comment from either the therapist or another group member will convince the client that he or she is being listened to and understood. The effect of empathy is to encourage this client to open up even more. PAE, used often in groups, will help build an atmosphere of safety and trust and will help the group progress toward a state of cohesiveness.

PAE is considered "primary" because it does not reach far below the surface. It reflects, but does not repeat, what the client has actually said. Empathy requires that the feeling of the client be recognized, and that may require careful observation of nonverbal cues as well as what the client actually says. (In the practice exercise, you'll just have to read between the lines.) The "accurate" part of empathy requires that the emotion be identified accurately. Emotions vary in both kind and intensity. Some psychologists have divided feelings into the categories of sad, mad, bad, and glad. It is not enough to just say "you feel angry." Anger varies from low intensity, like annoyed or perturbed, to very high intensity, like rage. Clients often do not have a very wide "feeling" vocabulary; many are not used to expressing their feelings in words. Often, clients need the help of the therapist to find right words to describe their feelings accurately. Worksheets 3-3 and 3-4 will help you to develop a better "feeling" vocabulary.

After expanding our knowledge of "feeling" words, we will apply them to the skill of PAE. When practicing PAE, we will use a sentence completion to facilitate finding the right feeling words. We will complete the sentence, "You feel _____ because _____ ." "You feel" refers to the feeling word that best reflects how the client is feeling. "Because" refers to the thoughts or behaviors that are seen to have caused the feeling. When leading a group, you will learn to use your own words to show empathy. Now, try Worksheet 3-5.

Stage II Skills

According to Egan (2001), the goal of Stage II in counseling is self-understanding. The middle stage of group development is more complex than this, with its subgroups, leadership struggles, and questioning of purpose/value, but the outcome is still a greater self-understanding. It is helpful to groups if the leader uses and teaches the skills of Stage II to get through this vital phase of group development. The skills of Stage II are immediacy, advanced accurate empathy (AAE), confrontation, and therapist self-disclosure.

Immediacy

Immediacy is the direct mutual communication between therapist and client. It enables the therapist to discuss openly and directly what is happening in the here and now of their interpersonal relationship. It is an invitation to process the relationship, and this is how it is best used in groups. When a group bogs down, and nothing seems to be happening, a question like, "What is happening right now?" or "What do you think the silence means?" will serve to refocus the group on its own process. The group's relationship to its leader is commonly a troubled one in Stage II, with which immediacy can help. For example, the leader can often sense anger, resentment, or rebellion in the members and invite the group to discuss it. He or she could ask, "Are you angry with me for insisting that you give each other constructive feedback?" This direct question encourages the members to examine their own feelings about the leader, an essential task in the "control" stage of groups. Trust is another important issue to help therapist immediacy. A comment like, "I can see that you're having a hard time trusting one another in this group today" will invite the group members to examine their relationships with one another. Now, try Worksheet 3-6.

Worksheet 3-2
Open-Ended Questions

Directions: In each of the following examples, respond to the client with an open-ended question that can do the following:

- Elicit more specific information
- Focus the discussion on a specific problem
- Help define the problem

1. "I'm always so unlucky!"
   Therapist response:

2. "No matter what I do, I can't win."
   Therapist response:

3. "I'm not thinking right today."
   Therapist response:

4. "Boy, did I have a boring weekend!"
   Therapist response:

5. "My doctor gave me new medication, and I'm just not myself."
   Therapist response:

6. "Life is so unfair. Do you think there's any justice in the world?"
   Therapist response:

7. "What good does it do to write down a schedule? When I go home, it's all for nothing."
   Therapist response:

8. "I'm really afraid to talk about how I feel."
   Therapist response:

9. "Just let well enough alone. I feel great today."
   Therapist response:

10. "Why should I care what my mother thinks?"
    Therapist response:

From Cole, M. B. *Group dynamics in occupational therapy: The theoretical basis and practice application of group intervention* (4th ed.). Thorofare, NJ: SLACK Incorporated. © 2012 SLACK Incorporated.

Worksheet 3-3
Developing Your Empathy Vocabulary, Part I

Directions: This exercise may be done as a group or individually. Take 10 or 15 minutes to list as many feeling words as you can think of in each category listed at the top of the first four columns. A fifth column is provided for those words that seem to defy categorization but are nevertheless expressive of feelings. You may use a thesaurus to form a more complete list (at least 20 words per column). When you are finished, go to Worksheet 3-4.

Mad	Sad	Bad (Fearful)	Glad	Other Emotions

Worksheet 3-4
Developing Your Empathy Vocabulary, Part II

Directions: From the list you made in Worksheet 3-3, sort the words in each column into the three levels of intensity described to the left: mild, moderate, or severe. For example, in the "Bad" column, a mild emotion might be "worried," a moderate emotion might be "fearful," and a severe one might be "petrified." Refer to your completed list when completing the Primary Accurate Empathy Worksheet (Worksheet 3-5).

	Mad	*Sad*	*Bad (Fearful)*	*Glad*	*Other Emotions*
Mild					
Moderate					
Severe					

From Cole, M. B. *Group dynamics in occupational therapy: The theoretical basis and practice application of group intervention* (4th ed.). Thorofare, NJ: SLACK Incorporated. © 2012 SLACK Incorporated.

Worksheet 3-5
Primary Accurate Empathy

Directions: After reading each client's comment in group, write a response that completes the sentence: "You feel _____ because _____ ." and communicates the following:

- What emotion that patient is feeling (as accurately as possible)
- A summary of the thoughts or behaviors that are seen to have caused the feeling

1. "I can't draw very well (shows a very faintly drawn picture to the group). This is supposed to be my sofa and my dog."
"You feel _____ because _____ ."

2. "He just accused me of being prejudiced! I say he's a moron!"
"You feel _____ because _____ ."

3. "Brian is doing so well. He's leaving tomorrow to start a new life, and here I am, still in the hospital."
"You feel _____ because _____ ."

4. "Can I leave now? This group is making me very upset, especially when Mark sounds so angry."
"You feel _____ because _____ ."

5. "This group just isn't helping me. None of you understand what I'm going through!"
"You feel _____ because _____ ."

6. "I didn't want to come to occupational therapy group today. Setting goals is too much work."
"You feel _____ because _____ ."

7. "When Laurie tells me I'm being insensitive, I don't know what she means."
"You feel _____ because _____ ."

8. "All I know is that I'm restricted to the ward again. They seem to like punishing me."
"You feel _____ because _____ ."

9. "My boyfriend always picks on me when he's had a bad day. Now I am too upset to participate in this group."
"You feel _____ because _____ ."

10. (Laurie crying) "I don't know why I'm so upset. Just hearing Roy talk about being old and alone. He reminds me of my grandfather who died 2 months ago."
"You feel _____ because _____ ."

Worksheet 3-6
Practice of Immediacy

Directions: In the following examples, respond with a direct question or statement that encourages the group to examine its here-and-now relationships.

1. Group of adolescents hospitalized for drug abuse.
   Tina: "If we discuss our problems in group, you'll just tell our parents. They're the ones who sent us here in the first place."
   Bob: "Yeah, how do we know you won't rat on us?"
   Mikki: "I'm not telling you nothin'. I may have to come to this group, but I don't have to talk."

Therapist response:

2. Group of clients with eating disorders working on vocational readiness. This group has chosen to do one small craft project after another. None of the members have opted to take on anything more challenging, yet three of the members face discharge with only three or four more occupational therapy sessions.

Therapist response:

3. Group of clients with arthritis attending the third session of a leisure planning group.
   Morgan: "What are we in this group for anyway? All I want to do is go back to work. Then I won't have any leisure time."
   Jackie: "I stopped participating in sports back in high school. Sure, it would be good for me, but it's just too much effort."
   Ellie: "Sure, my doctor told me I need to plan time for relaxation and enjoyment, but I'm not sure I need someone telling me how or when to do it."

Therapist response:

From Cole, M. B. *Group dynamics in occupational therapy: The theoretical basis and practice application of group intervention* (4th ed.). Thorofare, NJ: SLACK Incorporated. © 2012 SLACK Incorporated.

Advanced Accurate Empathy

AAE goes a step further than PAE. This skill enables the therapist to bring feelings and thoughts that the client may only be implying to the forefront. Therapists find AAE difficult because it involves forming a hypothesis about the underlying or hidden feelings/topics the client just hints at with his or her statements. Egan (2001) defines AAE as "...sharing hunches about clients and their overt and covert experiences, behaviors, and feelings which the therapist thinks will help clients see their problems and concerns more clearly, and in a context that will enable them to move to goal setting and action."

AAE helps the client in several specific ways. First, it can help him or her become aware of hidden or forbidden feelings. Male clients, for example, often try to hide their sad or hurt feelings because they consider them to be a sign of weakness. Second, the therapist can use AAE to help the client see patterns of behavior or general trends. A bad experience with one doctor, for example, may lead a client to mistrust all doctors. A third way that AAE can help a client is to help him or her draw logical conclusions to his or her behaviors or comments. An older teen who feels trapped by his parents' rules and says he is tired of his parents treating him like a child may be expressing a desire to leave home and become more independent. Actually moving out may be very scary to an adolescent who has never been on his own, but that is where his comments seem to be leading.

Because AAE is really the therapist's hypothesis or educated guess about the client's implications, it is best to present these ideas tentatively. Always leave yourself a way out by using phrases like "could it be that...," "it seems likely that...," or "I could be wrong, but...." The fact is, you could be wrong, and it should always be acceptable for the client to correct you if you are. Even if you are not wrong, if the client really is hiding a seething rage at his or her spouse, he or she may not be ready to face or accept such intense feeling. Tentativeness also leaves the client a way out without damaging the therapeutic relationship.

The easiest way to learn AAE is to begin with PAE. Practice AAE by doing Worksheet 3-7.

Confrontation

Confrontation involves the resolution of possible discrepancies, distortions, games, and smoke screens that clients use to avoid self-understanding and/or behavior change. It includes challenging the undeveloped, unused, or misused potentialities, skills, and resources clients may have as well. Confrontation as a technique is actually an extension of AAE or interpretation. However, whereas interpretation involves the therapist's understanding of a client's behavior, confrontation permits the client him- or herself to put his or her own meaning to the behavior. In confrontation, the therapist points out maladaptive behaviors or inconsistent actions and comments and invites the client to explain or make sense of them.

Confrontation has a reputation for being harsh and accusing. However, the skilled confrontation is not harsh, but an act of caring. It should offer genuine feedback to the client about his or her comments or behavior, while leaving the judgment of the behavior up to him or her. The tone of voice used by the therapist is very important here. The correct words, conveyed in an angry or accusing tone, will not achieve the desired result. What is hoped for is self-discovery on the part of the client, using the confrontation as a guide.

For example, when Ben expresses that he's "happy-go-lucky and able to cope with almost anything," the therapist might ask, "If this is true, what are you doing in a psychiatric hospital?" In this confrontation, it is Ben who has to explain the discrepancy between his healthy self-presentation and his psychiatric inpatient status. The therapist might say, "One doesn't get admitted to a psychiatric ward by being healthy and able to cope. How did a healthy person like you end up on a psychiatric ward?" There must be problems Ben is not talking about. However, the point of the confrontation is not to accuse Ben of having problems; the point is to get Ben himself to stop denying or hiding his problems and instead try to solve them.

Use Worksheet 3-8 to practice your skills in confrontation as an act of caring and promoting self-understanding.

Therapist Self-Disclosure

When a client discloses a difficult situation to us, it is hard to just listen without attempting to solve the problem. There are times, however, when it is appropriate for the OT to offer a different perspective or alternative approach to the client. The skill of therapeutic self-disclosure allows the therapist to share personal stories and professional experiences in therapy, which illustrate how the therapist handled a similar problem. This communicates to the client, "I know what you mean because I, too, had a similar experience and this is how I handled it." It is a respectful way to open up the clients' thinking about their own problems without jeopardizing the collaborative nature of the therapeutic relationship. Therapeutic self-disclosure may be defined as the therapist sharing his or her feelings, experiences, and behaviors with a client (or group of clients) in a way that will provide that client with a greater awareness and understanding of self and situation.

There are two levels of therapeutic self-disclosure: indirect and direct. Indirect self-disclosure refers to the impressions that the therapist conveys both consciously and unconsciously to the client. Examples are nodding, smiling, frowning, shifting body movements, laughing, etc. These responses convey genuine interest in the

Worksheet 3-7
Advanced Accurate Empathy

Directions: First, respond with a primary accurate empathy statement (PAE) to the client. Then, respond with some statement of advanced accurate empathy (AAE). Freely interpret so as to assist the client in taking a larger view of his or her situation, see the implications, or examine the logical conclusions of what is said or done.

1. Sam, age 54. Situation: This man has a variety of problems. This time he has just undergone surgery to repair a back injury. His tendency is to ruminate constantly on his defects.

"To feel bad, all I have to do is review what has happened in my life. This past year, I let my drinking get the best of me for 4 months. Over the years, I've messed up my marriage. Now, my wife and I are separated. I don't have the kind of income that can support two households, and the job market is really tight. I'm not so sure what skills I have to market anyhow."

Therapist PAE response:

Therapist AAE response:

2. Adele, age 44. Situation: This woman has been admitted for the third time with a bleeding ulcer.

"I'm completely depressed. I don't feel like working anymore. Actually, I work all the time. I can't think of any day I get up and don't intend to work. I think I begrudge myself the time I take for relaxation. There's been no day for the past 2 years when I said, 'Today's a day off.' I always feel so good about myself after I've worked hard, and after all, it's my choice to spend the time the way I want, isn't it?"

Therapist PAE response:

Therapist AAE response:

From Cole, M. B. *Group dynamics in occupational therapy: The theoretical basis and practice application of group intervention* (4th ed.). Thorofare, NJ: SLACK Incorporated. © 2012 SLACK Incorporated.

Worksheet 3-8
Practice in Confrontation

Directions: Respond to each of the following clients first with primary accurate empathy, then with confrontation.

Example: Sheila says, "Everything is fine" as she stares at the floor and looks sad.

Therapist confrontation: "You must feel sad, judging from the downcast look on your face. Yet you're telling me everything is fine. How do you see that?"

1. Mike, a spinal cord injured patient, age 25, comments after a visit from his wife. "It really hurts me when I think about what she said to me." He smiles and shrugs his shoulders.

Therapist confrontation:

2. Anne, age 35, is an arthritic patient who has become socially isolated except for a few friends. She is seeking ways of getting along better with others interpersonally. "I give a lot to my friends, but I expect a lot in return. Unfortunately, it seems like many of them don't recognize my caring and I react by getting angry with them."

Therapist confrontation:

3. Robert, a cardiac patient, is recently divorced, has lost his job, and is broke. He keeps joking about it.

Therapist confrontation:

client's disclosures and reflect our humanity as therapists. Direct self-disclosure, on the other hand, requires an ability to 1) verbally reveal a short story that has similar themes to the client and 2) clearly describe the strategies used to cope or resolve the situation. The primary reason for using therapeutic self-disclosure is to model how to deal with a challenging situation for the clients' sake. It is not meant as a venting opportunity for the therapist. The situations between therapist and client need not be exactly alike, just similar in topic or theme. Examples may include recovering from an injury or illness, overcoming significant barriers in life, pushing oneself to the limit, recovering from loss of a loved one, and endless other experiences. Direct self-disclosure stories should be kept brief and should always end with a question or statement that focuses attention back to the client. For example, "How does my experience relate to yours?" or "How do you think that strategy would work in your situation?" For practice in self-disclosure, try the exercise in Worksheet 3-9.

CLIENT-CENTERED GROUPS IN THE SEVEN-STEP FORMAT

The following section of this chapter elaborates upon how the general group format presented in Chapter 1 uses a client-centered approach.

Introduction

In client-centered groups, the purpose should be thoroughly explained, when member self-understanding and insight is possible. Care in this initial explanation will make it possible for the members themselves to strive to accomplish the purpose as they do the activity.

Activity

Selecting activities is guided by the therapeutic goals of the members. Activities will vary widely, depending on the frame of reference used and the interests and preferences clients have expressed. They may involve exploring interests, making choices, or developing new skills. Creative activities like drawing, painting, sculpting, and storytelling or drama often encourage the expression of hidden aspects of the self and are helpful in the goals of self-awareness and insight, as long as these activities are client directed. The therapist selects and structures the activity in collaboration with clients to maximize goal achievement.

For example, when clients express a need to improve their ability to express emotions in their relationships, the OT might suggest an activity called "Circle of Feelings." This requires each member to draw a circle in the center of a piece of 9- x 12-inch white drawing paper. Then, they use colored markers to indicate layers of feel-

ings. The outer edge of the circle represents the outer self, the feelings they show to others, while the center of the circle represents the inner core, those feelings kept well-hidden and seldom shown to others. Such an activity serves to focus and guide the group toward a frank discussion of their inner feelings, promoting the goal of greater self-understanding among members.

The time frame for such an activity should adhere to the rule of no more than one-third of the entire group time. Emphasis should always be on discussion and processing.

Sharing

In client-centered groups, feedback is the most vital therapeutic tool available and should be encouraged early in groups, beginning in the sharing stage. The purpose of feedback goes beyond the acknowledgment of member contributions. It is a skill to be taught to all the group members if they are to help one another. Considerable time should be taken with this stage to be sure each member's work is correctly understood and explored by the group. The therapist might ask questions of each member to help clarify and focus his or her issues. Leader skills in concreteness, PAE, immediacy, confrontation, and AAE can be used effectively in all of the discussion stages of client-centered groups. The OT can use client issues as examples to demonstrate the techniques of reality testing and consensual validation for the group.

In our example of the "Circle of Feelings" exercise, members may question one another about the meaning of color and about reported feelings. They may agree or disagree about the outer circle a client describes. If Ben draws an outer circle of yellow and reports feeling that others see him as cheerful and carefree, the statement invites other group members to comment. Some may agree with Ben, that he presents a jovial exterior. Others may see beyond this, to his inner pain and suffering. Ben and the group both benefit from a discussion of how he really comes across to others.

Processing

The potential of members sharing the leadership of groups is maximized in client-centered groups. Thus, the skill of giving and receiving feedback is further defined in the processing stage. As members discuss their feelings about the activity, the leader encourages them to also express feelings about one another. The best that we hope for is a genuine curiosity about one another, leading to concern and caring in the later stages of group development. The focus on feelings in the processing stage leads clients to think about their own subjective experience of engaging in occupation within a social context. The therapist can further maximize benefits of the group context by getting members to use their own experiences and capabilities to help one another.

Worksheet 3-9
Therapeutic Self-Disclose Practice

1. Take a few moments to write down a personal problem that you have solved with some success. Include both feeling and content. How did you solve the problem?

2. Then, imagine that your client has a similar problem. Write a statement you might say to a client, in which you briefly share your experience and then turn the focus back onto the client.

Example:
Problem—"My social life is not nearly as full as I would like it to be."

Feeling & content—"When I first went away to college, I felt a little lost. Even though I have good problem-solving skills, I didn't apply them to my social life situation. Instead of seeking new friendships, I'd wait around to see if someone would approach me."

Solution—"When I figured out that I could be the one to approach others, it opened a lot of doors for me."

Statement to the client—as above, but add, "How might my experience help you to liven up your social life?"

3. Take turns sharing your problem, solution, and client statements with the group. Discuss.

4. Now try responding to this client situation:
Receptionist, 54, recently hospitalized for a broken hip from slipping on a wet floor while rushing to answer a phone after hours: "I get all mixed up when there are so many people asking me to do things at once. Answer this letter! Fill out this form! Call so and so! It gets me all flustered, and look what happened this time. I guess it's really all my fault for letting the situation get the best of me."

1. Respond first with a primary accurate empathy statement:

   You feel _____ because _____ .
   Then respond with brief self-disclosure:

2. Describe your own similar problem and solution briefly.

3. Follow up with question to re-focus attention to the client.

Generalizing

In client-centered theory, the meaning of occupation is a central concern. The generalizing stage of the group is devoted to deriving the meaning of a small slice of life, the group experience. The therapist should encourage the members to verbalize the meaning of the experience for them. Looking at similarities and differences in what is meaningful will help reinforce the values of each member. Using our "Circle of Feelings" example, some members might find meaning in becoming more aware of their own inner feelings, while others might value the opportunity to learn how others really see them. It may surprise some members to find themselves able to express feelings verbally, while others may be more guarded and unwilling to disclose their inner feelings to others. Some people seek the understanding of others through self-disclosure, and these people find meaning in close relationships with others. For other people, the impression they leave with others might be more important—the "never let them see you sweat" approach. Therapists need to be careful not to judge any value as right or wrong. Accepting differences among members is an important norm to promote during this step.

Application

In this step, meaning is expanded and personalized. In client-centered groups, a connection needs to be made between the group activity and the goals of each individual member. The therapist asks each member in turn to discuss how he or she could apply this group experience to his or her own life. It will be important for the therapist to use concreteness and to get each member to give a specific example. This step provides an opportunity for therapist and clients to collaborate in identifying outcomes. These may take the form of greater self-awareness, new learning, skill development, greater self-understanding, new choices, or new solutions or strategies for stated problems. Enabling clients to verbalize the possible benefits or outcomes of group activities reinforces the value of occupational therapy group interventions. However, therapists should be careful to also accept negative or neutral comments and to use these as an opportunity to re-evaluate, problem solve, and collaborate with the group members to plan more relevant activities.

Summary

The summary, as with every step, should involve the group members whenever possible. They are presumed capable of analyzing the entire group experience and judging which parts are most significant. The therapist's role is to encourage them to do this, and not to do it for them. When the therapist asks for a summary of the group, about 5 minutes before it is time to end, members will quickly learn that this is what is expected and may eventually do it spontaneously.

DESIGNING CLIENT-CENTERED GROUP INTERVENTIONS

Yalom and Leszcz (2005) describes a basically existential humanistic approach. Clients are treated in groups not only because it is practical, but because of the many unique advantages that only a group can offer in treatment. The goals for an individual have mostly to do with increasing self-understanding, self-worth, and self-actualization. In the group setting, members are expected to discuss their own lives, their problems, and their successes. Through their self-disclosure, members develop relationships with one another and learn to trust one another. The feedback and support they give one another is of far greater value than what they can get from any individual.

Furthermore, many of the therapeutic factors described by Yalom (discussed in Chapter 2) will help the members achieve their goals. The therapeutic factors are those aspects of groups that make them therapeutic. Instillation of hope conveys the positive expectation members have at the outset of groups that the group experience will help them. Clients in group intervention often feel great relief when they discover that their problems are not unique, that others share their misery (universality). Altruism implies that clients benefit not only by receiving from others, but also from giving. Learning to give to others in the group may in fact be the most important lesson of all. Group cohesiveness has been described as the final and most desirable stage of group development. It is an attraction for each other that is shared by all its members. Cohesiveness makes possible all the positive, productive work that can be accomplished by the mature group described in Chapter 2. Interpersonal learning incorporates a broad range of factors about the give and take of emotional and social relationships to one another. Client-centered groups work best when members have a moderately high cognitive ability. It is the approach suggested for personal/professional growth of student groups or staff groups. A certain level of self-awareness is expected, and members should be able to communicate their self-perceptions to the group reasonably well. In short, members must be capable of insight. Insight means not only acknowledging one's own problematic behavior but having some understanding of the reasons behind it.

However, client-centered theorists warn that therapists should not underestimate the ability of cognitively disabled individuals to express their goals and preferences. Therefore, groups should be adapted to match the level of client understanding and insight, and therapists should enable whatever participation the members can contribute. For example, Ross (Ross & Bachner, 2004) uses five-stage groups with a sensory integrative focus for clients with severe cognitive disabilities. Regarding groups with institutionalized clients, she writes:

> Relating to others without the use of words is very interesting. A connection made between two persons when no words have been spoken but only action takes place is a golden moment, perhaps the more poignant because it feels so stark. It was observed whenever group members showed more awareness and shared or passed items to one another for the first time. It was seen when a man in a group, the victim of Alzheimer's disease, suddenly intercepted a large, soft ball before his male neighbor could reach it, but then handed it to a withdrawn woman sitting next to him so she would have a turn. It is observed in the sudden smile, the unconsciously straightened posture, or the unsolicited hug that comes for the first time from someone who avoided contact or response. When a string of such golden moments happens, a marvelous feeling occurs and illuminates my understanding of how to proceed further. It is easy to become addicted to encouraging the feeling of flow (Ross, 2009, p. 105).

The skilled group leader can adapt the seven-step format using a client-centered approach with many different levels of client ability, disability, and circumstance.

Activity Examples and Worksheets

The Activity Examples at the end of this chapter are designed for use in the evaluation process of occupational therapy. They may be used to help clients to identify and better define their occupational difficulties, to clarify and better communicate their goals and priorities, and to build trust and support within the safety of a therapeutic group. Some of the group activities help clients to explore contextual factors and/or to identify barriers to participation and use group feedback in developing strategies for the removal of barriers and the creation of enabling environments.

The Worksheets are designed for classroom use, to practice skills in therapeutic use of self. The principles they represent are described earlier in the chapter.

REFERENCES

American Occupational Therapy Association. (2002). The occupational therapy practice framework. *American Journal of Occupational Therapy, 56,* 609-639.

American Occupational Therapy Association. (2004). *The reference manual of the official documents of the American Occupational Therapy Association* (10th ed.). Bethesda, MD: Author.

American Occupational Therapy Association. (2008). *Occupational therapy practice framework: Domain and process* (2nd ed.). Bethesda, MD: Author.

Babiss, F. (2002). An ethnographic study of mental health treatment and outcomes: Doing what works. *Occupational Therapy in Mental Health, 18*(3/4), 1-147.

Banks, S., Crossman, D., Poel, D., & Stewart, M. (1997). Partnerships among health professionals and self-help group members. *Canadian Journal of Occupational Therapy, 64,* 259-269.

Baum, C. M., & Law, M. (1997). Occupational therapy practice: Focusing on occupational performance. *American Journal of Occupational Therapy, 51,* 277-288.

Black, R. M. (2005). Intersections of care: An analysis of culturally competent care, client centered care, and the feminist ethic of care. *Work, 24*(4), 409-422.

Black, R., & Wells, S. (2007). *Culture and occupation: A model of empowerment in occupational therapy.* Bethesda, MD: American Occupational Therapy Association.

Brown, J. B., McWilliam, C. L., & Weston, W. W. (1995). The sixth component being realistic. In M. Stewart, J. B. Brown, W. W. Weston, I. R. McWhinney, C. L. McWilliam, & T. R. Freeman (Eds.). *Patient-centred medicine transforming the clinical method* (pp. 102-113). London, England: Sage.

Canadian Occupational Therapy Association. (1991). *Occupational therapy guidelines for client-centered practice.* Toronto, Ontario: Author.

Canadian Occupational Therapy Association. (1997). *Enabling occupation: An occupational therapy perspective.* Toronto, Ontario: Author.

Cillers, P. (1998). Complexity and postmodernism: Understanding complex systems. London, England: Routledge.

Clark, F. (2010). High-definition occupational therapy: HDOT. *American Journal of Occupational Therapy, 64,* 848-854.

Cole, M., & McLean, V. (2003). Therapeutic relationships redefined. *Occupational Therapy in Mental Health, 19*(2), 33-56.

College of Health. (1999). *Patient-defined outcomes.* London, England: College of Health.

Corey, G. (1991). *The theory and practice of counseling and psychotherapy* (4th ed.). Monterey, CA: Brooks/Cole.

Corey, G. (1996). *The theory and practice of counseling and psychotherapy* (5th ed.). Monterey, CA: Brooks/Cole.

Corring, D. J. (1996). Client-centred care means I am a valued human being. *Canadian Journal of Occupational Therapy, 66,* 71-82.

Coulter, A., & Dunn, N. (2002). After Bristol: Putting patients' care at the center/commentary. *British Medical Journal, 324*(7338), 648-651.

Creek, J. (2010). The conceptual framework. In J. Creek (Ed.), *Core concepts of occupational therapy: A dynamic framework for practice.* London, England: Jessica Kingsley.

Crepeau, E., Cohn, E., & Schell, B. (Eds.) (2003). *Willard and Spackman's occupational therapy* (10th ed.). Philadelphia, PA: Williams & Wilkins.

Delbanco, T. L. (1992). Enriching the doctor-patient relationship by inviting the patient's perspective. *Annals of Internal Medicine, 116,* 414-418.

Dixon, S. (1987). *Working with people in crisis* (2nd ed.). St. Louis, MO: Mosby.

Dunton, W. (1919). *Reconstruction therapy.* Philadelphia, PA: Saunders.

Edgman-Levitan, S. (1997). On the value of patient-centred care. *Journal American Academy of Physician Assistants, 10*(3), 9-21.

Egan, G. (2001). *The skilled helper* (5th ed.). Monterey, CA: Brooks/Cole.

Ellers, B. (1993). Innovations in patient-centered education. In M. Gerteis, S. Edgman-Levitan, J. Daley, T. L. Delbanco (Eds.), Through the patient's eyes (pp. 96-118). San Francisco, CA: Jossey-Bass Publishers.

Fallowfield, L. (2001). Participation of patients in decisions about treatment of cancer. *British Medical Journal, 323(7322)*, 1144.

Fearing, V., Clark, J., & Stanton, S. (1998). The client-centered occupational therapy process. In M. Law (Ed.), *Client-centered occupational therapy*. Thorofare, NJ: SLACK Incorporated.

Fleming, M. H. (1994). The therapist with the three track mind. In C. Mattingly & M. Fleming, *Clinical reasoning: Forms of inquiry in a therapeutic practice* (pp. 239-269). Philadelphia, PA: F. A. Davis.

Geyer, R. (2004). *Europeanisation, complexity, and the British welfare state*. Liverpool, UK: Policy Press.

Gray, J. M., Kennedy, B. L., & Zemke, R. (1996). Dynamic systems: An overview. In R. Zemke & F. Clark (Eds.), *Occupational science: The evolving discipline*. Philadelphia, PA: F. A. Davis.

Hall, J. A., Roter, D. L., & Katz, N. R. (1988). Meta-analysis of correlates of provider behavior in medical encounters. *Medical Care, 26*, 657-675.

Harrison, J. (2001). Client-centered care: Transforming to the human becoming theory. *Perspectives, 25*(3), 4-8.

Hasselkus, B. (2002). *The meaning of everyday occupation*. Thorofare, NJ: SLACK Incorporated.

Iwama, M. K. (2006). The Kawa model: Culturally relevant occupational therapy. Toronto, Canada: Elsevier.

Jones, I. R., Berney, L., Kelly, M., Doyal, L., Griffiths, C., Feder, G., Hillier, S., ... Curtis, S. (2004). Is patient involvement possible when decisions involve scarce resources? A qualitative study of decision-making in primary care. *Social Science and Medicine, 59*, 93-102.

Kalmanson, B., & Seligman, S. (1992). Family-provider relationships: The basis of all interventions. *Infants and Young Children, 4*(11), 46-52.

Kielhofner, G. (2004). *Conceptual foundations of occupational therapy* (3rd ed.). Philadelphia, PA: F. A. Davis.

Landeen, J., Pawlick, J., Woodside, H., Kirkpatrick, H., & Byrne, C. (2000). Hope, quality of life, and symptom severity in individuals with schizophrenia. *Psychiatric Rehabilitation Journal, 23*, 364-369.

Law, M. (Ed.). (1998). *Client-centered occupational therapy*. Thorofare, NJ: SLACK Incorporated.

Law, M., Baptiste, S., Carswell, A., McColl, M., Polatajko, H., & Pollock, N. (2005). *Canadian Occupational Performance Measure* (4th ed.) Ottawa, ON: CAOT Publications ACE.

Law, M., & Mills, J. (1998). Client-centered occupational therapy. In M. Law (Ed.), *Client-centered occupational therapy* (pp. 1-18). Thorofare, NJ: SLACK Incorporated.

MacGill, V. (2007). *Complexity pages: A non-technical introduction to the new science of chaos and complexity*. Retrieved from http://complexity.orconhosting.net.nz

Mant, A. (1997). *Intelligent leadership*. Sydney: Allen & Unwin.

Maslow, A. H. (1968). *Toward a psychology of being* (Rev. ed.). New York, NY: Van Nostrand Reinhold.

Matheson, L. N. (1998). Engaging the person in the process: Planning together for occupational therapy intervention. In M. Law (Ed.), *Client-centered occupational therapy*. Thorofare, NJ: SLACK Incorporated.

Mattingly, C. (1994). The narrative nature of clinical reasoning. In C. Mattingly & M. Fleming, *Clinical reasoning: Forms of inquiry in a therapeutic practice* (pp.239-269). Philadelphia, PA: F. A. Davis.

Maxmin, J. S. (2002). Do we hear our patients? And would a patient's page help? *British Medical Journal, 324*, 684.

May, R. (1977). *The meaning of anxiety* (Rev. ed.). New York, NY: Norton.

May, R., & Yalom, I. (1989). Existential psychotherapy. In R. J. Corsini & D. Wedding (Eds.), *Current psychotherapies* (4th ed., pp. 363-402). Itasca, IL: F. E. Peacock.

McKinlay, E. M. (2001). Within the circle of care: Patient experiences of receiving palliative care. *Journal of Palliative Care, 17*, 22-29.

Neistadt, M. E. (1998). Teaching clinical reasoning as a thinking frame. *American Journal of Occupational Therapy, 52*, 221-229.

O'Reilly, M. (1994). Case example: The New York subway. In C. Mattingly, & M. Fleming (Eds.), *Clinical reasoning* (pp. 261-268). Philadelphia, PA: F. A. Davis.

Peloquin, S. M. (2002). Confluence: Moving forward with affective strength. *American Journal of Occupational Therapy, 56*, 69-77.

Powers, P. H., Goldstein, C., Plank, G., Thomas, K., & Conkright, L. (2000). The value of patient- and family-centered care. *American Journal of Nursing, 100*, 84-88.

Rimmington, G. (2001). Systems thinking and leadership in agricultural science. *Agricultural Science, 13*, 28-31.

Rogers, C. (1939). *The clinical treatment of the problem child*. London, England: George Allen and Unwin.

Rogers, C. (1961). *On becoming a person*. Boston, MA: Houghton Mifflin.

Rogers, C. (1967). The conditions of change from a client-centered viewpoint. In B. Berenson & R. Carkhuff (Eds.), *Sources of gain in counseling and psychotherapy*. New York, NY: Holt, Reinhart, and Winston.

Rogers, C. (1975). Empathic: An unappreciated way of being. *The Counseling Psychologist, 5*(2), 2-9.

Rosenbaum, P., King, S., Law, M., King, G., & Evans, J. (1998). Family-centered service: A conceptual framework and research review. *Physical and Occupational Therapy in Pediatrics, 18*, 1-20.

Rosenfeld, M. (1997). *Motivational strategies in geriatric rehabilitation*. Bethesda, MD: American Occupational Therapy Association.

Ross, M. (2009). *For the love of occupation: Reflections on a career in occupational therapy*. Bethesda, MD: American Occupational Therapy Association.

Ross, M., & Bachner, S. (Eds.) (2004). *Occupational therapy with the developmentally disabled*. Bethesda, MD: American Occupational Therapy Association.

Saleh, U. S., & Brockopp, D. Y. (2001). *Hope among patients with cancer hospitalized for bone marrow transplants*. Edinburgh: Churchill Livingstone.

Schell, B. B., & Schell, J. W. (2008). *Clinical and professional reasoning in occupational therapy*. Philadelphia, PA: Wolters Kluwer, Lippincott, Williams & Wilkins.

Schwartzberg, S. (2002). *Interactive reasoning in the practice of occupational therapy*. Upper Saddle River, NJ: Prentice Hall.

Sumison, T. (2005). Facilitating client-centred practice: Insights from clients. *Canadian Journal of Occupational Therapy, 72*, 13-21.

Sumison, T., & Law, M. (2006). A review of evidence on the conceptual elements informing client-centred practice. *Canadian Journal of Occupational Therapy, 73*, 153-162.

Taylor, R. (2007). *The intentional relationship*. Philadelphia, PA: Lippincott, Williams & Wilkins.

Taylor, R., Lee, S. W., Kielhofner, G., & Ketkar, M. (2009). Therapeutic use of self: A nationwide survey of practitioners' attitudes and experiences. *American Journal of Occupational Therapy, 63*, 198-207.

Townsend, E. (2003). Reflections on power and justice in enabling occupation. *Canadian Journal of Occupational Therapy, 70*, 74-87.

Townsend, E. A., & Polatajko, H. J. (2007). *Enabling occupation II: Advancing an occupational therapy vision for health, well-being, & justice through occupation.* Ottawa, ON: Canadian Association of Occupational Therapy.

Urbanowski, R., & Vargo, J. (1994). Spirituality, daily practice, and the occupational performance model. *Canadian Journal of Occupational Therapy, 61,* 88-94.

Von Guten, C. F. (2002). Discussion hospice care. *Journal of Clinical Oncology, 20,* 1419-1424.

Ward, J. D. (2003). The nature of clinical reasoning with groups: A phenomenological study of an occupational therapist in community mental health. *The American Journal of Occupational Therapy, 57,* 625-634.

White, R. (1959). Motivation reconsidered: The concept of competence. *Psychoanalytic Review, 66,* 197.

Whiteford, G., Klomp, N., & St. Clair, V. W. (2005). Complexity theory: Understanding occupation, practice and context. In G. Whiteford & V. W. St. Clair (Eds.), *Occupation & practice in context* (pp. 3-15). London, England: Elsevier, Churchill Livingstone.

Wilcock, A. (2001). *Occupation for health (Vol. 1): A journey from self health to prescription.* London, England: British College of Occupational Therapists.

Wilkins, S., Pollock, N., Rochon, S., & Law, M. (2001). Implementing client-centred practice: Why is it so difficult to do? *Canadian Journal of Occupational Therapy, 68,* 70-79.

World Health Organization. (1986). Ottawa charter for health promotion. Geneva, Switzerland: Author.

World Health Organization. (2001). International classification of functioning, disability, and health (ICF). Geneva, Switzerland: Author.

Yalom, I., & Leszcz, M. (1995). *The theory and practice of group psychotherapy* (4th ed.). New York, NY: Basic Books.

Client-Centered Activity Example 3-1
Self-Awareness

Directions: Fill out all the information listed on the worksheet. Then, select what parts you would like to share with the group.

I am (name you prefer):

Some of my needs are:

Some of my hopes are:

I would describe myself as:

Some things that are important in my life now are:

Some things that may become important to me are:

Three things I am trying to achieve are:

I am good at:

Some things I would like to improve about myself are:

I run away from:

I feel confident when:

I am proud of:

My most striking quality is:

From Cole, M. B. *Group dynamics in occupational therapy: The theoretical basis and practice application of group intervention* (4th ed.). Thorofare, NJ: SLACK Incorporated. © 2012 SLACK Incorporated.

Client-Centered Activity Example 3-2
Positive Attitudes

Materials: Magazines (at least two per client) with pictures on a variety of subjects.

Directions: Select from these magazines pictures of negative scenes, problems, or situations. There is no required number, so find as many as you like. You have 15 minutes for this task.

Procedure: Each member presents his or her pictures and describes the negative situation. Then, the group is asked to point out all the positive aspects of the pictures (For example, appearance or personal hygiene of the people, weather conditions, communication, and support available, etc.). Then, the group can choose a few situations to problem solve. Answer the question: "What can be done to give this situation a happy ending?"

From Cole, M. B. *Group dynamics in occupational therapy: The theoretical basis and practice application of group intervention* (4th ed.). Thorofare, NJ: SLACK Incorporated. © 2012 SLACK Incorporated.

Client-Centered Activity Example 3-3
Leisure Collage

Materials: Magazines on varied topics, scissors, glue, white paper, and markers.

Directions: Cut pictures of things you like to do from these magazines and then arrange and paste them on the paper. You have 20 minutes to do this task. After you have finished pasting, use a marker to label each picture with a word ending in "ing" (e.g., eating, talking, playing volleyball, singing).

From Cole, M. B. *Group dynamics in occupational therapy: The theoretical basis and practice application of group intervention* (4th ed.). Thorofare, NJ: SLACK Incorporated. © 2012 SLACK Incorporated.

Client-Centered Activity Example 3-4
Saying Goodbye

Materials: Writing paper and pens.

Directions: At some point in our lives, we have all had to leave someone we love. Either we left, or we got left behind (i.e., a best friend moving away, a lover finding a new love, a relative's death, a child going away to school). Often, we do not have the chance to say the things we want to say before the separation. So, here is another chance. Take the next 15 minutes to write a letter to a loved one, telling him or her the things you would like the person to know. Begin with "Dear _____ ," and end with some form of goodbye.

From Cole, M. B. *Group dynamics in occupational therapy: The theoretical basis and practice application of group intervention* (4th ed.). Thorofare, NJ: SLACK Incorporated. © 2012 SLACK Incorporated.

Client-Centered Activity Example 3-5
My House

Materials: Worksheets, rulers, colored markers, and pencils with erasers.

Directions: Imagine you are going on a 1-month vacation and will live in a small house on the beach by yourself. The beach has a path that leads to town where you can buy food or other supplies. Visualize what the house would look like. You arrive in a taxi with your bags. You step onto the deck, unlock the front door, and walk in. What would you like to see? Now, fill in the floor plan on the worksheet with whatever you would like in your house. Some suggestions are sofa, bed, dresser, rug, television set, bookshelf with books, refrigerator, stove, washer, dryer, bicycle, sailboat, etc. (Figure 3-2).

While doing this activity, think about what necessities you will need and also what items you would like to help you enjoy your vacation. You may assume there are other people to socialize with at the beach, but they will not be staying with you. You are the only one living in your house.

From Cole, M. B. *Group dynamics in occupational therapy: The theoretical basis and practice application of group intervention* (4th ed.). Thorofare, NJ: SLACK Incorporated. © 2012 SLACK Incorporated.

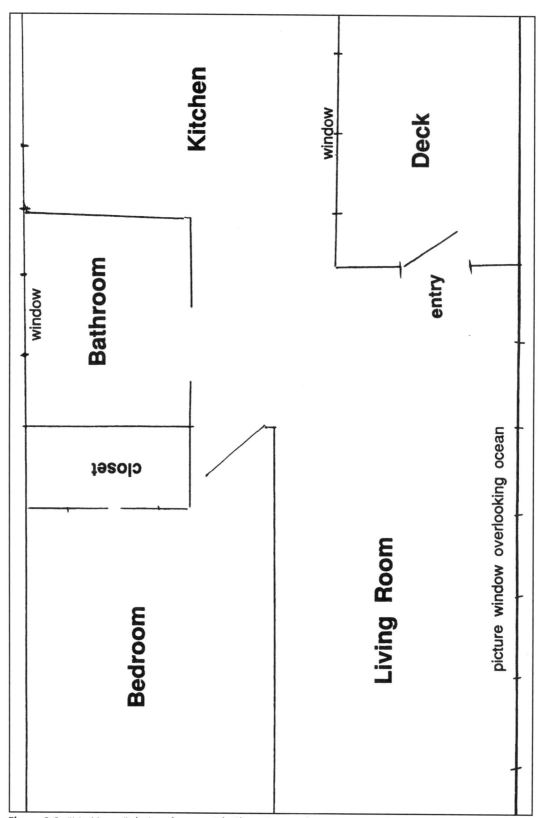

Figure 3-2. "My House" design (for use with Client-Centered Activity Example 3-5).

Client-Centered Activity Example 3-6
My Ideal Job

Materials: Worksheets and pencils.

Directions: Suppose you had the opportunity to be trained to do whatever job you want. What would be your ideal job? To help you define your ideal job, first circle your answers to the following questions. If you circle more than one, write "first choice" or "second choice" next to the answer.

1. What work setting do you prefer?
   Contemporary office
   Well-equipped workshop
   Home-like setting
   Outdoors
   Other

2. What other people would you prefer to work with?
   Work by yourself
   Be part of a working team
   Be the expert who gives help and advice to others
   Be your boss' right-hand man/woman

3. What skills do you prefer to use while working?
   Manual skills, work with hands or tools
   Artistic or creative skills
   Intellectual skills, knowledge, and ideas
   Political skills, strategies, or persuasion
   Technical problem-solving skills

4. What rewards would you seek from your job?
   Lots of money
   Satisfaction from helping others
   Having others recognize your skills
   Achieving your own potential

5. How much risk are you willing to take in your job?
   Prefer doing something familiar with regular pay
   Do not mind being paid on commission
   Willing to try new ideas, even if they are not a sure thing
   An element of danger might make work more exciting

From Cole, M. B. *Group dynamics in occupational therapy: The theoretical basis and practice application of group intervention* (4th ed.). Thorofare, NJ: SLACK Incorporated. © 2012 SLACK Incorporated.

Client-Centered Activity Example 3-6
My Ideal Job (Continued)

Now, consider your answers to those questions, and circle the jobs that might fit your criteria from the list below:

- Salesperson in a small clothing store
- Licensed electrician
- Mechanic
- Nursery school teacher
- Medical technician
- Nurse in a large hospital
- Medical receptionist in a doctor's office
- Advertising artist
- Newspaper reporter
- High school coach
- Hairdresser
- Interior decorator
- Telephone lineman
- Insurance claims adjuster
- Traveling salesperson for a large company
- Chef in an expensive restaurant
- Hostess in an expensive restaurant
- Manager of a small delicatessen
- Manager of an expensive antique shop
- Home health nurse
- Musician in a band
- Public relations representative for a hotel
- Counselor in a drug rehabilitation center
- Landscape designer

From Cole, M. B. *Group dynamics in occupational therapy: The theoretical basis and practice application of group intervention* (4th ed.). Thorofare, NJ: SLACK Incorporated. © 2012 SLACK Incorporated.

Client-Centered Activity Example 3-7
Draw Your Wall

Anne Golensky, MS, OTR, is acknowledged for creating this activity for use with recovering alcoholics.

Materials: White drawing paper and sets of colored markers.

Directions: The purpose of this activity is to discover the barriers we face that prevent us from moving toward self-actualization. Members introduce themselves, and each completes the sentence "Something I've always wanted to do is _____ ." Then, with paper and markers, members draw their "wall," which symbolizes the things that hold them back from achieving their dreams.

From Cole, M. B. *Group dynamics in occupational therapy: The theoretical basis and practice application of group intervention* (4th ed.). Thorofare, NJ: SLACK Incorporated. © 2012 SLACK Incorporated.

Client-Centered Activity Example 3-8
Primary Concerns

Materials: Three 3" x 5" index cards for each member, pens, and area telephone directories.

Directions: This activity is for acute inpatient groups. Members introduce themselves giving names and stating one reason they are in the hospital. They may briefly discuss where they intend to go when they leave, if known.

Write on each of three index cards the following information:
- Card 1—What are you most concerned about at this moment?
- Card 2—What are you most worried about after you leave the hospital?
- Card 3—Who can you count on to help you with your concerns after you leave this group? List names and phone numbers of your doctor, a pharmacy near your residence, your closest family members and friends, and any other resources available to you (phone numbers may need to be filled in afterwards).

From Cole, M. B. *Group dynamics in occupational therapy: The theoretical basis and practice application of group intervention* (4th ed.). Thorofare, NJ: SLACK Incorporated. © 2012 SLACK Incorporated.

Client-Centered Activity Example 3-9
Activities Wheel

Materials: Worksheet with two circles representing 24-hour days. A calculator on hand would be helpful.

Directions: For each hour, fill in the name of the activity you are typically doing at that time of day. Then, total the hours for each general category at the bottom of the circle. Finally, approximate the percentage of the total for each category.

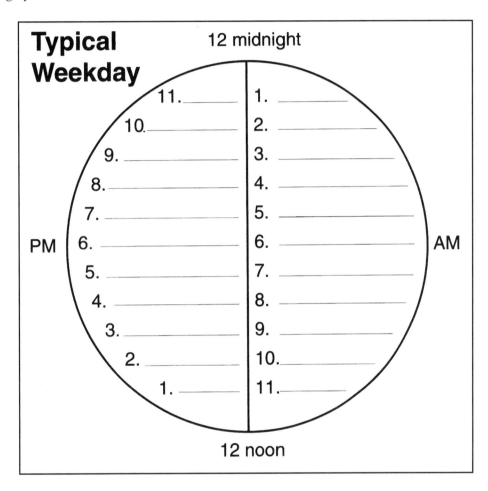

Work/Obligations: _____

Total Time: _____

Leisure/Relaxation: _____

Total Time: _____

Sleep/Rest: _____

Total Time: _____

Self-Care/Caregiving: _____

Total Time: _____

Other: _____

Total Time: _____

From Cole, M. B. *Group dynamics in occupational therapy: The theoretical basis and practice application of group intervention* (4th ed.). Thorofare, NJ: SLACK Incorporated. © 2012 SLACK Incorporated.

Activities Wheel (Continued)

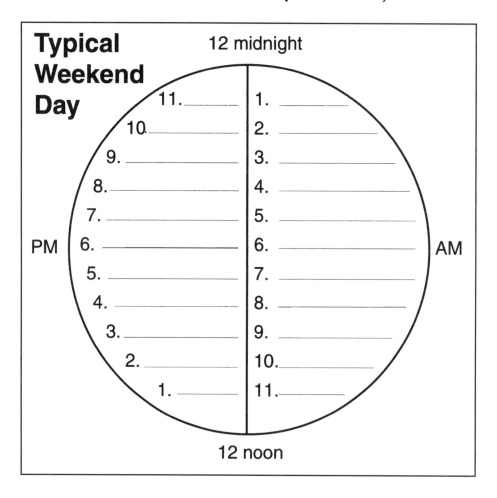

Typical Weekend Day

12 midnight

11. _____
10. _____
9. _____
8. _____
7. _____
6. _____
5. _____
4. _____
3. _____
2. _____
1. _____

1. _____
2. _____
3. _____
4. _____
5. _____
6. _____
7. _____
8. _____
9. _____
10. _____
11. _____

PM

AM

12 noon

Work/Obligations: _____
Total Time: _____

Self-Care/Caregiving: _____
Total Time: _____

Leisure/Relaxation: _____
Total Time: _____

Other: _____
Total Time: _____

Sleep/Rest: _____
Total Time: _____

Purpose in Life Chart

Things I love:

1.

2.

3.

4.

5.

Things I am proud of:

1.

2.

3.

4.

5.

Things I want to strive for:

1.

2.

3.

4.

5.

Things I can do today to feel better about myself:

1.

2.

3.

Things I hate:

1.

2.

3.

4.

5.

Things I am ashamed of:

1.

2.

3.

4.

5.

Things I never want to become:

1.

2.

3.

4.

5.

GROUPS AND THE
OT PRATICE FRAMEWORK-II

When the American Occupational Therapy Association (AOTA) first published the "Occupational Therapy Practice Framework: Domain and Process" in 2002, it truly ushered the profession into the 21st century. Much of the terminology has changed, and this fourth edition has changed with it. With the first version, the term *client* replaced *patient*, and the term *treatment* became *intervention*. In the second edition (Framework-II), this professional document continues to clarify and expand the scope of occupational therapy practice (AOTA, 2008). The framework does not identify specific models and frames of reference; it does not change the many areas of specialized expertise developed by the profession. Rather, the document reframes previously identified domains of concern and redefines the process of OT within a new health care paradigm, which is holistic, client-centered, and systems-oriented (Cole & Tufano, 2008). Therefore, our skills of therapeutic communication and group leadership, and our understanding of the dynamics of groups, remain basic competencies in the process of occupational therapy evaluation and intervention, but can now find applications in a broader range of settings and purposes. The framework's stated purpose is to provide consistency in OT focus and language (including the language of the *International Classification of Function* [ICF]) (WHO, 2001) and to outline the process of evaluation and intervention that "supports health and participation in life through engagement in occupation" (AOTA, 2008, p. 626).

CHANGES IN THE PROFESSION

This chapter explores how the Framework-II guides OT group leadership, professional leadership, and advocacy within a broad range of settings. It will review the expanded definition of client, as individuals (groups of individuals, families, caregivers), organizations (existing groups, community groups, agencies, and corporations), and populations (groups with common circumstances, health conditions, or risk factors). Next, it explores some of the ways that the major categories of the OT domains and process relate to group interventions, giving recent examples from the OT literature. It reviews some topics particularly relevant for groups in greater depth, including theories related to social participation (an area of occupation), role theory (an occupational pattern), culture change, and social support theories (occupational contexts). Third, it discusses how various parts of the Framework-II Process incorporate groups for evaluation and intervention in order to focus on a broad range of desired OT outcomes, including the newly defined areas of self-advocacy and social justice.

IDENTIFYING GROUPS IN
THE OT FRAMEWORK-II

The Occupational Therapy Practice Framework (2002) defined clients as "a) individuals (including others involved in the individual's life who may also be served

Cole M.B. *Group Dynamics in Occupational Therapy:
The Theoretical Basis and Practice Application
of Group Intervention (pp 103-124).*
© 2012 SLACK Incorporated.

indirectly such as caregiver, teacher, parent, employer, spouse), b) groups, or c) populations (i.e., organizations, communities)" (AOTA, 2002, p. 630). This expanded definition of the client allows occupational therapists to design group interventions on a variety of levels. In the Framework-II, the definition of client changes to: "1) persons, including families, caregivers, teachers, employers, and relevant others; 2) organizations, such as businesses, industries, or agencies; and 3) populations within a community, such as refugees, veterans who are homeless, and people with chronic health disabling conditions (Moyers & Dale, 2007)" (AOTA, 2008, p. 625).

The framework states, "the broader definition of client included in this document is indicative of the profession's increasing involvement in providing services not only to a person but also to organizations and populations" (2008, p. 647). It later continues, "rarely is an individual the exclusive focus of the intervention" and that "collaboration may include significant others, community members, and stakeholders who affect or are affected by the client's engagement in occupation, health, and participation" (AOTA, 2008, p. 647). Although the word *groups* no longer appears in the definition of client, groups as the focus of OT intervention are implicit in all three of the above categories.

Groups of Individuals

The occupational therapist identifies three to eight clients with common problems, disabilities, and/or goals to participate in a specific group or series of groups designed to meet one or more of the goals identified. In this type of group, individual goals will serve as the outcome measures, and the client members will actively participate in the task-selection process. The seven-step format described in Chapter 1 was designed for groups of individuals with similar goals. For example, a group of people with hemiparesis following stroke in a subacute care facility practiced upper extremity exercises while participating in a daily breakfast group. While each member may have needed different adaptations based on different levels of ability, all members recognized the added benefits of group participation: "increased practice, socialization, encouragement, and support from other clients, and the opportunity to work with a variety of (OT) therapists" (Capasso, Gorman, & Blick, 2010).

Family Groups: Clients in Context

An increasingly common group intervention is designed in collaboration with an identified client and the family members and significant others who participate in his or her care. Family-centered care parallels client-centered care, yet requires additional expertise in the dynamics of family groups. This new area of practice uses knowledge of group dynamics theory and research on social contexts to design interventions with entire family groups to assist them in making adaptations and planning activities to enable the identified client to participate in family life.

The disciplines of family therapy and family science have done substantial research on the family-centered approach, which views the family group as one entity rather than a group of individuals (Schaber, 2003, personal communication). Reviewing this extensive body of literature is beyond the scope of this chapter. The application of small group theory, the Fundamental Interpersonal Relations Model (FIRO), has been applied to families and has been redefined as the Family FIRO model and serves to inform occupational therapists intervening with families with Alzheimer's disease by highlighting the unique needs of the family member (Schaber, 2002). The FIRO model is based on the theory of Schutz (1958), who proposed that each individual has three interpersonal needs: inclusion, control, and affection that can be met through group membership. Earlier (see Chapter 2), these needs formed the basis of the developmental stages of groups. Here, the theory applies to the family member in the family group. "Families as context" serve as the needs satisfier in evaluating and working with clients who are dependent on their families for daily care. Schaber (2003, personal communication) points out that this application does not replace the family-centered care model, but offers an understanding of the function of the family and can enhance the interviewing process. It is not intended to replace family therapy and is not a social work approach. Rather, it provides a way to examine the social context in which an identified client engages in occupations and explores their meaning within the context of family relationships.

Practically speaking, the occupational therapy family intervention most likely begins with an identified client. We will use the example of a grandmother with dementia, living with her daughter who serves as the primary caregiver. From a systems perspective, the progression of chronic disease in one family member affects all of the other members in some way. Therefore, instead of focusing only on Grandma, the occupational therapist defines her client as a family with dementia. Schaber (2003, personal communication) suggests that the primary caregiver select the members who will participate in the occupational therapy group intervention. From Grandma's perspective, this group may include a son-in-law, several grandchildren, brothers or sisters who live nearby, nieces and nephews, or close friends and neighbors who are willing to participate. Schaber cautions that occupational issues do not always flow in a sequential manner and that issues of inclusion, control, and affection often need to be addressed simultaneously. Accordingly, the sequential structure described in the Family Group Protocol may need to be altered to address changing family priorities. A Family Group Protocol is described in Group Example 4-1 at the end of this chapter.

Caregiving Teams

The AOTA Framework-II specifies caregivers, teachers, employers, and relevant others within the definition of an individual client. An example might be a group of professionals in a school system who are dealing with problem behaviors of a child with autism or a group of professionals in a nursing home. Such teams often include both clients and family members as part of the caregiving team. OT practitioners as members of such teams may take a leadership role when dealing with issues involving the client's occupational performance. In less formal settings, the occupational therapist may collaborate with other professionals, caregivers, or family members in addressing identified problem areas concerning a client's occupational engagement.

Organizations

Organizations are defined in the Framework-II as "entities with a common purpose or enterprise such as businesses, industries, or agencies" (AOTA, 2008, p. 673). Occupational therapy consultants use group leadership skills in collaborating with organizations to identify problem areas, educate regarding evidence-based interventions, develop strategies for intervention, and enable and structure occupations related to targeted outcomes (e.g., fund raising, advocacy, mentoring, creating support groups). Some examples of organizational groups from the OT literature are group homes, rehabilitation departments or provider groups, public or private agencies, and corporations.

Existing Community Groups

Groups of clients in the community often have common occupational issues, such as clients with mental retardation who share a group home or a group of clients with dementia who attend a day-care program. In these groups, the occupational therapist evaluates the group as a whole and recommends and plans group interventions that address targeted outcomes. OT interventions may address the group as a whole, using shared activities such as meal preparation, home maintenance, or leisure participation as a focus. An example of group intervention in a community setting is the "successful student groups," designed to assist university students with multiple sclerosis to function effectively in an educational environment. This group, co-led by an occupational therapist, included strategies for studying, note taking, and test taking, as well as managing symptoms, disclosure of health issues to professors and other students, asking for help, and strategies for staying connected with others (Kalina, 2009).

Groups of Service Providers

These include caregivers and staff members working in hospitals, health care agencies, and nursing homes.

For example, in consulting with a 20-member occupational therapy department in a large inpatient rehabilitation hospital, Schwartz (2010) describes her group interventions as a product and education specialist for splinting materials and techniques for a manufacturing company. After conducting a needs assessment (survey, interviews, and observation) using all of the categories of the Framework-II domain, Schwartz designed a splinting workshop including education, therapeutic use of self, consultation, and occupation-based intervention. She encouraged workshop participants to offer input to the learning experience, acknowledging the variety of knowledge and experience of each member, so that the workshop content was relevant for them. During a hands-on splinting lab, group members worked in pairs, with more senior therapists partnered with novices, while Schwartz acted as a facilitator in problem solving.

Nonprofit Organizations

Research on volunteering has revealed that there are many issues regarding how volunteer jobs are structured and matched with personal interests and skills and how volunteer workers are supported and supervised (Cole & Macdonald, 2011). This area of practice seems to be a good fit for OT, yet there are no examples published.

Populations

Populations is defined by the Framework-II as "large groups as a whole, such as refugees, homeless veterans, and people who need wheelchairs" (AOTA, 2008, p. 673). The OT may be asked to evaluate an entire population and to design group interventions that address the population as a whole. An example of this might be designing wellness programs for elderly seniors living in a community. The community senior center might be the "client" with whom the occupational therapist collaborates in setting goals and selecting strategies. Community organizations whose purpose is to enhance the quality of life for underserved populations, such as people with AIDS, or other specialized groups may benefit from occupational therapy consultation.

Example: At-Risk Youth

For example, the Occupational Therapy Training Program (OTTP) provides mental health services to at-risk youth ages 11 to 18 years and transitional age youth between 16 and 25 years (Bream, 2010). The program is one division of Special Service for Groups, a Los Angeles-based nonprofit agency. Within this program, OTs design and facilitate groups in various schools, working on mental health goals of individuals within the context of the group. Examples of group activities are stress management, coping skills, work readiness, communication, anger management and conflict resolution, self-care, nutrition, cooking, banking, and budgeting. The OTs also provide family-based interventions and facilitate occupation-based groups for youth with more intensive mental health needs.

Example: People in Recovery

Gutman and colleagues (Gutman, Schindler, Furphy, Klein, Lisak, & Durhan, 2007) describe a supported education program for adults with psychiatric disabilities. Supported education helps people gain basic academic and social skills needed to successfully engage in student occupations at a university level. These OT researchers conducted the "Bridge Program" for 3 hours/week over 12 weeks in a university setting. Eighteen participants aged 24 to 50 years attended 2 hours of group education and 1 hour of individual mentoring each week. Of the original 18, 16 successfully completed the program, and 12 enrolled in further courses. All reported feeling better prepared and more comfortable in the student role. Additionally, OT students who instructed and mentored participants reported greater comfort in working with people with mental disabilities (Gutman et al., 2007).

Wellness and Prevention for Older Adults

Many OT initiatives in programming for populations have the goal of wellness and prevention (AOTA, 2008; Neufeld, 2004). An example of this is the federally funded Program of All-Inclusive Care for the Elderly (PACE) described by Leighty (2010). The San Diego-based PACE program, one of 70 nationwide, employs eight OTs working with an interdisciplinary health care team, whose goal is to provide nursing home-eligible older adults support for the skills of daily living (shopping, house cleaning, cooking, home adaptation) for frail elders to continue living independently. Two types of groups are described: educational and social group activities, and an action committee of 15 PACE members who wrote a letter to President Obama, advocating that PACE programs be expanded to meet the needs of the rest of the 70 million elders who will need holistic health services to keep them out of nursing homes (Leighty, 2010).

GROUPS BASED ON FRAMEWORK DOMAINS

AOTA's Framework-II outlines six interrelated categories of occupation with which OTs are concerned: areas of occupation, client factors, performance skills, performance patterns, context and environment, and activity demands. Any of these areas or a combination of areas can serve as the focus of group evaluation and intervention.

Areas of Occupation as Group Focus

Activities of daily living, work, or student roles might serve as the focus for group design. For example, in applying occupation-based models with groups, intervention focuses on the occupational roles that clients find meaningful. Occupations connected with valued roles clients identify coincide with the Framework-II's occupational performance areas. More frequently, the content for group intervention will be a combination of factors from several domain categories. For example, a work readiness group involves worker habits and roles (performance patterns), work task analysis and synthesis (activity demands), and the human and nonhuman contexts (environments) of the workplace.

Children's Play Groups

One example of a children's OT group occurred at a summer camp for students with disabilities. The focus of the group was to build social skills through participation in camp activities (Parke & Szymanski, 2010). The campers were placed in small groups according to grade level in school and met each morning to start their day, where they set goals for the activities they would participate in that day. Groups also engaged in social skills lessons "with the goal of meeting new friends in camp, learning to play in small groups, and winning/losing appropriately" (p. 36).

Education as Group Focus

Glennon and Marks (2010) identified some of the special needs of teens with high-functioning autism (HFA) and Asperger's syndrome (AS) transitioning to college. Topping the list of anticipated problems (identified by 51 student respondents aged 18 to 25 and their parents) were dating, managing intimate relationships, making friends, revealing their diagnosis to classmates, calling classmates on the phone, understanding nonverbal communication, and finding a group to work with on projects or study with. All of these issues might appropriately be addressed within a small group context in which the needed skills could be learned and practiced, and social and emotional components discussed within a supportive environment.

An after-school OT group program for at-risk youth was described by Bream (2010). Middle and high school students in urban Los Angeles who demonstrate behavioral or mental health issues participate in groups addressing stress management, coping skills, communication, anger management, conflict resolution, as well as self-care, work readiness, cooking, banking, and budgeting. These OT groups have the overall goal of helping students deal with some of the difficulties that prevent them from learning and achieving in the classroom.

Work and Volunteering as Focus

According to O'Brien (2010), "socialization is an aspect of work settings, and thus, helping clients return to work may require remediation of social participation skills. Role playing, practice, and cognitive awareness of social behaviors appropriate for work may help a client return to work successfully" (p. 211). Preparatory and simulated work activities that require cooperation, collaboration, and compromise might become the focus of client groups who anticipate obtaining or returning to valued work roles. For example, a preparatory group activity might have a goal of reducing stress or managing one's time effectively. Clients could potentially try out work roles through volunteering, for example, forming a community clean-up team or performing a service such as washing cars and using funds raised to purchase something for the entire group. Task-oriented groups, such as those described in Chapter 5, focus on building work skills such as cooperation, communication, decision making, and other basic social skills needed for successful participation in the workplace.

Social Participation as Focus

Social participation is a particularly relevant area for OT group intervention. In fact, one could argue that evaluation and intervention for this occupational performance area cannot be adequately accomplished outside of a group format. Social participation is an area of occupational performance defined in the Framework-II as "organized patterns of behavior that are characteristic and expected of an individual or a given position within a social system" (Mosey, 1986, p. 340, in AOTA, 2008, p. 633). Occupational therapy group interventions, with their multiple opportunities to develop and practice social interaction skills, are ideal for preparing clients for many levels of social participation. Groups that facilitate social participation, as guided by the Framework-II, also include contexts within which clients wish to participate. Social participation groups have a goal of developing, establishing, or maintaining clients' inclusion in some of the naturally occurring groups in which they wish to participate: families, peer or friendship groups, classes, sports teams or recreational groups, work groups, church groups, and community organizations.

OT theorists and scholars have developed considerable expertise in the area of social participation. Mosey (1986) addressed group behaviors through her recapitulation of ontogenesis theory, which outlined five subskills of group interaction skill. Group interaction involves the ability to be a productive member of a variety of primary groups, including taking appropriate group membership roles, engaging in decision making, communicating effectively, recognizing and behaving according to group norms, contributing to goal attainment, assisting in resolving conflicts, and working toward group cohesiveness (Mosey, 1986, p. 435). The five subskills are organized into a sequence of developmental groups, which are described more fully in Chapter 5 (also see Appendix B and C). They are as follows:

1. Parallel groups (18 months to 2 years)
2. Project groups (2 to 4 years)
3. Egocentric cooperative groups (5 to 7 years)
4. Cooperative groups (9 to 12 years)
5. Mature groups (15 to 18 years)

Donohue (1999) has reviewed and analyzed the theoretical foundations of Mosey's concepts of these five levels of group interaction skill and adds the following new assumptions: 1) most people function at two or more levels of developmental group interaction, 2) there is a relationship between the nature of the activity and the level of function, and 3) adults function at lower developmental levels of group interaction if the activity requires it (p. 35). Donohue also suggests extending the age range of the mature group to end in adulthood.

Context and Environment as Focus

In group work, the most relevant aspects of context for clients are social and cultural. The AOTA Framework-II defines social context as "constructed by presence, relationships, and expectations of persons, organizations, and populations:

- Availability and expectations of significant individuals, such as spouse, friends, and caregivers.
- Relationships with individuals, groups, and organizations.
- Relationships with systems (political, legal, economic, institutional) that are influential in establishing norms, role expectations, and social routines" (AOTA, 2008, p. 645).

There is some overlap with the definition of cultural context, which is defined as "customs, beliefs, activity patterns, behavior standards, and expectations accepted by the society of which the individual is a member. (Cultural context) includes ethnicity and values as well as political aspects, such as laws that affect access to resources and affirm personal rights. (It) also includes opportunities for education, employment, and economic support" (AOTA, 2008, p. 645).

Most occupation-based models recognize social and cultural (and other) contexts as highly influential aspects of the occupational environment (Dunn, 2007; Schultz, 2009). In the current ICF definition, "disability serves as an umbrella term for impairments, activity limitations, and participation restrictions" (WHO, 2001, p. 3). This definition implies that people and contexts together create disability; therefore, changes in context so as to remove barriers and create supports for engagement in occupation, participation, and inclusion now fall within the domain of occupational therapy intervention. "Occupational therapy practitioners are concerned not only with occupations but also the complexity of factors that make possible clients' engagement and participation in positive health-promoting occupations" (Wilcock & Townsend, 2008, in AOTA, 2008, p. 629).

Groups Based on Cultural Context

An example of the impact of cultural context is described by Ekelman (2010). Occupational therapists who are members of palliative care teams share in providing comfortable and supportive environments for people who are dying or terminally ill. In hospice and other settings, professionals along with the client, family, and others work together to maintain or improve quality of life through care when cure is no longer deemed possible. Central to palliative care is respecting the cultural and spiritual needs of the family (Chater & Tsai, 2009). When clients have less than 1 year to live, OTs may assume that they want to plan their lives differently in order to better prepare for death by making the most of their remaining time. Yet, for clients from non-Western cultures, including Chinese, Japanese, Native American, and Arab-American (Muslim) backgrounds, autonomy and truth telling are not always accepted beliefs. Often, in these cultures, families will request that medical truths be withheld from the client, and clients may prefer to delegate medical or other life decisions to their families (Wintzelberg et al., 2005). A culturally competent OT practitioner can avert this ethical dilemma through therapeutic use of self in family group leadership (Ekelman, 2010). The OT meets with client, family members, and others and facilitates a discussion to discover and understand the client's cultural experience. OT and the family group will then collaborate to incorporate individual and family values and beliefs into the OT intervention plan.

Culture Change as a Context-Focused Organizational Approach

Nursing homes provide some good examples of culture change affecting both clients and their institutional settings. Wilson (2009) reviews three new models for nursing homes: 1) the Eden Model, 2) Green House, and 3) Wellspring Initiative. In 2005, Medicare and Medicaid services included culture change principles in the scope of work assigned to state quality improvement organizations (Rahman & Schnelle, 2008), with a goal of creating a stronger focus on quality of life and person-centered care. Each of these models gives nursing home residents greater autonomy and opportunity for participation in the occupations of their daily lives.

The Eden Model

Designed by William Thomas in the 1990s, this model's goal was to change three common areas of complaint for nursing home residents: loneliness, helplessness, and boredom. The Eden Model creates "elder-centered habitats" that foster continued development of older adults through relationships with others, including plants, animals, and children. In this model, institutional housing is divided into "neighborhoods" of both staff and residents. This culture change required extensive staff training, introducing consistent staffing patterns and mechanisms for increasing group interaction and collaborative decision-making regarding daily schedules.

Green House Model

This model, also designed by Dr. Thomas, takes the philosophy one step further by breaking up larger institutions into separate "homes" for just 10 residents each. Universal workers consistent to each "home" provide not only personal care, but also meal preparation, cleaning, and group activity facilitation. The goal of this model is to promote resident autonomy and dignity. For both Eden and Green House models, research "found elders more engaged in everyday life, with making decisions, and in teaching staff how to prepare meals their way" (Wilson, 2009, p. 2).

Wellspring Initiative Model

The Wellspring alliance, initially including 11 nonprofit nursing homes, focused on staff education, data collection, and analysis. This effort included the goals for improving staff working environments as well as resident care. Among the research results for this initiative are higher quality care for residents, improved staff satisfaction, and cost-effectiveness (Stone et al., 2002; Wilson, 2009).

Implied within these models are roles for occupational therapists, including staff training groups and resident groups that facilitate autonomy and empowerment. The OT profession, according to Scaffa (2003), embraces the values of "competence, mastery, and independence," which counteract the helplessness, anger, fear, or depression that can be associated with institutional care. According to Wilson (2009), culture change for organizations takes both time and commitment because major structural changes to the management systems of the nursing home administrations are needed to create substantive change. In this regard, OTs and family members of nursing home residents may need to advocate for culture change in order to remove identified barriers to occupational engagement and participation for this population of older adults.

Groups Based on Social Contexts

Social contexts in everyday life include many types of groups, families, work teams, friendship clusters, community organizations, and many others. For clients, members of these groups can either facilitate or create barriers to occupational performance. Social groups and networks represent complex, dynamic systems. We can use systems theory to understand the operation of social systems on many levels. Bronfenbrenner (1977, 1993) is most often quoted by OT theorists when defining the multiple levels of social context and their influence on individual behaviors (Spencer, 1998; Stark & Sanford, 2005). His ecological model includes microsystems, mesosystems, exosystems, and macrosystems, each of which are described in terms of occupational influence:

1. Microsystems are immediate social environments, such as client and caregivers or household members. Not surprisingly, caregiver attitudes and values have the most powerful influence upon the occupational performance of people with disabilities (Mattingly & Fleming, 1994). Occupational therapists could create groups that include clients and their caregivers to help resolve cultural and ethical differences regarding occupational issues, such as which occupations the client can do safely and which require caregiver assistance.

2. Mesosystems, or proximal scale social contexts, include social environments frequented by the client outside the home, such as a classroom, workplace, or clinic. Occupational therapists need to understand the social systems in each of these settings, including roles, expectations, occupational patterns, and rules for interaction. Many cultural factors overlap these social factors. Occupational therapists can consult with groups of workers, students, or day-care attendees to facilitate communication; improve factors that enable occupational functioning of workers/clients; and minimize or recommend removal of barriers to social participation.

3. Exosystems, also known as community scale social contexts, include both social networks and multiple formal and informal services. Communities often provide services such as home-based medical services, transportation, delivery services, and senior services. Groups can explore community resources and share information. The occupational therapist should be prepared to recommend or facilitate access to community services that will enable social participation. For example, many churches offer assistance, visitation, and social activities for people seeking engagement in occupation at the community level. Community organizations may be viewed as potential "clients" for occupational therapists. Potentially, a need exists for most organizations to recognize and eliminate barriers to participation for people with disabilities.

4. Macrosystems are societal-level systems, including political, economic, legal, and institutional. The welfare system, for example, follows national policies in dispersing funds and benefits to those people who meet specific criteria, whether poverty or disability. States have different guidelines for services offered to welfare recipients, and cities have still different policies and procedures. Local officers assist potential recipients when entering the system, and certain rules need to be followed by recipients in order to remain in the system. Large bureaucratic systems like this can present problems for individuals. For example, once a person with a disability enters the system, he or she cannot secure paid employment without losing benefits. This fact provides little motivation for clients to participate in the worker roles of their peers, even if they find themselves capable.

At the proximal level, OTs often consult with employers, teachers and administrators, or community day-care staff regarding the occupational issues of a specific client. However, these entities may present challenges with the client-centered approach. In OT consultation, Townsend and Landry (2005) suggest the application of enabling guidelines in working with social groups, including the following:

- Participation: Invite recipients of service to be involved in the group process.

- Collaboration: Share the power of problem solving and decision making.

- Advocating for change: Involve group members in organizational change, such as changes in policy to prevent burnout or reduce stress.

- Empowerment and justice: Awareness of inequities and promotion of more inclusive communities.

Implied within these guidelines is the formation of small groups of workers, managers, or public service providers who have some interest or investment in an occupational goal. For example, an OT consultant and speech therapist began a group intervention in a group home for people with mental retardation, with a goal of increasing nutrition and fitness. Clients were enthusiastic at first and began eating more vegetables at mealtime and walking together several times a week. However, other staff continued to serve high-calorie snacks and encouraged clients to watch TV shows with them instead of walking. It became clear that the entire staff needed to be included in the planning and implementation of this new group. When the entire staff and resident group met, they were able to agree on the goals, list potential barriers to the program's success, and problem-solve ways to facilitate healthier lifestyles for residents.

When focusing on environments, the barriers to participation often fall outside the control of either clients or OT practitioners. Interventions might involve the need to change a rigid work schedule to allow a client more time to travel to work or to perform some work functions from home. Advocacy for change in company policy involves another set of skills, those of self-advocacy in order to promote inclusion for a disabled worker. Such efforts work best when both disabled and nondisabled workers approach management as a group, with suggestions for policy changes that will be fair for all sides.

Social Support Groups

Social support has been defined as the experience of being cared for and loved, valued and esteemed, and able to count on others should the need arise (McColl, 1997; Stark & Sanford, 2005, p. 315). Clients need different types of support at different times. McColl (1997) reviews the evidence on the usefulness of social support for people with disabilities. Three types have been identified by McColl (1997):

1. Practical: Tangible or instrumental tasks done for the client, such as fixing lunch or doing laundry. This type was reported as least helpful and tends to encourage dependence on others.

2. Informational: The type of support most often sought from formal or community and societal level sources, such as specific medical information, how to apply for Medicare, or where to find a good support group.

3. Emotional support involves providing the client with validation, a sense of belonging, or esteem. Emotional support usually comes from family members and peer groups, who provide "everyday opportunities to be a member of a group or provide moral support for difficult times" (Stark & Sanford, 2005, p. 315). Emotional support was found most helpful in crisis situations.

On a personal level, sources of this type of support may be perceived as coming from spouses, parents, or significant others. Some people need a great deal of support, and others have difficulty accepting or giving support. Social support is best thought of as a reciprocal process. People with mental illness often need excessive amounts of support but cannot offer anything in return to those who give it. Group interventions can provide training and practice in giving and receiving social support. Group interventions can deal with the above problems in two ways. The first uses the group format to assist clients in understanding the reciprocal nature of social support and providing opportunities to practice meeting each other's social and emotional needs. Another approach is to organize ongoing support groups for people with disabilities in the community. The "clubhouse" concept for people with mental illness and the 12-step recovery groups for alcohol and drug abuse survivors are examples of such support groups. However, there is a great need for organized support groups in addition to these. The "Healthy People 2010" initiative calls for the promotion of health for people with all types

of disabilities through social participation as well as surveillance and health promotion programs (U. S. Dept of Health & Human Services, 2000/2001). Occupational therapists have the knowledge and training in group facilitation needed to initiate community support groups for many different disability or at-risk populations.

Caregivers also need social support. For example, a study of young caregivers aged 10 to 25 years whose parent had multiple sclerosis reported lower life satisfaction and positive affect, more family responsibility, higher levels of perceived maturity, worry, activity restriction, and isolation (Miller, 2009; Pakenham, Bursnall, Chiu, Cannon, & Okochi, 2006). Occupational therapists can organize groups that support caregivers, provide needed education, and enable them to make environmental changes to increase safety, security, and occupational performance for the disabled client. Occupational therapists should also be knowledgeable about sources of social support in the larger community or through public or national sources. When gaps in available services are found, advocacy and political or community action may be needed to overcome barriers or meet specific needs.

The International Classification of Functioning, Disability, and Health (WHO, 2001) lists extrinsic sources of support and relationships (Table 4-1). Group interventions can be organized to include some of these potential supports, or clients can develop strategies for building their social networks in order to better meet their needs. Social support involves Yalom's therapeutic group factors of universality and altruism (Yalom & Leszcz, 2005). Groups can provide social support to clients in crises, comforted by the knowledge that they are not alone and drawing upon their own innate need to belong, to be needed, and to help others. Occupational therapy groups can focus on developing skills in forming closer, more meaningful relationships with others so that social support will be available for each member, should the need arise.

A significant body of evidence exists in the multidisciplinary literature favoring social and peer support group effectiveness. A review of the literature on social support in the elderly from 1985-2008 revealed strong positive relationships with functional skills, well-being, health-related quality of life, and survival (Dahan-Oliel, Gelinas, & Mazer, 2008). According to McColl (1997), people with disabilities tend to have smaller social networks and often rely on only a few individuals or one individual for most of their social needs. Evidence of the value of peer support groups in mental health was reviewed by Swarbrick (2009). Peer self-help is defined as "services that are planned, managed, staffed, and evaluated by mental health consumers (both as facilitators and members), and designed to address social and emotional needs of adult consumers and the social consequences of mental illness through a peer-support model" (p. 253).

Table 4-1

Extrinsic Sources of Support and Relationships

- Immediate family
- Extended family
- Friends
- Acquaintances, peers, colleagues, neighbors
- People in positions of authority

- People in subordinate positions
- Personal-care providers
- Strangers
- Domesticated animals
- Health professionals

Adapted from World Health Organization. (2001). *The international classification of functioning, disability, and health.* Geneva: Author.

Peer support groups focus on the dimensions of relationships, personal growth, and system maintenance and change. Consumers identified the best and worst aspects of their peer-support groups as follows:

- Best features of peer support experience are belonging and friendships, comfortable and accessible place to participate in group activities, personal benefits of increased feelings of self-worth, and educational opportunities.

- Worst features of current experience of peer-support services are not enough funding or hours, conflicts or arguments with peers or facilitators, facilities too small, stairs, lack of parking, etc.

This study concluded that 71% of studies supported the need for more peer-support services and resources. The author recommends possible OT roles to provide better leader training to develop cohesive groups, create welcoming environments, and provide a wider range of structured group activities that enable mental health consumers to form and sustain friendships and participate in therapeutic activities and programming (Swarbrick, 2009).

The idea of peer support has its roots in the recovery model, which began with the Alcoholics Anonymous and other 12-step programs during the mid-20th century. Recovery for people with various illnesses including addictions, mental illness, and other disabilities is "an individual's journey of healing and transformation to live a meaningful life in a community of his or her choice while striving to achieve maximum human potential" (U. S. Dept. of Health & Human Services, 2005, p. 4). (See Chapter 9 for a more in-depth discussion of OT's participation in this national recovery initiative. As a national movement, the recovery model offers many new opportunities for OTs to become involved in designing groups for community populations, using social context as a focus).

Virtual, a New Framework Context for Groups

Social networking Web sites and internet groups represent a recent addition to OT's domain. The virtual context is defined as an "environment in which communication occurs by means of airways or computers and an absence of physical contact. (It) includes simulated or real-time or near-time existence of an environment via chat rooms, email, video-conferencing, radio transmissions" (AOTA, 2008, p. 645). Bondoc, Powers, Herz, and Hermann (2010) discuss some of the virtual reality programs that can be experienced in groups. For example, the Wii-fit (Nintendo of America Inc., Redmond, WA) programs offer exercises and games to help people stay fit, and these programs can be seen in many senior centers where groups follow along with the runners, skiers, or surfers on the TV screen. "Many VR (virtual reality) games may be played by multiple users where communication, interpersonal skills, and social skills are intrinsically required. More specifically, users must take turns, cooperate, or compete and even follow VR game etiquette (i.e., sportsman-like behaviors) as they would in real-world activities" (p. CE-3).

Performance Skills and Client Factors as Group Focus

Most of the traditional, medically based domains of concern in occupational therapy fall within these categories, which include all physical and mental functions related to occupational performance. They include the following categories: motor and praxis skills, sensory perceptual skills, emotional regulation skills, cognitive skills, and communication and social skills. The AOTA Framework-II process lists the following categories for therapeutic use of occupation as 1) occupation-based interventions, 2) purposeful activity, and 3) preparatory methods. Preparatory methods are defined as "methods and techniques that prepare the client for occupational performance. Used in preparation for, or concurrently with purposeful and occupation-based activities" (AOTA, 2008, p. 674). For example, a group of children with attention deficit disorder may participate in guided movement and sensory exercises to increase alertness and prepare them for an academic learning activity. A group of veterans with upper extremity amputations may participate in skill building with their prostheses in preparation for playing a game of poker. Many OT frames of reference address specific client skill areas, and these can guide the design of OT groups as outlined in the next section (Section II) of this book. OT groups based on specific aspects of functioning, such as physical strength, cognitive problem solving, or social skills training, need to be connected and worked on within the context of valued life roles and the overriding goal of occupational engagement.

Performance Patterns and Task Demands as Group Focus

In applying a holistic, client-centered, and systems-oriented approach, performance skills and client factors should be addressed within the context of occupations or social and occupational roles. The AOTA Framework-II includes roles as one of the occupational performance patterns, along with habits, routines, and rituals. Roles are defined by the Framework-II as "set(s) of behaviors expected by society, shaped by culture, and may be further conceptualized and defined by the client" (AOTA, 2008, p. 643). In other words, roles provide a structure for organizing one's daily activities, and occupations take on meaning within the context of life roles.

Roles as Focus

The concept of roles comes from social psychology (Mead, 1934; Sullivan, 1953). They "form the nucleus of social interaction" by defining the rules and procedures. "Smooth social interaction requires role reciprocity, or the effective role performance of each member of a group" (Christiansen & Baum, 1997, p. 56). Three types of group roles described in Chapter 2 are task roles, group maintenance roles, and individual roles. Task roles help the group get its work done, while maintenance roles address psychosocial issues. Individual roles are viewed by Benne and Sheats (1978) as meeting individual needs while interfering with overall group cohesiveness.

Roles may also be viewed as prescribed sets of behaviors and expectations that situate the person structurally (meaning position in the unit) or functionally (meaning performance demands associated with that structural role) within the social entity (Schaber, 2003, personal communication). Family roles can include spouse, sibling, mother, father, daughter, son, and grandparent as well as extended family members. Each role implies a set of expectations coming from society, one's culture, and oneself. Each has a set of occupations that accomplish an agreed-upon function. For example, caregiving, feeding the family, doing laundry, and keeping a clean house are occupations typical of a mother. The performance of these occupations and how they are carried out is influenced by both self-expectations and cultural expectations.

Occupational therapy group interventions can use social context to support role competence and reciprocity among client members. Group activities that encourage role reciprocity involve all members taking different roles in a shared task, such as giving a holiday party, preparing a meal, or taking a trip. The task-oriented groups described in Chapter 5 are examples of enabling engagement in occupations through role reciprocity. Using this approach, clients engage in planning and preparation, implementation of their various roles, and evaluation of the group task. This type of group helps members work on issues such as decision making, planning ahead, problem solving, communication, and cooperation with others.

Role theory helps to explain a few problems with occupational performance, such as role conflict, role overload, and role confusion. Role conflict occurs when a person finds him- or herself having to choose between meeting one role expectation or another. The mother who is called home from work to care for a sick child is an example of a role conflict. She must either ignore the sick child or leave her work undone. Role overload can occur when a person takes on more roles than he or she can handle. For example, a "workaholic" might work night and day, yet never seem to be able to meet all of the obligations demanded by his or her multiple social roles.

Roles can provide scripts that define our social interactions and behaviors. For example, our occupations, mode of dress, and style of interaction will be different when we are at work than when we are home with our families. Role confusion can occur when a husband and wife start a business together or when a boss invites an employee out for dinner.

Roles serve as a basis of commonality in forming client groups. Clients who identify significant problems with work roles, for example, may be grouped together to deal with common areas of interest, such as accepting supervision, issues of authority, getting along with co-workers, or coping with job stress. Role identification occurs when a role is internalized. We call ourselves students, workers, or family members because we see ourselves occupying these social positions and performing the occupations associated with these roles (Kielhofner, 2002). Group interventions can help clients problem-solve role confusion, conflict, and overload as well as other role behaviors that are creating difficulty. Groups can be organized around enabling clients in choosing roles that are meaningful for them, performing roles more effectively, or preparing for roles they perceive as helping them to achieve valued goals. For example, a client might choose the role of a student because he or she perceives that role as a stepping stone to acquiring a better job. Some roles help us organize and sequence the occupations we need to perform in order to achieve a higher social status.

Habits, Routines, and Rituals as Focus

Habits, routines, and rituals also structure and organize daily activities, and these concepts inter-relate with aspects of social roles. Habits are defined as "automatic behavior that is integrated into complex patterns that enable people to function on a day-to-day basis..." (Neistadt & Crepeau, 1998, p. 869, in AOTA, 2008, p. 670). Habits, within this definition, can either facilitate or impede occupational performance. Routines are defined as "patterns of behavior that are observable, regular, repetitive, and that provide structure for daily life. They can be satisfying, promoting, or damaging. Routines require momentary time commitment and are embedded in cultural and ecological contexts" (Fiese et al., 2002; Segal, 2004, in AOTA, 2008, pp. 674-675). Rituals add a spiritual component, defined by the Framework-II as "symbolic actions with spiritual, cultural, or social meaning, contributing to the client's identity and reinforcing the client's values and beliefs" (Fiese et al., 2002; Segal, 2004; in AOTA, 2008, p. 674). Groups may focus on habits or routines when they create barriers for group members. For example, people with obsessive compulsive disorder (OCD) often repeat nonfunctional behaviors as a means of reducing their anxiety. An OCD group intervention may apply cognitive behavioral strategies through group education, self-exploration, and mutual support, with the overall goal of overcoming nonfunctional habits that create barriers to occupational engagement and successful role performance.

Groups may also focus on routines as a way to restore order and balance in their daily lives. For example, a group of recently unemployed workers who suddenly find their lives lacking the structure of work could benefit from OT intervention to create new job-seeking routines, voluntary work alternatives, and supportive social activities that help them maintain health and well-being until they become re-employed. Many life transitions require changes in life structure, such as older adults transitioning from work to retirement (see Chapter 8 for a fuller description of transitions in lifespan development). Many rituals are typically performed in groups. For example, groups of Chinese Americans sometimes gather at sunrise to perform Tai Chi movement sequences in unison, a ritual that has physical, mental, and spiritual meaning within their culture.

An example of routines and rituals supporting family health as a focus for intervention is described by Fiese (2007), in families of children with chronic health conditions such as asthma. Family health is defined as "ways in which the household as a whole engages in daily activities to promote well-being of its members and is emotionally invested in the maintenance of health over time" (p. 41s). Examples of family health routines and rituals are mealtimes, bedtime routines and sleep, and medication adherence. Routines have an external defined purpose with associated activities and roles, such as meal preparation and cleanup and taking out the trash. Rituals hold a deeper emotional meaning; for example, discussing the day's events during the evening meal conveys caring and belonging among family members. Thus, routines and rituals are inter-related concepts, and "the overall rhythms of a household are made up of coordinated routines of the residing members" (p. 41s).

Fiese gives examples of two different families involving a child with asthma. The first is lacking in preventive health routines and generates an emergent response to health issues. The child in this family complains of chest tightening and problems breathing, typical symptoms of asthma, but the parents do not take it seriously, assuming the child is looking for an excuse to stay home from school until a late-night emergency room visit becomes necessary. The child's mother conveys distrust and annoyance over the child's health issues. After the diagnosis of asthma, nothing much changes in the household routine, and the child continues to wake the family up at night with asthma attacks. The second family looks for every possible way to lessen their child's exposure to environments that cause asthmatic episodes, such as removal of carpeting and draperies from the child's room, frequent vacuuming and dusting, and nightly medication at bedtime, routines/rituals that make the child feel comforted and safe. There are structured times for meals, outings, and other family activities and regular medical checkups for all family members. This child maintains control over asthma symptoms and almost always sleeps through the night.

For families experiencing difficulty maintaining routines and rituals that support health and well-being, Fiese (2007; Fiese & Wamboldt, 2001) recommends four possible types of OT interventions:

1. Remediation will be required when the child's behavior can be altered to contain the problem, such as adding a daily medication routine and avoiding exposure to pollen, mold, or dust.

2. Redefinition is appropriate when the illness causes pre-existing routines and rituals to be disrupted, and every family activity has changed to accommodate the identified client. In this case, the family needs to re-center its routine activities to meet the needs of the entire family unit.

3. Realignment is needed when there is disagreement among family members about the importance of routines for prevention and maintenance of well-being. Without routines, family life can become chaotic, which happens when parents divorce, for example. Such families could use OT intervention to create routines that all might agree upon and preserve despite other disruptions.

4. Re-education is needed when no routines and rituals exist in the household. Many factors contribute to voids in family routines, including poverty, generational histories of abuse, neglect, exclusion, caregiver burden, and otherwise strained resources. When a client with a disability comes in one of these families, OTs may take the opportunity to work with the family group to create proactive and health-promoting routines. Children with disabilities, as well as others in the family, need the structure of routines and the safety, caring, and sense of belonging created by rituals in order to avoid many serious health risks.

GROUPS BASED ON FRAMEWORK-II PROCESS

The process of OT practice involves three basic categories: evaluation, intervention, and outcome, with an end goal of "supporting health and participation in life through engagement in occupations" (AOTA, 2008, pp. 647-648). Central to this dynamic process is the client-therapist collaborative relationship within which the client shares self-knowledge, life stories, and perceptions, and the OT frames these from an occupational perspective, using theory, knowledge, evidence, clinical reasoning, and therapeutic use of self. The evaluation consists of an occupational profile of the individual, organization, or population, along with an analysis of occupational performance.

Evaluation in Groups

The framework specifies that evaluation focuses on client goals and priorities, indicative of a client-centered approach. In working with groups, this information may be obtained in two ways: 1) each client member may be evaluated prior to becoming a member of a therapeutic group, or 2) the entire group may be evaluated as a group prior to designing an intervention plan. Traditionally, clinical settings favored the individual approach. However, focus groups (see Chapter 1 and 3) provide another model for evaluation using group interview strategies. This method has the additional advantage of offering the OT an opportunity to observe the social interaction skills of clients, and with the inclusion of a group task, the effects of the social context on occupational performance may be directly observed.

For populations in the community, focus groups can identify and clarify many problems with occupational engagement, participation, and inclusion for people with disabilities. One recent study explored the problems faced by clients with spinal cord injury (SCI) in finding personal care assistants needed for them to live independently

(Matsuda, Clark, Schopp, & Hagglund, 2005). These authors use five focus groups—three SCI consumer groups and two groups of personal-care assistants—to further explore the problem. Each group met once for 3 hours, with breaks and refreshments provided. Two facilitators for each group took turns leading and taking notes (also, groups were audio taped). Questions for the groups included:

- What barriers do consumers encounter obtaining and maintaining personal-care assistants?
- What barriers do personal-care assistants encounter in providing quality care?
- How satisfied are consumers with their personal-care assistants?
- How satisfied are personal-care assistants with their jobs?

Some of the problems identified by personal-care assistants were restrictions imposed by public health agencies on the scope of services assistants were allowed to provide, high turnover among assistants because of low wages, poor benefits, and high stress created by inflexible work schedules and conflicts between what consumers needed and what they could provide. Consumers reported issues with high turnover of assistants, with agencies randomly scheduling different assistants. Satisfaction with assistants occurred when the same assistant came regularly, allowing the pair to form a positive working relationship. Consumers felt they needed more input in training and directing assistants to meet their unique needs (consumer-directed personal assistant model). The study concluded with recommendations that consumers advocate for higher wages for personal assistants and increasing flexibility of personal assistance service policies. Authors suggested that OTs could provide training programs for both consumers and assistants, so that they might facilitate clients with disabilities to pursue educational, occupational, and social activities outside the home, as well as enabling them to live independently in the community (Matsuda et al., 2005).

Groups as Framework Interventions

Five types of intervention are listed in the Framework-II: 1) therapeutic use of self, 2) therapeutic use of occupations (occupation, purposeful activity, preparatory methods), 3) consultation, 4) education process, and 5) advocacy. One or more of these types may occur concurrently in group facilitation.

Therapeutic Use of Self

The OT forms a collaborative partnership with clients through therapeutic use of self. Skills in forming therapeutic relationships are discussed in Chapter 3, as part of client-centered practice. The same skills that enable rapport building with individuals are also applied in group leadership, but with an added component. The OT group leader also must have a good understanding of the dynamics of groups in order to make use of the therapeutic benefit for members that groups can provide. This type of intervention, therefore, always occurs simultaneously with other types of group interventions.

Therapeutic Occupation as Focus

Some of the groups using areas of occupation are examples of occupations as focus. Clients recovering from spinal cord injury, for example, might practice aspects of self-care (eating a meal) or instrumental activities (meal preparation and clean up, grocery shopping) in a group. According to a recent study, social support provides motivation and enhances the ability to participate in occupations for people with spinal cord injury (Isaksson, Lexell, & Skar, 2007). Needed support was identified by female participants as both physical and emotional and was accomplished through social support networks within which they gave and received support in a reciprocal fashion. For example, one woman needed the assistance of co-workers in order to try doing work tasks in a new way. When attempting to perform familiar everyday tasks post-injury, participants preferred the ongoing emotional support from peers or friends, not health care workers. This study provides evidence of the importance of social support for occupational engagement. In the absence of onsite family and friends during the acute and rehabilitative phases of recovery, OTs might organize and facilitate client peer groups engaging in therapeutic occupations together while providing needed support for each other.

Consultation

OTs consult with organizations and institutions in order to address occupational issues within these entities. In addition to meeting with organization leaders to define issues and set goals, OTs may also organize focus groups of representative clients or other stakeholders in order to better understand their needs and perspectives (see Chapter 1 for a fuller explanation of focus groups). In a nonprofit organization, for example, an OT may consult with managers concerning the recruitment, use, and supervision of volunteers. Focus groups involving both volunteers and paid employees could yield important information about how OTs intervene to create a better fit between workers, tasks, and environments (Cole & Macdonald, 2011).

Education

OTs may take an educational approach when designing interventions for many community populations. A good example of this approach is OT's role with the "Up to Date Club," a group of women in Danville, Indiana. The members began meeting as young mothers with a desire to continue learning and keeping up with current events. Now ages 65 to 93 years, their interests have turned to issues of productive aging. The OT prepared and presented topics related to "living gracefully," including maintaining physical fitness, joint protection and energy conservation, and using assistive devices during home maintenance activities. Educational sessions on home safety and modifying environments and strategies to prevent falls elicited many stories from members of their experiences with falls, balance problems, and other fears and concerns related to aging. These community-based OT educational interventions facilitated this independent group of older women in continuing their lifelong learning through social participation (Dale, 2008).

Advocacy

The Framework-II defines advocacy as the "pursuit of influencing outcomes—including public policy and resource allocation decisions within political, economic, and social systems and institutions—that directly affect people's lives (Advocacy Institute, 2001, as cited in Goodman-Lavey & Dunbar, 2003, p. 422)" (AOTA, 2008, p. 669). Advocacy for the profession at the federal level as described by Marks (2010) has taken the form of contacting congressmen and senators, compelling them to vote in favor of public policies that include and pay for OT services, for example, extending Medicare reimbursement for home health. Advocacy can take the form of letter writing, contacting legislators (in one's individual voting districts) by phone or e-mail. However, advocacy is more effective when performed in groups. American Occupational Therapy Political Action Committee (AOTPAC) is one such group, consisting of OT professionals who combine resources and raise money to support political candidates who favor the OT profession and its goals.

Advocacy as an intervention, however, has a much broader purpose, which is to influence public policies that create barriers to participation or limit occupational opportunities for our clients. Given the profession's recent emphasis on evaluating occupational environments and ideally altering them to facilitate occupational performance for clients, it is not surprising that advocacy has become a required professional role. Many of the barriers to occupational health and well-being have their origin in public policies that favor dominant cultures while marginalizing minorities, people with disabilities, and others. Barriers may also take the form of the absence of needed services, such as public transportation, or limited handicapped accessibility, and many other more subtle social barriers. Marks (2010) suggests that advocacy efforts work best in groups, and these groups should include both professionals and clients. OTs can help clients tell their stories at public hearings or in addressing appropriate governing bodies, such as town councils or institutional boards of directors. Real-life examples of how clients experience barriers and why they limit occupational participation can clarify the problem for listeners and make a powerful case for needed changes.

Outcomes as Focus

General outcomes of the OT process include health, participation, and engagement in occupation. Ideally, clients for whom we provide services will continue on after leaving therapy, fully participating in the roles, occupations, and life situations of their choosing. Some outcomes listed in the Framework-II are occupational performance, adaptation, health and wellness, participation, quality of life, and prevention. In AOTA's Framework (2008) update, client satisfaction was removed (from the older edition), and two new outcome areas were added: self-advocacy and occupational justice. This emphasizes outcomes where we, as service providers, can effect change (Roley & Delany, 2009). Outcomes do not guide group planning per se, but they do represent goals that can be anticipated and for which measures need to be selected early in the planning process. For these broadly defined goals, occupation-based models provide many appropriate measurement tools, including rating the performance of specific occupations and adapting to occupational contexts, new life circumstances, or the person's state of health, well-being, or life satisfaction. The measurement tool relates to the clients' occupational goals and typically comes from the model or frame of reference that served as the basis of the group design.

Additionally, every group (therapeutic, educational, or work-related) has a social interaction dimension that greatly affects occupational outcomes for members. After conducting a group intervention, how might the OT measure the level of participation achieved by the members? Donohue (2010) provides an overview of evaluations for social participation.

The Social Profile: A Measure of Social Participation

The Social Profile (Cole & Donohue, 2011; Donohue, 2003) is a good example of an assessment tool designed for evaluation of levels of activity group participation. Based on Parten's (1932) and Mosey's (1970) descriptions of levels of group interaction, the profile incorporates five levels of group function among members around the activity or task involvement (Donohue, 1999; Donohue & Greer, 2004). The Social Profile measures the five levels of group participation based on Mosey's (1986) group interaction skills mentioned earlier: 1) parallel, 2) associative, 3) basic cooperative, 4) supportive cooperative, and 5) mature.

The items of the Social Profile measure three categories of group participation:

1. Group membership

2. Group interaction

3. Group activity behavior

Groups usually interact at multiple levels of participation in one session and across sessions. To achieve a profile measurement of the range of participation, all of the level ratings observed during the group session are averaged. Various activities can influence the level or type of group participation, despite the group's highest potential or developmental level. A mature group may choose to perform exercises in a parallel mode while participating in an aerobics class. Groups can choose to interact at a range of levels of participation suitable for a given activity, depending on the goal. For example, a developmentally mature group may watch a movie together, express feelings or opinions about the movie, and share a bowl of popcorn, thereby demonstrating behaviors of parallel, associative, and supportive cooperative levels during the viewing. Because the activity selected affects the members' group role and interactive behaviors, the group activity's potential for stimulating behaviors at each of the five levels is also rated. In this case, the Social Profile may serve as a guide for planning therapeutic groups that encourage targeted levels of social participation skills among the members.

The Social Profile provides one of the first occupational therapy-based measures of social participation in groups. Students have used the profile with fieldwork I sites, family groups, self-help groups, and community groups to evaluate multiple factors that are observed simultaneously: activity, interaction, and leadership. This assessment tool has the potential to provide the basis for linking the interaction and process skills of individual clients with the naturally occurring groups available to such clients in their communities. Currently, the Social Profile is available at www.socialprofile.com. Examples of activities associated with group interaction levels of behavior are given in Table 4-2.

Occupational Therapy Team Interventions

Adult teams might be expected to operate at mature level, based on Mosey's highest interaction skill. However, when measured using Donohue's Social Profile, many teams in education, work or community organizations, and governing boards or committees whose job is to solve problems and make policy decisions fall short of mature group behaviors. Teams may benefit from consultation to help them improve communication and boost collaboration with one another through activities that build understanding and trust. A team may be defined as "two or more individuals working together toward the achievement of specific goals" (Latella, 2002, p. 96). Work teams, sports teams, research teams, and health care teams are examples. An occupational therapist consulting with work teams might use group problem

Table 4-2

Donohue's Social Profile (2011): Examples of Activities and Behaviors

Group Profile Levels	Examples of Activities and Behaviors
Parallel group level	3-year-olds playing separately next to each other in a sandbox Adults standing in rows next to each other doing movement to music in a movement group
Associative level group (project group)	4-year-olds playing telephone for 2 minutes 5-year-olds building blocks together to make a fort: 5-minute interaction Adults engaged in a "Pass the Ball" game identifying names of members: 15-minute interactive exercise
Cooperative level group (egocentric group)	7-year-olds role playing in costumes with mutually designed guidelines for role interaction Adults in an activities of daily living group washing, cutting, mixing, serving, and eating fruit in a salad
Cooperative level group	16-year-olds discussing feelings about musical lyrics while making decorations for a parade float Seniors discussing feelings about peers' illnesses, memories of the past, and process of dying
Mature level group	20-year-old college students take turns coaching each other in a computer science course 40-year-old parents of children with learning disabilities coach each other on methods of intervention for their children in a parents' support group

solving strategies to create social and physical contexts that enable occupation and prevent injury and stress. The Framework-II gives this example: "prevent social isolation of employees by promoting participation in after work group activities" (AOTA, 2008, p. 659). Workers can build social relationships through supportive cooperative groups, such as dining together, attending fitness centers, or playing informal sports. Formal team building activities outside the office might encourage co-workers to mentor one another and to collaborate rather than compete in the workplace. OT roles in many types of businesses or community organizations will likely involve group facilitation. The seven steps for group leadership may occur more informally in these types of groups, but can serve as a useful guideline in clarifying the purpose, meaning, and application of the group's work, encouraging full member participation and facilitating the application of client-centered principles required by the Framework-II (AOTA, 2008, p. 649).

Team Participation for Clients

Teams exist in many workplace, educational, and community settings. Gersick (2003) points out that most "organizations use teams to put novel combinations of people to work on novel problems and use committees to deal with especially critical decisions; indeed, organizations largely consist of permanent and temporary groups" (p. 59). Clients may have difficulties related to team membership. Deficits in communication and interaction skills, as well as poor self-social, or cultural awareness, may interfere with successful occupational performance related to team roles. Participation in occupational therapy groups may be structured so as to prepare clients to become better team members in whatever life contexts they choose.

From a business perspective, Luthans (1995) offers a somewhat different view of teams as "highly cohesive groups that... given positive leadership, will have the highest possible productivity" (p. 251). According to this author, teams differ from traditional work groups in several ways. Work groups have a strong leader who delegates the work to members and holds each individual accountable for what he or she produces. Meetings of work groups are marked by efficiency, low cohesiveness, and a focus on overall organizational goals. In contrast, teams use shared leadership and work together to produce collective outcomes. Team meetings are highly interactive, use group problem solving, and are mutually accountable for decisions and outcomes. Good teamwork depends upon maintaining group cohesiveness, honest feedback, and open communication within all levels of management. Teams work best when self-managed (no appointed supervisor in charge) and given responsibility for the real work of the organization.

Many parallels may be drawn between this view of teams in business and groups in occupational therapy. Both rely on skilled and well-trained leaders who value and enable the unique contributions of each member. While goals may vary, the process of facilitating sessions or meetings includes similar principles. The group interacts openly to deal with the issues of the day. Each member shares his or her perspective or expertise, problems are defined and clarified, and the group reflects upon possible solutions or outcomes.

Health Care Team Membership and Leadership

Occupational therapists often work as members of health care teams. From a medical perspective, the purpose of the team approach is to discuss client problems from several perspectives and to coordinate a treatment plan. Health care teams may be understood in terms of the people who are members, the purpose, the team's place or position within the system, the power structure, and the plan (Latella, 2002). The team's purpose is its vision of what is to be achieved, which usually reflects an organization's mission statement. In the case of health care teams, the vision includes holistic, high-quality assessments and interventions for clients. Place refers to the relationship of the team to the entire organizational structure. A health care team is one part of the structure of a hospital or home care agency, for example. Power refers to leadership style and degree of shared leadership among members. In a medical model, health care teams are usually led by a physician, psychiatrist, or medical director, with input from members structured around each case/client. Plan refers to the structure of the team and how members work together.

Cohn (2009) describes three approaches used by health care teams:

1. *Multidisciplinary*: Members of various disciplines work together but maintain separate and distinctive roles. Collaboration and coordination are not typically a part of this approach. Members perform separate assessments but coordinate overall client-care plan and goals. OTs are most often a part of this type of team structure, which may include shared or rotating team leadership.

2. *Interdisciplinary*: This approach allows more flexibility in member collaboration and shared assessments, reports, goals, and intervention plans.

3. *Transdisciplinary*: This approach involves all team members "blurring" roles by crossing boundaries predetermined by their disciplines. This model

maximizes the effectiveness of each member, and leadership rotates according to client needs and priorities (Latella, 2002, p. 97).

People are the members of the team. Typical health care teams average five members and may include doctors, nurses, social workers, speech therapists, physical therapists, and occupational therapists. Team membership may be stable within an organization or may shift according to needs, goals, or other criteria. Occupational therapists can combine this model with their knowledge of group dynamics to better understand the interactions of teams in their own practice.

Interdisciplinary teams demonstrate the same group dynamics as other groups. They go through a developmental process to create cultural norms, shared language and meaning, and collective reasoning, which Cohn calls a "constructionist process" (2009, p. 398). Members of the team begin by defining their various roles and areas of expertise within the work setting, and eventually they come to value each other and think about issues from multiple points of view. Moyers (2005) has suggested that effective participation on a health care or educational team be recognized as a core OT professional competency. She identifies key competencies for team participation: cooperating, collaborating, communicating, and integrating to ensure that client care is continuous and reliable. OT practitioners should become competent in leading as well as participating on interdisciplinary teams, "directly assuming the responsibility of developing teams, when needed, to address the occupational performance needs of clients" (Moyers, 2005, p. 19). In current practice, clients and their family members or caregivers are also included as members of the team. OTs often assume the role of case manager for a specific client, which includes team leadership when that client's case is discussed, communicating directly with the client, family, and others involved, and advocating for the client when necessary (Cohn, 2009).

SUMMARY

The purpose of this chapter is to broaden the student's perspective on the kinds of groups that might now be included in occupational therapy's domain of concern. Groups form an integral part of our clients' participation in daily life. This chapter reviews both occupational therapy approaches to working with groups from the perspective of the AOTA Framework-II (2008) and theoretical perspectives regarding some of the naturally occurring groups in which our clients participate, including family groups, community organizations, and work teams. It is hoped that when students become entry-level graduates, they will help to define and expand some of the new roles suggested in this chapter for occupational therapists dealing with groups in community settings.

REFERENCES

American Occupational Therapy Association. (2008). Occupational therapy practice framework: Domain and process, 2nd ed. *American Journal of Occupational Therapy, 62,* 625-683.

Benne, K., & Sheats, P. (1978). *Functional roles of group members.* In L. Bradford (Ed.), Group development (2nd ed.). La Jolla, CA: University Associates.

Bondoc, S., Powers, C., Herz, N., & Hermann, V. (2010). Virtual reality-based rehabilitation. *OT Practice, 15,* June 28, CE 1-8.

Bronfenbrenner, U. (1977). Toward an experimental ecology of human development. *American Psychologist, 32,* 513-531.

Bronfenbrenner, U. (1993). The ecology of cognitive development: Research models and fugitive findings. In R. H. Wozniak & K. W. Fisher (Eds.), *Development in context: Acting and thinking in specific environments.* New York, NY: Erlbaum.

Bream, S. (2010). Meeting the mental health needs of adolescents. *OT Practice, June 28,* 15-18.

Capasso, N., Gorman, A., & Blick, C. (2010). Breakfast group in an acute rehabilitation setting: A restorative program for incorporating client's hemiparetic upper extremities for function. *OT Practice, 15*(8), 14-18.

Chater, K., & Tsai, C. (2009). Palliative care in a multicultural society: A challenge for western ethics. *Australian Journal of Advanced Nursing, 26,* 95-100.

Christiansen, C., & Baum, C. (1997). *Enabling function and well-being* (2nd ed.). Thorofare, NJ: SLACK Incorporated.

Cohn, E. (2009). Team interaction models. In E. Cohn, E. Crepeau, & B. Schell (Eds.), *Willard & Spackman's Occupational Therapy* (11th ed., pp. 306-402). Philadelphia, PA: Williams & Wilkins.

Cole, M., & Donohue, M. (2011). *Social participation in occupational contexts: In schools, clinics, and communities.* Thorofare, NJ: SLACK, Incorporated.

Cole, M., & MacDonald, K. (2011). Retired occupational therapists' experiences in volunteer occupations. *Occupational Therapy International, 18,* 18-31.

Cole, M., & Tufano, R. (2008). Applied theories in occupational therapy. Thorofare, NJ: SLACK Incorporated.

Dahan-Oliel, N., Gelinas, I., & Mazer, B. (2008). Social participation in the elderly: What does the literature tell us? *Critical Reviews in Physical and Rehabilitation Medicine, 20,* 159-176.

Dale, L. (2008). Healthy aging through social participation. *OT Practice, Dec. 15,* 24-26.

Donohue, M. (1999). Theoretical bases of Mosey's group interaction skills. *Occupational Therapy International, 6*(1), 35-51.

Donohue, M. (2003). Group profile. Studies with children: Validity measures and item analysis. *Occupational Therapy in Mental Health, 19,* 1-23.

Donohue, M. (2010). Evaluation of social participation. In K. Sladyk, K. Jacobs, & N. MacRae (Eds.), *Occupational therapy essentials for clinical competence* (pp. 151-160). Thorofare, NJ: SLACK Incorporated.

Donohue, M., & Greer, E. (2004). Designing group activities to meet individual and group needs. In J. Hinojosa & M. L. Blount (Eds.), *The texture of life: Purposeful activities in occupational therapy.* Bethesda, MD: American Occupational Therapy Association, Inc.

Dunn, W. (2007). Ecology of human performance model. In S. Dunbar (Ed.), *Occupational therapy models for intervention with children and families* (pp. 127-156). Thorofare, NJ: SLACK Incorporated.

Ekelman, B. (2010). Palliative care ethical dilemmas in a multicultural society. *Home & Community Health Special Interest Section Quarterly (AOTA), 12*(2), 1-3.

Fiese, B. H. (2007). Routines and rituals: Opportunities for participation in family health. *Occupational Therapy Journal of Research, 27,* 41s-49s.

Fiese, B. H., Tomcho, T., Douglas, M., Josephs K., Poltrock, S., Baker, T. (2002). Fifty years of research on naturally occurring rituals: Cause for celebration? *Journal of Family Psychology, 16,* 381-390.

Fiese, B. H., & Wamboldt, F. (2001) Family routines, rituals, and asthma management. A proposal for family based strategies to increase treatment adherence. *Families, Systems, and Health, 18,* 406-418.

Gersick, C. (2003). Time and transition in work teams. In R. Hirokawa, R. Cathcart, L. Samovar, & L. Henman. (Eds.), *Small group communication: Theory and practice.* Los Angeles, CA: Roxbury Publishing Co.

Glennon, T. J., Marks, A. (2010). Transitioning to college: Issues for students with an autism spectrum disorder. *OT Practice, 15,* 7-9.

Goodman-Lavey, M., & Dunbar, S. (2003). Federal legislative advocacy. In G. McCormack, E. Jaffe, & M. Goodman-Lavey (Eds.), *The occupational therapy manager* (4th ed., pp. 421-438). Bethesda, MD: American Occupational Therapy Association, Inc.

Gutman, S. A., Schindler, V. P., Furphy, K. A., Klein, K., Lisak, J. M., & Durhan, D. P. (2007). The effectiveness of a supported education program for adults with psychiatric disabilities: The Bridge Program. *Occupational Therapy in Mental Health, 23,* 21-38.

Isaksson, G., Lexell, J., & Skar, L. (2007). Social support provides motivation and ability to participate in occupation. *Occupational Therapy Journal of Research, 27,* 23-30.

Kalina, J. T. (2009). Role of occupational therapy in a multiple sclerosis center. *OT Practice, June 28,* 9-13.

Kielhofner, G. (2002). *The model of human occupation* (2nd ed.). Baltimore, MD: Williams & Wilkins.

Latella, D. (2002). Teams and teamwork. In K. Sladyk (Ed.), *The successful occupational therapy fieldwork student* (pp. 95-101) Thorofare, NJ: SLACK Incorporated.

Leighty, J. (2010). Keeping PACE: OTs play key roles in programs that keep seniors out of nursing homes. *Today in OT, June 21,* 12-13.

Luthans, F. (1995). *Organizational behavior* (7th ed.). New York, NY: McGraw Hill, Inc.

Marks, E. (2010). Advocacy. In K. Jacobs & K. Sladyk (Eds.), *Occupational therapy essentials for clinical competence* (pp. 507-574). Thorofare, NJ: SLACK Incorporated.

Matsuda, S. J., Clark, M. J., Schopp, L. H., Hagglund, K. J., Mokelke, E. K. (2005). Barriers and satisfaction associated with personal assistant services: Results of consumer and personal assistant focus groups. *Occupational Therapy Journal of Research, 25,* 66-74.

Mattingly, C., & Fleming, M. (1994). *Clinical reasoning: Forms of inquiry in a therapeutic practice.* Philadelphia, PA: Davis.

McColl, M. (1997). Social support and occupational therapy. In C. Christiansen & C. Baum (Eds.), *Enabling function and well-being* (2nd ed., pp. 411-425). Thorofare, NJ: SLACK Incorporated.

Mead, G. (1934). *Mind, self, and society.* Chicago, IL: University of Chicago Press.

Miller, B. (2009). Young caregivers: What can OT offer? *OT Practice, Aug. 10,* 9-12.

Mosey, A. C. (1968). Recapitulation of ontogenesis: A theory for practice of occupational therapy. *American Journal of Occupational Therapy, 22,* 426-433.

Mosey, A. C. (1970). *Three frames of reference for mental health.* Thorofare, NJ: SLACK Incorporated.

Mosey, A. (1986). *Psychosocial components of occupational therapy.* New York, NY: Raven Press.

Moyers, P. (2005). Working in teams. *OT Practice, Feb. 7,* 19-20.

Neufeld, P. S. (2004). Enabling participation through community and population approaches. *OT Practice: 9,* August, CE1-CE8.

O'Brien, J. (2010). Interventions of social participation. In K. Sladyk, K. Jacobs, & N. MacRae (Eds.), *Occupational therapy essentials for clinical competence* (pp. 207-216). Thorofare, NJ: SLACK Incorporated.

Pakenham, K., Bursnall, S., Chiu, J., Cannon, T., & Okochi, M. (2006). The psychosocial impact of caregiving on young people who have a parent with an illness or disability: Comparisons between young caregivers and non caregivers. *Rehabilitation Psychology, 51,* 113-126.

Parke, J., & Szymanski, M. (2010). Working and playing together: A social skills program. *Advance for Occupational Therapy, October 11th,* 36.

Parten, M. B. (1932). Social participation among pre-school children. *Journal of Abnormal and Social Psychology, 27,* 243-269.

Rahman, A., & Schnelle, J. (2008). The nursing home culture change movement: Recent past, present, and fugure directions for research. *Gerontologist, 48,* 142-148.

Roley, S. S., & Delany, J. (2009). Improving the occupational therapy practice framework: Domain & process. *OT Practice, Feb. 2,* 9-12.

Scaffa, M. (2003). Competence, mastery, and independence: Our cultural heritage. *AOTF Connection, 10,* 1, 6-7.

Schaber, P. (2002). FIRO model: A framework for family-centered care. *Physical & Occupational Therapy in Geriatrics, 20*(4), 1-18.

Schultz, J. (2009). Theory of occupational adaptation. In E. Crepeau, E. Cohn, & B. Schell (Eds.), *Willard and Spackman's occupational therapy* (11th ed, pp. 462-475). Philadelphia, PA: Lippincott, Williams, & Wilkins.

Schutz, W. (1958). The interpersonal underworld. *Harvard Business Review, 36*(4), 123-135.

Schwartz, D. A. (2010). My turn at applying the occupational therapy practice framework. *OT Practice, April 5,* 22-23.

Spencer, J. (1998). Evaluation of performance contexts. In E. Crepeau, E. Cohn, & B. Boyt Schell (Eds.), *Willard & Spackman's occupational therapy* (pp. 427-448). Philadelphia, PA: Lippincott, Williams & Wilkins.

Stark, S. L., & Sanford, J. A. (2005) Environmental enablers and their impact on occupational performance. In C. Christiansen & C. Baum (Eds.), *Occupational therapy: Performance, participation, and well-being* (pp. 299-327). Thorofare, NJ: SLACK, Incorporated.

Stone, R., Reinhard, S. C., Bowers, B., Zimmerman, D., Phillips, C. D., Hawes, C. ... Jacobson, N. (2002). *Evaluation of the wellspring model for improving nursing home quality.* New York, NY: Commonwealth Fund.

Sullivan, H. S. (1953). *Conceptions of modern psychiatry.* New York, NY: W. W. Norton.

Swarbrick, M. (2009). Designing a study to examine peer operated self-help centers. *Occupational Therapy in Mental Health, 25,* 252-299.

Townsend, E., & Landry, J. (2005). Interventions in social context: Enabling participation. In C. H. Christiansen, C. M. Baum, & J. Bass-Haugen (Eds.), *Occupational therapy: Performance, participation, and well-being.* Thorofare, NJ: SLACK Incorporated.

U. S. Dept. of Health & Human Services. (2000). *Healthy people 2010* (2nd ed.). Retrieved November 3, 2003 from http://www.healthypeople.gov/2010/Document/pdf/uih/2010uih.pdf.

U. S. Dept. of Health & Human Services. (2005). Substance abuse and mental health administration, center for mental health services. *Mental Health Transformation Trends: A Periodic Briefing, 1*(July/Aug), 4.

Wilson, K. (2009). Culture change: Definition and models. *Gerontology Special Interest Section Quarterly (AOTA), 32*(3), 1-2.

Wintzelberg, G., Hanson, L., Tulsky, J. (2005). Beyond autonomy: Diversify end of life decision-making approaches to serve patients and families. *Journal of the American Geriatrics Society, 53,* 1046-1050.

World Health Organization. (2001). *The international classification of functioning, disability, and health.* Geneva: Author.

Yalom, I., & Leszcz, M. (2005). *The theory and practice of group psychotherapy* (4th ed.). New York, NY: Basic Books.

Client-Centered Activity Example 4-1
Family Group Protocol

The following is a proposed structure for six weekly occupational therapy sessions with a hypothetical family group, using the group protocol method described in Chapter 11. The sessions will include all seven steps of group facilitation, but the occupational therapist shifts their order, dealing with feelings, ideas, and practical applications repeatedly throughout the session. Working with families in the home environment, the activities (or occupational interventions) may not take place during the family session at all. In this example, the occupational interventions are collaboratively planned during the sessions, but occur at other times and are processed after the fact the following week. Each session, therefore, begins with sharing how the "homework" activity went, and processing (i.e., how they felt about it), generalization (i.e., what they learned from it), and application (i.e., how they might alter strategies or plan additional changes) flow naturally through facilitated discussion. Each session ends with an outcome, which serves as an occupational intervention for the family to try out during the following week. In other words, the "activity" that was described in Chapter 1 as Step 2, actually occurs before each session begins.

Session 1: Inclusion

The initial session serves as an evaluation of the entire family system in regards to the occupations of Grandma. What are the ways that Grandma is included or excluded from participation in family life? What are the barriers to inclusion from various members of the group? What are Grandma's feelings about inclusion or exclusion? Which member of the family best represents Grandma's wishes and preferences if she cannot voice them herself? Using the client-centered approach, the family collaborates with the occupational therapist to identify some specific occupations that address the need to belong. The group chooses an experimental activity for the following week and discusses ways the family members might enable Grandma's participation through occupations. For example, Grandma might help prepare a Sunday family dinner by using routines with which she is already familiar, such as setting the table or peeling apples for pie.

Session 2: Enabling Control

After reporting on the experimental activity and problem solving as needed, this session focuses on additional areas in which assistance is needed to enable autonomy in daily care. What occupations can Grandma continue to perform on her own with some assistance from family members? Using specific activities selected by the client and family, therapist expertise may be shared with the family regarding what is possible for Grandma to do for herself safely and ways that caregivers could facilitate Grandma's continued independence in self-care or contribute to performance of instrumental activities of daily living. The session might include watching Grandma perform one task while the occupational therapist models the use of appropriate cues to enable autonomy and choice over activity involvement. The group will problem solve around what assistance is needed and which family member will provide it. The outcome of this session may be a schedule of supervision or assistance involving different family members.

Session 3: Balancing Control and Safety

In the case of dementia, safety concerns may arise regarding which occupations Grandma wants to do versus what she is able to do safely. Here again, therapist expertise may be shared regarding the effects of moderate-stage dementia. She might use an Allen's Cognitive Levels Screen to evaluate Grandma's cognitive level and use this theory to predict potential safety issues. For example, if Grandma wants to cook, she needs to be able to understand the consequences of unsafe use of a stove and remember to take safety precautions. Family members may report problems like letting things burn or forgetting to use a potholder. Problem solving might include home adaptations to address specific safety issues involving Grandma. In recommending changes made to the environment, the occupational therapist considers the needs of the entire family. For example, disconnecting the stove will probably not be an option because the rest of the family uses the same stove for cooking. Restricting access to the kitchen during periods when Grandma is unsupervised might be more workable. A house tour and a list of possible adaptations for safety and to maximize Grandma's opportunities for choice may be an outcome of this session.

From Cole, M. B. *Group dynamics in occupational therapy: The theoretical basis and practice application of group intervention* (4th ed.). Thorofare, NJ: SLACK Incorporated. © 2012 SLACK Incorporated.

Family Group Protocol (Continued)

Session 4: Control, Resolving Conflicts

Review the past week in which family members have rearranged environments and made home modifications as discussed during the previous week. What tasks can family members help Grandma do, and which are still causing problems? Some areas to explore are the following:

- Who provides care and when?
- What self-care routines can Grandma learn to do independently?
- What are some attitudes toward giving/receiving assistance?
- What expectations have been met/not met?
- How is care being received? Are caregivers feeling appreciated?
- What might be some financial issues regarding paid caregiving or supervision?
- What barriers to inclusion in family life still exist?
- Any other problem areas client and family members bring to the table.

Family members need to discuss strategies for resolving the most important conflicts as a family group. Collaborative decision making can be facilitated by the occupational therapist around the activities that are posing problems for family members. Some of the following strategies may be suggested:

- Deferring to Grandma when the risk is low
- Giving Grandma a realistic role to play in family activities
- Using environmental adaptation to manage risk
- Giving choices and/or making compromises
- Allowing Grandma to express self/emotions in nonverbal and verbal ways
- Getting Grandma her own pet
- Finding ways to communicate with Grandma during times she is left alone
- Allowing noninvolvement of members or relief of overburdened members

An outcome might be each member thinking of one way to show respect and affection for Grandma or to modify nonproductive responses while engaging in occupations with Grandma during the upcoming week.

Session 5: Expressing Affection Through Occupations

Problem-solving issues of control pave the way for the family to resolve conflicts that interfere with the expression of affection between Grandma and members of her family. This session centers on occupations that help family members learn from Grandma. Family members can learn from Grandma, drawing on her life skills and accomplishments to raise the status and respect she enjoyed before the cognitive decline. Some examples might be writing down family recipes, retrieving photographs of ancestors and writing or tape recording stories about them, reframing old photos, or making scrapbooks. Recalling family history through reminiscence serves several purposes. It reaffirms Grandma's ties with family members, giving her a unique role as family historian, while providing a context of positive interactions with children and grandchildren. Whatever Grandma's special experiences and interests were, these can be shared through storytelling and sharing expertise (worker roles, living in another country, living in a specific period in history, doing needlework, cooking, gardening, or singing). In later-stage dementia, family photographs can be labeled in clear letters to remind Grandma of each person's name, relationship, and approximate date. This is especially helpful for people with large families and assists nonfamily caregivers in understanding the older client's stories or clearing up confusion about when in her life history different events occurred. An outcome of this session might be a schedule when each interested family member might share a chosen reminiscence activity with Grandma during the following week.

Family Group Protocol (Continued)

Session 6: Measuring Outcomes

This session will review all of the previous sessions. What were the desired outcomes with regard to inclusion, control, and affection? What has changed since the first session? What problems remain? A review of self-care routines and participation in family activities may be compiled. A tour of the house to observe environmental adaptations might be useful in confirming what was changed and its effect on Grandma's occupational performance and avoidance of problems. The occupational therapist might share expertise about the progression of dementia, its current severity, and what the subsequent stages are likely to entail. Possible preventive strategies may be discussed, such as Grandma wearing a "safe return" bracelet with her name, address, and telephone number engraved on it if she becomes prone to wander. Possible supports in the community might be identified, both social activities for Grandma and respite for caregivers. Finally, a plan for follow-up or a way to identify need for future intervention can be discussed.

From Cole, M. B. *Group dynamics in occupational therapy: The theoretical basis and practice application of group intervention* (4th ed.). Thorofare, NJ: SLACK Incorporated. © 2012 SLACK Incorporated.

GROUP GUIDELINES FROM SIX FRAMES OF REFERENCE

Once the basics of group dynamics and client-centered practice have been mastered, the therapist can modify Cole's seven steps to fit different clinical situations. The American OT Association (AOTA) Framework-II (2008) suggests that the OT select and apply "various theories and frames of reference" to guide clinical reasoning during both evaluation and intervention (AOTA, 2008, pp. 649, 655). Thus, when planning groups for the purpose of evaluation or intervention within selected occupational domains, the OT must apply the theories, models, and/or frames of reference that best fit the needs of a group of clients. This section reviews five frames of reference and five occupation-based models that can guide clinical reasoning about group approaches and illustrates how each might adapt the group structure using Cole's seven steps.

FRAME OF REFERENCE VERSUS MODEL

Multiple levels of theory exist in the OT literature. The current OT paradigm was earlier described in terms of three theoretical trends: holistic, client centered, and systems oriented (Cole & Tufano, 2008), and these trends are confirmed by AOTA's Framework-II (2008). Theory contributes to the OT paradigm by attempting to explain the relationship between people, health, environment, and other factors, "making it possible for OTs to understand the complexity of occupation and the optimal participation in daily life" (Dunbar, 2007, p. 2). Scientifically derived theories come from various disciplines and contribute concepts to the various OT models and frames of reference. Dunbar (2007) acknowledges the confusion in defining the terms, theory, model, and frame of reference in the OT literature. She corroborates the following differentiation. Models take a broad perspective, explaining how OT works. These models tend to be generic, applicable across age groups and practice areas, explaining how the concepts of person, environment, and occupation inter-relate as a system, but do not provide much direction for actual practice (Reed & Sanderson, 1999).

Frames of reference, on the other hand, address specific disabilities that cause problems with occupational performance. They draw upon interdisciplinary knowledge and research and offer specific techniques and strategies for OT evaluation and intervention within specific areas of OT's domain of concern. In Dunbar's view, and mine, both occupation-based models and frames of reference are needed in combination to produce the best OT outcomes for our clients (Cole & Tufano, 2008; Dunbar, 2007).

SELECTION AND ORGANIZATION OF OCCUPATION-BASED MODELS

In the past decade, OT frames of reference have all but disappeared from the OT literature, mirroring the profession's advancement to more occupation-centered trends (Polatajko, Mandrich, & Martini, 2000). It seems that the long-revered OT frames, such as psychodynamic, cognitive disabilities, sensory integration, and the biomechanical/rehabilitative approaches have now relocated to the basement and have become the underground practice of the 21st century. This is unfortunate because much of the collective OT wisdom, techniques, and evidence that has accrued within them remains just as valid and effective today as ever. Occupation-based models contribute the broad, holistic picture of the client in context and provide a heterarchical (Kielhofner, 2008), top-down (Baum, Bass-Haugen, & Christiansen, 2005), ecological (Dunn, 2007), and/or client-centered (Law & Dunbar, 2007) approach for OT evaluation and intervention. But these models do not replace frames of reference. The Model of Human Occupation (MOHO), for example, "was always intended to be used alongside other OT models.... MOHO rarely addresses all of the problems faced by a client, which requires therapists to actively use other models (frames of reference)" (Kielhofner, 2008, p. 4).

In this fourth edition, MOHO has been elevated to its rightful place, the first of several occupation-based models to emerge in recent decades. The guidance given OTs for designing groups by MOHO and other such models is given in broad strokes, with the intent of focusing intervention on the central concept of our profession, occupation. Within these models, groups use everyday activities as both means and end, and groups occur within or parallel with natural settings and contexts. Chapter 10, while still focusing on MOHO, also reviews four additional frequently used and cited occupation based models: Ecology of Human Performance (Dunn, 2007), Occupational Adaptation (Schultz & Schkade, 2003), the Person-Environment-Occupation Model (Stewart, Letts, Law, Cooper, Strong, & Rigby, 2003), and the Kawa Model (Iwama, 2006).

Each of the occupation-based models, while addressing similar broad concepts, has a unique focus. OTs need to understand their differences in order to select the model most appropriate for their specific clients, settings, and situations. Models are organized in the same way as frames of reference, first defining the basic concepts, function and dysfunction, change and motivation, and, finally, assessment and intervention. Because these models are so broad and inclusive, they work well in guiding interventions with not only groups of individuals, but also for OT group programming for organizations and populations within the community.

SELECTION AND ORGANIZATION OF FRAMES OF REFERENCE

Practice models (which I will call *frames of reference*) "are used to explain how the ideas of the theoretical model can be implemented into a plan of action to provide services to clients" (Reed & Sanderson, 1999, p. 201). Mosey (1981) preferred the term *frame of reference* to describe this concept, which may be defined as "a set of compatible concepts from theory which together guide the therapist toward a specific focus, view of function and dysfunction, explanation for how change occurs, and strategies for evaluation and intervention." Mosey writes that "many authors…recognize that no theory can be directly applied. A theory must first be transformed through a linking structure into usable information" (1989, p. 195). Mosey suggests that our research should focus on the development, refinement, and evaluation of the effectiveness of frames of reference. OT uses a method called *extrapolation* (Mosey, 1989, p. 197) to make theory usable, involving several steps as follows:

- Identification of appropriate theories
- Selection of useful concepts from theory
- Combining concepts and postulates from various compatible theories
- Reformulating of the selected concepts and postulates to provide guidelines for treatment (intervention)

In addressing the problem of planning and leading OT groups, I have used a similar technique in applying theory within the frames of reference reviewed here. Compatible concepts are combined from various theories to formulate a point of view on function, dysfunction, change, and motivation. A frame of reference should guide our understanding of illness and disability in our clients. Before jumping into group intervention, OTs should have some understanding of the state of health of the group members, and this understanding is different in each frame of reference. The definition of dysfunction can range from neurological malfunctioning in the sensorimotor frame of reference, to the presence of unconscious conflicts in the psychodynamic frame, to the lack of adaptive skill development in the developmental frame. Principles or postulates regarding change (Mosey, 1981) are the assumptions derived from theory that help us formulate how intervention will work. These are the "principles by which prevention of dysfunction occurs, function is maintained, interfering behavior is managed, and an individual is assisted in moving from a state of dysfunction to a state of function" (Mosey, 1981, p. 141). The AOTA Framework-II might call this "promoting health and participation in life…through engagement in occupation" (AOTA, 2008, p. 626).

Mosey (1981) further suggests that principles of intervention begin with the function to be developed (e.g., trunk balance, self-esteem) and end with the nature of the external environment that is likely to enact this therapeutic change. In other words, these principles help us predict how change will occur and guide our designing of OT activities that will facilitate the development of function or occupational performance. For example, in using a developmental frame of reference for a group of older adults with Parkinson's disease, the postulate regarding intervention may be as follows: A sense of integrity and acceptance of one's life and death may be facilitated by participation in group activities where past accomplishments are the focus. In a behavioral cognitive frame of reference for the same clients, socially acceptable eating habits may be learned through the use of weighted utensils combined with peer examples. Each of these frames of reference suggests a different definition of function and dysfunction, different goals to be addressed, and a different kind of activity. Thus, the important parts of OT group evaluation or intervention are addressed in the different frames. Within each chapter on frame of reference, concepts are applied to group structure, limitations, role of the leader, appropriate goals, and suggested activities as examples. The following five frames of reference have been retained in this fourth edition, and each has been updated with current changes, evidence, and published group examples.

- Chapter 5—Psychodynamic
- Chapter 6—Behavioral cognitive

- Chapter 7—Cognitive disabilities
- Chapter 8—Developmental
- Chapter 9—Sensorimotor

These are not the only frames of reference that could potentially be used, and this list is not intended to be all-inclusive. Most of the theoretical concepts that make up OT frames of reference have also been researched and applied in other disciplines. What makes these frames of reference different from similar theories in psychology, basic science, and medicine is that the concepts were reorganized in a way that can guide us in planning and leading OT groups.

Theory-Based Occupational Therapy Groups Using Frames and Models

The relationship of the concepts for each model and frame to OT groups is facilitated through examples and learning exercises.

To provide the student with a concrete idea of how OT frames of reference and models change the way OT groups are designed, structured, and led, the seven-step format for group leadership described in Chapter 1 has been adapted at the end of each chapter on frames of reference and models. Suggested modifications to the introduction, use of activity, sharing, generalizing, application, and summary are described at the end of each chapter in this section. A chart reflecting differences in the structure of groups based on these frames of reference and models may be found in Appendix E. It is hoped that, with this breakdown, the application of theory will be, at least partly, demystified.

References

American OT Association. (2008). OT practice framework: Domain and process, 2nd edition. *American Journal of OT, 62,* 625-683.

Baum, C., Bass-Haugan, J., & Christiansen, C. (2005). Person-environment occupational performance: A model for planning interventions for individuals and organizations. In C. Christiansen, C. Baum, & J. Bass-Haugen (Eds.), *OT: Performance, participation, and well-being* (pp. 373-392). Thorofare, NJ: SLACK Incorporated.

Cole, M. B., & Tufano, R. (2008). Applied theories in occupational therapy. Thorofare, NJ: SLACK Incorporated.

Dunbar, S. B. (2007). Theory, frame of reference, and model: A differentiation for practice consideration. In S. B. Dunbar (Ed.), *OT models for intervention with children and families* (pp. 1-10). Thorofare, NJ: SLACK Incorporated.

Dunn, W. (2007). Ecology of human performance model. In S. B. Dunbar (Ed.), *OT models for intervention with children and families* (pp. 1-10). Thorofare, NJ: SLACK Incorporated.

Iwama, M. K. (2006). *The Kawa Model: Culturally relevant OT.* Toronto, Canada: Churchill Livingstone.

Kielhofner, G. (2008). *A model of human occupation: Theory and application* (4th ed.). Baltimore, MD: Williams & Wilkins.

Law, M., & Dunbar, S. B. (2007). Person-environment-occupation model. In S. B. Dunbar (Ed.), *Occupational therapy models for intervention with children and families* (pp. 27-49). Thorofare, NJ: SLACK Incorporated.

Mosey, A. (1981). *OT: Configuration of a profession.* New York, NY: Raven.

Mosey, A. (1989). The proper focus of scientific inquiry in OT: Frames of reference. *OT Journal of Research, 9,* 195-201.

Polatajko, H. J., Mandich, A., & Martini, R. (2000). Dynamic performance analysis: A framework for understanding occupational performance. *American Journal of Occupational Therapy, 54,* 65-72.

Reed, K., & Sanderson, S. (1999). *Concepts of OT* (4th ed.). Philadelphia, PA: Lippincott, Williams & Wilkins.

Schultz, S., & Schkade, J. (2003). Occupational adaptation. In E. Crepeau, E. Cohn, & B. B. Schell (Eds.), *Willard & Spackman's OT* (10th ed.). Philadelphia, PA: Lippincott, Williams & Wilkins.

Stewart, D., Letts, L., Law, M., Cooper, B., Strong, S., & Rigby, P. (2003). The person-environment-occupation model. In E. Crepeau, E. Cohn, & B. Schell (Eds.), *Willard & Spackman's Occupational Therapy* (10th ed.). Philadelphia, PA: Lippincott, Williams, & Wilkins.

Chapter 5

PSYCHODYNAMIC APPROACHES

In previous editions, this frame of reference has been called *psychoanalytic*. The term *psychodynamic* expands the conceptual base of this as an OT frame of reference to encompass concepts from ego psychology, humanism, and human spirituality (Bruce & Borg, 2002). Historically, OT theorists have been acknowledging the usefulness of various forms of psychoanalytic theory in guiding our interventions with clients with mental illness. Diasio (1968) explores the psychoanalytic view of motivation and the environment. Fidler and Fidler (1963) point out the importance of the unconscious and view activities as part of a communication process with human and nonhuman objects to effectively gratify instinctual needs. Mosey (1986), in considering analytical frames of reference, emphasized the "structure for linking psychoanalytic theories, the symbolic potential and reality aspects of activities, and the process of altering intrapsychic content in the direction of providing a more adaptive basis for interaction with the environment." Llorens and Johnson (1966) refer to "socially acceptable, ego-adaptive functioning" in describing the effects of client involvement in activity groups, thus focusing on OT techniques that help develop and strengthen the functions of the ego. Fidler and Velde (1999) refer to the "dynamic of congruence, or match, of an activity with the nature and characteristics of the person" (p. xi). In recent years, both Fidler and Velde (1999) and Hasselkus (2002) have looked beyond the "purposeful" nature of activities and focused on their symbolic and metaphorical meaning in the dimension of spirituality.

Nicholls (2007) writes "psychoanalysis is a language of understanding one's feelings through the process of thinking, a process that I have termed 'being concerned with matters of the heart'" (p. 55). She focuses on two areas of psychodynamic theory that remain important for OT: the unconscious and the symbolic meaning of activities/occupations. Many parts of our clients' behavior can be observed and explained using rational, scientific approaches, but how do we understand clients' irrational behavior? Why do they take drugs, cut themselves, deprive themselves of food, or let their anger destroy the very human relationships upon which they depend? Why do they view suicide as the only option when faced with oppression, bullying, chronic pain, or the loss of significant others? These may only be understood through the exploration of the unconscious, where emotional conflicts, failed relationships, unspeakable trauma, fear of inadequacy, or uncontrollable hostility continue to operate below the level of awareness, compelling our clients to make self-destructive choices and sabotaging OT's best efforts to help them.

The other important area for OT that Nicholls describes is the symbolic meaning of occupation. She uses the example of mountain climbing, a high-risk occupation to which some are drawn again and again despite near-tragic experiences. The compulsion to keep climbing can be better understood as a defense against "the internal experience of human vulnerability" (2007, p. 60). Many clients also use occupations as a way to earn the respect of others, refute the criticism of others, prove one's own

Cole M.B. *Group Dynamics in OT:*
The Theoretical Basis and Practice Application
of Group Intervention (pp 129-154).
© 2012 SLACK Incorporated.

worth, or defend against the passage of time or void of meaninglessness. As such, the psychodynamic frame of reference views occupation as a primary path to a meaningful life and a necessary building block to satisfying human relationships.

WHY STUDY PSYCHOANALYTIC THEORY?

Psychoanalytic theory has been out of favor for several decades, even in the field of mental health from which it originated. This fact is generally attributed to the lack of efficacy research and the slowness and abstractness of the therapeutic process itself. As an OT approach, it is probably due for a comeback, perhaps in a redefined form. One sign of this comeback is the emergence of spirituality as a concern in OT. This spirituality is not defined as religion, but as belief in the human spirit. The spirit, essence, or soul of the person is really not so different from the "ego" or conscious self discussed in psychoanalytic theory. Furthermore, the complexity of the psychoanalytic theory provides an explanation for many of the irrational, even bizarre behaviors we observe in people with a variety of illnesses (e.g., suicide attempts, risk-taking behaviors, paranoia, self-starvation, or obsessive compulsive behaviors) that are otherwise unexplainable.

Following the early theorists, two general goals of OT groups will be considered: alteration of personality and development of ego skills. This chapter will first review the basic assumptions of psychoanalytic theory, which are useful in planning OT groups. Ego functions and their relevance to OT will then be reviewed. Finally, contributions from the OT literature will be summarized, and group leadership guidelines will be derived from these psychodynamic theoretical concepts.

Psychoanalytic theory, based on the work of Sigmund Freud in the late 19th and early 20th centuries, has had a profound influence on all theories of group intervention. Corey (1991) describes Freud as an "intellectual giant" whose work represents "the most comprehensive theory of personality and psychotherapy ever developed." In the 1990s, there was a tendency to underestimate the influence of psychoanalytic theory because many subsequent theorists have either developed it further or reacted against it. The current emphasis on brain biochemistry as a determinant of human behavior has overshadowed the importance of personality dynamics in our understanding of mental illness. New technology has enabled researchers to observe the physiological and biochemical functioning of the brain in ways never before possible, and thus new genetic links have been discovered.

However, for OTs, these new scientific discoveries do not alter the fact that there are many mental illnesses currently being diagnosed for which psychoanalytic theory offers the only plausible explanation. For example, there is a growing interest in borderline personality disorder (BPD), which is thought to originate from a failure to separate from parents and achieve an autonomous sense of self at around age 2. If parents do not allow their children to explore their environment and do activities of their own choosing in a safe environment, then, as adults, they are unable to derive any satisfaction from activities. Knowing this, the OT can offer clients with BPD an opportunity to explore activities according to their own interest. Recent research shows that for some clients with BPD, it is possible to strengthen autonomous functioning through participation in task-oriented OT groups (Greene & Cole, 1991).

For OTs, psychoanalytic theory is also useful in the physical disability areas of practice. The concept of self-worth and the many defenses of the ego can help us understand why some of our clients use denial of their illness or resist our suggestions for intervention. It is important for OTs to determine the symbolic meaning of illness or trauma in the structure of personality and how symptoms are incorporated into the client's perception of him- or herself. For example, Julia, an 83-year-old woman with osteoporosis and chronic arthritis, was in and out of doctors' offices all her life, with many failed attempts to increase her independent functioning in OT. Only at age 79, after her husband died, did she learn to perform self-care independently. In her earlier years, Julia's many illnesses symbolized her helplessness. Her dependency on her husband for personal self-care fulfilled her need for attention and love. The client's sense of self is vital to her acceptance or rejection of OT intervention, whether the illness is mental or physical.

The original form of psychoanalytic theory, sometimes called *id psychology* (Fine, 1979, p. 319), has been widely criticized by psychologists, social scientists, and OTs during the past 20 years for its vagueness and its unsuitability for research. The link with psychoanalysis and its questionable appropriateness for treating many types of mental illness has added fuel to the fires of discontent. Psychoanalysis is a therapeutic approach developed by Freud in which individual clients are assisted in uncovering their unconscious conflicts by conversing with a therapist, a process that could take many years. Critics feel that one cannot research the unconscious because it is not observable or measurable.

A more current emphasis on ego psychology focuses on the conscious rather than the unconscious aspects of the personality and is therefore, by definition, more observable and measurable. The ego is best understood as the "self." A client's sense of self, his or her self-concept, can determine his or her degree of involvement in OT intervention. If a client sees him- or herself as a capable and worthwhile individual, he or she will be motivated to overcome disability. If Dean defines himself as an accountant, he will make the effort to overcome his depression to return to that occupation. In this frame of reference, the ego is seen as a powerful motivating force that can either resist or facilitate therapeutic change.

Bellak, Huruich, and Gediman (1973) operationalized the functions of the ego, making them more amenable for research purposes. They define 12 ego functions:

1. Reality testing
2. Judgment
3. Sense of self and the world
4. Control of drive, affect, and impulse
5. Object relationships
6. Thought processes
7. Adaptive regression in service of the ego
8. Defensive functioning
9. Stimulus barrier
10. Autonomous functioning
11. Synthetic integrative functions
12. Mastery/competence

Those ego functions most applicable to OT will be further defined later in this chapter.

FRAMEWORK FOCUS

Psychodynamic theory addresses a person's ability to love and to work. It includes both self-identity and interpersonal relationships, which impact the performance in areas of occupation in the American OT Association's (AOTA) *Practice Framework-II* (2008). The context areas have a special importance as these environmental factors continue to shape the "self." It would be a mistake to limit the use of this approach to treating those with primarily mental illness. Psychodynamic approaches are especially useful in dealing with human emotions and motivational issues for all clients, as well as exploring the symbolic meaning of occupations. Groups that use creativity as a projection of the self to promote self-awareness and insight are best understood from a psychodynamic perspective. The initial use of expressive groups as a way to help clients to better define their occupational problems and to overcome internal barriers to engagement in occupation has also been used in combination with a client-centered approach (see Chapter 3).

BASIC ASSUMPTIONS

The following is intended as a brief review of the original concepts of Freudian psychoanalytic theory. A more thorough understanding may be obtained by referring to other basic psychology texts. Psychoanalytic theory is exceedingly complex, and there are many variations currently in use. It must be remembered that Freud's theory provides an intellectual understanding of the personality and its development. The parts described as id, ego, and superego do not parallel structures or functions of the brain, nor do they represent distinct developmental stages. The purpose for which psychoanalytic theory will be used in this text is to define those concepts that help us understand the dynamics of illness, both mental and physical, and to develop intervention techniques to address these dynamics. Because of the focus on group intervention, many important aspects of Freudian theory will be left out.

Freudian Concepts

Personality Structure

Freud organized personality into three parts: the id, the ego, and the superego. This structure is still accepted by many psychotherapists regardless of their discipline or theoretical preferences. While a balance of these components is considered ideal, the functions of the ego in this text will be emphasized because of their direct relevance to OT groups.

The Id

The id is seen as largely unconscious. It is the part of the personality that houses primitive drives and instincts, needs, and conflicts that the ego is unable to integrate. The id is the biological component of the personality and is thought to operate through primary process thinking. Primary process thinking is the earliest to develop in the infant. It is illogical and undisciplined and operates on the pleasure principle, demanding immediate gratification of needs and drives.

The Ego

The ego is the psychological component and has contact with the external world. It functions logically and works to achieve a balance between internal drives and external expectations. The ego operates through a secondary process, one that is learned through experience in reaching compromises and applying logic and discipline in an attempt to adapt to the environment.

The Superego

The superego is the social component of the personality that serves as an individual's moral code, his or her sense of good and bad, right and wrong. The superego is often illogical and unrealistic in its quest for idealism and perfection. The superego is the last part to appear in the developmental process, and its beliefs are learned from parents and from society.

Table 5-1

Freud's Psychosexual Stages

Age (Years)	Stage (Source of Gratification)	Fixation Characteristics (Potential Problem Areas)
Birth to 1 year	Oral stage Early: Sucking Late: Biting	Theme: Trust, dependency Regression: Psychosis
1 to 3 years	Anal stage Early: Excreting Late: Retaining	Theme: Control, autonomy Regression: Neurosis, character disorders
3 to 5 years	Phallic stage Genital interest Penis envy	Theme: Oedipal/Electra complex
5 to 12 years	Latency stage Sublimation of sexual drive Superego develops	Theme: Skill development, social role development, emergence of guilt
12 to adulthood	Genital stage Puberty Capacity for intimacy	Theme: Sexual identity, adult responsibility for love and work

Psychosexual Stages

Freud believed that personality is largely determined by one's early childhood experiences. Psychosexual stages of development, spanning a range of 18 years from birth to maturity, are differentiated by changes in the objects that potentially provide need satisfaction. An object is someone or something that gratifies or frustrates a need; objects can be human or nonhuman. The classic example of an object in the oral stage is mother's breast. A nonhuman substitute for mother's breast is the bottle. When a child's needs are gratified, he or she thrives and is able to develop and move on to the next stage. However, when the child's needs are continually frustrated, he or she develops a fixation that can remain in the unconscious and cause many of the problems in adulthood that we know as symptoms of illness. Freud's psychosexual stages of development are outlined in Table 5-1.

The psychosexual stages are critical to our understanding of mental illness. In spite of current discoveries of the genetic and biochemical origins of some illnesses, most psychopathology is still explained in terms of Freud's levels of personality organization. In general, the earlier the conflict occurs, the more severe the illness. While there are not rigid parallels between the stages and the development of certain illnesses, fixations in the early stages are likely to result in faulty or incomplete development in later ones. For example, failure to develop self-control in the anal stage may result in the overdevelopment or misuse of defense mechanisms as the ego's attempt to compensate for lack of self-control in later stages.

When we, as OTs, observe clients in our therapeutic groups who are unable to work together and get along with one another, a knowledge of how the clients have progressed through the psychosexual stages may help us understand the reasons why. In addition, the stages may offer guidelines as to what type of therapeutic intervention is needed. For example, trust is an issue dealt with in the oral stage. Groups in which members seem to lack a basic trust of one another might benefit from activities that assist clients in feeling more comfortable with self-disclosure. This self-disclosure can form the basis of establishing trusting relationships with the therapist and with one another.

Psychic Energy, Libido, Aggression, and Anxiety

In Freud's view, the amount of psychic energy is limited and must be shared by all three parts of the personality. This explains why people cease to function when too much energy is being used up in trying to deal with unresolved conflicts from the past. A healthy individual is able to resolve conflicts as they arise and therefore keep psychic energy available for the ego to grow and develop and interact effectively with the environment. In mental illness, psychic energy may be trapped in the id and may produce nonadaptive behaviors, which we call symptoms.

Two specific forms of psychic energy are described by Freud: the libidinal and the aggressive drives. Libido is the sexual energy that represents the urge to perpetuate life, to be intimate, to love, and to reproduce. This is also called the life-force and is demonstrated by a person's tendency to form relationships with other people. The aggressive drive is equated with the death-force and is associated with hostility, hatred, and the urge to destroy. It is expressed in the tendency to be self-sufficient and to keep others at a distance. Both the libidinal and the aggressive drives are part of the id, and both seek expression through objects. It is a function of the ego to control these drives and to allow their expression in ways that are socially acceptable. It is a function of the superego to guide an individual's libidinal and aggressive drives toward constructive and morally acceptable expression.

Anxiety, in Freud's view, is defined in relation to both drives and the ego's control function. Anxiety is an alerting response that lets us know that something is wrong and needs to be changed and that some action needs to be taken to get us out of danger. However, unlike the existentialists who view anxiety as a normal condition of life, Freud views anxiety as pathological. Freudian anxiety develops out of the conflicts over control of the available psychic energy within the personality itself. This anxiety goes beyond fear of realistic danger from the external world. It is the fear that the id may take over, forcing the individual to act irrationally or in ways that are morally wrong, or that the superego may take over, causing a pervasive sense of guilt and self-punishment. As long as the ego maintains control, anxiety can be safely held in check and dealt with realistically. High levels of neurotic anxiety, however, may necessitate the unconscious use of ego defense mechanisms to help reduce the tension and protect the survival of the ego. These mechanisms will be reviewed later in this chapter.

OTs may facilitate the expression of psychic energy through activities. This helps the client in a variety of ways. Through activities, the aggressive drive can be directed toward productive work, constructive homemaking, or toward competition in sports. The libidinal drive can energize the client to the development of social skills, nurturing skills, and cooperation with others. Various ego functions might be encouraged in OT groups, such as appropriate expression of feelings, both loving and aggressive, or the sharing of perceptions to help members develop a realistic sense of self.

Symbols, Projections, and Communication With the Unconscious

Rarely, except in episodes of psychosis, does the content of the unconscious become known. Psychoanalytic therapy's main thrust is to help an individual become aware of his or her unconscious conflicts and fixations, so that the mature ego can deal with them effectively and resolve them. However, the nature of primary process makes awareness of unconscious material very complex. Primary process is not organized or logical and is not remembered in words or complete thoughts. Highly emotional material may take the form of symbols that represent experiences that originally produced them. For example, a child who experienced the violent death of a parent in an automobile accident may have repressed the original memory. If, as an adult, he or she draws a car as part of an OT activity, he or she may suddenly re-experience an overwhelming feeling of grief and loss without knowing why. It is the therapist's role to help the adult client to interpret the meaning of the symbols he or she produces and, with the help of a psychiatrist, remember and work through the original traumatic experience.

Object Relationships

Object relationships were previously mentioned as the organizing principles of the psychosexual stages. Freud viewed object relations as the foundation of an individual's capacity to love and to work. Fidler and Fidler (1963) define OT in terms of the development of relationships with human (therapist) and nonhuman (environment) objects. In human relationships, the client develops the ability to satisfy some of his or her basic needs, such as recognition, self-esteem, and belonging, through a therapeutic relationship with the OT. In the safety of a therapeutic environment, the client uses realistic feedback from the therapist or other clients to correct his or her unrealistic concepts and expectations of self and others. Nonhuman objects are related to the client's ability to work. The client can learn, in OT, to use the symbolic as well as actual properties of objects to help satisfy instinctual drives and needs. For example, Bob can satisfy his need to express hostility by flattening a ball of clay or sawing a piece of wood. Mary can express her compulsive needs by maintaining a perfectly clean and organized kitchen. Using this principle, OT activities can be selected according to the instinctual needs of group members.

Assumptions of Ego Psychology

Alfred Adler is credited with making the first significant break with Freud over the nature and importance of the ego (Fine, 1979). He believed that the ego is responsible for shaping the personality, rather than the person being shaped by biological forces and early childhood experiences. Another theorist who recognized the importance of the ego was Heinz Hartmann. Hartmann (1939) looked at the process of psychoanalysis and suggested that it was not a reconstruction of what once existed buried in the unconscious (the Freudian view). He saw that psychotherapy requires that the mature ego establish correct causal relationships and judgments of the emerging memories. The significance of Hartmann's work is in establishing the autonomy of the ego as separate from the id in psychoanalytic theory. Ego psychology has been developing since 1923 and has had many spokesmen, including Adler, Sullivan, Hartmann, Erikson, Lewin, and Rapaport (Fine, 1979). The common element is an emphasis on the ego. For the sake of brevity, not all the functions of the ego can be reviewed. Those selected for emphasis are as follows:

- Reality testing
- Sense of self
- Thought processes
- Judgment
- Self-control
- Defensive mechanisms
- Competence/mastery

Reality Testing

Reality testing is perhaps the most important function of the ego in therapy. It is the ego's ability to use perception and judgment to differentiate between internal needs and external demands. This process involves the use of interaction with the environment and with others in shaping and reshaping one's views of self and the world. It is precisely this process that is responsible for adaptation to the environment. The ego becomes aware of needs and drives from the id, but delays their gratification until they can be satisfied in ways that are socially acceptable.

Consensual Validation

Reality testing is an integral part of the therapeutic use of groups. As members share their perceptions of themselves and the world with others in the group, they have the advantage of hearing the responses of others. It is through this feedback that group members gather evidence to support their self-other perceptions. When perceptions of others are clearly different from one's own, then one needs to question whether his or her own perceptions are realistic. The process of integrating one's own perceptions, views, or beliefs with those of others is called consensual validation.

For example, Lisa shared with the group a painful experience involving her father's rejection of her. Lisa believed she had to live with this rejection and was powerless to change it. Several other members recounted similar feelings about their own fathers, based on similar experiences. This feedback helped validate Lisa's feelings of rejection. Based on clear evidence, she had a right to feel rejected; in her situation, anyone would. However, another member of the group, Roberta, also told Lisa how she had begun speaking to her father after a 7-year period of silence. Roberta was able to significantly improve her father-daughter relationship through some more adult conversations and sharing of feelings. This feedback made Lisa reconsider her position; perhaps she

was not as powerless as she believed herself to be. The group helped Lisa to see which parts of her self-perception were real (being rejected) and which were not real (being powerless).

Exploring Outer Reality

OT groups involving the use of concrete tasks provide another kind of reality testing, one on a sensory level. Manipulation of objects and materials provides sensory input: taste, touch, smell, vision, hearing, and proprioception (position, pressure, balance, etc.), which can lead one to challenge internal perceptions. Robert felt he had no energy and therefore could not complete a woodworking project. When the group members persuaded him to try it, however, the sensory stimulation provided by sawing and hammering the wood (proprioceptive and auditory) helped release the needed energy. Robert learned through experience that by engaging in appropriate motor activities, he was able to direct his energy to produce a positive effect on the environment (a completed project). If the group then also provides positive feedback on his wood project, Robert is further inclined to change his view of himself from ineffectual, "I can't," to effective, "I can!" It is important here for the OT to be aware of Robert's abilities in choosing a task, ensuring that his experience is likely to be a successful one.

Sense of Self

Many aspects of sense of self appear in the literature, and their meaning can be somewhat confusing. Three discrete aspects will be defined here:

- Self-concept
- Body image
- Self-esteem

Self-Concept

Self-concept or self-identity is sometimes used interchangeably with the word *ego*. Developmentally, the idea of self originates when the infant begins to differentiate self from mother and then from the environment in general. Psychotic individuals are understood by ego psychologists to have regressed beyond the point where they are able to differentiate self from others. These psychotic individuals are said to have "poor" or "loose" ego boundaries. This factor makes psychotic clients particularly sensitive to their environment. When someone in the group is angry, for example, it is often the psychotic client who is first to notice it, although he or she may not express his or her awareness realistically or appropriately.

Following Freud's original formulations, the attempt was made to correlate the various clinical entities with the points of fixation in psychosexual development. Primarily, the oral stage is associated with psychosis, the anal stage with neuroses, and the phallic stage with hysteria. Ego psychologists have elaborated and changed this original oversimplified concept of mental illness but have retained the idea that the ego or self-concept is fundamentally different in these three levels of psychiatric diagnosis. Psychological testing such as word association (Jung, 1910), interpretation of inkblots (Rorschach, 1921), and association with photographs (Murray, 1951) are a few of the earliest attempts to measure ego functions with particular regard to self-concept.

The idea that concept of the self is a common problem area for mentally ill individuals has led OTs to make self-concept and its related ideas—body image, self-esteem, and self-perception—the focus of OT intervention. Groups using movement, dance, or physical sports and exercise may be helpful to clients in developing a realistic body image. Drawing and word association activities, often taking their cue from the various psychological tests, have been useful in promoting knowledge of the self. Self-esteem is better approached in OT through successful experiences and feedback from others. Person drawings in particular are a useful therapeutic tool for both evaluation and intervention in OT.

Body Image

Body image is the perception of one's physical self that forms the basis of self-awareness. According to theories of child development, the earliest learning involves the association and differentiation of somatosensory sensations. These provide a kind of geographical knowledge of the body and how it works that defines "me." Body sense, according to Allport (1958), allows a child to develop a sense of personhood. It is the sensorimotor exploration of early play that helps the child define the boundaries of his or her body and distinguish "me" from "not me." In adulthood, body sense continues to provide a basic reference point from which environmental interactions take place. The sensory systems, for example, help people know how they feel. Influences from the body guide day-to-day behavior. For example, you may stay home from work because you feel fatigued, or you may go for a walk because you feel restless. The child achieves a sense of control over his or her body by reaching out to the environment to satisfy body needs: a bottle satisfies hunger, a toy satisfies need for pleasure, mother satisfies the need for comfort. As adults, we continue to reach out to the environment and to others based on our perceptions of our bodies and what we need.

Illness tends to produce distortions in body image, and this may be the source of problem behaviors. As OTs, one of our goals is to determine whether our client's body image is realistic. Using activities that encourage clients to become aware of their feelings and sensations can help to correct body image distortions. Movement activities and person drawings are two examples of this.

Self-Esteem

Self-esteem describes the subjective feelings of one's own ability. As with sensorimotor, perceptual, and cognitive processes, feelings are innate and develop as the child matures. However, feelings or affects are intricately tied to objects, and their expression determines how people relate to one another and to their world. The idea that affects our ego states comes from Freud's 1926 work *Inhibitions, Symptoms and Anxiety* (Bellak et al., 1973). Rapaport (1953) attempted to articulate a theory of affect, suggesting that affect originates as psychic energy and is seen as a signal emitted by the ego to indicate an internal feeling state needing to be noticed. Spitz (1959) offered a theory of affect development in the infant as the following:

- Crying
- Smiling
- Stranger distress or fearfulness

Language development then allows the child to express a multiplicity of feeling states of increasing complexity.

The expression of affect or emotion is an important function of the ego. As suggested by Rapaport, it is one of the ways the ego has to control and direct energy from the id. Acting out has been described earlier as a more primitive, less socialized form of expression of affect through action. Those with special talents are able to express affect through artistic media, such as painting, music, or poetry and drama. While these ways are socially acceptable, the most commonly acceptable way to express affect is by describing it verbally with words.

As OTs, we often observe in our clients (and sometimes in ourselves) a lack of ability to communicate emotions to others. In the ego adaptive frame of reference, a common goal of OT groups is the appropriate expression of emotions.

Thought Processes

Thought processes are the cognitive functions of the ego having to do with the following:

- Attention
- Memory
- Learning and logical thought
- Compromise
- Problem solving

Attention

Attention is the ability of the ego to focus on something for a period of time. It requires not only alertness of the mind, but a readiness to take in new information. Information coming in through the sensory systems is screened for relevance, and the brain focuses on aspects of the environment to which a response is appropriate. Sustained attention, or concentration, is needed for the individual to participate in OT groups.

Memory

Memory is central to psychoanalytic theory, as seen in Freud's persistent efforts to recapture early childhood events. Rapaport (1942) recognized the relationship between memory and emotional factors. The ego was thought to censor memory in accordance with the intensity of associated emotional factors. In other words, events that were extremely painful are repressed; the ego stores them below the level of consciousness, and they cannot be remembered at all. Or, the ego can alter the perception of a traumatic event so that the senses are numbed and the brain will not receive more stimuli than it can handle. In this case, the memory of the event would be inaccurate or unrealistic. The current metaphor most closely associated with memory is that of the computer, with information storage and retrieval as the primary activities. It is believed that one's memory process reflects individual styles of secondary process functioning. In other words, what someone remembers is dependent upon how he or she perceives and understands an event in the first place.

When an OT hears a client report a remembered event in a group, it becomes the task of the therapist to listen not only for the facts, but also for the emotional bias the client expresses. This is particularly important if the client's emotional response is problematic. For example, Shelley reported at the beginning of the group that something about the last group had been bothering her all week. Last week, during a serious discussion among several group members, Shelley had gotten up from her chair and stepped into the center of the group to kill a spider that was crawling on the floor. She felt "terrible" that her action would be viewed as a violation or mocking of the members whose discussion she had disrupted. The group's response to this confession was surprising. Two or three members remembered the incident in passing, but said it was "no big deal." The three members who were involved in the discussion had no recall of the event at all. The facts of the spider killing event were the same for everyone, but Shelley remembered them in the context of a strong emotional bias that put herself in a negative light. It was only with the feedback of the other group members that she was able to shed the bias and put the event in a more realistic perspective.

With most significant events in our lives, we do not have the advantage of the feedback of the others to help us correct our emotional bias. Hence, when past events not witnessed by the group are reported to the group, it is difficult for members or the therapist to separate the facts from the emotions involved. It is only in the context of "here and now" events that groups can be helpful in this way. This is one reason that it is suggested that our OT groups have a "here and now" focus.

Learning and Logical Thought

Learning is a skill of the ego that has been given little attention by followers of psychoanalysis, yet it is central to the notion of making therapeutic change. It has been noted by ego psychologists that intellectual development (learning) occurs most favorably in a warm, secure environment. This observation is helpful to OT so we can recognize the importance of creating and maintaining this kind of safe environment in our groups. Physical safety should be a given; this means that the OT removes any dangerous objects or factors from the environment (e.g., sharp objects, loose wires, wet or slippery floors). Psychological safety is provided when the OT maintains control through the establishment of group norms, such as mutual respect and prevention of verbal attacks on one another.

Problem Solving

The kind of thinking attributed to the ego is secondary process thinking. This is also called *reasoning* or *logical thought*. It is the ability of the ego to consider facts in the light of reality and put them to use in guiding behavior. Problem solving is a cognitive skill that requires the use of logical thought. In fact, all of the functions of the ego contribute to problem solving: accurate perception and reality testing, memory, and control of impulses as well as appropriate use of defenses. The process of solving problems is quite complex, but the ability to do so is often a deciding factor in whether our clients are considered to be competent in activities of daily living. OTs are often asked to evaluate a client's problem-solving ability. Observation of the client in a group activity is one way to determine this skill. For example, Rich, a client in a cooking group, was unfamiliar with the process of peeling and slicing carrots for a salad. However, because he had arrived late, that was the only job available. Rich picked up the knife and proceeded to chop the carrot, leaving the skin on and cutting only part way through with each chop. When another client handed Rich a vegetable peeler, Rich turned on the would-be helper and waved the knife at him in a somewhat threatening way. After a few more attempts to cut the skin off the carrot with the knife, Rich put down the carrot and abandoned the task. After observing Rich's behavior, the OT discussed the situation with Rich and determined that Rich's ability to solve problems was poor.

How can OT groups be helpful to Rich in learning to solve problems? Clearly, teaching him to use a vegetable peeler will only help temporarily in the specific situation. In general, Rich's tendency to act alone and reject help are the real issues that need to be dealt with. Group discussion following the cooking task helped Rich to understand what his options were in solving the carrot problem. Asking for help and being able to accept it in a nonthreatening way were agreed upon as goals for Rich in future group tasks.

Judgment

Judgment is another function of the ego that is often the focus in OT groups. Good judgment requires the following cognitive processes:

- Accurate and realistic perception of the situation
- Identification of intended behaviors and likely consequences
- Prediction of the behaviors' effect on others
- Control of response until options are considered
- An appreciation of what it takes to accomplish something

On a well-known psychological test, the client is asked the question, "What is the thing to do if you find an envelope in the street that is sealed, addressed, and has a new stamp?" The most acceptable answer is, "mail it" (Wechsler, 1981, p. 126). How one arrives at this response requires a complex process of perception, reasoning, and anticipation of consequences. Judgment is a cognitive skill of the highest order and one of the most difficult to learn or teach.

Self-Control

Control was the earliest of the ego functions to be recognized, when Freud conceptualized the ego's main function to control the instinctual drives from the id. Impulse control may be seen as a derivative of this earlier conceptualization.

In OT groups, we often encourage impulse control in a number of ways. We expect group members to arrive on time and to remain attentive for the length of the group, usually 50 to 60 minutes. We expect members to consider others in the group, listening to them, waiting their turn to speak, sharing tools and materials, passing the glue or the scissors. In a cooking group, we would ask members not to taste the food with their fingers and to wait to begin eating until the whole group is seated. On a shopping trip, we ask our clients not to taste items in the store, not to buy items impulsively, and to wait to light their cigarettes until they have finished shopping. Following social norms and interacting effectively in groups requires good control of impulses.

Defense Mechanisms

Defenses are broadly understood as a way of warding off anxiety and ensuring the safety and preservation of an intact ego. The strengthening of healthy defenses is a common goal in OT groups. In addition, the concept of defenses helps us as OTs to understand better our clients' responses to activities. Through our recognition of defenses in our clients, we as OTs are better able to plan activities and make therapeutic interventions in our groups to help clients achieve a healthy balance in their lives. Defense mechanisms are an important part of the structure of the ego. Early psychologists focused on this aspect when developing the techniques of psychoanalysis. The goal of psychoanalysis was to break through a person's defenses so as to uncover the memory of critical childhood events.

Kaplan and Sadock (2003, pp. 208-209) have classified defense mechanisms into four categories:

1. *Narcissistic defenses:* Projection, denial, and distortion
2. *Immature defenses:* Acting out, blocking, hypochondriasis, introjection, passive-aggressive behavior, regression, schizoid fantasy, and somatization
3. *Neurotic defenses:* Controlling, displacement, dissociation, externalization, inhibition, intellectualization, isolation, rationalization, reaction formation, repression, and sexualization
4. *Mature defenses:* Altruism, anticipation, asceticism, humor, sublimation, and suppression

The contemporary ego psychologists view mature defenses as performing a healthy adaptive function, and these will be most relevant to our work in OT. Those defenses that are dealt with most often in OT are reviewed here. The reader is referred to Kaplan and Sadock (2003) for a more thorough description of the above defenses.

Sublimation

Sublimation was identified by Anna Freud in 1936 as a healthy and acceptable rechanneling of libidinal and aggressive drives into constructive activity. While sublimation is no longer a focus in psychological literature, the concept remains central to OT because of its implications regarding activity, creativity, and tasks or work. As OTs using a psychoanalytic frame of reference, we continue to see clear evidence of this rechanneling of energy. The concept allows us to understand why work is such a central part of living and why the loss of the work role produces both aggressiveness and anxiety and a sharp decline in one's self-worth. Neutralization (Hartmann's updated substitute for sublimation) refers to the de-energizing of the libidinal and aggressive drives. It is the "successful defense" by which the mature ego masters reality.

Projection

Projection is another defense, originating with Freud (1914), that continues to hold value in OT. The modern-day variation was described by Melanie Klein (1948) as projective identification. In this mechanism, parts of the self are split off and projected onto an external object or person. Projection provides the ego with a means of getting rid of bad parts of the self. Sam is angry with his boss, but he believes the anger is bad, so he projects the anger onto his boss. Now, Sam can like himself and feel justified in believing his boss is the bad guy who gets angry. Good parts of the self may be projected also, to avoid separation or keep them safe from the bad parts. Projection at higher levels leads to misinterpreting the motives, feelings, attitudes, or intentions of others.

Projection as a concept is used extensively in OT in the form of projective techniques. Projective techniques are generally creative modalities, such as drawing, sculpture, poetry, creative writing, or drama, that allow/ encourage a person to express the hidden parts of the self. A client is said to project parts of him- or herself, particularly affects such as anger or love, in the form of symbols or shapes in art or characters and situations in writing or drama. When done in adulthood, these images or fantasies are then open to interpretation by the mature ego. As therapists, we encourage our clients to apply logic and mature judgment to the products of their projective creations when we ask them to explain them to their fellow group members. One Vietnam veteran participating in an OT projective arts group was asked to explain his elaborate drawing of the atrocities of war. The guns, the dead body parts, and the destructive remains of buildings symbolized for him the bad parts of himself, which he found so hard to accept.

Regression

Regression was also an emphasis of Freud's early work as it helped to explain "fixations" as a cause of mental illness. Regression is going backward from a later to an earlier stage of development. In 1964, Arlow and Brenner defined regression as "the re-emergence of modes of mental functioning characteristic of earlier phases of psychic development." They further state that regressions are usually transient and reversible.

Pathology is not determined by the depth of the regression (oral, anal, etc.) but by its irreversible nature, by the conflicts that it engenders, and by its interference with the process of adaptation. The importance of regression has recently been enhanced by its relation to borderline and psychotic conditions. Psychotic individuals are said to be regressed to the oral stage (birth to 1 year), the earliest stage in Freud's psychosexual stages of development. Borderline (character disorder) individuals are thought to be regressed to the anal stage (1 to 3 years) and fixated there. This view of regression may help to explain the behavior of our clients with these diagnoses in terms of the functioning of the ego. To do so, however, would require a thorough understanding of Freud's psychosexual stages of development.

Regression has another implication that is important for the OT in planning intervention. This is the concept of "regression in the service of the ego." Ernst Kris (1936) first used this term to imply a purposeful regression to earlier modes of functioning without the loss of overriding ego control. The artist who smears paint on a canvas to express extreme affect but retains the control to return to the normal world (while the psychotic client cannot) is a good example. The technique of "free association" or the uncensored, often illogical associations of words and images has been cited as another example.

The therapeutic usefulness of regression to the ego lies in its contribution to a clearer self-understanding.

When we ask our clients to wedge clay or use finger paints, these processes reflect the typical (sometimes forbidden) fascination of the anal stage (smearing feces). Our therapeutic purpose for doing this is not to encourage regression, but to free the individual to express affect in an uninhibited way, with the hope of recapturing the innate urge toward mastery that may be trapped there. The client, after engaging in such a creative process, returns to a more mature level of functioning, but he or she retains an awareness of the affect discovered during the regression. This affect is essential if the client is to change the way he or she understands and uses activity as a part of his or her return to healthy functioning.

Acting Out

Acting out can best be defined as an action, usually repetitive and compulsive in nature and often self-destructive, that serves the unconscious purpose of resolving a repressed internal conflict by external means. This is a popular way to explain self-destructive behavior in analytical terms. It reflects a primitive lack of control over actions that are typical of the infant and regressively present in psychosis and character disorder.

In groups, we often see emotions being "acted out" instead of talked about. For example, anger at someone in the group is expressed by walking out of the room and slamming the door. An action is substituted for a mature verbal description of a feeling state. OT group leaders should discourage acting out responses. These are inappropriate and unproductive for both the client and other group members. The more mature ego skill of verbal expression of affect should be encouraged.

Identification

Identification, as a defense described by Freud, was meant quite literally as the taking onto oneself the characteristics of another. The concept originated as a logical outcome of the Oedipal conflict, in which sexual desire for the opposite-sex parent is replaced by identification with the parent of like sex. Anna Freud (1936) described this phenomenon as "identification with the aggressor." The child's identification with the feared "aggressor" is used, in part, to explain the repetition of behavior patterns in families. Child abuse is an example when the abused child grows up to abuse his own children. Erikson (1950) contributed greatly to the popularity of this concept in his extensive discussion of the identity crisis occurring in late adolescence.

Competence/Mastery

Bellak and colleagues (1973) define this function of the ego as adaptive performance in work and relationships and the subjective feelings of competence. R. H. White (1967) defines competence as "an organism's capacity to interact effectively with its environment..." (Bellak et al., 1973, p. 260). "Fitness to interact with the environment" in White's view, includes language and motor skills, cognition, and higher thought processes. The affect or feeling of efficacy is what White called "effectance motivation" (Bellak et al., 1973, p. 260), referring to the individual's tendency to put more effort and energy into producing responses that will have a desirable effect on the environment. The feelings of competence are the result of a well-developed ego and include a history of successful experiences in coping with the environment.

The ego's ability to cope is what rescues a person in times of illness or crisis. In an emotional crisis, many of the ego defenses described earlier may be viewed as coping mechanisms, protecting the ego from destruction by diverting psychic energy. In the case of physical trauma, the ego uses body sense and reality testing to determine what functions of the body remain intact. The ego's sense of self will often provide the motivation to find ways to compensate for lost functions. For example, a client with right-sided hemiplegia will learn to write with his or her left hand. Compensation is a coping strategy.

Another example of a coping strategy is energy conservation. When physical and mental deterioration occur, energy for use in everyday activities is severely limited. Careful planning before embarking on a task can prevent the client from wasting energy in needless movements. For example, after I had an operation, I was only able to stand up or walk for 15 minutes before stopping to take a rest. When preparing a meal, I had to learn to use the 15 minutes to gather absolutely everything I needed to make meatballs, then assemble them while sitting at the kitchen table. The cooking had to be done in an electric frying pan on the table, rather than at the stove. I had to learn to be satisfied with accumulating a mess around me, rather than cleaning as I went along, and to use a wet sponge to wipe my hands, rather than washing at the sink every few minutes. For clients with chronic disability, conserving energy is a coping skill that is absolutely essential for continued functioning at a level that is consistent with the client's self-identity.

FUNCTION AND DYSFUNCTION

A functioning adult is free of conflicts and fixations and is able to satisfy his or her needs and direct his or her drives in ways that fit in with the social environment and culture. A balance exists in the functioning individual that allows the psychic energy to flow freely between the id, ego, and superego. The ego is in control, and defense mechanisms are not exaggerated, so that the individual with a healthy ego can use most of his or her energy to grow and develop and interact effectively with others. In Fidler's model, the healthy person is able to work productively with others to accomplish a task. As an adult, he or she has acquired all six of Mosey's adaptive skills (Mosey, 1970a, 1981; see Appendix A). The defenses the individual uses are mature ones, like

sublimation of aggression in work, identification with idealized others, and the suppression of immediate gratification. A healthy ego is synonymous with a strong sense of self; body image, self-identity, and self-esteem are realistic and can serve as the basis of adaptive function.

Dysfunction in the psychodynamic frame of reference is defined in terms of inadequate psychosexual development, the presence of conflicts and fixations, and the imbalance of psychic energy among the three parts of the personality. These abnormal states can produce symptoms of neurosis, psychosis, or character disorder, which imply a disturbance in the ability to carry out activities of daily living.

Dysfunction can be seen as a lack of ego skills. This can take the form of poor reality testing, poor or unrealistic body image, poor self-identity, poor self-esteem, impulsiveness or passivity, unbalanced use of defenses, and an inability to cope. Assessment of the ego functions will guide our goal-setting in OT. Clients with similar goals may be treated together in groups.

CHANGE AND MOTIVATION

Change occurs through the learning and performance of adequate ego adaptive skills. These skills can be learned within the social context of therapeutic groups, where the consequences of problem behaviors can be readily seen and discussed. Foundation skills can be worked on through simple, well-structured, reality-oriented tasks that focus on the development to sensorimotor, perceptual, and cognitive skills. Motivation can be enhanced through success experiences in OT. Nicholls (2007) looks at occupations as creative expression and reparative representation. Occupation, in the psychodynamic view, facilitates change through its symbolic power to resolve unconscious intrapersonal conflicts and clarifying the "dreadful complexity of relationships that are often charged with ambivalence" (Craib, 1994, p. vi).

Motivation comes from the directing of psychic energy toward the mastery of ego skills. When energy is bound up in dealing with conflict, people may not be motivated to develop ego skills. As the ego is available to help reduce tensions and to satisfy needs through mature relationships and meaningful work activities, people will be motivated to increase ego skill development. The OT can set up therapeutic groups that allow clients to practice adequate ego skills and experience successful and satisfying consequences for clients. A strong self-concept and high self-esteem are also motivating; these foster a sense of control and lead people to direct their energy toward even greater skill development. Creative occupations that ease tensions can have a cathartic effect. Thus, the need for reducing anxiety can become a powerful motivator for occupational engagement.

REVIEW OF THE OCCUPATIONAL THERAPY PERSPECTIVE

The next portion of this chapter will review three authors from OT whose work has reflected the principles of the psychoanalytic frame of reference: Gail Fidler, Lela Llorens, and Anne Mosey. OT groups using this frame of reference became popular during the 1960s and 1970s, and consequently many of the published works of these authors began about then. While this historical perspective may seem irrelevant today, an understanding of the psychodynamic approach to occupation used by these OT scholars adds much to our own clinical interpretation of client behaviors and the outcomes of engagement in occupation to client sense of self and well-being.

An important influence in OT at the time of the early writings of Fidler, Llorens, and Mosey was an intervention approach begun in England by Maxwell Jones (1953) known as the therapeutic community. The therapeutic community represented in the 1960s and 1970s a fundamental change in approach to interventions with mental illness. Both psychodynamic theories of personality and theories of sociology contributed to this unique approach, which called for the client role to change from a "sick role" to that of a responsible community member. Hospitals and institutions all over Europe and America began therapeutic communities on their psychiatric units, and OTs were an integral part of this new approach.

Prior to the 1960s, OT, although administered in groups, had a task skill focus with an emphasis on the use of crafts and productive work skills. The rise of therapeutic communities called for OTs to incorporate milieu principles into their intervention approach. Examples of these principles are the following:

- Those most affected by a decision should be involved in making it (Jones, 1953).

- "In the context of responsibility for self and others, clients will alter their self-perception from that of subordinate to that of peer group member" (Fairweather, 1964).

- Clients learn best when they are allowed to experience the consequences of their own actions.

Fidler's Task-Oriented Group

In keeping with the times, Gail Fidler published her classic article, "The Task-Oriented Group as a Context for Treatment" in 1969 (see Appendix A). She mentions several spokesmen for ego psychology in her rationale, such as Sullivan and Lewin, and points to the "emerging focus on ego functions and adaptive skills" (Fidler, 1969, p. 43). Fidler also alludes to a focus on the use of groups in therapy as "a dynamic force in facilitating learning and behavior change" (Lewin, 1945).

Fidler, in incorporating OT principles with those of the therapeutic milieu, pointed out the value of observing clients doing tasks. She noted that "as clients engaged in activities or created objects, they expressed characterological difficulties, and that attention to these problems as they emerged and were operant in the here and now, seemed to be of benefit to the client" (Fidler, 1969, p. 45). There appeared to her to be a relationship between problems encountered by a client in his or her activity experiences and those difficulties he or she encountered in the outside world. The assumption here is not unlike one made by the ego psychologists. If the client's difficulties either interpersonally or in task performance are made conscious, whether by experience itself, group feedback, or feedback from the therapist, the client can use ego skills to cope with the difficulties. The strengthening of ego skills, then, becomes the goal of the task-oriented group.

Although the task is defined as either an end-product or a service that is done by the group as a whole, Fidler points out that task accomplishment is not really the purpose. Rather, the task is intended to "provide a shared working experience wherein the relationship between feeling, thinking and behavior, their impact on others and on task accomplishment and productivity can be viewed and explored" (Fidler, 1969, p. 45). Through the task group experience, ego skills and deficits can be observed in the client. Clients demonstrate, in the process of participating in the group, their problems in interaction and in doing, and these problems can then be the focus of group problem-solving. Through both therapist and group feedback, "alternate patterns of functioning can be considered and tested within the context of the here and now, to the end that such learning may induce ego growth and improve function" (Fidler, 1969, p. 45).

In other words, clients are expected to reflect on their behavior in the group and to come to some understanding of its consequence on other members and on task accomplishment. Behavior that is disturbing to others or counterproductive is identified as such, and presumably more adaptive modes of behavior are suggested and tried. The OT facilitates this process during the group; he or she intervenes as problems arise, points them out to the group, and helps the group problem solve. (See Appendix A for Fidler's article.)

Llorens' Occupational Therapy in an Ego-Adaptive Milieu

Lela Llorens (1976) also wrote about OT programming using the psychoanalytic frame of reference. Her article "OT in an Ego-Oriented Milieu" with Johnson (1966) and her book *Developing Ego Functions in Disturbed Children* with Rubin (1967) present useful OT assessment and intervention ideas using this practice model. Llorens writes that "a program of OT designed to enhance and support adaptive functioning must provide for the development of ego skills, opportunities for practice, and support for mastery" (Llorens & Johnson, 1966, p. 179). She describes OT groups in three phases of treatment:

1. Evaluation
2. Convalescence
3. Rehabilitation

In the evaluation phase, observation is emphasized. The group meets 3 consecutive days for 1 hour each day, and activities include orientation to OT, written completion of a background information sheet, and completion of a small mosaic tile tray. This small sample of behavior allows the OT to observe the client's mood, relationships, motivation, performance, and skills. Results of the evaluation show how well the client's ego is functioning in helping him or her adapt to the environment. Those whose egos are functioning less than normal are assigned to the convalescent phase of treatment.

The goals of the convalescent phase are to promote increased feelings of adequacy and to encourage independence in functioning. Modalities suggested to achieve these goals are sewing, needlework, art, leather work, metal work, and woodwork. Convalescent groups consist of five to 15 clients with two therapists. Some ego skills worked on in this phase include the following:

- Expression or sublimation of needs in an acceptable manner
- Attention span and work tolerance
- Reality testing and orientation
- Verbal and nonverbal communication of feelings

The therapist takes responsibility for planning in these groups according to the client's ability.

Clients whose egos are more highly functional are placed in the rehabilitation phase of OT treatment. Modalities for groups in this phase include more interaction: male and female interest groups, activities of daily living discussion group, graceful living, typing, and cooking. A less authoritative leadership style is used in these groups. Mastery is both the motivation and the goal.

Mosey's Adaptive Skills and Developmental Groups

Anne Cronin Mosey's concept of adaptive skills is also useful in the psychoanalytic frame of reference. While she frames the adaptive skills in a developmental context (recapitulation of ontogenesis), the skills themselves closely resemble many of the functions of the ego described earlier. According to Mosey (1970b):

> ...the term adaptive is used to indicate that these skills are acquired and utilized by the individual so that he may satisfy his inherent needs and the needs of others, interact with the environment in order to attain personal goals, and knowledgeably select those environmental demands he wishes to meet (p. 134).

Mosey acknowledges the influence of psychoanalytic theory on the adaptive skills by accepting the concepts of conscious, preconscious, unconscious, complex formation, and regression, but adds the need for mastery as an important component. She proposes that fixation may be the result of deficient adaptive skill learning. She identifies six adaptive skills, which are learned in sequence, with some overlap and interdependence as the child matures:

1. Perceptual-motor skill
2. Cognitive skill
3. Dyadic interaction skill
4. Group interaction skill
5. Self-identity skill
6. Sexual identity skill

The idea that group interaction skill precedes and therefore needs to be mastered before self-identity or gender identity is possible is significant. For an elaboration on these, the reader is referred to Mosey's *Psychosocial Components of Occupational Therapy* (1986). (See Appendix C for a complete list of Mosey's adaptive skills and subskills.)

Leadership Roles in Mosey's Developmental Groups

Of particular interest to OTs working with groups are the components of group interaction skill described by Mosey. She suggests five types of nonfamily groups that simulate those that may be encountered in normal development. The intention of these groups is to provide opportunities to develop group interaction skills in the correct developmental sequence. Group interaction skill is "the ability to participate in a variety of groups in a manner that is satisfying for oneself and for one's fellow group members" (Mosey, 1970b, p. 273). The five types of groups are as follows:

1. Parallel
2. Project
3. Egocentric-cooperative
4. Cooperative
5. Mature (Mosey, 1986)

(See Appendix B for Mosey's article describing these groups.)

Parallel Groups

Parallel groups are the lowest level, made up of clients doing individual tasks side by side. Preschool children may be observed in a similar process on a playground, one swinging, another climbing, another digging in the sandbox. Little interaction is required, and the OT leader defines the task and provides clients with the necessary assistance and emotional support.

Project Groups

Project groups emphasize task accomplishment. Some interaction may be built in, such as shared materials and tools and sharing the work. Social interaction outside of the task is not expected. The OT leader structures the group with tasks that require interaction of two or more people to complete.

Egocentric-Cooperative Groups

Egocentric-cooperative groups require the members to select and implement the task. Tasks are longer term, and social interaction is expected. Although the task serves to organize this group, members are expected to respond to one another's social and emotional needs. The OT leader provides appropriate activity choices and facilitates this process.

Cooperative Groups

Cooperative groups require the OT leader only as an advisor. Members are "encouraged to identify and gratify each other's social and emotional needs in conjunction with task accomplishment" (Mosey, 1970b, p. 273). The task in the cooperative group may be secondary to social aspects.

Mature Groups

In mature groups, the OT leader is a co-equal member. The group members take on all the necessary leadership roles in order to balance task accomplishment with need satisfaction of the members.

GROUP INTERVENTIONS

OT writers have implied that ego functions can be both evaluated and developed (learned) in the context of task-focused groups. The task, in groups using a psychoanalytic frame, takes on greater importance than in humanistic groups. Even when the task is not the focus, it is the context in which discussion, problem solving, and therapeutic change take place. Therefore, the structure of the OT group in this frame is fundamentally different.

Structure and Limitations

After the introduction, the task predominates the group session, providing both the structure and the time-frame for the group. Tasks can last for part of one session or can go on for several sessions. A task might take 3 hours at one time. Discussion depends on problems that arise and how the therapist chooses to intervene. Evaluative discussion is left for the last 15 minutes of each session, with a longer evaluation reserved following the end of the task. This alternative structure is primarily based on Fidler's task-oriented group but has

been expanded and further defined. Mosey's concept of developmental groups is reflected in the changing role of the leader. The leader gives more help and structure to groups that are less capable and less help to groups that have a higher level of ego functioning. The task group is not limited to high-functioning clients. It can be adapted to fairly low levels of group interaction skill, with some changes in structure and the amount of help given by the leader.

Role of the Leader

Fidler defines the role of the OT as one of a facilitator. The leader's major goal is to make learning possible and not to take over the group. Facilitation, then, requires that the therapist maintain and communicate a basic belief in the group's capacity to be "constructively self-determining" (Fidler, 1969, p. 46). This means he or she does not make decisions for the group or rescue the group from its difficulties. Rather, he or she intervenes in the group's process in ways that encourage the group to make its own decisions and solve its own problems. The therapist decides how much freedom he or she will allow the group to be self-determining, based on his or her assessment of the level of ego functioning of group members. There is a delicate balance between success and failure, and he or she should not permit the group to become immobilized with frustration when it is truly incapable of doing a task or solving a problem without his or her help. This kind of leadership requires a thorough understanding of group dynamics.

Goals

The goals of groups in the psychoanalytic frame are for clients to develop and practice ego skills. These skills, reviewed from the beginning of the chapter, are reality testing, body image, self-identity, self-esteem, sense of control, and the use of healthy defenses and coping strategies. Providing the foundation for these skills are cognitive, perceptual, and sensorimotor skills. Clients can be encouraged to develop and practice these skills within the group context through the shared working experience of tasks.

Examples of Activities

The group itself should decide on the task, using the resources of its members. Some of the successful task groups are reviewed here. Most tasks offer many opportunities to develop and reinforce ego skills. A few of these are highlighted for each group, but it is likely that many others are also possible.

A Group Newspaper

The group consisted of six Vietnam veterans who exhibited symptoms of substance abuse and post-traumatic stress syndrome. This was significant in their choice of a task. They decided that what was most meaningful to them was to "tell the world the truth" about Vietnam veterans. The group took a trip to the library, where books and articles on the Vietnam war and on post-traumatic stress syndrome were read and notes taken. From the notes, articles were written. Group members added their own stories, poems, and drawings, as well as old newspaper articles they had saved. The result was a 20-page booklet that was typed, copied, collated, and widely distributed to VA hospital clients and staff by the group members.

In this group, members' common self-identity as "the unsung heroes" was reinforced. The task facilitated a sense of control by giving members a vehicle for expression of feelings and opinions that was acceptable in the social environment. Self-esteem was increased by the recognition of their work by others.

Easter Chocolates

The chocolates were really a combination of a product and service project. The group knew of a local residential school for handicapped children and wanted to do something for them. Because Easter was the next holiday, they decided to give them Easter candy. But they were on a limited budget, so they came up with the idea of making candy instead of buying it. Candy molds, baker's chocolate, sugar, and tin foil were the only purchases. Members were able to collect enough old Easter baskets to hold the wrapped candy. The candy was made in the shapes of eggs, chicks, and small bunnies. Members wrapped each piece in foil and placed them in the baskets. Two of the group members delivered the baskets to the staff of the residential school the week before Easter. A week later, they were very proud to receive a big thank you letter from the children.

Self-identity and esteem were reinforced in this group through doing for others. Members learned that they were capable of producing a product that brought pleasure to others and were recognized for their altruism. Identification as a healthy defense was encouraged through nurturing the children (by giving candy) as perhaps they might have wished to be nurtured themselves.

A Walk to the Pet Store

The most important factor to this group was to get away from the hospital. They were psychiatric clients and were not even allowed to walk around the grounds unescorted. In the task group, walking to the pet store gave them a way to go out as a group during scheduled group time, escorted by the OT staff. They decided on the destination because it was only a 15-minute walk, it was always interesting to see, and it would not cost any money. This task group gave them the opportunity to plan something together to meet their needs, restoring in them some sense of control. The sensory stimulation of walking and being in the outdoor environment also increased sensorimotor skills.

Cooking a Spaghetti Dinner

Almost every group seems to enjoy a cooking task. It is relatively short-term, provides enough work for all the members to participate, and satisfies a basic need for everyone—the need to eat. If possible, the group can do the menu planning and shopping, as well as the actual meal preparation. Because spaghetti and salad can feed the whole group for relatively little money, the group was able to afford soft drinks and dessert as well. This group made brownies from a mix before beginning the main course. Members were divided into salad makers, spaghetti makers, dessert makers, and table setters. The meal was enjoyed by the whole group, and everyone was expected to help clean up.

This group requires many adaptive ego functions. Members identify with different roles to work on a realistic goal. They use their skills to cope with their part of the task and receive feedback from others about their performance (reality testing). All of the senses are stimulated through the cooking task, and impulse control is necessary when using the tools and equipment (knives, stove).

Group Car Wash

This task required the cooperation of the hospital or sponsoring institution to provide permission, a space to work, and a source of water. At the VA Hospital, the group took on the responsibility of writing letters to the various hospital administrators asking for permission. The letters were followed up with phone calls from the OT and other staff. Supplies included buckets, soap, rags, sponges, and a nozzle for the hose, most of which were borrowed from relatives and friends. Members prepared for the car wash 1 week ahead by making signs to post all over the hospital. On the day of the car wash, a few group members, accompanied by staff, went outside to post signs and arrows on the street and in the parking lot directing customers to the car wash location. Clients and staff took shifts of 2 hours each for 6 hours. At $3 a car, the group made almost $200, which they spent on a videotape player so the whole ward could watch movies on weekends.

Patience and perseverance were required in the planning of this extended task. There were many opportunities to reality test and reinforce body image (gross motor actions), self-identity (through working roles), and self-esteem (through the concrete result of their effort).

GROUP LEADERSHIP

In this frame of reference, as suggested earlier, the structure of the group is modified to include most of the discussion areas in the context of the activity or task. The activity, sharing, processing, generalizing, and application are not done as separate phases of the group, but are incorporated into the process of doing the task. Because the goal is to develop ego skills, the leader may stop the group whenever an opportunity for members to learn becomes evident. The evaluation portion should include all of the discussion phases of the group and should end with a summary.

Introduction

This part of the group can dispense with the warm-up and replace it with choosing a task. In beginning a task-oriented group, it is helpful for the leader to set forth some ground rules. Some of these will be specific, such as when and where the group will meet, for how long, and the practical limitations to their choice of task, such as availability of supplies. The leader also needs to set forth the expectation that the group will choose a task that they can all work on together and that, once decided, every member of the group is expected to contribute to task accomplishment. Three phases of a task group are introduced:

1. Planning
2. Doing
3. Evaluating

The timeframe may vary according to the task, and a thorough discussion will be delayed until the task itself is finished.

Phase 1—Planning (Step 2: Activity, Part 1)

After a brief introduction by the facilitator, the planning phase begins with brainstorming.

Brainstorming

Brainstorming involves the suggestion of possible tasks for the group by all members. Cooking a meal, planning a group walk, learning to do needlepoint, and making Easter baskets for the pediatric ward are some examples of group tasks. It is often useful for a member of the group to record the ideas. The therapist should caution the group not to make judgments of the ideas suggested during brainstorming, but just to collect a list of ideas.

Persuasion

The next step in planning is persuasion. Members consider the pros and cons of each suggestion and attempt to persuade the group to do one of them. Here, the therapist may need to introduce the idea of meaningfulness. A task that is likely to succeed is one that has meaning for its members. It is very tempting for some groups to plan something easy to accomplish, but often the easy tasks hold little value for the members. This results in member residence in the doing phase. While the therapist should not under any circumstance influence the decision of the group, he or she should perhaps point out that a better decision will be made when the opinions of every member have been voiced and considered.

Interventions of the leader should be carefully thought out so as not to exert more authority than is necessary. Groups with poor ego skills will need more help than those with stronger ego skills. When in doubt, it is best to allow the group to experience the consequences of its actions and then to find something to be learned from whatever happens. OTs often have difficulty with allowing groups to "fail" or to turn out badly. In the task-oriented group, however, it is often from the "failures" that clients can learn the most. Successful groups are of benefit in many ways also, but it is often the failures that promote real therapeutic change.

For example, I have sometimes observed in task-oriented groups with members of varied diagnoses, ages, and functioning levels an inability to make a group decision, even after 45 or 50 minutes of group discussion. Nothing is more frustrating to a group than sitting and doing nothing for an hour because nothing was planned. It is a mistake that groups usually do not make twice. The planning session following such a group usually turns out to be quite productive.

Decision

After more or less persuasion, the group is expected to reach some kind of decision. Group decisions are made in several ways. Someone in the group can take a vote, with the majority ruling. Perhaps a consensus will be reached on the last suggestion discussed; if no one voices an objection, it may be assumed that everyone agrees. A client leader might emerge in the group whose preference might be deferred to by the other members, or a decision can be made by a process of elimination. However the decision is made, it must be considered at some point during planning to be final. Often, the group needs for the decision to be acknowledged and approved by the leader in order to proceed.

Specific Planning and Division of Labor

Once a decision is made, how the task will be accomplished should become the topic of discussion. Questions about what equipment and supplies are needed, how these will be obtained, where the group should be held, and how necessary procedures will be learned are addressed. The facilitator, in this phase, often needs to be a resource to the group, offering his or her knowledge of supply sources, procedures, and space availability. In lower-functioning groups, this information should be offered more readily; in higher-functioning groups, the therapist may offer information only if asked. The discussion of procedures naturally leads to the division of labor (who will do what). It is best when all the planning and preparation can be done by group members. Often, each client is charged with the responsibility of obtaining some item and bringing it to the group. Each member bringing one ingredient for a fruit salad or a pizza is an example of this. In this way, it is easily seen that the success of the group task is dependent on each member of the group remembering and carrying out his or her responsibility.

Phase 2—Doing (Step 2: Activity, Part 2)

It is usually most practical for the doing phase to be done at least a day or two later than the planning. This gives members a chance to prepare adequately. On the day of the activity, gathering and organizing is best left up to group members, although they may need some help. If moving right into activity is something that works for the group, then the leader should allow this. Generally, if careful planning has been done, then not a great deal of time is needed to organize the doing. As members proceed with doing the activity, the facilitator's role may expand to include consulting, advising, and providing information. The leader should be careful to offer these services only when asked or when group disorganization is imminent. It is the role of the facilitator, however, to look for problems and to bring these to the attention of the group along the way. As problems arise, the leader may apprise the group: "Mary seems to be feeling left out" or "Sam seems to be doing all the work." Care should be taken not to suggest solutions until it is evident that the group cannot cope with the problem on its own.

Phase 3—Evaluating (Steps 4 Through 7: Processing, Generalizing, Application, Summary)

Doing is not complete until the task is finished. However, evaluation of the group should be done before the end of every session. Sessions should be sufficiently long to allow for this process to occur. It is usually necessary for the leader to let the group know when it is time to stop doing and start talking. Discussion should focus on the process of the group and the role each member has chosen to play. The discussion phases of processing, generalizing, and application are incorporated into this evaluation phase of task groups.

Reflection of Behavior and Its Consequences

This should be verbalized if members are to learn from their experiences. Why was Mary feeling left out? Did she withdraw because she is shy? Was she seeking attention through nonparticipation? Was she uncertain about how to do her part of the task? Was she threatened by the perceived dominance of another member? How well did the group cope with Mary's problem? How did Mary feel? How did others feel about her? What other choices did the group have regarding Mary? These are the types of issues that should arise in evaluation of the group.

Feelings of Members About the Group

This "processing" aspect is an important part of evaluation. If Sam feels really good about the group, but Mary feels terrible, what are the reasons for this? Could Sam be feeling good because he is doing the whole thing himself and not allowing Mary an opportunity to contribute? How do other members see this? Suppose most of the members are bored with the task. What do they think makes it boring? How are they responsible for the boredom? What can they do about it? A leader should be very reluctant to allow a group to abandon a task partway through. Opportunities to learn should determine what is to be gained or lost from the abandonment. Most of the time, the group can learn more from following through on a task, even if to do so is frustrating and problematic. However, if the group is overwhelmed by frustration, the members' anxiety may interfere with their ability to learn. This is another judgment call that may be difficult for the leader to make.

Evaluation of Task Accomplishment

Finally, an overall evaluation of task accomplishment is in order. How does the group feel about the result? How does it compare with what they hoped for/expected? What did each member contribute to its accomplishment? To what extent did planning affect outcome? It is in this phase that the relationship between thinking, feeling, and behavior is most evident, and the therapist should never miss an opportunity to emphasize it. Good planning (thinking) generally produces successful action (behavior) and results in good feelings about oneself and the group. Concurrently, bad planning often produces an unsuccessful outcome and promotes bad feelings about self and the group. Individual examples of this process might also be pointed out. In all cases, learning from mistakes should be emphasized, so that members develop the strength and skill for making things turn out better next time.

Expressive Therapy Groups

Task-oriented groups are an excellent example of OT intervention using the psychodynamic frame of reference. It is a context in which all of the ego skills discussed can be evaluated and worked on. However, it should be noted that it is not the only approach that works in this frame. Groups that use the symbolic meaning of activities or encourage self-expression through art, poetry, drama, dance/movement, or creative writing are alternative group goals. OT groups that encourage exploring the unconscious and uncovering painful or conflictual memories to be resolved remain a less popular, but an equally legitimate, application of psychodynamic theory.

Art as Therapy

Painting, drawing, and sculpture have traditionally been used as nonverbal projections of the inner self. Many OT evaluations have these media to evaluate internal processes such as self-image, emotions, and perceived relationships with others and with elements of the outside world. For example, if a client with depression draws a volcano erupting, what might that suggest about the client's emotional state? In OT, therapists always ask clients to interpret their own artistic productions, rather than interpreting the content itself. Drawings can become a tool for therapeutic communication in groups, and self-interpretations can be shared as a way of building trust among the members.

Drama as Therapy

Psychodrama was developed by Moreno in the mid-20th century and was considered by some as a powerful therapeutic tool. Clients choose others to play themselves and significant others with whom they have problematic relationships, and the client who is the "protagonist" or main character describes then directs a scene from his or her own life. The techniques for psychodrama are complex and require special training, because the re-enactment of difficult life episodes can open old wounds and leave clients vulnerable to strong emotions. However, there are some dramatic techniques that can be safely used in OT groups, such as role-playing assertiveness skill exercises, conflict-resolution techniques, job interviews, or discussion of interpersonal problems with relatives or friends. Another common dramatic technique is the empty chair. A person who has unfinished business with someone in his or her life imagines that person sitting in the chair opposite them, and speaks as if they were there. This can be especially emotional when the client is saying goodbye to someone who has died or expressing remorse to someone who they have hurt in some way. These techniques should only be tried with groups that have already developed a degree of cohesiveness, and the clients who volunteer to enact a life episode should have adequate time for the group to process the experience. OT leaders who wish to use these techniques should first do further research and/or obtain additional training and be sure they understand how to bring about closure of emotional issues for the client and other group members. People need a high degree of self-awareness to benefit from psychodrama techniques.

Poetry and Creative Writing

One way to encourage spiritual expressions is through the activities involving writing. Poetry can convey the symbolic meaning of occupations and activities. Groups sometimes write a poem together, such as paying tribute to someone leaving the group or expressing feelings about an experience that the group has shared. Writing short poems on greeting cards to send to significant others can be a meaningful group activity using poetry. An example of the therapeutic use of poetry is the expression of emotions by clients with substance abuse, a population that typically has difficulty identifying their own feelings. Letter writing or journal writing are alternate ways that writing can be used as a form of emotional expression. Sharing and discussing one's writing with the group can also help establish trust between members, and they can benefit from giving feedback to one another about the messages conveyed through their stories, letters, and journal entries.

Pet Therapy

One up-and-coming group intervention based on object relations theory is pet therapy. Johnson (2001) defines a pet (animal companion) as "a being whom we have a significant relationship and close connection with, and who lives, works, and plays with us on a daily basis" (p. 201a). People create relationships with animals in order to satisfy needs, use skills, socially engage, and find meaning in life. From an attachment theory perspective, animals provide a means by which individuals can love and be loved unconditionally. The interactive nature of caring for animals is deeply satisfying to many individuals. Pets provide affirmation of the self and an unconditional source of need gratification. Animals can provide a sense of security through their protective nature. Furthermore, service animals have been shown to improve self-esteem, internal locus of control, and psychological well-being in individuals with severe ambulatory diseases (Latella, 2003). There is a growing body of evidence of the benefits of pet ownership as an occupation. Older adults experience attachment, increased self-worth, social integration, and opportunities for nurturance and guidance (Enders-Slegers, 2000). In a descriptive study of pet owners with mental illness, Zimolag and Krupa (2009) looked at the connection between pet ownership and community integration. They found that pet owners demonstrate better social community integration and a higher likelihood of engagement in occupations than non-pet owners. In this sense, pets can facilitate social relationships with other people and can help people with serious mental illness to grow their social networks and to forge community connections that could provide needed social support. The ICF refers to pets as "animals that provide physical, emotional, or psychological support..." (WHO, 2001, p. 188). Pet therapy in groups provides a focus for social interaction as well as physical interaction with a friendly animal such as the dog, Griffin, in Figure 5-1.

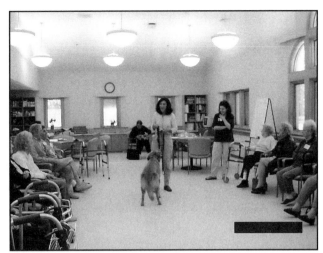

Figure 5-1. Professor Donna Latella conducts a pet therapy session for an older adult day-care group. Baldwin Senior Center, Stratford, CT, reprinted with permission.

REFERENCES

Allport, G. (1958). *Becoming: Basic considerations for a psychology of personality.* New Haven, CT: Yale University Press.

American Occupational Therapy Association. (2008). OT practice framework II: Domain and process. *American Journal of OT, 62,* 625-683.

Arlow, J., & Brenner, C. (1964). *Psychoanalytic concepts and the structural theory.* New York, NY: International University Press.

Bellak, L., Huruich, M., & Gediman, H. (1973). *Ego functions in schizophrenics, neurotics and normals.* New York, NY: Wiley & Sons.

Corey, G. (1991). *Theory and practice of counseling and psychotherapy* (4th ed.). Monterey, CA: Brooks/Cole.

Craib, I. (1994). *The importance of disappointment.* London: Routledge.

Diasio, K. (1968). Psychiatric OT: Search for a conceptual framework in light of psychoanalytic ego psychology and learning theory. *American Journal of OT, XXII*(5), 50-57.

Enders-Slegers, M. J. (2000). The meaning of companion animals: Qualitative analysis of the life histories of elderly cat and dog owners. In A. L. Podberscek, E. S. Paul, & J. A. Serpell (Eds.), *Companion animals and us* (pp. 237-256). Cambridge, England: Cambridge University Press.

Erikson, E. (1950). *Childhood and society.* New York, NY: Norton.

Fairweather, G. W. (1964) *Social psychology in treating mental illness.* New York, NY: Wiley & Sons.

Fidler, G. (1969). The task-oriented group as a context for treatment. *American Journal of OT, XXIII*(1), 43-48.

Fidler, G., & Fidler, J. (1963). *OT: A communication process in psychiatry.* New York, NY: Macmillan Co.

Fidler, G., & Velde, B. (1999). *Activities: Reality and symbol.* Thorofare, NJ: SLACK Incorporated.

Fine, R. (1979). *A history of psychoanalysis.* New York, NY: Columbia University Press.

Freud, A. (1936). *The ego and the mechanisms of defense.* New York, NY: International University Press.

Freud, S. (1914). History of the psychoanalytic movement. In J. Strachey (Ed.), *The standard edition of the complete psychological works of Sigmund Freud.* London: Hogarth.

Greene, L., & Cole, M. (1991). Level and form of psychopathology and the structure of group therapy. *International Journal of Group Psychotherapy, 41*(4), 499-521.

Hartmann, H. (1939). *Ego psychology and the problem of adaptation.* New York, NY: International University Press.

Hasselkus, B. (2002). *The meaning of everyday occupation.* Thorofare, NJ: SLACK Incorporated.

Johnson, C. M. (2001). *Relationships with animals as a component of the healing process: A study of child abusive survivors.* Doctoral dissertation, Union Institute Graduate College, Cincinnati, OH.

Jones, M. (1953). *The therapeutic community: A new treatment method in psychiatry.* New York, NY: Basic Books.

Jung, C. (1910). The association method. *American Journal of Psychology, 21,* 216-269.

Kaplan, H., & Sadock, B. (2003). *Synopsis of psychiatry* (9th ed.). Baltimore, MD: Williams & Wilkins.

Klein, M. (1948). *Contributions to psychoanalysis 1921-1945.* London: Hogarth Press.

Kris, E. (1936). The psychology of characterature. *IJP, 17,* 285-303.

Latella, D. (2003). *Animals as a therapeutic modality: A curriculum model for OT.* Bridgeport, CT: University of Bridgeport Press.

Lewin, K. (1945). *Dynamic theory of personality.* New York, NY: McGraw Hill.

Llorens, L. (1976). *Application of a developmental theory for health and rehabilitation.* Rockville, MD: American OT Association.

Llorens, L., & Johnson, P. (1966). OT in an ego-oriented milieu. *American Journal of OT, XX*(4), 178-181.

Llorens, L., & Rubin, E. (1967). *Developing ego functions in disturbed children.* Detroit, MI: Wayne State University Press.

Mosey, A. (1970a). *Three frames of reference for mental health.* Thorofare, NJ: SLACK Incorporated.

Mosey, A. (1970b). The concept and use of developmental groups. *American Journal of OT, XXIV*(4), 272-275.

Mosey, A. (1981). *OT: Configuration of a profession.* New York, NY: Raven Press.

Mosey, A. (1986). *Psychosocial components of OT.* New York, NY: Raven Press.

Murray, H. A. (1951). Uses of the thematic apperception test. *American Journal of Psychiatry, 107,* 577-581.

Nicholls, L. (2007). A psychoanalytic discourse in OT. In J. Creek & D. Lawson-Porter (Eds.), *Contemporary issues in OT: Reasoning and reflection.* Hoboken, NJ: Wiley.

Rapaport, D. (1942). *Emotions and memory.* New York, NY: Harper.

Rapaport, D. (1953). On the psychoanalytic theory of affects. *IJP, 34,* 177-198.

Rorschach, H. (1921). *Psychodiagnostics: A diagnostic rest based on perception.* New York, NY: Grune & Stratton.

Spitz, R. (1959). *A genetic field theory ego formation: Its implications for pathology.* New York, NY: International University Press.

Wechsler, D. (1981). *Wechsler Adult Intelligence Scale* (Rev. ed.). New York, NY: The Psychological Corporation.

White, R. (1967). *Competence and the growth of personality. In Science and psychoanalysis: Vol. XI: The ego.* New York, NY: Grune & Stratton.

World Health Organization. (2001). *International classification of functioning, disability, and health (ICF).* Geneva, Switzerland: Author.

Zimolag, U., & Krupa, T. (2009). Pet ownership as a meaningful community occupation for people with serious mental illness. *American Journal of OT, 63,* 126-137.

Psychodynamic Activity Example 5-1
Out on the Town

Materials: Colored crayons or pastels and 9- x 12-inch white drawing paper for each member.

Directions: Imagine that it is Saturday night and you have big plans. Choose anyone you like to be your companion—a significant other, a relative, a friend, even someone you have not yet met. Write the name of this person at the top of the paper.

Next, think about where you would like to be going—a romantic dinner, a concert, a play or movie, a sports event, a social event—really anything you can imagine.

Now, draw yourself, as you imagine, ready to go out for the evening. Pay attention to how you would look, what you would be wearing, and what would be your emotional state. Choose colors that represent your emotions as well as your outward appearance. You have 20 minutes to complete this drawing, so do not worry about artistic perfection.

Psychodynamic Activity Example 5-2
My Room

Materials: 8½- x 11-inch white paper, pencils with erasers, and rulers for each member. Colored pencils may also be used.

Directions: Introduce yourself by saying your name and recalling a name your parents called you before you were 5 years old or recalling a toy you remember playing with as a child.

Use the paper, pencil, and ruler to draw the floor plan of the room you slept in as a child. Try to remember as much about the room as you can.

- What was its size and shape?
- Whom did you share it with, if anyone?
- What color was it (paint, wallpaper)?
- Where was the bed? The window? Other furniture?
- Where did you keep your clothes and belongings?
- How old were you when you began sleeping there?
- What do you remember doing in this room besides sleeping?
- What else was in the room (carpets, curtains)?
- How did the bed look (bedspread, pillows, stuffed toys)?
- How did it feel to be in the room (sunny, dark)?
- What did it smell like?
- What was on the floor?

When you feel that you have a sense of this memory, begin drawing. You have 25 minutes to complete this floor plan.

From Cole, M. B. *Group dynamics in OT: The theoretical basis and practice application of group intervention* (4th ed.). Thorofare, NJ: SLACK Incorporated. © 2012 SLACK Incorporated.

Psychodynamic Activity Example 5-3
Pass the Hat

Materials: A collection of various hats (e.g., sun visor, cowboy, baseball, ski hat, beret, etc.).

Directions: Choose a hat from the center of the circle and try it on. Think about who might wear this hat. As you introduce yourself, describe for what occasion you might wear a hat like this, if ever.

Put the hats back in the center of the circle. Now ask someone to volunteer to begin a story about a character wearing one of these hats. If no one volunteers, the leader may begin the story. After 1 minute, the first person stops and passes the hat to the next person in the circle. That person continues the story for 1 minute, and on around the circle. At any time during the storytelling, a member may choose to change the main character or add a new character by choosing a different hat. Ask members to describe interaction between the characters.

Discussion centers around the fantasized characters.

- Who did you like or dislike?
- Who do you know that any imagined characters reminded you of?
- Who are you versus who you might rather be?
- How would you change if you could?
- Which hat fits most comfortably?
- What does your imagination say about yourself?

From Cole, M. B. *Group dynamics in OT: The theoretical basis and practice application of group intervention* (4th ed.). Thorofare, NJ: SLACK Incorporated. © 2012 SLACK Incorporated.

Psychodynamic Activity Example 5-4
A Poem for Myself

Materials: Pens and paper for each member and an assortment of used greeting cards (e.g., birthday, anniversary, wedding, sympathy, get well, friendship) that contain some form of a short poem.

Directions: Ask members to choose a greeting card and read the poem to the group. Collect the cards, and put them away. Give out pens and paper. Ask members to think about how they are feeling right now and what kind of card they might like to receive from someone. Ideas for this may be shared and discussed.

You have 15 minutes to write the first draft of a poem to yourself. This may be written as if it were from someone specific or may be anonymous. The poem does not have to rhyme. It does not have to be in complete sentences. However, it should contain some words of inspiration relating to your current emotional state. Possible themes include the following:

- Needing a friend
- Sharing a joy
- Feeling alone
- Praying for guidance
- Missing someone
- Wishing to be healed
- Finding something (or someone) that was lost
- Discovering the truth about yourself

From Cole, M. B. *Group dynamics in OT: The theoretical basis and practice application of group intervention* (4th ed.). Thorofare, NJ: SLACK Incorporated. © 2012 SLACK Incorporated.

Psychodynamic Activity Example 5-5
Introducing the Empty Chair

Materials: 3- x 5-inch index cards and pens. Members sit in a circle with one extra chair in the center.

Directions: Everyone has troubled relationships in their lives. Is there someone you wish you could become emotionally closer to or have more supportive of you? As you introduce yourself, say a few words about someone in your life with whom you might like to have a better relationship.

Now, on the index card, write the name of one such individual. Then, write the answers to the following questions:

- How is this person related to you (relative, spouse, friend, parent, neighbor)? Write a few sentences about the quality of this relationship.
- Where and when did the relationship begin?
- How many years have you known this person?
- What activities did you share with this person? Describe one such activity.
- When and where was your last meeting?
- Describe the nature of your most recent interaction.
- What about your relationship with this person do you wish to change?
- What would make the relationship better?

Sharing: When members have finished writing, ask them to focus on the empty chair in the center of the circle and imagine the person each member has chosen seated in it. Members then take turns standing behind the chair and introducing their significant person to the rest of the group, giving details from their writing.

Discussion: Focus on mutual support and give-and-take of relationships. Encourage feedback and suggestions.

From Cole, M. B. *Group dynamics in OT: The theoretical basis and practice application of group intervention* (4th ed.). Thorofare, NJ: SLACK Incorporated. © 2012 SLACK Incorporated.

Psychodynamic Activity Example 5-6
Paint Your Day

Materials: Roll of bond paper large enough to cover the center of a 72-inch oblong table, 12 poster paints in a variety of colors, a paintbrush for each color, large jars of water, and sponges for cleaning up. No chairs are allowed.

Directions: Group members (no more than eight) introduce themselves and describe how they are feeling today. They are then instructed to do a group mural. The group members take a few minutes to organize how they will do the painting, such as if there will be a "top" and a "bottom" and how space will be divided. Members are encouraged to move around the table as they paint and to exchange colors as they wish. The subjects should relate to the feelings presented and should not be reality oriented (e.g., garden scene, ocean scene). Abstract shapes and symbols are best. About 20 minutes usually suffices to cover most of the surface of the paper.

Discussion: This centers around how members interacted with each other, as shown in the group mural. Sharing will reveal each member's painted creations, as well as what they might mean to that individual. Overassertive or bold painting, color choices, and shapes and lines all reveal emotional states as well as personality traits. Group roles may also be identified this way (e.g., imitator, follower, orienter, elaborator, etc.). Refer to Chapter 2 for a review of potential group roles.

From Cole, M. B. *Group dynamics in OT: The theoretical basis and practice application of group intervention* (4th ed.). Thorofare, NJ: SLACK Incorporated. © 2012 SLACK Incorporated.

Chapter 6

The Behavioral Cognitive Continuum

From a historical perspective, most of the cognitive frames of reference in OT are derived from "learning theory," which grew from the roots of behaviorism in the 1930s and 1940s. The works of Skinner, Pavlov, and others revolutionized the field of psychology by applying the scientific method to human behavior. This idea was directly opposed to the concept of the unconscious in psychoanalytic theories because behaviorists believed that only what was "observable and measurable" could legitimately be the subject of scientific study. Modern-day thinking has mellowed the radical thinking of early behaviorism. Most current theories include cognition in the definition of observable behavior and acknowledge the internal control of the individual. However, some concepts from behaviorism remain useful and may be recognized in the OT practice of today. Therefore, this chapter begins with an overview of those behavioral concepts that still apply to group leadership in OT: behavioral objectives, conditioning and habits, shaping and chaining, rehearsal and practice, modeling, and reinforcement.

Next, the biomechanical approach is briefly reviewed. While this frame is not usually included in a behavioral or cognitive context, therapy in the biomechanical frame of reference relies on behavioral concepts such as practice and repetition, behavioral objectives, and the formation of good habits of posture and body mechanics and often requires external reinforcement. The biomechanical frame of reference also provides the background for certain cognitive-behavioral techniques, such as biofeedback, progressive relaxation, and systematic desensitiza-

tion, which are useful in groups when addressing issues like stress management, the management of pain, or the modulation of emotions. Frames previously described as rehabilitative or acquisitional, including those of Denton, Mosey, and Trombly, are briefly included as their concepts contribute to group intervention.

Several different cognitive approaches are then described in this chapter. The first is "cognitive rehabilitation," including Giles' (2005) neurofunctional model, Auerbuch and Katz's cognitive retraining, Abreu and Peloquin's quadraphonic model, and the cognitive perceptual model developed by Abreu and Toglia (1987) and its various updates—the "multicontextual approach" (Toglia, 1991; Toglia, Golisz, & Coverover, 2009) and the "dynamic interactional approach" (Toglia, 1997, 2005). Toglia's theory has recently moved away from its original focus on separate and distinct cognitive subskills toward a more integrated systems approach. This model uses the works of Luria, a noted Russian brain physiologist, and other current brain research to develop a more holistic approach to perception and cognition that focuses on self-awareness and generalization of learning. This theory, as updated, is particularly well-suited to group intervention, especially as it impacts "metacognition," or the ability to monitor, regulate, and predict one's own functional performance.

The second set of concepts discussed in this chapter is cognitive-behavioral therapy (CBT). Duncombe (2005) has presented this approach as a legitimate OT frame of reference, which uses principles similar to those used in its psychological counterpart. Cognitive behaviorism is

Cole M.B. *Group Dynamics in OT:
The Theoretical Basis and Practice Application
of Group Intervention (pp 155-192).*
© 2012 SLACK Incorporated.

Table 6-1

Summary of Behavioral Cognitive Continuum

	Behavioral, Behavior Modification	Biomechanical, Rehabilitative	Cognitive, Rehabilitation, Multicontextual	Cognitive-Behavioral Dialectical
Theorists	Skinner, Pavlov, Bandura	Trombly, Denton, Mosey, Fidler	Toglia, Giles, Abreu, Peloquin, Averbuch, Katz	Beck, Ellis, Lazarus, Linehan
Client Applicatons	All populations	Physically disabled	Brain injury, stroke, mental illness	Mental illness, emotional aspects, character disorders
Concepts and Techniques	Goals and objectives, conditioning and habits, shaping and chaining, reinforcement, rehearsal and practice, role playing and role reversal, systematic desensitization	Strength, ROM, endurance, positioning, prevention, restoration, compensation, adaptation, skill acquisition, lifestyle performance, biofeedback	Orientation, attention, neglect, motor planning, visual processing, self-awareness, executive functions, metacognition, generalization, transfer of learning	Social learning, modeling, self-regulation, cognitive distortions, automatic thoughts, disputing irrational beliefs, cognitive restructuring, dialectical strategies
OT Group Themes	Graded tasks, social skills training, assertiveness, relaxation, stress, time or emotion management, coping skills training, conflict management	Group exercise, group games involving movement, graded strength and endurance, prevention education, social ADL activities, work readiness, work hardening	Strategies for all cognitive areas, multiple contexts, group discussions of strategy generalizations, self-skill assessments, community integration	Psychoeducational groups, reading, films, discussion, role-playing groups, worksheets and discussion, interpersonal effectiveness, emotion regulation, distress tolerance, mindfulness

one of the most frequently used in mental or behavioral health settings for several reasons. It sounds simple and logical, it easily lends itself to advances in technology, such as computer programming and biofeedback, and it is appropriate and useful in short-term intervention. OTs use the psychoeducational approach from cognitive behaviorism in treating clients on a verbal and symbolic level. To benefit from this approach, it is suggested that clients be capable of learning through logic and reasoning. The principal spokesmen for the cognitive-behavioral therapies in psychology are Aaron Beck, Albert Ellis, and Albert Bandura. A more recent outgrowth of cognitive behaviorism used by OTs, called "Dialectical Behavior Therapy (DBT)" developed by Linehan (1993a), is described. This approach is widely used and is a basis of group intervention with psychiatric populations. Both CBT and DBT share the guiding principle that therapy should focus on the cognitive process and that changes in thinking will produce adaptive changes in client behavior.

FRAMEWORK FOCUS

This group of approaches, some more behavioral, others more cognitive, were all developed through application of the scientific method to human behavior. They can be expressed in a continuum as shown in Table 6-1.

Behavioral approaches are most ideal when addressing the need for learning or changing client performance patterns in the *OT Practice Framework-II* (AOTA, 2008). Contexts will be examined in identifying "cues," which can either facilitate function or trigger maladaptive behaviors in any of the areas of occupation. Cognitive-behavioral approaches are the top choice when self-control and self-management are primary concerns. This approach includes theories of learning, which are especially useful in promoting client performance skills, whether motor, process, or communication/interaction skills.

BASIC ASSUMPTIONS

Behavioral Concepts

This section selects for review those behavioral concepts that still appear as an integral part of OT: behavioral goals and objectives, conditioning and habits, shaping and chaining, reinforcement, and rehearsal and practice.

Behavioral Goals and Objectives

One of the most fundamental contributions of behaviorism is the concept of behavioral goals. Only observable behavior was thought to be an appropriate focus for intervention. Therefore, behavioral goals and objectives should always be observable and measurable. The early behaviorists taught us to identify problems narrowly and specifically, so that focused intervention could be designed and its effects measured. The goals for our OT groups should be written in specific, measurable terms, so that necessary documentation of progress is possible. Often, these goals are set by the clients and therapist together, and progress toward the goals is openly discussed with the group. In cognitive-behavioral groups, an evaluation of the group should be set up to see if goals are met. Worksheets 6-1 through 6-3 are designed to help students learn how to write behavioral goals.

Long-term goals are not always measurable. Sometimes, when we set lifetime goals, such as "Be successful at my job," it is not clear what it is that success really means. Even when these goals are measurable, such as "become a millionaire by age 40,"' how these goals will be accomplished remains unplanned. Until these goals are broken down into smaller, doable steps, they will remain only dreams. Short-term, measurable goals are the actions and behaviors that help us and our clients make dreams a reality. A measurable goal is one that describes behavior that can be observed. For example, your goal might be to improve self-esteem. How can you tell when self-esteem has improved? What behaviors would you look for? What actions could you take? Some possibilities might be standing taller, taking more care in dressing and hygiene to look your best, and verbalizing several positive aspects of yourself.

The measurable goals in Worksheet 6-2 are 2, 4, 9, 10, 12, 14, 15, 17, and 18. One key to writing a measurable goal is the language used. Words like *learn, understand, encourage, improve, handle,* and *manage* are vague because they do not specify how these things can be accomplished. Measurable goals are usually specific, and they incorporate behaviors that can be observed. Words like *define, list, discuss,* and *complete* refer to either words or actions that can be readily observed, heard, or read. In the cognitive-behavioral frame of reference, thoughts are also considered to be behavior. However, thoughts must be verbalized in order to be measurable.

Conditioning and Habits

Pavlov has been credited with identifying classical conditioning as a process through which much of human behavior is learned. When a piece of chocolate candy is placed in the mouth, the mouth waters, and the person experiences a pleasant taste sensation. The autonomic response is soon associated with the visual stimuli, so that it only takes a glance at the candy bar in the store window to make the mouth water. Likewise, many associations in the brain are formed that attach meaning to incoming stimuli. Pavlov was able to recreate this phenomenon in the laboratory, and he called it "classical conditioning." Much of today's advertising uses this principle (Corey, 1996).

Skinner (1953) identified a more complex, but less controlled form of learning, which he called "operant conditioning." According to this principle, behavior that is reinforced by the environment tends to be repeated, while behavior that is discouraged or ignored tends to become extinct or disappear. Humans are continually subjected to random or chance reinforcement as they go through life, causing maladaptive as well as constructive learning. Therapy, therefore, must involve the identification and control of environmental factors that reinforce a behavior, so that the stage can be set for positive behavior change.

The development of habits is explained by the principle of operant conditioning. People repeat behaviors that are reinforced repeatedly until they become habitual, but once a habit is formed, reinforcement is no longer necessary. Habits are routine or customary ways of doing things. James (1985) explains that an "acquired habit, from a physiological point of view, is nothing but a new pathway of discharge formed in the brain, by which certain incoming currents ever after tend to escape" (p. 55). This statement implies that certain stimuli, when encountered in the environment, evoke predictable responses that have been "conditioned" or learned. Waking up in a familiar environment, most people can wash, dress, eat breakfast, and otherwise get ready for the day, without much conscious thought. James writes that "habit diminishes the conscious attention with which our acts are performed" (1985, p. 59). In the above example, the familiar objects in the environment serve as stimuli for the habitual performance of these necessary tasks, so that brain energy is reserved for the more challenging tasks at work or school. Using this principle, cognitive rehabilitation seeks to re-establish habitual ways of performing functional tasks after brain trauma. When familiar ways of accomplishing a task are no longer possible, new pathways must be formed through the rehearsal and practice of the most efficient alternative strategies.

Worksheet 6-1
Writing Long-Term Goals

Directions: Begin by writing your lifetime goals for yourself. Write at least one goal for each of the following categories.

1. Professional

2. Educational

3. Monetary

4. Family

5. Health

6. Social

7. Spiritual

8. Emotional

9. Recreational

10. Creative

Worksheet 6-2
Recognizing Measurable Goals

Directions: From the list below, circle the goals that you find measurable.

1. Encourage decision making.

2. List one strength and one weakness.

3. Develop a better self-concept.

4. Discuss feelings about parents.

5. Relate better to authority figures.

6. Manage time better.

7. Conserve energy in cooking a meal.

8. Handle frustration.

9. Demonstrate pride in personal accomplishment.

10. Plan a weekend activity and carry it out.

11. Define assertive behavior.

12. Complete a task within time limit.

13. Relieve stress.

14. Eat a well-balanced diet.

15. Plan time to study for a test.

16. Take responsibility for behavior.

17. Attend school regularly.

18. Stay on a diet 80% of the time.

19. Understand yourself better.

20. Strengthen feminine/masculine identity.

Worksheet 6-3
Making Our Lifetime Goals Measurable

Directions: In Worksheet 6-1, we wrote down some lifetime goals. First, go back to that list and check off which of those goals are measurable. Next, choose three goals from your list that are not measurable, and write them down below. For each one, list several measurable short-term goals or steps to be completed.

Lifetime Goal 1
1.

2.

3.

4.

5.

Lifetime Goal 2
1.

2.

3.

4.

5.

Lifetime Goal 3
1.

2.

3.

4.

5.

From Cole, M. B. *Group dynamics in OT: The theoretical basis and practice application of group intervention* (4th ed.). Thorofare, NJ: SLACK Incorporated. © 2012 SLACK Incorporated.

Shaping and Chaining

Skinner once demonstrated, before a large audience, teaching a live pigeon to turn around using the technique of shaping. The pigeon's cage was set on the stage, where it could be readily seen. Using the principle of operant conditioning, he waited until the pigeon turned slightly in the desired direction and reinforced this behavior with a pellet of food. Each time the pigeon turned a little farther in the desired direction, it was reinforced again with a pellet of food. Within 2 or 3 minutes, the pigeon had learned to turn a full 360 degrees before being reinforced. The technique of shaping requires that each step in a sequence be reinforced until the entire task is learned. When OTs analyze activities, we break them down into component parts, or steps. Instructing a client in using a reacher, for example, we may begin with the correct grip, then practice the movements of the handle and, finally, practice picking up first lighter, then heavier objects. We may use approval or praise after each step is done correctly, without even realizing that we are using reinforcement to shape the client's behavior.

Chaining refers to the learning of steps in a specific sequence, so that each action serves as the stimulus to provoke the next action (James, 1985). When a sequence follows along smoothly, A-B-C-D, without hesitation or making a decision among alternatives, then the sequence has become a habit. James suggests that it is the sensation of the movement just finished that provides reinforcement and signals readiness for what comes next.

Reinforcement

From the discussion of behavioral concepts so far, it is evident that reinforcement comes in many forms. Early behaviorists identified reinforcement as external to the individual. Positive reinforcement is a reward, something desirable to the individual: an edible treat, a gold star, a hug, words of praise, a paycheck. In negative reinforcement, something desirable is removed: privileges, freedom, participation in a social or recreational activity, a holiday. Later behaviorists believed that reinforcement can also be internal. Bandura, a cognitive-behavioral theorist, identified two kinds of internal reinforcers: vicarious and self-produced. Vicarious reinforcers are symbolic, such as a person's learned images of success and failure or reflections of his or her values and ideals. Self-produced reinforcers come from the person's sense of competence, efficacy, and self-control. In other words, feeling good about oneself is reinforcing.

Bandura's hierarchy of reinforcement is helpful in understanding and planning learning experiences for our client groups. The levels of reinforcers progress from simple to more complex as they parallel the developmental sequence:

- Initial reinforcers refer to the external ones such as food, attention, and approval.

- Symbolic reinforcers are internal images or messages regarding probable consequences of behavior. An example of this is a child refraining from going outside in his or her yard because he or she remembers how angry his or her mother got the last time he or she did it.

- Social contract refers to more complex or role-dependent behavior such as performing a job or honoring one's marriage vows.

- Personal satisfaction is the best and most effective reinforcer in Bandura's opinion because it is the least dependent upon external circumstances, and therefore the least vulnerable to extinction. When feelings of self-satisfaction or self-worth result from particular behaviors, those behaviors tend to be repeated.

Because reinforcement is what motivates learning, the OT seeking to motivate a group of clients must decide what level of reinforcement the group members can respond to. Even when treating adults, we may need to fall back on external reinforcement when motivation for therapy is found lacking.

Rehearsal and Practice

A popular technique associated with the behavioral approach is assertiveness training. This group activity requires the rehearsal and practice of newly learned assertive behaviors through group role playing and, subsequently, trying out the new behaviors in real-life situations. The leader first uses self-awareness exercises to help the members analyze their own habitual responses to difficult situations as either passive, aggressive, or assertive.

- *Passive:* The individual does not state his or her feelings or stand up for his or her rights, and usually does not get what he or she wants.

- *Aggressive:* The individual insists on his or her rights, lets his or her feelings explode, and gets what he or she wants by abusing the rights and hurting the feelings of others.

- *Assertive:* The individual expresses his or her feelings and requests that his or her rights be honored. He or she may not always get his or her way, but his or her behavior encourages mutual respect and open communication.

Hypothetical situations may be presented by the leader, which are likely to be familiar, such as

- Just as you reach the ticket counter at the movies after a 20-minute wait, someone cuts ahead of you in line.

- A group of friends with whom you are talking decide spontaneously to meet at an unfamiliar restaurant for coffee. You'd like to join them, but you do not know how to get there.

- You receive a credit card bill for an item you did not buy.
- While driving you to an unfamiliar doctor's office for an appointment, your friend makes a wrong turn and becomes lost. He or she refuses to stop to ask directions.
- You have made your spouse (significant other) a special birthday dinner, and he or she shows up an hour late, with no explanation or apology.

The group discusses each situation with regard to the following: What would I typically do? Is my response passive, aggressive, or assertive? What would be an appropriate assertive response? The exact words of an assertive response are then practiced by each member. The key is to focus on the verbal expression of feeling or statement of legitimate rights, followed by a request for change or action. Using incomplete sentences and asking each member to fill in the blanks might be a good place to start: I feel ____ when you ____ . I request that you ____ . Hypothetical and real situations are rehearsed and practiced through role playing, group discussion, giving and receiving feedback, and homework. Most people have difficulty behaving assertively, and people with disabilities are especially vulnerable. Assertiveness group members should be encouraged to provide one another emotional support when attempts at assertive behavior outside the group do not bring expected results. Reinforcement for assertive behavior must initially come from the group leader and members, until it is practiced often enough, and with enough success, to become a part of the individual's habitual response repertoire. (For further ideas on assertiveness groups, see Posthuma, 2002.)

Many functional skills addressed in OT require rehearsal and practice. The cognitive rehabilitation approach stresses the rehearsal of cognitive strategies in a variety of clinical contexts and practice of skills over a range of possible applications. Giving groups specific homework assignments encourages the practice of skills in real-life contexts. Discussion of the results of practice allows the group leader and members to provide "reinforcement" in a controlled and predictable way.

Role Playing

According to Posthuma (2002), role playing evolved from the practice of psychodrama, in which the client (protagonist) directs his or her own real-life situation by choosing other members of the group to play the roles of significant others. As a behavioral technique, the structure of role playing remains the same, but the focus is slightly different. In OT groups, playing roles provides a forum for practice and rehearsal of new behaviors within a safe and supportive therapeutic environment. Members recall or anticipate difficult situations in their own lives and bring them to the therapy setting in constructing the role play. Each role play has four parts, according to Posthuma (2002):

1. Definition of the problem
2. Assuming the roles
3. Enactment
4. Discussion

For example, a client anticipating a return to work after a long absence may choose others to play co-workers, supervisors, or clients/customers. The client (protagonist) tells each member how to play his or her role, and the furniture in the room can be rearranged to resemble the work setting for a more realistic effect. Although the protagonist may play him- or herself the first time through, it is often helpful for another member to play that role or to reverse roles. As a learning tool, role reversal has the advantage of helping the protagonist to see the situation from the other's point of view. The purpose of role playing is to practice new behaviors, develop insight into a situation, develop empathy with others, anticipate consequences, increase self-confidence, and/or decrease anxiety. A discussion of the role play allows the other members of the group to give feedback and support to the protagonist and reveals its meaning for all the group members. Role plays are also models for social learning (described later in the section on cognitive-behavioral therapies).

Systematic Desensitization and Biofeedback

These techniques have elements of both behavioral and cognitive theory. Systematic desensitization has been used successfully by clinical psychologists in interventions with phobias, such as fear of flying, and has been less successfully used to control addictions, such as drinking or smoking. The first step in desensitization is to evoke a state of relaxation, usually using some form of progressive muscle tension and release sequences combined with visualization. The "progressive" part involves the introduction of images of the feared object/situation in graded degrees of severity. For example, the person with fear of flying would begin by visualizing the drive to the airport and gradually work up to the plane taking off, while maintaining a state of relaxation. The entire process requires a series of sessions, often over a period of several months. Psychologists are required to get special training before attempting this technique. However, the same concepts form the basis of many group activities used in OT. Progressive muscle relaxation takes on many forms and may be used in OT groups dealing with stress management or as a coping strategy when faced with any situation that tends to evoke anxiety. Guided fantasy is a form of visualization that is useful for group intervention. Although feared images should be avoided, pleasant ones may be very powerful motivators. For example, the group may begin by closing their eyes, breathing deeply, and imagining themselves lying on a sunny beach, listening to the rhythm of the ocean waves as they break along the shore. This visual image sets the stage for relaxation and prepares them for learning other useful strategies for the control of anxiety, anger, frustration, and other causes of distress.

Biofeedback refers to the monitoring of bodily functions, such as pulse, respiration rate, heart rate, and body temperature. Stein and Nikolic (1989) suggest using biofeedback in conjunction with other stress-management techniques. Mechanical monitoring devices are used to give clients information about how their mental state affects them physically. Various mental strategies can then be learned to help people gain control over their own physiological responses to stress. Biofeedback is often combined with visualization and relaxation techniques. It is also used in the biomechanical approach to monitor the effects of movement and exercise and as a safety precaution to prevent overexertion in any physically strenuous activity.

Biomechanical Approach

Note: This approach overlaps with the sensorimotor approaches covered in Chapter 9. It is included here because of its reliance on theories of learning.

This approach is primarily appropriate for clients who lack range of motion (ROM), strength, and endurance to perform daily life tasks (Trombly & Radomski, 2002). The whole is considered to be the sum of its parts: single muscles making up muscle groups or synergies, tasks divided into force and resistance, angles and directions, and rearranged into positions and movement sequences. Therefore, behavior can be broken down into its component subskills for the purpose of easier learning. The theory draws upon the kinetic principles of human movement, and its goals are to prevent injury, restore function, and/or compensate for lost function. These are some of the same principles of strength and effort that are presently associated with work hardening.

The biomechanical frame of reference is included here because it uses the behavioral principles of conditioning, habit formation, shaping and chaining, and rehearsal and practice with the goal of restoring function. Adaptation and compensation are often required when injury or illness results in chronic physical disability. Behavioral goals and objectives are set, and effects of intervention are carefully measured. Because recovery from physical loss often requires multiple repetition, building these repetitions into meaningful group activities can be helpful and motivating.

Range of Motion

The maximum motion of every joint in every possible direction is called its ROM. Average ROMs for each joint in each direction have been calculated, so that deviation from the norm, or limitation of ROM, can be determined. There are many causes of limitation in ROM; some are head injury, stroke, burns, fractures, arthritis, and peripheral nerve injury. ROM is measured with a goniometer, which, when applied to the joint, determines the angle or number of degrees the joint can move. For example, the typical ROM of the elbow joint is 0 to 150 degrees. The ROM can be measured actively—"Lift your arm high over your head" (AROM)—or passively—"Let me flex and extend your shoulder" (PROM). Specific guidelines for measuring ROM for each joint may be found in Trombly and Radomski (2002).

In OT, activities are devised to encourage the client to increase and/or maintain range of motion. Particularly in groups of clients who are at risk, such as those with arthritis, multiple sclerosis, or post-head trauma or stroke, exercise "classes" to maintain/extend range of motion are common. Crafts and games can be adapted by positioning them in a way that forces the client to reach, bend, push, pull, or grasp in order to accomplish the goal. Care should be taken to plan the right amount of movement, because overestimating it can easily cause injury. A creative activity using this approach is the "Range of Motion Dance," a supportive exercise group format for clients post-stroke to maintain their range of motion (Harlowe & Yu, 1997; Van Deusen & Harlowe, 1987).

Strength

Muscle weakness is another common problem treated in OT with physical disabilities. When illness or injury results in specific muscle weakness, or when weakness can potentially cause deformity, activities can be devised to increase muscle strength. Strength can be increased in several ways. Stress is applied to a muscle or muscle group by increase in load or weight. Lifting objects of gradually increased weight will strengthen the muscles. Duration of muscle contraction also influences strength. Holding a position or lifting and holding a heavy object for longer and longer intervals can increase strength. The rate and frequency of the contraction also affect strength; faster or more frequent exercise increases strength, even when lighter weight is used. Any combination of these parameters when applied to exercise has been found to increase strength. The challenge for the OT is to find activities that can be graded in load, duration, rate, and frequency, so that strength can be increased gradually and without injury. Craft activities, such as sanding wood or weaving on a loom, have traditionally been adapted to accomplish these goals. When treating in groups, work activities such as gardening and landscaping, cleaning and moving furniture, or stocking shelves might accomplish the goals of increasing strength.

Endurance

Endurance refers to the length of time muscles can continue to work without becoming fatigued. A person can sustain isometric contraction equivalent to 50% of maximum voluntary contraction (MVC) up to 1 minute. In normal subjects, contraction time and percentage of

MVC are inversely related (Trombly & Radomski, 2002). For example, if Sally carries a 50-pound bag of dog food from her car up three flights of stairs to her apartment, she will need to sustain a 50% MVC for 2 minutes. Chances are it will be necessary for Sally to stop and rest after 1 minute before continuing. However, if she carries a 25-pound bag of dog food, she can sustain a 25% MVC for the 2 minutes it takes her to walk all the way to her apartment without resting.

In OT, endurance may be increased by using moderately fatiguing activities for progressively longer periods of time. In groups, the OT can offer activities that sustain interest over the needed increases in duration. Many active games and sports can be adapted to the goal of increasing strength and endurance. Tug of war, for example, can be timed so that the length of effort progressively increases with each round. Relay races, perhaps carrying progressively heavier items, can be graded also.

Prevention, Restoration, and Compensation

Particularly in the workplace, prevention of injury and maintenance of health are important areas for OT intervention. Insurance companies, worker's compensation, and other third-party payers are hiring OT consultants to organize educational groups in the use of correct body mechanics, positioning and seating, environmental adaptations, and energy-saving strategies to help save the cost of worker absence and medical intervention due to preventable injuries. In addition, educational groups for people with specific injuries, such as carpal tunnel syndrome or osteoarthritis, will help them learn good health maintenance strategies.

Restoration of function is defined within the context of developing client competence in performing occupational roles. The client should identify the roles he or she will continue (e.g., worker, spouse, club member, friend). The roles played, in turn, help define the tasks the individual must learn or relearn. The goals are specific, and OT intervention centers around accomplishing those specific goals or tasks that the client has identified as his or her preferences.

The OT uses a compensation strategy for clients who need to live with a disability on a temporary or permanent basis. Using this approach, the client with physical disability uses his or her remaining abilities to perform needed tasks. OT helps the client to develop strategies or use adaptive equipment that can compensate for the loss of physical capacities in order to accomplish activities of daily living. The OT organizes the environment, then motivates and reinforces the client toward successful completion of the task. Adaptations, compensations, and adaptive equipment may be incorporated. Competence in doing the task is achieved through repetition and practice.

Acquisitional Approaches— Mosey, Denton, Trombly

The above approach to the rehabilitation of physical disabilities has previously been called "acquisitional" by Mosey (1986) and others. Denton (1987) called it "functional performance," and Trombly called it simply the "rehabilitative approach" (Trombly & Radomski, 2002). This refers to the process of relearning lost skills in activities of daily living and other areas of occupation due to physical disability. Rehabilitation in OT occurs on a continuum of restoration-adaptation-compensation. That is, foundation skills of movement, strength, endurance, and perception are remediated or brought to the highest level of recovery possible within the limitations of the illness or injury. Adaptations in everyday functioning are then made to maximize that level of recovery through using special equipment, changing the task demand, or altering the environment. When full recovery is not anticipated, compensatory strategies are then substituted for skills that have been lost or compromised. This practical approach to rehabilitation is so well-known in OT that it has not really needed an official "name." However, the 2002 edition of Trombly and Radomski elaborates on the approach using many names. One of these, the task-oriented OT approach, is described in Chapter 9.

Two related approaches worthy of mention here are Mosey's "role acquisition" and Fidler's "lifestyle performance profile" (Robertson, 1988).

Role Acquisition

Mosey addresses the role acquisition approach to those individuals whose disability has stabilized and who continue to have difficulty in performance of tasks of their major social roles (Robertson, 1988). She identifies the basic skills common to all social roles as task skills and interpersonal skills. These basic skills are necessary building blocks for the performance of self-care (activities of daily living), family interaction, recreation, and work. Temporal adaptation, or skill in the perception and use of time, serves to organize and balance the tasks of occupational roles on a daily basis. Table 6-2 lists task and interpersonal skills that may be helpful in setting group goals. Skills are separately defined for family interaction, activities of daily living, leisure, and work. Temporal adaptation, the ability to perceive and manage time, is defined as orientation, organization, planning, goal setting, and establishing a schedule. Mosey suggests that interventions in task skill development begin on an individual basis. Group interventions can be effective in learning the more advanced task skills and in working on interpersonal skills. She suggests topical or thematic groups be designed to address specific skills.

Table 6-2

Mosey's Role Acquisition: Task and Interpersonal Skills

Task Skills
1. Willingness to engage in tasks
2. Adequate posture for tasks
3. Physical strength and endurance
4. Gross and fine motor coordination
5. Interest in task
6. Rate of performance
7. Ability to follow oral, demonstrated pictorial, and written directions
8. Use of tools and materials
9. Acceptable level of neatness
10. Attention to detail
11. Ability to solve problems
12. Ability to organize task in logical manner
13. Ability to tolerate frustration
14. Ability to be self-directed

Interpersonal Skills
1. Initiate, respond to, and sustain verbal interactions
2. Express ideas and feelings
3. Be aware of needs and feelings of others
4. Participate in cooperative and competitive situations
5. Compromise and negotiate
6. Assert self
7. Take on appropriate group roles

Table 6-3

Fidler and Velde's Four Domains of Occupation

1. *Self-care and self-maintenance*—Manner determined by personal needs and capacities

2. *Intrinsic gratification*—Pursuit of pleasure and enjoyment

3. *Societal contribution*—Contribute to need fulfillment and welfare of others

4. *Reciprocal interpersonal relatedness*—Developing and sustaining relationships with others

Velde and Fidler's Lifestyle Performance Profile

This OT model and assessment tool was developed by Beth Velde and Gail Fidler (2002). In it, skills for self-care and maintenance, self needs/intrinsic gratification, and service to others are listed and assessed within the framework of age, culture, and biology (Table 6-3). Fidler (1996) says

Each individual, over time, develops a configuration of activity patterns that can be described as a lifestyle. These patterns of doing, of being engaged, emerge through the interplay of a person's intrinsic needs, desires and capacities, and unique expectations of the environmental context of a person's living (p. 140).

Three contributing factors to lifestyle are motivation, well-being and quality of life, and the environment. An individual's motivation is strongest when engaging in occupations that are personally and socially relevant.

Success may be seen in a satisfying end product. Concepts of well-being and quality of life include the following:
- Satisfaction is one's cognitive appraisal of one's lifestyle
- Quality of life is higher when the individual can personally exert control over the environment
- Occupations that produce a sense of well-being and quality of life must be defined by the individual.

The environment may be structured to respond to individual needs and interests. Elements of the environment can clarify reality and define expectations for occupational performance. An ideal environment supports autonomy, individuality, affiliation, volition, consensual validation, predictability, self-efficacy, adventure, accommodation, and reflection.

In the lifestyle performance model, intervention is required during the following:
- When illness or trauma affects occupation in any lifestyle domain

- When lifestyle changes become necessary
- When individuals desire to establish a more satisfying lifestyle.

This profile can serve as an alternative basis for grouping clients with similar lifestyles, situations, and concerns, as well as similar deficits. Lifestyle changes and adaptations may be made more easily within a supportive, therapeutic group context.

Cognitive Rehabilitation Approaches

Cognitive rehabilitation models were originally designed for people with traumatic brain injury or stroke, both sometimes referred to as acquired brain injury. Various frames of reference have been developed and studied, all having a strong scientific basis in neurophysiology and neurobiology. In recent years, the approaches have also been used successfully for some mental health populations. The frames of reference reviewed here are Toglia's multicontextual model, Giles' neurofunctional approach, Averbuch and Katz's cognitive retraining model, and Abreu and Peloquin's quadraphonic approach. Toglia and colleagues (2009) also include Allen's cognitive disabilities model in this group of OT cognitive approaches. However, in this text, Allen is covered in Chapter 7. Toglia's multicontextual approach, the most widely researched of these, is presented in greater detail because of its applicability with groups. A large body of evidence supports this approach, also known as the dynamic interactional model (Zlotnik, Sachs, Rosenblum, Shpasser, & Josman, 2009).

Functional Brain Areas

Cognitive rehabilitation with brain-injured adults involves the reorganization of functional systems so that new methods of performing old behaviors are acquired. The retraining seeks to maximize the efficiency of information processing and involves repetitive exercises that place demands on the individual to perform skills of graded difficulty. Russian physiologist Aleksandr Luria (1973, 1980) identified six cognitive deficit areas: orientation, attention, visual processing, motor planning, cognition, and occupational behavior. In an approach called cognitive-perceptual retraining, Abreu and Toglia (1987) referred to Luria's brain region classifications in their organization of perceptual and cognitive deficits. The first brain area described includes the brainstem and the old cortex, containing the midbrain, thalamus, hypothalamus, uncas, reticular formation, and cerebellum. These are the innermost portions of the brain and are responsible for attention, wakefulness, arousal, and response to stimuli. The second brain area Luria defines includes the backmost areas and is responsible for analysis, coding, and storage of information. It receives raw data from sensory systems and assigns meaning to it.

Luria's third functional area includes the frontal portions of the brain and is responsible for intentions, programs, and problem solving.

A distinction is also made between the right and left hemispheres of the brain in terms of function. The right hemisphere is responsible for diffuse representation, gestalts, and organized wholes. It deals in concepts rather than specifics and processes visual-spatial data and nonverbal sounds. Body scheme and tactile, somatosensory integration are primarily attributed to the right side of the brain. The left hemisphere is analytic and sequential, concerned with language, specific details, and mathematical operations. While there are discrete characteristics for the two sides of the brain, functionally they work together to perform daily life tasks. Often, it is through clinical work with brain-damaged clients that we learn what types of functions are lost when certain parts of the brain are damaged.

Accidents and illness that cause damage to discrete areas of the brain are the most likely candidates for cognitive and perceptual retraining. "Cognitive impairments can result in significant activity limitations and participation restrictions in all aspects of a client's life" (Toglia et al., 2009). Toglia presents an updated list of cognitive impairments that commonly occur in acquired brain injury:

- *Orientation*—Able to identify self and surroundings, including time, place, person, and situation.
- *Attention*—Including detection, selective attention, sustained attention, shifting attention, and mental tracking.
- *Neglect*—Failure to orient to stimuli on the contralateral side of the brain lesion, not due to visual or motor deficits.
- *Visual processing*—Includes reception, organization, and assimilation of visual information.
- *Executive function*—Includes volition, planning, purposeful action, self-monitoring, and problem-solving.
- *Motor planning*—Praxis, positioning, using body to perform skilled activities.
- *Awareness*—Metacognition, ability to identify one's errors and accurately predict occupational performance (adapted from Toglia et al., 2009).

REVIEW OF OCCUPATIONAL THERAPY COGNITIVE APPROACHES

Several current approaches address these cognitive deficit areas, using varying degrees of behavioral and cognitive theory and techniques.

Giles (2005) describes a neurofunctional approach to cognitive rehabilitation, focusing on functional skills and habits and task retraining within natural settings. This approach uses task-specific training (not underlying skills) through the application of behavioral techniques, including breaking down tasks into steps, using vanishing cues, chaining and reinforcement, and practice.

The cognitive retraining model (Averbuch & Katz, 2005) integrates remedial training with strategy use and awareness of abilities, drawing upon neurophysiological, neurobiological, and neuropsychological theories. The training sequence begins with impaired cognitive functions such as visual scanning, categorization or classification, and sequencing. Complexity gradually increases to encompass planning, problem solving, and other mental operations in the clinic, followed by practice in real-life situations. These authors use a combination of paper and pencil exercises, computer and tabletop tasks, and functional activities.

The quadraphonic approach (Abreu & Peloquin, 2005) provides a holistic perspective using both micro and macro "quadrants." Discrete skill practice based on biomechanical, neurodevelopmental, and information processing theory provide micro guidelines for teaching-learning, which includes postural control and motor planning. The macro perspective embraces the client-centered model of therapist-client collaboration and individualizes OT to support engagement in valued occupations. The fluid movement between micro and macro perspectives acknowledges the dynamic interactions of multiple systems and levels of functioning and recovery.

The Multicontextual Approach

This approach will be more fully described because of the multiple applications of cognitive strategies with groups. Toglia has expanded her dynamical interaction model, now renamed the "multicontextual approach" with the addition of self-awareness and metacognition retraining and graded criteria for transfer of learning (Toglia, 2004). These additions do not abandon the original delineation of cognitive deficit areas, but they do alter the approach to their treatment. Toglia's recent work acknowledges the dynamic, interactive, and holistic nature of brain functioning and maximizes the likelihood of generalization of newly learned strategies or compensatory measures in restoring occupational performance (Toglia, 2004; Toglia et al., 2009).

Toglia contends that simply practicing each skill separately does not result in the generalization of skills to life in the real world (1997, 2005). Once cognitive strategies are relearned, they must be practiced and applied over a wide range of functional tasks, in a variety of social and situational contexts, in order to facilitate generalization of skills. For example, a client needs to learn to monitor time during task performance so that he or she can complete tasks more quickly and be on time to appointments. He or she may begin with an individual task, writing down the time in the margin after each paragraph he or she reads in a magazine. In a group setting, members may complete a series of word puzzles, noting the time they started and completed each, and comparing with each other to check for accuracy. Clients with acquired brain injuries may be assigned homework such as timing each morning task, washing, dressing, eating breakfast, and shaving or applying make-up. Estimating the time it takes to get ready for an appointment may be the topic of discussion in the next OT group. In the group, time-saving ideas can be shared, and clients can learn new strategies from each other. Multiple contexts used during interventions encourage an understanding of the significance of a strategy and a recognition of properties of situations in which the strategy is applicable. The multicontextual approach does not distinguish between remediation and compensation. Rather, it focuses on a person's awareness of the need to use a selected processing strategy.

Self-Awareness Training

Toglia and Kirk (2000) identified two types of awareness, self-knowledge and online awareness. Self-knowledge refers to the clients' awareness of their own strengths and limitations, sometimes referred to as insight. Online awareness refers to the metacognitive ability to accurately judge task demands; anticipate the likelihood of problems; and change, adapt, or fine tune one's behaviors during the performance of an activity or occupation. Online awareness changes with each task, while self-knowledge builds from a variety of experiences over time. A significant number of brain-injured clients are unaware of their limitations in occupational performance, causing them to attempt activities that are beyond their post injury capability and raising issues of judgment and safety. Bandura (1997, 1999) notes that self-efficacy, or a belief in one's own ability or control over a situation, is necessary in order to sustain motivation to work toward a goal. Errors in judgment and lack of self-awareness can lead to unexpected consequences and erode a person's self-efficacy.

Awareness training begins with familiar tasks and contexts that present a just-right challenge. In performing familiar occupations, clients can more easily compare previous experience with current occupational performance, therefore discovering for themselves their own areas of difficulty. Zlotnick and colleagues (2009) used a combination of Toglia's awareness training and multicontextual approaches with adolescents with TBI; results showed that participants gained full awareness of their own limitations and made significant improvement in mobility, self-care, and graphomotor ability using these approaches.

Metacognition

Toglia (1991) defines metacognition as "insight, or the degree of awareness one has regarding one's cognitive or physical capacities." Impairment in metacognition results in a misjudgment of the tasks one may attempt. This misjudgment may expose clients to significant danger, such as driving with a visual impairment, or failure to use a needed cane or walker when walking outdoors. Training increases self-awareness by a) acquiring knowledge of one's own processes and cognitive capacities and b) by developing self-monitoring strategies. Metacognitive skills include the ability to do the following:

- Evaluate task difficulty
- Predict consequences of action
- Formulate goals
- Plan for anticipated problems
- Monitor one's own performance
- Recognize errors
- Demonstrate self-control

Toglia stresses that without metacognition, people are unable to initiate and use either remedial or compensatory strategies. Therefore, these skills should be worked on significantly during therapy. Some suggested techniques for increasing metacognition are

- Self-instruction—Person verbalizes plan before execution, then verbalizes speed and accuracy of performance during and afterwards.
- Self-estimation—Person rates task difficulty on a scale of 1 to 5 (very easy to very hard), then compares estimate to actual performance.
- Role reversal—Client watches therapist making errors while doing the task; client must identify errors and hypothesize why they occurred.
- Self-questioning—At intervals during actual performance, person stops and asks, "How am I doing? Am I using (specific strategy)? Have I followed directions accurately?"
- Self-evaluation—After completion, persons asks, "Have I checked work for accuracy/completion? Have I paid attention or maintained focus? How confident do I feel about the results?"

Toglia suggests that metacognition has such a profound effect on new learning that this ability should be addressed in groups first before attempting to teach remedial or compensatory strategies. In one experiment on memory training for people with traumatic brain injury, group discussion and education about awareness of one's own performance increased accuracy of predictions by 50% on a recall task (Toglia, 1991). New research on the process of adaptation to disability suggests that, for some clients, a series of shock waves and adjustments to the reality of chronic disability, taking several months (or years), may be necessary before the kind of insight or "metacognition" Toglia suggests is actually possible (Macdonald, 1998).

The nature of metacognitive training makes it especially well-suited to group interventions for several reasons. The obvious reason is that one's performance in a group is observed by others and has the advantage of multiple opportunities for observations and feedback. The company of others who also need to work on metacognition increases the level of support and encouragement if performance is poor, while decreasing the possibility of minimizing or denying one's difficulties. Applying the above skills to any processing task in a group context can be easily planned by the OT using Toglia's guidelines.

Generalization and Criteria for the Transfer of Learning

Using Toglia's dynamic interactional model, cognitive strategies are always taught in the context of an activity. The initial demonstration of a strategy may be simple and designed for clinical use. For example, an organizational strategy might be presented to the group that involves 20 picture cards in four different categories (e.g., dishes, clothing, office supplies, and furniture). Each of the people in the group chooses one category and takes turns picking up the cards belonging to that category. The strategy of sorting can be applied to putting away laundry (things to hang up, things for the drawer, things for the linen closet, things for long-term storage). Sorting incoming mail then follows (bills, read now, read later, throw away). Next, the group may be given a grocery list that may be sorted according to the signs in the aisles of a local grocery store, which have been photographed with a camera. This one might be followed up with an actual trip to the grocery store to check for accuracy.

Different applications of a processing strategy represent different levels of generalization or transfer of skills. The therapist can identify a graded series of tasks that display decreasing degrees of physical and conceptual similarity to the original situation. To do this, potential tasks must be analyzed. The similarity of tasks depends on both surface characteristics and underlying concepts. Surface characteristics are as follows:

- Type of stimuli
- Presentation mode
- Variables of size, color, shape, etc.
- Stimuli arrangement
- Movement requirements
- Environmental context
- Rules or directions, number of steps

The underlying concepts of tasks are as follows:

- Underlying skills required (eye-hand coordination)
- Nonsituational strategies (planning)
- Situational strategies (grouping, visual imagery)

Transfer of skills may be near, intermediate, far, or very far. The closer the practice task resembles the training task, the easier the transfer. Clients in the sorting group example had a fairly easy time understanding how to sort the laundry items presented as pictures. They may have more difficulty if a basket of laundry is dumped on the table in front of them because the mode of presentation and task requirement (hanging, folding) is different. The picture categories and pictures of laundry items might be considered near transfer because only two characteristics have changed (subject of pictures and categories). In intermediate transfer, three to six characteristics have changed. Actually sorting items and putting them away adds the characteristics of three dimensions—color, texture, and necessity of manipulation and movement. If the group takes a trip to the grocery store, they will be faced with a far transfer. Far transfer tasks are conceptually similar to the initial task, but the surface characteristics are either completely different or have only one surface similarity. In the grocery store exercise, the physical surroundings, number of people, number of steps, and variety of object properties make the application of sorting by aisle and finding items on the grocery list a much more challenging task. Very far transfer refers to "generalization" or spontaneous application of what has been learned to everyday functioning (Toglia et al., 2009, p. 753). After discharge from treatment, a person might be able to demonstrate the sorting strategy in cleaning out the attic or garage.

Dynamic Nature of Cognition

Grouping people with brain dysfunction is based on Toglia's dynamic interactional assessment, which includes both the structural and functional capacity of each individual. Standardized pencil and paper or simulated tasks are not considered adequate for assessment. Processing skills in the six brain areas—orientation, attention, visual processing, motor planning, cognition (organization, memory, problem-solving), and activity of daily living functions—are examined and evaluated in the context of the physical, social, and cultural environment and within the parameters and variables of everyday task performance. Often, the functional capacities of brain-damaged individuals can be greater in familiar social and physical contexts than it appears in the clinic. This is because a person's capacity for cognitive functioning changes in different contexts. A person's cognitive functioning is largely dependent upon familiar cues from the environment and the expectations of one's social and cultural roles.

Therapy goals are set to match, as closely as possible, the expected roles and requirements of the discharge environments. People with similar learner capabilities are grouped together for learning selected strategies that are estimated to be within their capabilities. Metacognition and multicontextual strategy training

are then worked on simultaneously in these homogeneous groups. Multiple contexts for the strategy are used during interventions to encourage understanding of the significance of the strategy and a recognition of the properties of situations in which the strategy is appropriate. For example, estimating the time needed for task performance may be applied to a variety of tasks. The group might begin by estimating the time it will take them to read a one-page article, then reading the article and monitoring the time elapsed after each paragraph is completed and totaled at the end. Estimated times are compared with actual times.

Cognitive-Behavioral Concepts

Just as ego psychology was an outgrowth of psychoanalytic theory, cognitive behaviorism has advanced from the original behavioral theories. Cognitive behaviorists basically accept the principles of early behaviorism but have added thinking to the repertoire of human behavior that can be learned and modified. The fundamental change these psychological theories have made from their predecessors is their rejection of determinism. Behavior modification is an outdated technique by which behavior of the individual is essentially controlled by the therapist through the use of external reinforcement. This technique is seldom used nowadays, except for individuals with such a low level of self-control that self-reinforcement is not possible. Just as the concept of ego autonomy implies that man can adapt and change according to his own will, cognition in the cognitive frame allows man to regulate his own behavior. This concept has important implications for intervention.

Unlike behavior modification, which puts the control in the hands of the therapist and external forces, cognitive-behavioral therapies seek to modify how a person thinks. Rather than just a stimulus and response continuum, thought processes are inserted between the two. The stimulus involves a situation and an emotion or feeling state; then, an analysis of both the situation and the feeling occurs in which various response behaviors are considered and their consequences anticipated. Only after such an analysis does a behavioral response occur. Cognitive therapists seek to discover the thought processes of clients and to help clients use their own cognitive abilities to dispute thinking patterns that lead to problematic behaviors.

Cognitive-behavioral therapy has become firmly planted in the field of OT, as most recently described by Duncombe (2005). In reviewing the literature, Duncombe has found that the role of OT is described by Aaron Beck and three other psychologists as follows:

Occupational therapists who work in a psychiatric setting are primarily concerned with teaching skills to promote self-reliance and independence. These therapists have received extensive training on how to deal with actual physical, intellectual, or social deficits. In fact, they are probably better prepared than most psychiatrists, psychologists, or social workers to teach adaptive skills to persons with significant handicaps.... The OT uses psycho educational procedures, demonstrations, and in vivo rehearsal to build functional ability and self-esteem (Duncombe & McCraith, 1997; Wright, Thase, Ludgate, & Beck, 1993).

Three major contributors to the psychological cognitive-behavioral theory are identified by Bruce and Borg (2002) as Albert Bandura, Aaron Beck, and Albert Ellis.

Bandura's Social Learning Theory

Bandura's best-known contribution to cognitive-behavioral theory is his social learning theory (1977, p. 78). The following are major areas of focus in Bandura's work:

- The role of internal and external reinforcers
- Mediating environment and person interactions
- Modeling and observation learning
- Self-control and self-regulation
- Alternative sources of motivation

Bandura's hierarchy of reinforcement, mentioned earlier, spans a range of both external and internal reinforcers. Regarding reinforcement, Bandura contends that the person as well as the environment determines behavior. A social learning interaction involves three factors: person, behavior, and environment. External reinforcers are measurable outcomes from the environment, such as getting a grade on a test. The person's interpretation and expectations are considered equally important; these are the internal reinforcers. Examples of external reinforcers are money, material goods, social approval or privileges, and penalties. Self-reinforcement develops with maturity and the enactment of internal values and self-expectations.

Person-Environment Interactions

The role of cognition in mediating environment and person interactions is another important component in social learning theory. Bandura contends that behavior is an interacting determinant of the outcome or response. For example, a group member's behavior might elicit anger in the other group members. Cognition affects the person in his or her beliefs about him- or herself and the group. Sam believes he is not an alcoholic, but that others in the group are alcoholics. This belief leads him to reflect an aloof attitude toward other members. When they ask him to participate, he refuses, and he will not respond to the comments of others. The group members interpret his behavior as critical of them—"He thinks he's better than we are." This makes them respond to Sam with anger. Sam hears their angry comments and

feels rejected; he logically concludes that the group is not interested in him or able to help him. All of these processes, beliefs, attitudes, interpretations, and logical conclusions are cognitive processes that influence the person-environment interaction. In using this concept with clients, group leaders can design activities that facilitate an analysis of social interactions that encourages the uncovering of underlying beliefs and attitudes. These clients may be able to use this process to question their own attitudes and change beliefs that are troublesome.

Modeling and Observation Learning

Modeling and observation learning are types of social learning that all people engage in throughout life. Yet, people do not imitate every behavior they see. Cognition plays a major role in the analysis of observed behavior and the selection of which behavior to model. Bandura (1977) contends that this selection depends upon anticipated consequences. This means that individuals seek to model behavior that they have observed to have positive consequences. A recent study of motor neurons in the brain supports this concept. Researchers discovered the existence of "mirror neurons," which fire just by watching someone else perform a skilled action, and imprinting new learning in the brains of vicarious learners (Colletti, 2010; Iacoboni, 2009). OT group leaders can use this process to great advantage. Leaders can model positive responses to others, effective interactions, and successful problem solving, for example. This technique helps clients to increase their own interactional and problem-solving skills. An important advantage of group intervention is the learning that takes place from watching and imitating each other.

Self-Control and Self-Regulation

Self-control and self-regulation are desired outcomes of therapy. The basic assumption is that people are in control of their own behavior and can influence the outcome of their treatment. Cognition influences their motivation, selection of goals, and the ability to achieve them. Goals can serve as guides for self-regulation. People can measure their own progress in terms of desired goals. Goals are always central in a cognitive-behavioral approach to group intervention. The goals of the group are shared with clients and are agreed upon at the outset. Activities of the group are directed toward the goal(s), and members often evaluate the group in terms of progress toward the goal. Because goals are clearly stated, progress can be easily tested and reported by the therapist. This is partly what makes this approach so useful in acute-care settings where gains are expected to be made quickly and progress is evaluated on a daily basis. This concept begins to apply at Allen's cognitive level 4, for which goal-directed behavior is possible.

Cognition also influences the development of insight or self-understanding. Educating clients about how they might analyze their own attitudes, behavior, and consequences will enhance their ability to regulate their own behavior. When an anxious client understands the forces in the environment and the beliefs in him- or herself that contribute to his or her anxiety, that client can more easily exercise self-control. He or she can regulate the situation by reconsidering the reality of his or her beliefs or removing him- or herself to a less stressful environment. For example, Amy, a college student, studies in her room where her roommate constantly irritates her by playing loud music. Amy believes she cannot study with loud music playing. If she changes her attitude, she may learn to enjoy the music, or she may be able to view it as a screen for other more distracting noises. If Amy cannot do this, she may choose to study in the library.

Beck's Cognitive Distortions and Automatic Thoughts

Aaron Beck developed his methods of cognitive-behavioral therapy in the 1960s and 1970s through his work with clients with depression. His approach is founded in empirical investigation: he treats the client's maladaptive interpretations and conclusions about events as hypotheses to be tested. Beck collaborates with the client in conducting behavioral experiments, verbal examinations of alternative interpretations, reality testing, and problem-solving, with the goal of correcting cognitive distortions of reality.

From his clinical findings, Beck concludes that psychological disturbances frequently stem from automatic thoughts, which reflect habitual errors in thinking (Beck, 1976). This cognitive model does not assume that the cognitions operate exclusive of biochemistry or behavior symptomatic of psychopathology. Cognition is considered the problem and not the cause. The structure and process of cognitive therapy includes setting the agenda for the session, eliciting feedback, setting goals for therapy, operationally defining problems, testing hypotheses, problem-solving techniques, and assigning homework. This structure lends itself very well to OT groups, which can address through activities the cognitive roadblocks to functional performance.

Ellis' Exposing Irrational Beliefs

Albert Ellis is well-known for his work in rational emotive therapy (RET). Although Ellis and Beck developed their techniques over approximately the same time period, each has his own somewhat eclectic basis of which traditional behavior therapy is only a part. Like Beck, Ellis considered thinking to be a legitimate behavior that could be learned and modified using behavior modification techniques. A distinguishing feature of RET is its systematic exposition of irrational beliefs that

result in emotional and behavioral disturbances. Ellis spends most of his energy looking for "unconditional shoulds" and "absolute musts." He contends that clients take "simple preferences" such as desire for love, approval, and success and make the mistake of thinking of them as dire needs.

Ellis' view of human nature is somewhat humanistic: he believes people have inborn tendencies toward growth and actualization. He takes for granted, however, that humans are fallible and often make mistakes resulting in "crooked thinking" and "self-defeating" behavior (Ellis, 1973). RET has developed into a kind of structured challenging and disputing of irrational beliefs. Its confrontive methodology, such as the use of exaggeration, absurdity, and humor, is not at all humanistic.

Cognitive Restructuring

Ellis suggests a philosophical restructuring process involving a series of steps (Ellis & Harper, 1975), all of which require high-level thinking. This method reflects both humanistic self-determination and the supremacy of rational thinking in controlling and directing human behavior:

- Acknowledging our responsibility for creating our own problems
- Accepting our ability to change our own problems
- Seeing that emotional problems stem from irrational beliefs
- Clearly perceiving our beliefs
- Rigorously disputing beliefs
- Working hard to change beliefs resulting in disturbed emotion and behavior
- Continued cognitive monitoring and restructuring over our lifetime.

Cognitive restructuring includes the process of questioning our decisions and life structures and considering alternatives. It is very much a skill development process to be used over one's lifetime. When emotional problems are identified, therapy consists of defining problems in thinking that contribute to the distressing emotions or behaviors and finding alternative, more realistic, and pragmatic ways of conceptualizing those life circumstances. The therapist acts as an educator-facilitator in collaborating with the client to achieve specific goals.

Building Self-Efficacy

In OT groups, when we use a psychoeducational approach, our role as educator-facilitator is similar to that outlined by Ellis and Beck. Within the context of activities, OTs can use cognitive restructuring principles to teach clients how to apply a scientific approach to thinking. Our goal is to teach skills that can be generalized by clients after they leave therapy groups. Groups that focus on pain management, time management, leisure planning, and health education/prevention are examples of OT groups using a cognitive-behavioral approach. Discussion of the problems clients have in the performance of activities often leads to exposure of faulty thinking. In our higher-functioning client groups, OTs can help the clients change their attitudes toward disability or ability as it affects performance. We can teach our group members to challenge each other and to encourage their use of rational thinking to solve problems.

Linehan's Dialectical Strategies

Dialectical behavior therapy (DBT) was developed by Dr. Marsha Linehan (1993a) over the past 15 years as an intervention specifically for borderline personality disorders (BPD). People with this disorder are frequently seen in hospitals (19% of mental health inpatients, 11% of mental health outpatients); they are burdensome to the health-care system because there is no effective medical treatment. It is suspected that many more "undiagnosed" BPD patients enter hospitals with a host of other diagnoses because of their tendency to exaggerate symptoms and their proneness to substance abuse and suicide attempts. Dr. Linehan translates the core of the disorder into cognitive-behavioral terms, by emphasizing its "pattern of behavioral, emotional, and cognitive instability and dysregulation" (1993a, p. 11). Dialectic is defined by Webster's College Dictionary (1991) as "pertaining to logical argument" and includes "conversation revealing the truth through use of logic, juxtaposition of conflicting ideas, or forces (and) debate over a constantly changing reality." Those who are familiar with BPD will recognize immediately why this term was chosen. Hallmark symptoms of this character disorder include a tendency to distort reality, to either idolize or condemn others, to create drama and conflict in relationships, and to continually redefine their own identity. Acceptance of the nature of life as a constant struggle involving balance and imbalance of opposites is an important part of DBT. The dialectic approach to intervention meets the person with BPD on his or her own turf and teaches a logical approach to self-regulation.

FUNCTION AND DYSFUNCTION

Adaptation to the environment is the common measure across behavioral and cognitive theories. Behaviorists use the terms *adaptive behavior* and *learning* and attribute dysfunctional behavior to maladaptive learning. The emphasis is placed on concrete, observable behavior.

In the biomechanical and rehabilitation frames, a person is fully functional when he or she has no restrictions in range of motion, strength, and endurance and maintains the ability to perform the tasks necessary for work, play/leisure, self-care, and social roles. Function also includes the practice of good health maintenance habits.

Function in the cognitive rehabilitation frames of reference refer to information processing skills and their flexible use across task boundaries (generalization). Toglia and Abreu (1987) look at brain functioning as the behavior to be measured and evaluate the outward manifestations of orientation, attention, neglect, visual processing, motor planning, executive functions, and self-awareness. However, Toglia rejects the notion of assessing these skills in isolation and has designed and researched several "dynamic" assessments that measure these cognitive processes during functional task performance (Toglia, 1997; Toglia et al., 2009). Dysfunction in cognitive rehabilitation is characterized by limitations in the brain's ability to process information efficiently. Symptoms of poor efficiency become obvious during the performance of everyday activities when there is a mismatch between the task and the skill level of the individual. Dysfunction in metacognition is significant in that the client's inaccurate self-perceptions cause him or her to misjudge the difficulty of tasks and the appropriateness of processing or compensatory strategies. Unawareness of one's own deficits prevents one from learning from mistakes and using feedback to modify behavior. Inefficiencies in organization, setting priorities, and shifting one's mental perspective or viewpoint are common areas of dysfunction to be treated from a cognitive rehabilitation perspective.

In cognitive behaviorism, a well-functioning individual has the ability to think logically and to form accurate perceptions of the self and the environment. He or she can use deductive reasoning to cope with problems and can logically regulate his or her own thoughts, feelings, and behavior. Dysfunction may be defined as faulty thinking, inaccurate self-perception, and the inability to handle one's affairs competently. Failure to adapt to the environment and to function independently in society in this frame of reference is seen as a product of cognitive disability. Therefore, it is cognitive impairments in attention, sensory awareness, perception, memory, and other thought processes that prevent efficient problem-solving, interfere with learning and application of new coping strategies, and cause problems in doing functional activities. These cognitive functions, therefore, should be the focus of intervention in OT.

In designing groups with people of similar cognitive ability, many assessments are available to use as guidelines. Claudia Allen (1997, workshop materials) has prepared a comparison chart of some of the most commonly used assessment scales, which may be helpful in selecting group membership (Table 6-4). Allen's Cognitive Levels are further defined in Chapter 7. The Medicare Physical Assistance and Cognitive Assistance Scales are taken from Medicare Part B Guidelines.

Table 6-4

Comparison of Various Medical Studies

Allen Cognitive Level/Mode	Medicare Cognitive Assistance %	Medicare Physical Assistance %	Global Deterioration Scale (dementia)	Rancho Head Trauma	DSM-IVR Global Assessment of Functioning (GAF) Axis 5	Bayley Maturation Approximate Age
0.8	100	100		I		
1.0	99			II		0 to 1 mo.
1.2	98			III		1 to 5 mo.
1.4	96	75				4 to 8 mo.
1.6	92					4 to 10 mo.
1.8	88	50				6 to 12 mo.
2.0	84	25	7	IV		9 to 17 mo.
2.2	82	15				10 to 20 mo.
2.4	78	10				
2.6	75					12 to 23 mo.
2.8	70				1-10	
3.0	64			V	11-20	18 to 24 mo.
3.2	60					
3.4	54		6		21-30	
3.6	50					3 yr.
3.8	46				31-40	
4.0	42	8	5	VI		4 yr.
4.2	38					5 yr.
4.4	34					6 yr.
4.6	30		4	VII	41-50	
4.8	25					
5.0	22	6				7 to 10 yr.
5.2	18	4				11 to 13 yr.
5.4	14	2	3		51-60	14 to 16 yr.
5.6	10	0	2	VIII	61-80	17 yr.
5.8	6				81-90	
6.0	0		1		91-100	18 to 21 yr.

© Claudia Allen, conference materials, 1997. Adapted with permission.

Global Assessment of Functioning (GAF) comes from the American Psychiatric Association (APA) (2000). For other scales, readers can refer to Katz (2005).

CHANGE AND MOTIVATION

Following the guidelines of learning theory, the basic strategy for change is reinforcement. Change occurs when behavior is reinforced in some way. In behavior modification, behavior may be controlled and shaped by the therapist (or other person) using external reinforcement. The type of reinforcement that can be effective will vary from client to client. Some clients do not seem to have the internal motivation to learn new skills. For these clients, external reward is most appropriate. This can be anything the client is willing to work for, such as praise, extra attention, candy, cigarettes, or privileges. Bandura (1999) expanded the definition of reinforcement to include a range of internalized reinforcements.

Some clients respond to social reinforcement, such as the praise and acceptance of their peers, family, or friends. At a higher level, clients will strive to learn skills or improve functioning in order to gain the approval of society or meet the expectations of their cultural group. The highest form, self-reinforcement, spontaneously emerges as the individual strives to measure up to his or her own internal standards. In OT, simple skills are mastered before more difficult ones are attempted. Thus, the clients can develop a feeling of competence as each new skill is mastered. The feeling of competence gained from successful occupational performance, in itself, provides reinforcement (White, 1967). This is known as self-reinforcement, the highest form of motivation clients can achieve.

In the cognitive-behavioral approaches, people change by changing the way they think. For adults with acquired brain injury, cognitive rehabilitation produces change by training in the use of remedial or compensatory processing strategies in the context of a broad range of tasks. To the extent that they are capable, people use metacognitive strategies, increasing awareness, and monitoring of their own cognitive capacities and limitations. The OT can use a psychoeducational approach to teach clients to apply logic to produce adaptive change in people with intact processing skills (e.g., people with disorders of substance use, eating disorders, obsessive compulsive disorders, or personality disorders). In DBT, becoming aware of beliefs and attitudes that result in problem emotions and behaviors is the first step. Clients are sometimes asked to sign a contract, agreeing to try out new thinking and self-regulation strategies for a defined period of time. Challenging their "faulty thoughts" can often convince clients to change or replace them, and this will lead to a change in behavior.

Current cognitive approaches assume that people have a natural drive toward competence and mastery and to achieve a better position in life. People wish to be self-directed and to have an effect on others and on the environment. To achieve these goals, most people are willing to learn and try new coping strategies for problem-solving and for self-improvement/regulation. A difficulty with this approach may be to find effective reinforcements for those clients who do not seem to be motivated or are unaware of a social pressure to improve their status.

GROUP INTERVENTIONS

Groups are homogeneous in this frame of reference. This does not mean, however, that all the members have the same diagnosis. Because a broad range of functional levels, verbal and reasoning abilities, and diagnostic categories is being addressed, assessment of the critical abilities for group involvement is an important prerequisite. In planning group intervention, clients with similar needs or deficits are usually grouped together, and goals are set to address their common issues. Groups of no more than eight members focus on learning specific skills or strategies. Members should be at approximately the same cognitive level so that they will be able to learn at the same pace and through similar modes of presentation. Groups working on perception and memory skills in cognitive rehabilitation, for example, might be given several memory games during a therapy session. All the members should be able to understand the verbal directions if the activity is to be successful in accomplishing its goal. In a psychoeducational problem-solving group, the goals might be to master each step in the problem-solving process. Clients will be able to do the following:

- Clearly state the desired outcome of the problem

- Gather relevant information

- Analyze and interpret the data

- Devise a plan to solve the problem (describe actions and sequence of steps)

- Implement the plan

- Evaluate the outcome

The goals in the behavioral-cognitive frames of reference are always very specific, observable, and measurable. This is because the intervention approach is very goal directed. Problems are generally addressed narrowly and specifically, and the learning, rehearsal, and practice of specific skills is usually the goal. The most closely aligned to behavioral theory is the biomechanical/rehabilitative frame of reference. When planning groups in this model, exercises to increase range of motion, strength, and endurance are demonstrated, imitated, and practiced in the groups within the context of functional activities. Groups may be designed around the need for training in the use of adaptive equipment or in techniques of energy conservation. Biofeedback and monitoring techniques during exercise groups allow individual members to participate at different levels, while having the advantage of group support and socialization. For the sake of clarity, any group examples that include elements of physical rehabilitation or the monitoring of physical attributes, such as relaxation, will be called biomechanical/rehabilitative, even though it may also draw upon behavioral techniques.

Cognitive Rehabilitation Groups—Toglia

In cognitive rehabilitation, Toglia's cognitive deficit areas—orientation, attention, neglect, visual processing, executive functions, motor planning, and awareness—may be used as guidelines for the selection of group activities. People who share similar functional problems may be treated in groups of three to six, or up to eight with a co-leader. The group should be structured so that several different contexts are presented for using the same strategy. For example, attention-sustaining strategies may be practiced with pencil and paper tasks, like alternating numbers and letters in a sequence when connecting dots on a page. Done in a group, partners can take turns monitoring and giving each other cues. Attention must be used when playing group board games, card games, or word games. Likewise, many visual processing, motor planning, memory, and problem-solving strategies may be learned and practiced in the context of group activities. There are numerous workbooks and collections of exercises that exist in the literature that are most helpful in planning groups (Dougherty & Radomski, 1987; Toglia, 2004). Some of the advantages of working on cognitive strategies in groups are as follows:

- Group "games" can be motivating and fun.
- Groups provide a real-life context for the use of skills.
- Therapeutic groups allow practice with guidance and safety.
- Feedback on performance from others increases self-awareness.
- Observation of a variety of group responses encourages generalization of skills.
- Possible applications of skills in the lives of each member can be discussed and explored.

Psychoeducational Groups

Psychoeducational groups, based on behavioral and cognitive behavioral principles, may be designed for skill training, such as assertiveness, social skills, or stress management. OTs often use a psychoeducational approach involving the imparting of information and the use of structured learning exercises. The OT Framework-II includes educator as one of the OT roles in current practice (AOTA, 2008). An example is the Bridge Program, a supported education program for people with severe mental illness (Gutman, Kerner, Zombek, Dulek, & Ramsey, 2009), in which OT students provided weekly group instruction on topics related to success in a higher educational setting. Clients completing the program reported feeling better prepared for classes, and many enrolled in college courses after completing the program, demonstrating successful participation/engagement in occupation as outcomes.

Due to changes in federal regulations by the Department of Mental Health and Addiction Services (DMHAS) limiting the use of restraint methods and expanding the rights of people with mental illness and/or addiction, many states have initiated community programs based on a recovery model. These state-mandated programs offer integrated, person-centered, and holistic treatment for people with persistent mental illness or addictions, including evaluation and intervention for the development and maintenance of life skills. In Connecticut, a comprehensive rehabilitation evaluation involves the following areas for potential OT evaluation and intervention: independent living skills, personal care, safety, money management, interpersonal communication skills, health awareness, coping, stress management, impulse control skills, cognitive functioning, vocational (employment and education), leisure, and awareness of legal rights (CT-DMHAS, 2008) (Assessment revised July 2010). The assessment tool uses the Medicare ratings of (5) maximum assistance, (4) moderate assistance, (3) minimum assistance, (2) standby assistance, (1) independent, or (0) unable to assess. In Massachusetts, LeBel, Champagne, Stromberg, and Coyle (2010) report a similar initiative using sensory and trauma-informed interventions. They write, "through the use of preparatory, purposeful, and occupation-based interventions, sensory approaches are used to foster feelings of safety and support development and engagement in meaningful life roles, routines, and activities" (p. 2). Sensory modulation guidelines have also been developed, although many of these are for children's groups, such as, How does your engine run? (Williams & Schellenberger, 1994). Lebel and colleagues (2010) suggest combining sensory modulation and self-regulation strategies such as DBT in recovery programming for adult mental health populations. Similar initiatives in other states are already underway, presenting a unique opportunity for OT to get involved in creating group programs of recovery with mental health, veterans, prisoners, and other "in recovery" populations under the auspices of all publically funded treatment facilities affected by the federal restraint reduction regulations.

Dialectical Behavior Therapy Groups

In DBT, Dr. Linehan has identified specific issues that need to be addressed by people with borderline personality disorder (BPD), which she defines as a "disorder of self-regulation" (1993a). These are dysregulation of emotions, interpersonal relationships, behavior, cognition, and sense of self.

Group intervention has traditionally been the treatment of choice for individuals with BPD because of their difficulty with authority, their need for peer feedback, and the desirability of avoiding the power struggles that are inevitable in one-on-one relationships, therapeutic or otherwise. Linehan (1993b) has designed a workbook for psychosocial skills training, which outlines specific group exercises in four major categories:

1. Core mindfulness
2. Interpersonal effectiveness
3. Emotion regulation
4. Distress tolerance

Babiss (2002) has applied DBT principles extensively with OT groups in mental health settings. She highlights the importance of the therapeutic relationship in creating an environment of validation, then walks a fine line between acceptance of individual members, and at the same time encouraging them to change. Babiss suggests the following group guidelines:

1. First listen intently to client stories—That alone is a form of validation.

2. Communicate empathy—Acceptance of feelings and perceived reason for the feelings.

3. Cautiously ask clients how happy they are with the results of their responses to life situations. Ask clients what they wish had happened and what they might do differently next time.

4. When clients do not acknowledge their own unsatisfying responses, make sure to structure groups so that they can hear how other group members can confront their own behaviors.

5. Clients who resist change (as many clients with BPD do) NEED groups that focus not on what happened, but on identifying and naming emotions. "This can be accomplished through expressive groups" (art, music, writing, movement) with facilitated expression of feelings through occupation" (2002, p. 119).

An example of an expressive group Babiss designed is a group art show, in which clients created self-portraits and then wrote essays about their portraits. An important application of DBT in such groups is making the connections between thinking, feeling, and behavior during the facilitated discussion. Babiss sees DBT and OT goals as similar, in that they both encourage "engaging in daily lives in spite of their disorders" (2002, p. 118). She creates groups to educate clients about their disorders, to teach functional skills and strategies to cope with their emotional extremes and distorted thinking, and to communicate effectively with their peers and families, groups she dubs "studying at the university of me" (p. 121).

Core Mindfulness

This teaches the mind to focus on one thing at a time, to pay attention to all the information available in a situation, and to refrain from quick judgments, jumping to conclusions, or acting on the basis of emotional responses. A useful technique is writing; taking time to describe conflict situations in words delays the response and leads away from the emotional and into the rational, analytical mind. Awareness of beliefs and attitudes one typically uses and analyzing these applying logic, labeling behaviors, and emotions as harmful and destructive or helpful and productive in accomplishing one's objectives in the conflict situation are also a focus of group exercises in the mindfulness category.

Interpersonal Effectiveness

Skills for achieving specific objectives in relationships, getting and keeping good relationships, and maintaining self-respect in relationships are learned and practiced in these group exercises. Recognition of the factors that interfere with relationships, strategies for challenging these negative factors, and self-reinforcing positive responses are also included. Exercises for expression of feelings and opinions, negotiating, reciprocating, and making specific requests help to build a repertoire of skills for building and maintaining healthy interpersonal relationships.

Emotion Regulation

This series of exercises begins with challenging beliefs about emotions and their importance. Describing and naming the emotions (love, joy, shame, fear, sadness, and anger are major categories) becomes the first step toward a rational approach, reducing vulnerability to the negative effects of emotions. Exercises in effective self-interventions when emotions threaten to overwhelm or take over include strategies for evoking positive emotion, building positive experiences, and steps to reduce painful emotions.

Distress Tolerance

These exercises for groups teach techniques for crisis survival. The goal is to stop the negative behavioral responses typical of BPD, such as substance abuse and self-destructive or suicidal acts. Strategies for distracting, self-soothing, and improving the moment (prayer, relaxation, deep breathing, brief escape) allow time for reason to gain control. Attitude change from "This is awful" to "I can survive this" is practiced. This is followed by exercises in the application of logic: listing the pros and cons for tolerating the distress and directing "willfulness" (imposing one's will on reality) toward what works and not what interferes with survival. Developing an awareness of the pleasures of ordinary tasks and cultivating a "half-smile" of acceptance leads group members toward the expectation that it is OK for life to be ordinary and that life circumstances are not always going to be ideal.

Care is taken to address each of these psychosocial skill areas in positive terms, avoiding the least hint of criticism (which commonly evokes anger and thus interferes with learning). The exercises use a variety of cognitive restructuring techniques to modify dysfunctional assumptions and beliefs and other behavioral and cognitive techniques mentioned earlier, including practice and rehearsal, therapist reinforcement, feedback and coaching, modeling and role playing. Groups of six to eight members are suggested for skill training, and these are offered in 8-week modules, complete with worksheets, handouts, and homework. Linehan offers workshops for training in DBT, which are open to OTs as well as other professionals. Her *Skills Training Manual for Treating Borderline Personality Disorder* includes handouts that may be photocopied for use with client groups (Linehan, 1993b).

Role of the Leader

The OT's role is more directive in this frame of reference than it is in most others. In a clinical setting, the focus is often on evaluation. The therapist typically chooses the activity or task and structures the group for concentrated work toward a specific goal. Efficiency in goal attainment is all-important, and the OT structures the group and the environment with this in mind. The therapist's role is active during the group, giving assistance, providing cues, and asking questions that will guide group members to improve their performance. Discussion may require frequent redirection to remain focused, with the guiding principle of reinforcing the learning of specific skills and achievement of specific goals. The OT should carefully monitor interaction to make sure the feedback given by members to each other is of a therapeutic nature.

Goals of the Group

Goals are behaviorally defined, specific, observable, and measurable. OT goals are practical in nature, focusing on increasing functional performance. This fact alone makes the behavioral cognitive approach the best fit in the current health-care atmosphere. Measurable goals are easy to document and justify the need for intervention. In working with the physical or cognitive perceptual dysfunction, the therapist sets goals for the group based on his or her best assessment of the client's potential. Norms are helpful in setting goals in the biomechanical areas (e.g., "resume normal strength in the injured right leg," "increase range of motion from 160° to 180° in a spastic elbow"). In clients with temporary cognitive impairment, Allen's Cognitive Level 6 or Rancho Los Amigo's head trauma level VII may be an appropriate goal. For clients with the capacity for rational thought, the goal is insight. Only when a client understands the impact of his or her cognitive distortions and irrational beliefs is he or she able or willing to change them. It is assumed that a change in thinking will produce a change in behavior. Therefore, goals will generally address the thought processes rather than the affective or overt behavioral components.

Current literature in OT has emphasized the importance of culture and individual values in goal selection. For this reason, the client's own preferences and social expectations will play a part in determining the goals. Research has shown that a meaningful task increases motivation and elicits a client's best effort. Long-term goals may be set collaboratively with each client, based on his or her expected environment, culture, and social roles. Within the group, limited choices can be offered, so that individual interests and preferences may become incorporated into the group experience.

Activity Examples

In psychoeducational groups, OTs use and adapt many specific behavioral techniques to enhance group learning. Some of these techniques should be recognized as very powerful and therefore dangerous to use without specific training. Some of the techniques OTs should avoid unless specifically trained are flooding, paradoxical intention, and systematic desensitization. These techniques involve vivid imaging of much-feared and disturbing situations, and the management of clients who have been so aroused requires more advanced therapeutic skills.

However, in moderation, imaging and visualization may be incorporated into a structured activity or may be expanded into drawing, sculpture, or dramatic role play. The use of images or visualization is a technique many OTs have found helpful. For example, the guided fantasy can enhance relaxation and foster creativity and self-awareness. Once goals are set, visualizing images of their successful achievement is often motivating. Drawing images of various kinds is one way to structure our groups to work on specific goals.

The concepts of group problem solving, keeping journals, and giving homework are also useful ideas in OT groups. Behavior rehearsal may be useful in the learning and practice of social skills. Some other techniques are contracts with oneself or with the group to change certain thoughts and behaviors; self-reward or self-punishment; writing beliefs in words and then deciding if the statements are true or false; and positive or negative labeling of thoughts, feelings, and behavior. The reader is referred to McMullin's *Handbook of Cognitive Behavioral Techniques* (1986), Linehan's *Skills Training Manual for Treating Borderline Personality Disorder* (1993b), Moyers' *Substance Abuse: A Multi-Dimensional Assessment and Treatment Approach* (1992), and Precin's *Living Skills Recovery Workbook* (1996) for more ideas.

At the end of the chapter are some examples of cognitive-behavioral groups (Activity Examples 6-1 through 6-8). They will be identified as belonging to one of the following categories: biomechanical/rehabilitative, cognitive rehabilitative, or psychoeducational. All of these categories use behavioral and cognitive principles, techniques, and strategies.

GROUP LEADERSHIP

The seven-step group format is not changed in structure. If anything, in this frame of reference, groups become even more structured. The beginning of the group places an emphasis on defining specific problems and collaborative goal setting. The therapist may do this individually with each member before the group begins.

Introduction

This kind of group will dispense with the warm-up and get right down to business. A more complete explanation of the goals and purpose will substitute. Expectations are spelled out in behavioral terms, and the group is told how their progress will be evaluated. The timeframe of the group should coincide with the members' level of cognitive functioning.

Activity

Cognitive-behavioral groups focus on learning coping skills and improving task performance. There is usually didactic instruction given in the form of short lectures or demonstrations of the steps in doing a task. The activities are learning experiences and opportunities for practice. In a leisure skills group, for example, members learn to do a series of specific activities: how to knit, how to cook, how to catch a fish, how to play card games. In a stress-management group, the OT gives mini-lessons in cardiovascular fitness, high nutrition diets, and progressive relaxation in conjunction with activities. The experience may take longer, up to two-thirds of the session, leaving the rest for discussion/demonstration.

Sharing

If members have done an individual activity, such as a worksheet, this is the time for reading it aloud or holding it up for the group to see. The leader should give recognition and feedback and encourage other group members to do the same. In the cognitive rehabilitation groups, this is an opportunity to discuss self-evaluations and compare results. Leaders should be cautious not to encourage competition, but to place emphasis on how well each member was able to predict and monitor his or her own performance. For cognitive-behavioral and psychoeducational groups, feedback from others is an important social reinforcement to learning and should be offered to all members. Feedback comes mostly from the therapist in the lower-level groups and from fellow members in higher-level groups.

Processing

Discussion of the underlying dynamics of the group is also not an area of focus. Most of the interaction should be between the leader and each member, just as a teacher interacts with a class. However, when the feelings or the implicit forces of the group begin to interfere with group learning, then the therapist must temporarily make group process the focus. This is not to say, however, that feelings about the activity should be ignored. This part of the discussion should invite honest expression of emotions, both positive and negative, as they pertain to the issues addressed by the activity. The group energy may be rallied in support of members who are discouraged with their progress or are having difficulty adapting to residual or permanent dysfunction. Group leaders need to beware of the offering of false hope or flattery by members, and discussion should be kept focused and controlled.

Generalizing

Inductive reasoning is encouraged in the members to come up with general principles to be learned from the experience. Inductive reasoning involves collecting evidence from many specific examples to build a general principle or theory. Members can do this best when they have heard several responses to the experience from other members, which has hopefully been done in the sharing and processing steps. In a well-planned group, the general principles suggested by the members will coincide with group goals. If this does not happen spontaneously, the therapist should help the group to make the connections. In cognitive rehabilitation groups, for example, members may take this opportunity to verbalize the specific strategies on which they have worked, take note of what they learned about their own ability to process information, and summarize insight they have gained.

Application

There is more emphasis here than in any other part of the discussion. An effective group will include a carry-over of behavior change from the clinic to the community environment. An open group discussion of how newly learned strategies may be concretely applied in everyday life will increase the likelihood of carryover. Members should know before they leave the group exactly how they will apply their new knowledge or skill. Application requires deductive reasoning, the application of theoretical ideas to specific, individual situations. Often, the therapist must structure this reasoning with thought-provoking discussion questions and concrete examples. Members may then share ideas on how to do this. The activities done by the group are usually planned to address specific problems, so the application is generally built into the group experience at the outset. If clients leave the group consciously aware of the usefulness of certain skills, they may communicate this to family members and caretakers, and they may initiate the process of self-reinforcement. Homework may be given by the therapist to support the application of what is learned. When homework is given, a timeframe should be included, and members should know when and where they will be asked to report on the results of the homework activity.

Summary

A verbal summary by the therapist is a tradition to be continued throughout the frames of reference. In this one, its major purpose is to reinforce learning. It is best done by the therapist in most cases. Emphasizing the important points of the session and giving positive feedback to members are the important elements. The few minutes it takes to summarize may make the difference between forgetting and remembering what was learned. Reminders about homework and announcements about what is planned next are also appropriate.

REFERENCES

Abreu, B., & Peloquin, S. (2005). The Quadraphonic approach: A holistic rehabilitation model for brain injury. In N. Katz (Ed.), *Cognition and occupation across the lifespan* (2nd ed., pp. 73-112). Bethesda, MD: American OT Association.

Abreu, B., & Toglia, J. (1987). Cognitive rehabilitation: A model for OT. *American Journal of OT, 41*, 439-448.

Allen, C. K. (1997). Cognitive disabilities: How to make clinical judgments. In N. Katz (Ed.), *Cognitive rehabilitation: Models for intervention in occupational therapy.* Bethesda, MD: AOTA.

American OT Association. (2008). OT practice framework: Domain and process. *American Journal of OT, 62*, 625-683.

American Psychiatric Association. (2000). *Diagnostic and statistical manual* (4th ed., revised). Washington, DC: Author.

Averbuch, S., & Katz, N. (2005). Cognitive rehabilitation: A retraining model for clients with neurological disabilities. In N. Katz (Ed.), *Cognition and occupation across the lifespan* (2nd ed., pp. 113-138). Bethesda, MD: American OT Association.

Babiss, F. (2002). An ethnographic study of mental health treatment and outcomes: Doing what works. *OT in Mental Health, 18*(3/4), 1-123.

Bandura, A. (1977). *Social learning theory.* Englewood Cliffs, NJ: Prentice-Hall.

Bandura, A. (1997). *Self-efficacy: The exercise of control.* New York, NY: W. H. Freeman.

Bandura, A. (1999). Social cognitive theory: An agentic perspective. *Asian Journal of Social Psychology, 2,* 21.

Beck, A. (1976). *Cognitive therapy and emotional disorders.* New York, NY: International University Press.

Bruce, M., & Borg, B. (2002). *Psychosocial frames of reference: Core for occupation-based practice.* Thorofare, NJ: SLACK Incorporated.

Colletti, M. (2010). Monkey see monkey do: Motor planning, mirror neurons and imitation of actions in task completion. *Advance for OT, Oct. 11th,* 28-29.

Corey, G. (1996). *Theory and practice of counseling and psychotherapy* (5th ed.). Monterrey, CA: Brooks/Cole.

Denton, P. L. (1987). *Psychiatric OT: A workbook of practical skills.* Boston, MA: Little, Brown, & Co.

Department of Mental Health and Addiction Services, Connecticut (DMHAS-CT) (2008). *Practice guidelines for recovery-oriented care for mental health and substance use conditions* (2nd ed.). Prepared for DMHAS by Yale program for recovery and community health. New Haven, CT: Yale University Press.

Dougherty, P., & Radomski, M. V. (1987). *The cognitive rehabilitation workbook.* Rockville, MD: Aspen.

Duncombe, L. (2005). Cognitive behavioral model in mental health. In N. Katz (Ed.), *Cognition and occupation in rehabilitation: Cognitive models for intervention in OT* (2nd ed., pp. 187-210). Bethesda, MD: American OT Association.

Duncombe, L., & McCraith, D. (1997). *Cognitive approaches for psychosocial evaluation and intervention, AOTA, SIS Practice.* Phoenix, AZ: Paper Presentation.

Ellis, A. (1973). *Humanistic psychology: The rational emotive approach.* New York, NY: McGraw-Hill.

Ellis, A., & Harper, R. (1975). *A new guide to rational living.* North Hollywood, CA: Wilshire Book Co.

Fidler, G. (1996). Lifestyle performance: From profile to conceptual model. *American Journal of OT, 50,* 139-147.

Giles, G. M. (2005). A neurofunctional approach to rehabilitation following severe brain injury. In N. Katz (Ed.), *Cognition and occupation across the lifespan* (2nd ed., pp. 139-165). Bethesda, MD: American OT Association.

Greenfield, J. M., & Godinez, M. (1989). *Stroke patients learn independence by leading their own therapy group.* Bethesda, MD: American OT Association.

Gutman, S. A., Kerner, R., Zombek, I., Dulek, J., & Ramsey, C. A. (2009). *Supported education for adults with psychiatric disabilities: Effectiveness of an occupational therapy program.* American Journal of Occupational Therapy, 63, 245-254.

Harlowe, D., & Yu, P. (1997). *The ROM dance: A range of motion exercise and relaxation program.* Madison, WI: Uncharted Country Publishing.

Iacoboni, M. (2009). Imitation, empathy, and mirror neurons. *Annual Review of Psychology, 60,* 653-670.

James, W. (1985). Habit: Its importance for psychology. *OT in Mental Health, 5*(3), 55-67.

Katz, N., Ed. (2005). *Cognition and occupation in rehabilitation: Cognitive models for intervention in OT* (2nd ed.). Bethesda, MD: American OT Association.

LeBel, J., Champagne, T., Stromberg, N., & Coyle, R. (2010). Integrating sensory and trauma-informed interventions: A Massachusetts state initiative, Parts 1 & 2. *Mental Health Special Interest Section Quarterly, 33*(1 & 2), 1-4.

Linehan, M. (1993a). *Cognitive-behavioral treatment of borderline personality disorder.* New York, NY: The Guilford Press.

Linehan, M. (1993b). *Skills training manual for treating borderline personality disorder.* New York, NY: The Guilford Press.

Luria, A. (1973). *The working brain.* New York, NY: Basic Books.

Luria, A. (1980). *Higher cortical functions in man.* New York, NY: Basic Books.

Macdonald, K. (1998). *Adaptation.* In Dissertation Abstracts. New York, NY: New York University.

McMullin, R. E. (1986). *Handbook of cognitive behavioral techniques.* New York, NY: Norton.

Mosey, A. (1986). *Psychosocial components of OT.* New York, NY: Raven.

Posthuma, B. (2002). *Small groups in counseling and therapy: Process and leadership* (4th ed.). Boston, MA: Little, Brown & Co.

Precin, P. (1996). *Living skills recovery workbook.* Boston, MA: Butterworth Heinemann.

Robertson, S. (1988). *Mental health focus.* Rockville, MD: American OT Association.

Skinner, B. F. (1953). *Science and human behavior.* New York, NY: Macmillan Co.

Stein, F., & Nikolic, S. (1989). Teaching stress management techniques to a schizophrenic patient. *American Journal of OT, 43,* 162-169.

Toglia, J. (1991). Generalization of treatment: A multicontext approach to cognitive perceptual impairment in adults with brain injury. *American Journal of OT, 45,* 505-516.

Toglia, J. (1997). A dynamic interactional approach to cognitive rehabilitation. In N. Katz (Ed.), *Cognition and occupation in rehabilitation: Cognitive models for intervention in OT.* Bethesda, MD: American OT Association.

Toglia, J. (2004). *The multicontext approach to awareness, memory, and executive function impairments.* Medfield, MA: Education Resources, Inc.

Toglia, J. (2005). A dynamic interactional approach to cognitive rehabilitation. In N. Katz (Ed.), *Cognition and occupation across the lifespan: Models for intervention in occupational therapy.* Bethesda, MD: AOTA.

Toglia, J., & Abreu, B. (1987). *Cognitive rehabilitation.* New York, NY: Authors.

Toglia, J., Golisz, K., & Coverover, Y. (2009). Multicontext treatment approach. In E. Crepeau, E. Cohn, & B. B. Schell (Eds.), *Willard & Spackman's OT* (11th ed., pp. 739-776). Philadelphia, PA: Lippincott, Williams & Wilkins.

Toglia, J., & Kirk, U. (2000). Understanding awareness deficits following brain injury. *Neurorehabilitation, 15,* 57-70.

Trombly, C., & Radomski, M. V. (Eds.). (2002). *OT for physical dysfunction* (5th ed.). Philadelphia, PA: Lippincott, Williams & Wilkins.

Van Deusen, J., & Harlowe, D. (1987). The efficacy of the ROM dance program for adults with rheumatoid arthritis. *American Journal of OT, 41*(2), 90-95.

Velde, B., & Fidler, G. (2002). *Lifestyle performance: A model for engaging the power of occupation.* Thorofare, NJ: SLACK Incorporated.

Webster's College Dictionary. (1991). New York, NY: Random House.

White, R. H. (1967). Competence and the growth of personality. In *Science and psychoanalysis, vol. XI, The ego.* New York, NY: Grune and Stratton.

Williams, M. S., & Shellenberger, S. (1994). *How does your engine run?* Albuquerque, NM: Therapy Works Inc.

Wright, J., Thase, M., Ludgate, J., & Beck, A. (1993). *The cognitive milieu: Structure and process in cognitive therapy with inpatients.* New York, NY: Guilford.

Zlotnik, S., Sachs, D., Rosenblum, S., Shpasser, R., & Josman, N. (2009). Use of the dynamic interactional model in self-care and motor intervention after traumatic brain injury: Explanatory case studies. *American Journal of OT, 63,* 549-558.

Behavioral Cognitive Activity Example 6-1
I Can Remember (Cognitive Rehabilitation)

Materials: Twenty objects on a tray, selected from three different categories (e.g., things normally found in the kitchen, things normally found in an office, and grooming items normally found in a bathroom cabinet), towel to cover items from sight, pencils and paper for each member, and a printed list of 10 commonly known names of objects (e.g., telephone, ruler, picture frame, mailbox, baseball, lamp, pitcher, teddy bear, stool, boat) for each member.

Strategies: Repetition and rehearsal, grouping and counting.

Directions: There are many reasons why we might need to be able to remember things. What are some things that are important for you to remember? Today, we will practice two strategies to assist you in remembering things.

Repetition and Rehearsal

When you encounter something you want to remember, say it over and over to yourself. For example, when you meet someone new, say the person's name to yourself four or five times. Look at the person as you are doing this so that the name and the face will be connected in your brain. To practice this, turn to the person next to you and introduce yourself. (If they already know each other, making up a new name or using their middle names may suffice.) Using his name in the next sentence of conversation is another way to practice: "Nice to meet you, Henry" or "Henry, how are you feeling today?"

Next, we will use the same strategy to memorize a list of words. (Give out printed list.) You will note that the worksheet lists common objects numbered 1 to 10. Before we start, I would like you each to predict how many of these items you think you will be able to remember after 1 minute of practice. Write this number down on the top of your paper. Now begin memorizing, using repetition and rehearsal, repeating the words over and over. (Time for 1 minute.) Time is up. Please turn your paper over and write on the back as many words as you can remember. No looking at each other's papers is allowed. How does the result compare with your prediction? Look back at the list, and correct your errors. This can be repeated if desired.

Next, we will practice remembering objects that we see. I will show you a tray full of objects, and you will have 1 minute to look at them. During that minute, you should say the name of each object to yourself. When I cover the tray of objects, you will write down as many names of objects as you can remember, so get your pencils out. Paper will be given out as soon as the objects are covered. No note-taking is allowed. (Place the tray in the center of the table, uncover it for 1 minute, then re-cover it.) How did everyone do? How many objects did you list? How many were there all together? Did anyone count?

Behavioral Cognitive Activity Example 6-1
I Can Remember (Cognitive Rehabilitation) (Continued)

Grouping and Counting

The second strategy we will use is counting the items you wish to remember and then grouping them into categories. When we try this again, count the objects first, then try to remember items together that are associated in some way. This strategy is used in addition to the repetition and rehearsal we have already practiced. There are objects from three categories on this tray. Did anyone notice what those might be? (Discuss and clarify the strategy as needed. Give out blank paper.) Before we begin, we will predict how many items we can remember this time. Write that number down in the corner of your paper. Now we will begin. (Uncover tray and time for 1 minute, then re-cover.) Write down as many as you can remember. (Pause.) How many items were there? (20) How many were in each category? Let's make a master list. (Have someone volunteer.) Write the three categories, then have group list the items. When finished, uncover tray once again to self-correct errors. How did people do in comparison with last time? Did the grouping help you to remember more items? Now compare with your predictions. Application discussion follows, in which members discuss two or three ways they can use these strategies during the next week. Homework may be given as needed.

From Cole, M. B. *Group dynamics in OT: The theoretical basis and practice application of group intervention* (4th ed.). Thorofare, NJ: SLACK Incorporated. © 2012 SLACK Incorporated.

Behavioral Cognitive Activity Example 6-2
Setting Priorities (Psychoeducational)

This activity has been used as the first session of a time management workshop for clients with substance abuse. It serves as an ice breaker for clients who do not know each other well and also helps the therapist to formulate goals for the group.

Materials: Values Survey Worksheets (p. 184) and pencils.

Directions: Often, the things we spend our time doing are not the things we want most to do. Setting priorities means deciding what is important to us and doing that first. As a first step in helping to plan our time better, we will look at what we value.

(Pass out Values Survey Worksheet.) Take the next 10 minutes to think about the values listed, and number them according to their order of importance to you. Put number 1 next to the most important item, number 2 for the next level of importance, and so forth, up to number 8 for the least important. Do not use the same number more than once.

(Ask each member to share their top three values and discuss in what way these values are a part of his or her life right now.)

Write your top three values on the lower section of the Values Survey Worksheet, and below each, write one specific goal that reflects that value. For example, if "freedom to do what I want" is one of your values, your goal might be to move out of your parents' house and get your own apartment. You have 5 minutes for this part.

Looking at your goals, choose one to work on this weekend. At the bottom of the worksheet, write down one activity that you can plan this weekend to help you accomplish the goal.

From Cole, M. B. *Group dynamics in OT: The theoretical basis and practice application of group intervention* (4th ed.). Thorofare, NJ: SLACK Incorporated. © 2012 SLACK Incorporated.

Value Survey Worksheet

Directions: Eight commonly held values are listed here. Think about your own life in relation to these values. Then, give each a number, beginning with number 1 for the most important to you, number 2 for the second most important, and so forth, up to number 8 for the least important. Do not use any number more than once.

___ A good love relationship
___ Financial security
___ A satisfying religious faith
___ Freedom to do what I want
___ Meaningful family life
___ Success at my chosen career
___ Excitement and adventure
___ Making lots of money

First most important value:

Goal:

Second most important value:

Goal:

Third most important value:

Goal:

Planned activity to work on goal:

From Cole, M. B. *Group dynamics in OT: The theoretical basis and practice application of group intervention* (4th ed.). Thorofare, NJ: SLACK Incorporated. © 2012 SLACK Incorporated.

Behavioral Cognitive Activity Example 6-3
Telling Others About Your Illness (Psychoeducational)

This behavioral cognitive activity has been part of a client group on coping with illness. The group is given short lectures each week on a different aspect of coping with illness, followed by participation in a related activity. This one uses role playing and behavioral rehearsal, and the support of the group serves as social reinforcement.

Materials: Two chairs placed in the center of the group.

Directions: Each patient will take a turn sitting in the chair in the center. First, the client will tell the group what his or her illness is and why it is difficult to talk to others about it. Then, the client will choose another member to play the part of a relative or friend. The therapist is the "director" and directs as follows:

Friend or relative: Ask how the patient is and ask follow-up questions.

Client: Answer him or her as if it were a real conversation.

Client: Now, change places with your friend and respond for him or her. Now, change places again and be yourself again. Try to tell your friend how you "feel" about being ill. Try to keep each conversation going for about 5 minutes. Members should volunteer for this, and no one should be forced.

After each discussion, the group is asked to respond and to discuss the role play. Were the players being "genuine"? Were feelings being expressed freely? What are other ways to make the discussion helpful?

From Cole, M. B. *Group dynamics in OT: The theoretical basis and practice application of group intervention* (4th ed.). Thorofare, NJ: SLACK Incorporated. © 2012 SLACK Incorporated.

Behavioral Cognitive Activity Example 6-4
Relaxation Fantasy Activity (Biomechanical/Rehabilitative)

This activity has been a part of a stress management group in which members use the techniques of visualization and guided fantasy to control their state of tension.

Materials: Carpeted open space, patients wearing sweat suits and sneakers or other comfortable clothing, and pillows for each person.

Directions: Members sit in a circle on the floor, pillows in their laps. They should be far enough apart that all can lie down and reach out their arms without touching one another.

1. Introduction—Relaxation is as much in your mind as in your body. Therefore, if you want to be relaxed and free your body from stress, your mind must take the lead. It is very difficult to feel relaxed when your mind is preoccupied with worry. As you do this exercise, try to concentrate on the visual images that come into your head. Instructions will be given for you to move your physical position as well as parts of your body. Try to do these with your eyes closed, so you will not lose the mental images created.

2. You are about to take a 30-minute relaxation break from your busy, stressful, or boring day. Maybe you have a lot of work to do or a difficult situation to face. Put that out of your mind for the next 30 minutes. Afterward, when you are relaxed, you will have more energy to cope with life's hassles.

3. Begin by reaching both arms up over your head in a big stretch. Open your mouth wide and yawn. Now, place the pillow behind your hips and lean back on your elbows. Close your eyes and imagine a door far across the room in front of you. Without moving your position, imagine yourself walking toward the door. Move your feet, your ankles, your knees, and your hips as if you were walking. When the right leg is tense, allow the left one to relax. Now, point your toes each time you take a "step." Slow down your steps and inhale as you tense your right leg, then exhale as you tense your left leg. As you approach the door, your steps become slower and slower (2 minutes). When you reach the door, stand in front of it and continue breathing slowly.

4. Push yourself up with your arms to a sitting position. With your eyes still closed, lean forward and peek through a small hole in the door. You see a welcome view. It is a lovely, sunny patio with a sparkling in-ground pool. It is surrounded by clean, comfortable lounge chairs. Keep your hands behind you on the floor as you lean forward to get a better view. Stretch your back and push yourself forward with your arms until you feel the stretch behind your thighs. Keep breathing slowly.

5. With eyes still closed, bend your knees up to your chest. With one hand gripping each knee, imagine that your knees are the handles of the door. Pull gently on the "handles," straightening your back as you pull. Then, let go as the door opens wide. As you pass through the door, you leave behind all the worries of the day. On the other side of the door, there are no worries, no stress, so let them all go.

6. Without opening your eyes, straighten your legs and move the pillow under your head as you lie down on one of the comfortable lounge chairs. The sun feels good as it warms you. Imagine you are wearing a bathing suit under your sweatshirt. While still lying down, pretend to take the sweatshirt off. First, put hands near hips and push down on elbows to raise hips slightly off the floor. Then, raise hands up to chest level, elbows still on the floor. Push head back into the pillow as you raise shoulders slightly off the floor. Pause here and breathe. Now, raise your head off the pillow as you pretend to lift the sweatshirt off over your head and let it drop to the ground behind your pillow. This done, slowly return arms to your sides while breathing out slowly. Just lie there breathing slowly, enjoying the warm sun (2 minutes).

Relaxation Fantasy Activity (Biomechanical/Rehabilitative) (Continued)

7. Check your body to be sure it is relaxed. Wiggle your fingers and your toes. Roll your head to the right, then roll your head to the left. If there is tension anywhere, shake it out. Put your hand behind your neck and massage your neck muscles. Keep breathing slowly. It feels so relaxing to lie here in the warm sun (2 minutes).

8. The sun is getting hot now. Maybe it is time to go for a swim. Raise yourself up to a sitting position again, and bring your knees up to your chest. Now, imagine you are sitting on the edge of the pool. Dangle your legs into the pleasantly cool water. Turn around to the left and look behind you; turn around to the right and look behind you. The signs say "Good Swimming Today," so turn over slowly onto your stomach as you lower yourself into the water.

9. As you float on your stomach, your pillow has become a life preserver. Hold onto the pillow as you kick your legs slowly, floating around the pool. Your feet need not even leave the floor. It takes almost no effort at all to move you through the water. Your body does not feel heavy. Now inhale as you kick your right leg, exhale as you kick your left leg. As you reach the edge of the pool, push away again, continuing to hold onto the life preserver with one hand, then the other.

10. Now, lift up on your elbows and push the pillow down under your ribcage, so it supports your chest as you lean on your elbows. Continue to breathe slowly. Shrug your shoulders up toward your ears, then release. Shrug away your last bit of tension. Now you are relaxed, refreshed, and energetic. Now, you are capable of resuming your day without feeling tension and stress. Miraculously, you are out of the pool, dry and dressed again, standing in front of the door. Now, you feel prepared to go back through that door and take on the world. When you are ready, open your eyes.

Behavioral Cognitive Activity Example 6-5
Building Our Community (Psychoeducational)

This activity is part of a psychoeducational group focusing on independent living skills with clients who have mental health issues. The goal of this session is to help the group become aware of community resources. My thanks to D. M. Hancock, OT student at Quinnipiac College, for this creative idea.

Materials: One square of ¼-inch plywood, approximately 30 x 30 inches, a variety of small blocks of scrap wood with rough edges and splinters sanded off, jars of poster paint in several colors, brushes, and wood glue. This project may take two sessions to complete.

Directions: The group begins by discussing the communities in which they live and what services and resources are available there. The OT helps the group develop a list of services that members need to have available in their community. A typical list includes a hospital, grocery store, department store, drug store, police department, fire department, school, and movie theater. Why they need each one and how they would use it is discussed.

Next, the group members build from the blocks a community they would like to live in. Each member chooses one or more community resources to build and constructs a school, a movie theater, etc., by gluing blocks together. The "buildings" are then painted, and colored signs are painted on to label them. Buildings are then placed and glued onto the plywood square, something like an architect's model city. Streets, parking lots, parks, or bodies of water may be painted directly on the plywood if desired (Figure 6-1).

Discussion/Summary: Sharing has already been done during the activity. Members are asked how they felt about doing the activity and about the result. Some generalization was done earlier in the choices of structures and organizations to be included in the community and their uses and importance. This may be reinforced and elaborated here, with an emphasis on how to contact and use community resources appropriately to meet one's needs. Each member then compares the "model" he or she has built to his or her own neighborhood or community. Application includes each member's plans for using his or her own community resources, now and in the future.

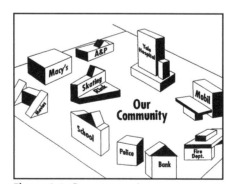

Figure 6-1. Our community.

Behavioral Cognitive Activity Example 6-6
Exercise Groups (Biomechanical/Rehabilitative)

Exercise to music and dance activities have good potential as therapeutic tools. Circle or group dancing is usually best suited to our purpose in OT. In physical disability areas where goals involve maintaining and increasing strength and ROM, group activities that accomplish these goals are more enjoyable and motivating than individual exercise programs. A good example of this type of group is the "Range of Motion Dance," an exercise program for patients with rheumatoid arthritis developed by Diane Harlowe and Patricia Yu at St. Mary's Hospital Medical Center in Madison, Wisconsin (Van Deusen & Harlowe, 1987). This is a guided fantasy done with groups of arthritis clients seated in chairs. The exercises, while following the story, go systematically through the ROM for nearly every joint in the body. Once the sequence of motions is learned, it can be repeated by the patients at home by listening to the story on an audiotape.

Greenfield and Godinez have introduced a similar group for people recovering from stroke, called "Self Range of Motion Exercises" (1989). They have defined eight skill levels for these exercises, ranging from complete dependence on the therapist leader to independence in performing the exercises.

In doing such groups, it is important to use the potential of the group to provide mutual support, encouragement, and feedback. Do not let the activity speak for itself; combine it with verbal reinforcement, progress checks, and education about how and why it is helping. It is generally the social and emotional aspects of a group that keep members coming back.

From Cole, M. B. *Group dynamics in OT: The theoretical basis and practice application of group intervention* (4th ed.). Thorofare, NJ: SLACK Incorporated. © 2012 SLACK Incorporated.

Behavioral Cognitive Activity Example 6-7
Map Reading (Cognitive Rehabilitation)

A group of clients with cognitive impairments has the goal of improving skills in visual processing and verbal communication. They are given a map of their community and a worksheet with a list of 10 locations. The following are examples of their tasks:

1. Write directions from Merritt Park Way to the Trumbull Shopping Mall on Main Street.
2. Write directions from the corner of Madison and Stonehouse Roads to Trumbull High School on Stroebel and Daniels Farms Roads.
3. Describe two alternate routes to get from the golf course on Tashua Road to Main Street at the Bridgeport line.
4. Direct someone from Teller and Whitney to the dog pound on Church Street.
5. Plan a route to pick up three friends, on Indian Ledge Road, Brittany Road, and Autumn Ridge Road, and take them to the Town Hall meeting room on Quality Street.

To change the context, other maps or diagrams can be introduced and directions given verbally or in writing. Each client in the group should have at least one location to find on his own, and then communicate the directions to the rest of the group. The therapist should encourage members to give each other feedback about the accuracy of the directions and clarity of communication.

From Cole, M. B. *Group dynamics in OT: The theoretical basis and practice application of group intervention* (4th ed.). Thorofare, NJ: SLACK Incorporated. © 2012 SLACK Incorporated.

Behavioral Cognitive Activity Example 6-8
Design Duplication (Cognitive Rehabilitation)

This activity appears in *The Cognitive Rehabilitation Workbook* by Dougherty and Radomski (1987). The goals are to give and follow verbal directions. The objectives are to develop vocabulary to give precise directions, increase accuracy in conveying detailed information, and develop a tolerance for the pitfalls in making oneself understood. Followers of directions are expected to increase their accuracy, develop skills in clarification and confirmation, and increase speed of processing verbal directions.

A group of six is divided into pairs. One from each pair acts as the direction giver and holds a line drawing of several lines and shapes. The other half of each pair sits with his or her back to his or her partner and holds a clipboard with blank paper and a pencil with an eraser. Both partners are provided with rulers. Partner 1 must verbally describe the line drawing so that Partner 2 can draw an exact duplicate of the drawing being described. Attention must be paid to shapes, spacing, and dimensions. The pair has 20 minutes to accomplish the task. Then, a new drawing is given to each pair, and roles are reversed.

It is very important that a feedback session follows each trial. The pairs should discuss the results and analyze any errors in communication in order to correct these on the next trial. This activity can be fun as well as useful, and the therapist should try to create a relaxed atmosphere for the group.

From Cole, M. B. *Group dynamics in OT: The theoretical basis and practice application of group intervention* (4th ed.). Thorofare, NJ: SLACK Incorporated. © 2012 SLACK Incorporated.

ALLEN'S COGNITIVE DISABILITIES GROUP

The group approach discussed here is the cognitive disabilities theory of Claudia Allen. Allen has been developing this theory since the early 1970s. Her basic premise is that functional behavior is based on cognition and that, in order to produce a more functional behavior, the thinking process must change. Group activities combine assessment and intervention in this approach, and these usually occur concurrently. Therapist observation of behavior during group activities leads to new assumptions about how information is being perceived and processed. Allen has developed a hierarchy of six cognitive levels and has described typical behaviors of each based on clinical observation. Using her guidelines, we can easily evaluate our clients and place them in activity groups that are appropriate for their cognitive level.

Many of the clients we will treat in occupational therapy are cognitively disabled. Examples of some disorders that involve a cognitive disability are stroke, traumatic brain injury, schizophrenia and other psychotic disorders, anxiety and substance abuse disorders, personality disorders, Alzheimer's and other dementias, mental retardation, autism, and learning disability. Some of these disorders can be successfully treated. For those cases, Allen groups provide one of the most accurate measures we have for documenting progress. However, for many people with these disorders, a plateau will be reached beyond which no further cognitive development is possible. These clients need ongoing care, protection from danger, and assistance with many activities of daily living. For these clients, an assessment of cognitive level during a group activity will provide useful guidelines for the level of assistance that will be needed after discharge.

FRAMEWORK FOCUS

The cognitive disabilities theory is broadly applicable for both chronic and acute-care settings. This theory is best applied when there is a need to measure and monitor a client's problem-solving ability and safety while performing daily activities in any of the "areas of occupation" listed in the *Occupational Therapy Practice Framework* (American Occupational Therapy Association [AOTA], 2008). Clients with health conditions that affect their cognition may be grouped together according to the Allen levels and may be re-evaluated and monitored as a group, saving valuable time for the occupational therapist. Caregiver groups or "families with dementia/traumatic brain injury, etc." may be guided to facilitate the client's best ability to function using Allen principles. Guidelines for assistance at various cognitive levels fit the *Occupational Therapy Practice Framework's* definition of "facilitating engagement in occupation" (AOTA, 2008). The primary features of intervention are adaptation of contexts and task demand (Toglia et al., 2009). Adaptation of the "physical" and "social contexts" are a focus in the Allen approach as the occupational therapy structures the materials, assistance, and "activity demands" to provide a "just-right challenge." Allen's task analysis considers all aspects of "activity demands" listed in the *Occupational Therapy Practice Framework*. Routines of daily occupation may be equated to "performance patterns" in the *Occupational Therapy Practice Framework* domain (AOTA, 2008). Levy and Burns (2005), using Allen's perspective with older adults with dementia, stress the importance of habits and routines in

Cole M.B. *Group Dynamics in Occupational Therapy:*
The Theoretical Basis and Practice Application
of Group Intervention (pp 193-216).
© 2012 SLACK Incorporated.

maintaining independence in self-care and engagement in the normal everyday activities, including a balanced schedule of mealtimes, social activities, and hours of rest and sleep.

Allen provides a pragmatic approach to living with the consequences of illness or injury. Some theorists have been critical of the Allen approach because it focuses on "disability" and seems to emphasize weaknesses rather than strengths. This is a misinterpretation. In fact, it is by acknowledging and understanding disability that Allen gives us the profession's most precise guidelines for using a client's remaining ability to maximize function. "Therapists should identify the person's best ability to function and select intervention goals that maximize these abilities" (Allen, Blue, & Earhart, 1995, p. 1). The focus of therapy is on assessment and enabling best ability to function.

Assessment

Perhaps Allen is best known for the Allen's Cognitive Levels Screen (ACLS), which uses leather lacing to assess the precise cognitive level of the client (from 3.0 to 5.8). This test has become increasingly standardized over the past decade and is widely used by occupational therapists as a screening tool. It gives a quick estimate of the client's current capacity to learn (Allen, 1999). Other standardized tests of cognitive level developed by Allen are the Routine Task Inventory (RTI; Heinmann et al, 1989; Josman & Katz, 1991) and the Cognitive Performance Test (CPT) (Allen & Earhart, 1992; Burns, 2003; Katz, 2008). These assessments use everyday activities to determine the cognitive level. The Allen Diagnostic Module (ADM), the most recently developed test, takes motivation and socialization into account and uses a dynamic approach to assessment of cognitive level. (The latest updates of these assessments may be obtained from S & S Worldwide at 1-800-288-9941.) The ADM uses a group format to observe performance while doing a variety of standardized craft activities. Crafts make an effective evaluation at levels 3.0 to 5.8 and are motivating because they are meaningful across the spectrum of cultures. Observation of an individual's response to instructions and sensory cues from the materials and tools of the craft provide the basis for predictions about many other aspects of human performance. Examples of these crafts are given later in the chapter in the section on activities.

Allen's assessment tools have been extensively researched and found to be highly valid and reliable (Ikiugu, 2007). However, in today's evidence-based scientific standards, therapists should use caution in making judgments about cognitive level based on the observation of these activities. Allen's levels and modes should never be considered labels, which prejudice others and limit the person's options or autonomy. Rather, they should be used as guidelines, upon which to plan initial

activities or make tentative discharge arrangements, which will only become valid when the person with cognitive disability has an opportunity to demonstrate his or her best ability to function.

Because the Allen approach advocates that clients be treated in groups of similar cognitive level, the initial screening becomes an important part of group planning. The approximate cognitive level must be determined in order to place clients appropriately in occupational therapy intervention groups.

Enabling Best Ability to Function

Once the client's best ability to function (ACL) has been determined, decisions about lifestyle and discharge placement need to be made. The occupational therapist's role is to make recommendations about the level of assistance the client will need in the immediate future. Enabling a client's best ability to function involves two aspects: 1) assistance from caregivers and 2) adaptation of the environment. The guiding principles for management come from the cognitive modes of functioning within each level. Goals for expected behaviors in activities of daily living are defined, along with the amount of physical and cognitive assistance needed at each mode/level (Allen et al., 1995).

Environmental adaptation flows from the amount of conscious awareness the client has at his or her disposal. To elicit his or her best effort in doing a task, the usable task environment must be defined. Supplies needed for a task to be done must be placed within the limits of conscious awareness, for example, within arm's reach at Level 3. Concurrently, all distractions and unsafe items should be removed. Think about how hard it is to get anything done when your desk is piled high with junk mail or your kitchen is stacked with dirty dishes. Our clients need our help to remove the clutter and help them focus on what is necessary to perform essential tasks.

Another essential component of client management is providing needed assistance. Allen also builds into the cognitive levels and modes the quality and quantity of assistance needed. To elicit the client's best performance, the caregiver must first observe the client's response to the task environment and then intervene as needed in a variety of ways. Four of the possible ways to give cognitive assistance suggested by Allen are as follows:

1. *Facilitate*—Give sensory cues appropriate to the level.

2. *Probe*—Ask focused questions to encourage problem solving.

3. *Observe*—Allow client time to process cues and questions and try out new behaviors.

4. *Rescue*—When frustration arises, correct error or do a step for the client.

The experienced therapist should never do for clients what they can do for themselves. For example,

Table 7-1

Allen's Cognitive Assistance for Levels 1 Through 6

Level	Cognitive Assistance Needed	Compensation Provided for the Following Cognitive Functions, Which Are Lacking
1	Total	Sensory stimulation (and 2 to 6)
2	Maximum	Prevent getting lost or into unsafe areas (and 3 to 6)
3	Moderate	Help with self-care (and 4 to 6)
4	Minimum	Maintaining the home (and 5 and 6)
5	Standby	Planning, advising, supervision
6	None necessary	None

© Claudia Allen, conference materials, 1997. Adapted with permission.

the person at Level 3 responds best to tactile cues. The caregiver, therefore, facilitates by using touch to get the client's attention and demonstrates the use of necessary objects. To assist with dressing, the caregiver hands the client a shirt and touches the right hand to be inserted in the sleeve. Probing or asking questions that suggest the next step might then be tried (e.g., "How can you get your arm in the sleeve?"). Observing the response determines if more assistance is needed. If the response is unproductive, a third attempt might be a direct verbal instruction, accompanying the demonstration, "Hold it by the collar with this hand, and put the other arm in here." The "rescue" is always a last resort; if the client shows significant signs of frustration, put the arm in the shirt for him or her.

In general, the amount of assistance needed to do a task decreases as the cognitive level increases. Table 7-1 is a general guideline for the amount of cognitive assistance needed at each level.

BASIC ASSUMPTIONS

Cognitive Disability Defined

Allen (1987a) defines cognitive disability as "a limitation in sensorimotor actions originating in the physical or chemical structures of the brain and producing observable and assessable limitations in routine task behavior." Allen accepts the concept that a person's cognitive level has biological and chemical determinants resulting from one or more health conditions. However, she maintains that engagement in activities and participation can be maximized by assessing activity limitations and adapting both task demand and contextual factors. Applying the framework of the *International Classification of Functioning, Disability, and Health* (World Health Organization [WHO], 2001), assessment and enabling best function in occupational therapy involve assessing the cognitive impairment, using assistance and environmental adaptation to compensate for activity limitations, and promoting routines that allow continued participation in the occupations of daily life (Table 7-2). Allen's theory provides a way for occupational therapists to predict the activities clients with cognitive disabilities will be able to participate in competently and safely.

Being unable to work, care for others, and maintain a home are some of the roles that are commonly lost as a result of cognitive disability. However, there are other roles that may be acquired, such as volunteer, hobbyist, family helper, and organization participant, with the appropriate cognitive assistance.

Allen's Task Analysis

Task analysis is defined as a method of determining the functional complexity of an activity by separating the activity into steps and determining the physical and cognitive functional abilities required to do each step. In recent years, Allen has developed a more dynamic approach to task analysis, which includes factors like culture, motivation, and situational context, as well as the basic ability to process information. This approach is visually outlined in Figure 7-1, and this serves as the basis for planning and interpreting craft activities such as those used in the ADM. In 1999, Allen updated her information processing theory by making a distinction between working memory and procedural memory. Working memory is what we use when we are actively processing information. It is necessary for the continual orientation to time and social context as well as new learning. Procedural memory is what we use for our habitual actions done without conscious awareness (Allen, 1999). This type of memory may be useful when well-learned self-care habits and routines remain in memory even when new learning and problem-solving ability is impaired.

Table 7-2

International Classification of Functioning, Disability, and Health: Overview of ICF Components (2001)

- Body functions: Physiological functions of body systems, including psychological function
- Body structures: Anatomical parts of the body, such as organs, limbs, and their components
- Impairments: Problems in body function or structure, such as significant deviation or loss
- Activity: Execution of a task or action by an individual
- Participation: Involvement of a life situation
- Activity limitations: Difficulties an individual may have in executing activities
- Participation restrictions: Problems individuals experience in life situations
- Environmental factors: Physical, social, and attitudinal contexts in which people live

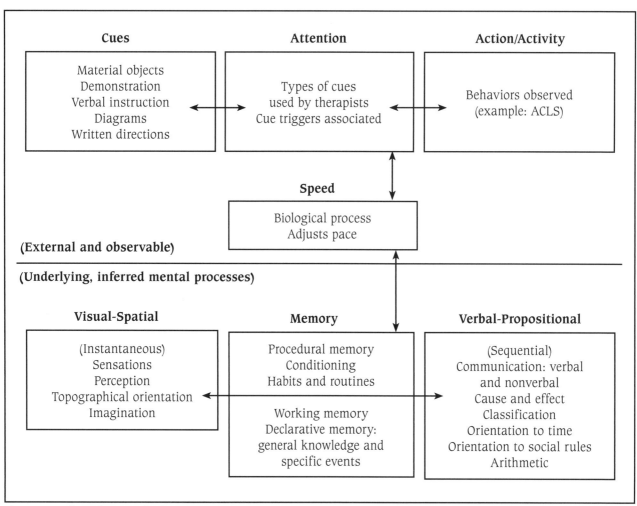

Figure 7-1. Allen's functional information processing system.

Cues

Cues consist of the environment itself; the materials needed for a task; and all forms of verbal, written, or demonstrated instruction. In normal everyday activity, when we find ourselves in a kitchen at mealtime, the cues we use are the food in the refrigerator or cabinets, the recipe or preparation we have in mind, and the equipment available for preparing a meal (e.g., bowls, baking pans, dishes, knives). Visual, olfactory, and gustatory memories may guide and motivate us.

Attention

Attention to cues is necessary for functional activity to occur. How our brain receives or screens out cues may depend on many psychological, physiological, social, and cultural factors. In cognitive disability, the limitations of attention and sensory screening need to be evaluated in order to plan appropriate intervention. When using cues in intervention, Allen advocates careful planning of the environment (clinic or home setting), thoughtful selection and placement of supplies and equipment to be used for a task, and varying the amount and type of assistance given, according to the specific guidelines at each cognitive level or mode.

Action/Activity

The combination of cues and a person's ability to attend and focus will hopefully result in an action or response (the performance of functional activity). Continuing the kitchen analogy, when I go home to my kitchen after a hard day's work, my meal preparation task will be greatly enhanced by how well I have prepared ahead. If I bought the right ingredients at the grocery store, if the pots and pans and dishes are clean and ready to be used, and if I remember or have easy access to the recipe or procedure to be used, the meal will be prepared correctly and in a timely manner. All sorts of things can go wrong, even in the absence of disability—telephone calls, unexpected company, key ingredients being eaten by another family member, the right size baking pan borrowed and not returned. Problem solving is needed to cope with unexpected obstacles.

When therapists select tasks to be performed by clients in the clinical setting, the client's problem-solving ability may be observed and evaluated. Allen has given us specific guidelines for making these observations and for interpreting them. The six cognitive levels are based on compiling typical behaviors at each cognitive level (and subsequently, each mode) in response to a variety of tasks (cues). From these sample behaviors, cognitive disability theory makes inferences about the thinking processes that produced them. These inferences explain how the person's brain processes the information being presented.

Speed

The speed of response depends upon the speed with which the brain processes information. Biological factors, such as brain chemicals, are responsible for setting the rate of thinking and behavior. People functioning below Level 5 generally have a difficult time adjusting the speed of their performance.

Underlying Mental Processes—The Evidence

Levy and Burns (2005) have used recent developments in cognitive information processing research to update Allen's original conceptions of how cognition impacts task performance. They applied research findings with the stages of dementia, which are largely determined by everyday task behaviors (Reisberg, Franssen, Souren, Auer, & Kenowskky, 1998). Remarkably, they found that most of the recent research developments correspond with, and therefore serve to validate, Allen's six cognitive levels. The following is a summary of research related to Alzheimer's disease, which accounts for about two-thirds of older adult dementias. Information processing involves three brain functions that interact to produce occupational performance: sensory perception, working or short-term memory, and long-term memory.

Sensory perception includes awareness of environmental cues, pattern recognition, filtering out irrelevant information, and selection of which cues to attend to (automatic attention). Second, short-term, working memory includes conscious attention to relevant cues, executive functions such as planning, sequencing, problem solving, judgment, reasoning, goal formulation, and organization, and the quantity and speed of information processing. Long-term memory has two categories, implicit and explicit. Implicit long-term memory operates mostly at an unconscious level and includes procedural memory (how to do a task [i.e., riding a bike]), perceptual priming, in which associations are activated by internal or external cues, and motor and emotional conditioning. Explicit memory requires awareness and also has two parts: episodic and semantic. Episodic memory stores personally relevant facts and events over a lifetime, including both recent and remote events. Semantic memory is language based and includes visual spatial and perceptual memories. Recalling explicit long-term memories involves a process of search and retrieval and is often triggered by associational cues, either internal or external. Levy and Burns note that typical tests of cognition are usually limited to episodic and explicit memories, ignoring procedural or sensory categories, which may, in fact, be quite important in retaining occupational performance capability.

Comparing this with dementia research, the brain areas damaged in the mild stages of Alzheimer's are

Table 7-3

Comparison of Allen's Cognitive Levels With Global Dementia and Medicare Assistance Levels

ACL Level	Global Dementia Level	Cognitive Assistance
ACL 6.0 (Competent)	Level 1	None
ACL 5.6	Level 2	10%
ACL 5.4	Level 3	14%
ACL 4.6	Level 4	30%
ACL 4.0	Level 5	42%
ACL 3.4	Level 6	54%
ACL 2.0	Level 7	84%

Adapted from Allen, C. K. (1997). Cognitive disabilities: How to make clinical judgments. In N. Katz (Ed.), *Cognitive rehabilitation: Models for intervention in occupational therapy*. Rockville, MD: American Occupational Therapy Association.

the hippocampus, residing in the temporal lobes, which are responsible for short-term, working memory. Mild dementia also affects the synaptic connectivity where working memory operates, causing many potential sensory cues to be lost in the reasoning process. The next brain area to be affected by Alzheimer's is the frontal lobes, which are responsible for executive functions to activate and synthesize relevant information. Examples of limitations in activities are failures in reading comprehension (understanding/following written directions) and complex visual spatial patterns (recognizing faces and places). These deficits are typical of mild dementia and also of Allen's Level 5 behaviors and limitations.

Moderate Alzheimer's is associated with loss of parietal brain lobes, which control spatial orientation, recognition of familiar objects, and body sensory awareness such as stereognosis. The speed of working memory processing is also affected, causing errors in reasoning and judgment based on incomplete information or inappropriate timing. The behaviors in moderate Alzheimer's closely resemble Allen's Level 4 (mild-moderate) and Level 3 (moderate) behaviors. Some typical task behaviors are loss of time orientation, inappropriate use of tools, and inability to choose and put on appropriate clothing. (More specific behaviors are later described in sections on each Allen level.)

The success of Allen's techniques of assistance, cueing, and environmental adaptation for people with dementia can largely be attributed to the relative resistance of occipital lobes (where long-term memory is stored) and of the cerebellum and basal ganglia, where procedural memory is spared until the final stages of Alzheimer's disease. The habits and routines of self-care, for example, are mainly stored in procedural memory and can be activated with appropriate cueing, coupled with environmental adaptation. Walking, eating,

brushing teeth, toileting, and many other familiar routines can therefore be retained well into the moderate-severe stages of Alzheimer's, especially when these activities are performed using familiar objects and in familiar contexts. OTs can teach caregivers how to best assist people with dementia to remain independent in self-care for as long as possible.

When comparing the progressive stages of brain deterioration to Allen's six stages in reverse, there is a remarkable similarity, as detailed by Levy and Burns in their comparative analysis, which they have titled "cognitive disabilities reconsidered" (2005, p. 347). Through many years of careful observation, Allen has analyzed the cognitive components for each level and mode (Table 7-3). While many subtle differences are too detailed to describe here, their contribution to the functional performance we observe in our clients during group activities should not be underestimated. In activity selection, a therapist should consider the client's prior knowledge, experience, and preferences, as well as sensorimotor and verbal abilities.

Six Cognitive Levels

Allen divides cognitive disabilities into six well-defined cognitive levels and provides several assessment tools to help occupational therapists evaluate the cognitive level. Assessment and intervention are based on how the client learns and performs tasks. Originally, the six levels were derived from Piaget's work on intellectual development. However, based on Allen's clinical observation, the cognitive levels are largely presented as descriptions of typical behaviors at each level. In consideration of cognitive impact on task performance, three categories were proposed: 1) attention, 2) motor actions, and 3) conscious awareness. Table 7-4 provides an overview of how these three features appear and guide behavior

Table 7-4

Allen's Cognitive Levels 1 Through 6

	1. Automatic Actions	2. Postural Actions	3. Manual Actions	4. Goal-Directed Actions	5. Exploratory Actions	6. Planned Actions
Attention to sensory cues	Subliminal	Proprioceptive	Tactile	Visible cues	Related cues (all senses)	Symbolic cues
Motor actions						
Spontaneous	Automatic	Postural	Manual	Goal-directed	Exploratory	Planned
Imitated	None	Approximations	Manipulations	Replications	Novelty	Unnecessary
Conscious awareness						
Purpose	Arousal	Comfort	Interest	Compliance	Self-control	Reflection
Experience	Indistinct	Moving	Touching	Seeing	Inductive reasoning	Deductive reasoning
Process	Habitual or reflexive	Effect on body	Effect on environment	Several actions	Overt trial and error	Covert trial and error
Time (attention span)	Seconds	Minutes	Half hours	Hours	Weeks	Past/future
Occupational therapy activities	Sensory stimulation	Gross motor, games, dance	Simple, repetitive tasks	Several-step tasks	Concrete tasks	Conceptual tasks

© Claudia Allen, conference materials, 1997. Adapted with permission.

at each Allen Cognitive Level. Information for this table represents many combined sources (Allen, 1982, 1987a, 1987b, 1991, 1994, 1997; Allen & Allen, 1987; Levy, 1997).

Attention

In observing people interacting with their environment, the first thing noted is what sensory stimuli capture their interest. The sensory systems most used at each cognitive level seem to more or less follow a developmental sequence, beginning with body sensation (position and movement), proceeding to incorporate touch and vision, and then integrating these and using them together.

Motor Actions

Second, motor actions are observed in the context of task performance. The therapist uses observations of a person's movements and verbalizations to make some assumptions about his or her perception, understanding, and intention, all a part of cognition.

Conscious Awareness

Finally, conscious awareness of the surroundings is observed. The scope or range of awareness and the

ability to use that awareness to determine appropriate action increases with each level. See Table 7-4 for a simplified description of attention, motor actions, and conscious awareness at each of the six levels. For a more complete understanding of these levels and their assessment, the reader is referred to Allen's books (Allen, 1985; Allen & Earhart, 1992).

Allen Cognitive Level (ACL) Descriptions

Level 1—Automatic Actions

In most cases, clients at Level 1 are bedridden. They are conscious but respond mainly to internal or subliminal cues (sensations from within the body), such as hunger or pain. Behavior is largely habitual or reflexive. Arousal and response to others may be elicited for a few seconds at a time. Most daily needs (dressing, grooming, feeding) have to be done by caregivers. Occupational therapists at this level are most helpful in providing appropriate sensory stimulation and attempting to elicit motor responses of any kind.

Level 2—Postural Actions

At Level 2, clients can be stimulated to perform postural actions (changes in position) in response to proprioceptive (sense of motion and position) cues. Clients can imitate gross motor actions and can assist a caregiver in bathing, dressing, and grooming. Usually, clients at Level 2 can feed themselves, although this may be messy. Twenty-four-hour nursing care is required. Engaging the client in any self-care tasks is an appropriate intervention at this level. Movement or exercise groups using imitation of position can be done. However, clients cannot benefit from interactive group intervention until they are at Level 3. A good quick test to determine whether a client is a Level 2 or 3 is to administer the Lower Cognitive Level (LCL) test. Ask the client to watch you while you clap your hands three times loudly (approximately one clap per second). If the client starts before you finish three, stop him or her and ask him or her to watch you first. If the client is able to imitate three claps, he or she is probably a Level 3 and therefore should be considered for group intervention.

Level 3—Manual Actions

At this level, clients perform manual actions (movements with their hands) in response to tactile cues (touch). Actions based on interest in objects found within arm's reach may be repeated many times. Attention can be maintained up to 30 minutes. Basic daily grooming tasks may be done independently with reminders; clients can walk to familiar places but get easily lost in new surroundings. Repetitive work tasks can be done at Level 3. Some of the tasks requiring supervision are care of belongings and clothing, money management, preparing meals, following a schedule, and using a telephone. Care should be taken to place potentially dangerous items out of reach or locked away, as a person at Level 3 cannot discriminate items by their intended use (e.g., paper napkins in the toaster). Tool use must be supervised, as it may be inappropriate (e.g., using a hammer to shut a window). However, with proper instruction, familiar repetitive actions can be fairly skilled, such as using a peeler to peel a potato or a paring knife to cut an apple. Tools that are an "extension of the hand," such as a fork, paintbrush, or nail file, are usually safe to use with supervision at Level 3. Steps in a task can be imitated one at a time, when demonstrated.

Level 4—Goal-Directed Actions

Becoming goal directed represents a major step toward independent functioning. It is goal directedness that makes activity purposeful; therefore, actions below this level are generally random or habitual. At Level 4, basic living skills are intact: grooming, dressing, toileting, bathing, and feeding. In addition, clients at Level 4 perform goal-directed actions in response to visual cues. In other words, if they see a toothbrush, toothpaste, and a cup next to the bathroom sink, this visible cue will remind them to brush their teeth. These clients are able to complete short tasks such as making a sandwich or washing the dishes. Attention is up to 1 hour, and steps toward a goal can be imitated in short sequences. Clients perform most daily self-care activities but need assistance in coping with new events, anticipating needs, and managing money. Visual stimuli are the focus, but nonvisible properties in the environment, like heat and electricity (e.g., a hair dryer near the bathtub or paper towels near a hot stove), may pose a danger. Directions for getting places or doing tasks must be demonstrated visually because verbal and written directions are not followed. Familiar routine tasks should be reinforced as new routines are established only by repetitive "drilling." Because people at Level 4 are aware of the goal, they are able to ask for assistance, and this plays a major role in keeping them safe and functional.

Level 5—Exploratory Actions/Independent Learning

Use of trial and error is the hallmark of Level 5. Here, for the first time, people use inductive reasoning and are capable of new learning. Clients at Level 5 can imitate new procedures and remember several steps at a time. In task performance, novelty is sought and variation explored. In choosing group projects, this is the first level at which choices may be given.

Deficits at Level 5 are in functions that require anticipation and planning. People at Level 5 are concrete thinkers primarily and have trouble imagining the long-term consequences of their actions or inactions. Hence, preventative measures are often not taken. In the home, for example, needed repairs may be neglected (a broken step is neglected until someone trips and falls). Cooking presents a problem when timing is involved (e.g., burning is not anticipated). Money management is a major problem because clients at Level 5 seldom save for emergencies or anticipate future expenses. Also neglected are purchasing needed items for a meal, cleaning or laundering clothing, and getting prescriptions refilled. The lack of abstract thinking prevents these clients from understanding the nature of their illness or the effects of medication. Jobs and social relationships may suffer because of failure to anticipate the consequences of self-centered behavior. Positive interventions at this level are activities that increase social awareness, reciprocation in relationships, and accepting the supervision of others in helping to avoid negative consequences.

Level 6—Planned Actions

This is the highest level and represents the absence of disability. The main distinguishing characteristic is the ability to use deductive reasoning and to plan ahead.

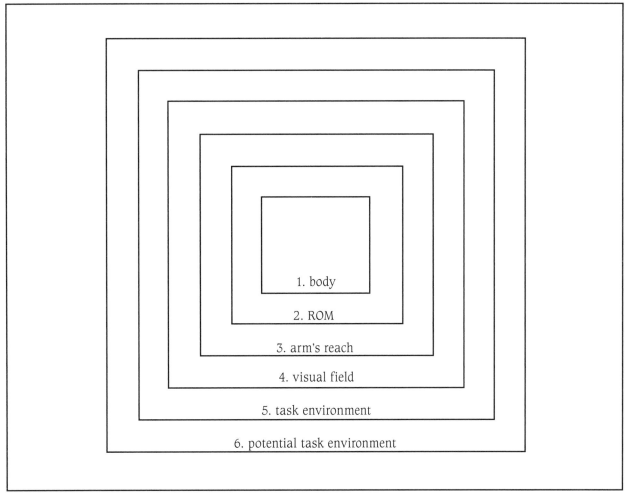

1. body
2. ROM
3. arm's reach
4. visual field
5. task environment
6. potential task environment

Figure 7-2. The usuable task environment. (Adapted with permission from Allen C. K. [1985]. *Occupational therapy for psychiatric diseases: Measurement and management of cognitive disabilities.* Boston, MA: Little, Brown and Co.)

Future events are anticipated, and behavior is organized. Verbal and written directions can be followed without demonstration, and the person is able to use symbolic cues (Allen, 1988).

The Principle of Brain Conservation

It is natural to think of ourselves as Level 6, which is Allen's representation of "normal." However, everyone has a flow of effort within the entire range of cognitive levels over the course of the day. We may indeed be functioning at Level 6 when we are listening to a lecture and rapidly taking notes in class. But there are many tasks we engage in that do not require that much effort. Bathing and dressing for the day are routine activities that may only require a Level 3 effort. Jogging around a track for exercise allows our brain to take a break and sink to a Level 2. Our brains have a tendency to conserve energy whenever possible. The difference between "normal" and "disabled" is that, in disability, no amount of effort can evoke a higher level of cognitive functioning. This limitation is what puts cognitively disabled people

at great risk when they encounter unexpected problems in everyday life. For example, Margaret, at Level 4, can drive a car from her home to a familiar nearby grocery store. But when road construction necessitated a detour, she ended up lost. She was unable to alter her usual route or to locate the necessary resources to find her way home. She wandered around on unfamiliar streets until someone noticed and called a policeman to escort her back home.

The Usable Task Environment

Allen's theory tells us that, as the cognitive level increases, awareness of the environment also increases. Specific guidelines are included in Figure 7-2.

For example, a new client, Sam, is being observed eating a meal. If he is being fed by an aide at his hospital bed, most likely he is at Level 1. If a piece of bread is placed in his hand, and he brings it to his mouth and takes a bite, he is at least a Level 2 because he is able to use movement functionally. If Sam reaches for the pitcher of juice in the center of the table, an Allen therapist knows he is at least a Level 3 because his attention extends to everything within arm's reach. If Sam asks that the catsup on the opposite side of the table be passed, the therapist will know immediately that Sam is at least a Level 4. He is using his visual system to look for what he wants, and his attention is projected beyond arm's reach. If he likes barbeque sauce, and he gets up and goes to get it out of the refrigerator, he is probably at least a Level 5. He looks for items he cannot see in places where they are typically kept, an action that integrates sensation, perception, and memory. At Level 6, Sam may remember he is out of milk and go to buy some next time he's out shopping. At each level, Sam's usable task environment has expanded.

Principle of Task Equivalence

Many people wonder why Allen uses crafts in her group assessment activities (ADM). The answer lies in the principle of task equivalence. The cognitive processing necessary in doing a craft activity is presumed to be equivalent to a variety of everyday tasks that a client will choose to participate in after discharge from an acute setting. The careful observation of the client doing a craft activity in a group allows the trained occupational therapist to determine the client's level of cognitive processing. A client who paints a wooden box on the top and three sides, but does not turn the project to paint the back, the bottom, or the inside, is showing some important limitations in his or her ability to process information and apply it to task performance. This client is only attending to what is immediately visible. Before he or she goes home, the therapist will be able to predict equivalent tasks that are likely to be problems for him or her there, such as personal grooming, keeping clothing clean, appropriate food preparation and storage, and many other aspects of home safety and maintenance. Because of task equivalence, recommendations for the level of assistance, supervision, and environmental adaptation needed for the best function and safety of the individual at home can be made more accurately. The usefulness of task equivalence, however, depends on the accuracy of the therapist's task analysis, using Allen's principles.

FUNCTION AND DYSFUNCTION

Allen gives the profession its best-defined system for measuring the impact of cognitive dysfunction. Not only are there six levels, ranging from comatose (1) to highly functional (6), but there are 52 modes of performance in between. Modes are identified by the decimal points after the level. Scores on the ACL Test are expressed as 3.0, 4.4, 5.8, etc. Each mode has implications that guide the occupational therapist in observing a progression of cognitive skills from one level to the next. A recent Allen publication, *Structures of the Cognitive Performance Modes* (1999), describes each mode from 1.0 to 6.0 with regard to expected cognitive abilities, functional goals, intervention methods, and safety. This text incorporates the most current research on cognition and provides excellent guidelines for accurate assessment, caregiver education, and discharge planning or placement. It requires some training and experience to learn to use the modes in assessment, intervention, and documentation.

For the purposes of students and therapists who are not previously familiar with cognitive disabilities theory, just identifying the low and high end of each level makes a good starting point for placing clients in groups. Table 7-5 outlines some simple behavioral observations that can be used to approximate the cognitive level for the purposes of group placement and initial activity selection. The level can then be confirmed by observation of task behaviors during the group itself.

The function-dysfunction continuum of cognitive abilities fluctuates in every individual, including those without a diagnosed disability. For this reason, intervention in the cognitive disabilities frame of reference cannot really be separated from ongoing evaluation. Intervention groups are primarily used, not so much for cognitive skill training, but as an opportunity for the client and therapist to discover the optimal environmental conditions necessary for the client to safely engage in purposeful activity. The client's response to a group activity may be understood as one example of the way he or she will respond to similar activity situations outside the intervention environment. The observation of group behaviors, together with Allen's modes of performance, allows the occupational therapist to make reasonable predictions about the difficulties clients are likely to encounter in everyday activities. This information is invaluable to medical teams who must document the need for services, as well as to families who must take appropriate safety precautions and provide needed guidance. In this regard, Allen uses group intervention as an ongoing evaluation.

Allen has been concerned with competence, which legally means the ability to handle one's own affairs. There is no cut-off cognitive level for defining competence. Determination of competence or incompetence is generally based on the ability to make sound judgments and reasonable decisions about those activities that the individual intends to do.

CHANGE AND MOTIVATION

Cognitive change occurs when the brain physiology or chemistry changes. We see an increase in cognitive level through activity when 1) the brain recovers from acute illness or 2) the brain chemistry is affected by a change in activity level, hormones, diet, or medication.

Table 7-5

Quick Overview of the Allen Cognitive Modes

ACL	Common Behavioral Descriptions
1.0 to 1.4	Bedridden; stimulus/response of head
1.6 to 1.8	Sits with support; moves trunk/limb; says "no"
2.0 to 2.4	Stands, righting actions, walks; names body parts, bed, toilet
2.6 to 2.8	Steps up/over; pushes/pulls; holds for support; sings; names target of action
3.0 to 3.4	Spontaneous grasp/release; repetitive actions; speaks in short phrases
3.6 to 3.8	Looks at effects of actions and follows cues to do the next step in self-care; understands waiting a minute, being done (finished with activity)
4.0 to 4.4	Independent in doing routine activities; identifies and sustains goals for 1 hour; speaks in sentences
4.6 to 4.8	Looks around and gets supplies; learns new procedure inflexibly; "Is this right?"—needs help now!
5.0 to 5.2	Discovers how to improve actions through overt trial and error; normal intonation and expression in speech; impulsive and poor judgment
5.6 to 5.8	Understands safety precautions; uses information gained by reading; compares hypothetical plans, anticipates consequences

© Claudia Allen, conference materials, 1997. Adapted with permission.

Using Allen's Cognitive Levels, the therapist verifies the presence or absence of a functional disability. If a client's cognitive ability stabilizes below Level 6 ("normal"), the occupational therapist assists the client and caregivers in making the necessary adjustments in daily living required by a residual cognitive disability. However, even when cognitive processes are irreversibly damaged by trauma or disease, Allen suggests that we can still produce changes in adaptive functioning by manipulating the environment. Allen's updated writings and presentations acknowledge the importance of culture and context in motivating a client to put forth his or her best effort. Offering a choice of craft projects, as well as including socialization in the selection of activities, helps to engage clients in group intervention. In doing a task, there are several factors to be manipulated. The task environment includes the placement and storage of materials, lighting, seating, facilities available, and assistance available. The task demand is the supplies, steps and instructions, and physical and cognitive abilities necessary to complete the task. Allen suggests that both the task environment and the task demand can be altered in ways that allow the client to perform more independently within his or her cognitive level. In planning activities, therapists should give group members a "just-right challenge" (i.e., the task should match, but not exceed, the members' capabilities). For example, clients at Level 4 can reach their maximum adaptive functioning when presented with a three- or four-step task, setting out all the necessary materials within their visual field, demonstrating the instructions, and providing a completed sample for them to copy. Successful performance of a task that is perceived as socially positive will reinforce the client's sense of well-being and increase motivation. Clients at Level 4 will be motivated to perform most self-care tasks at home with appropriate assistance and a suitable and safe environment.

COGNITIVE DISABILITIES GROUP INTERVENTION

Intervention group membership in occupational therapy is based on cognitive level. Clients are treated in homogeneous groups of similar cognitive level. Level 2 is the lowest that can be treated effectively within a group. Level 3 is the lowest level at which group interaction can be expected. Earhart (Allen, 1985) suggests that, in a large facility, a variety of groups should be offered for Levels 2 through 6. Some clients will move up a level or two as their acute symptoms remit. Others will stabilize at a lower level and will require a variety of tasks within that level. Activities appropriate for each level are suggested. Table 7-6, which describes the cognitive abilities of clients at each of the six levels, can serve as a guide for planning activities. The table is based on an earlier chart by Allen, revised by Mary Brinson and Mary Ann Mayer.

Role of the Leader

The leader must be more directive in this approach than in most others. In a hospital setting, the focus is

Table 7-6

Task Analysis for Cognitive Disabilities

	Level 1: Automatic Actions	Level 2: Postural Actions	Level 3: Manual Actions
Setting	Reduce the number of stimuli when possible. Patients do not screen out external stimuli.	Open space. Patients enjoy planned gross motor actions.	Clutter free. Patients are engaged in doing simple tasks that have repetitive actions.
The Therapist's Directions			
Demonstrations	Looks at demonstrated directions but does not imitate them.	The therapist may need to physically guide the action.	Patients will follow a demonstration of a familiar action on an object.
Verbalizations	Verbs, introjections	Pronouns, names of body parts, simple verbs reinforce demonstration.	Names of material objects, repeated simple nouns and verbs.
Number of directions	One action or direction, repeated.	One action or direction, repeated.	One action or direction, repeated.
Task Selection			
Structure of the activity	Alerting stimuli. The most important tasks are eating and drinking.	Familiar, repetitive gross body movements.	An activity that has one step or scheme repeated.
Choice and sample provided	N/A	The therapist plans movements and demonstrates actions. The therapist may respond to patient's suggestions or actions.	Activity is preplanned by therapist. Choices limited to two or three material items/objects.
Tools	Stimulated use of body parts.	Spontaneous use of body parts. Objects that are associated with gross body movement (e.g., softballs, jump ropes).	Hands: Some use of familiar tools.
Storage of materials/projects	Taken care of by the therapist	Taken care of by the therapist	Taken care of by the therapist
Preparation by the therapist	Provide materials for planned stimulation of sensory systems	Plan movements and obtain any needed equipment.	Supplies are laid out in advance. Do any preliminary or finishing steps that are not repetitive or familiar.

(continued)

Table 7-6 (continued)

Task Analysis for Cognitive Disabilities

	Level 4: Goal-Directed Actions	Level 5: Exploratory Actions	Level 6: Planned Actions
Setting	Other patients working on the same task, a shared goal. Setting conducive to production of immediate end product.	Clutter can be present, and other performing variations on similar tasks. Setting fosters exploration, trial and error.	Free access to materials and supplies to stimulate covert problem solving, sharing of plans with others.

The Therapist's Directions

Demonstrations	Patients will imitate single steps in a series and moderately novel actions that expand familiar schemes.	Patients can learn through serial imitation, so a number of steps may be demonstrated. Unfamiliar steps assimilated.	Not required. Patients learn through serial limitations so directions may be retained.
Verbalizations	Simple adjectives, adverbs, nouns, and verbs; avoiding open-ended questions or discussions.	Adjectives and prepositions may be used in explaining variations.	Conjunctions, conjectures, images.
Number of directions	One step at a time.	Several steps at a time.	Unlimited. Images, diagrams, written directions may be followed.

Task Selection

Structure of the activity	Simple quick tasks with a tangible end product. Avoid childish connotations.	An activity that permits variation, and that allows results to be easily seen and corrected.	An activity that permits variation in the selection and planning of steps.
Choice and sample provided	Avoid confusion by limiting the decisions and materials. The opportunity for exact replication of a sample is present.	Several choices in materials, tools, and activity selection. Demonstrate and clarify tangible possibilities.	Several choices in materials, tools, and activity selection. Discuss the hypothetical possibilities.
Tools	Hand tools limited to familiar objects. No power tools.	Simple tools that are linear extensions of the hand and arm.	Patients learn how to use unfamiliar machines and tools.
Storage of materials/projects	Patients will place and/or find supplies when clearly visible or very familiar.	The patient will search for things in probable locations and can place/find things in labeled drawers or cabinets.	The patient will follow verbal directions to place or find materials.
Preparation by the therapist	Supplies are laid out in advance. Provide an exact sample of the end product. Do those steps that require unfamiliar tools or schemes.	The sample of the finished product need not be exact. Patterns and procedures are supplied by the therapist.	Materials, designs, and/or pictures are provided to assist covert problem solving.

often on evaluation. The therapist typically chooses the activity or task or limits choices. The occupational therapist must use expertise in activity analysis, controlling or adapting the environment, and instructing the group members in the procedures of the task. The therapist's role requires skill in assisting clients in acquiring/demonstrating cognitive skills at increasing cognitive levels. The size of groups should not exceed eight members when led by one occupational therapist. However, when assisted by one or more occupational therapy assistants, groups of up to 12 members can still be effective. One occupational therapist assisted by one or more occupational therapy assistants may be ideal in using the Allen approach, because skilled observations of task performance are necessary for ongoing assessment. The most significant factor in determining group size is the members' need for assistance. The lower the cognitive level, the more frequently members need assistance with the task. However, at Levels 4 and 5, verbal interaction consumes a larger portion of group time, and more individual attention is needed for social and emotional support. For higher cognitive levels, groups should be limited to eight members so that group leaders can facilitate group discussion to reinforce learning. Therefore, the occupational therapist needs to weigh several factors before deciding on the size of an Allen group.

Structure and Goals

Allen's goals for clients have to do with function and adaptation. Specific goals might be set to encourage a client to progress to a higher level or to provide the ideal environmental support and assistance so that a client can maximize function within a given cognitive level. Allen has designed several excellent evaluation tools and specified many behaviors that indicate progress toward higher cognitive levels.

The structure and goals for an Allen group are different for each level. For this reason, groups at each level will be discussed separately, with examples of appropriate activities.

Level 2 Groups

Movement activities are suggested to meet the needs of Level 2 clients (clients at Level 3 may also be included). Activities consist of imitation of gross body movement, such as clapping, bending over to touch toes, and passing or tossing a large, soft ball. Simple movement games such as bean bag toss or Nerf basketball may be useful, although clients at Level 2 are apt to disregard directionality. Setting limits in Level 2 groups may be difficult because disruptive behaviors of clients at Level 2 or 3 are oblivious to verbal direction (but are often responsive to demonstrated direction). Movement at this level provides a pleasurable sensory experience, as well as needed stimulation and exercise. However, motor skill is likely to be limited.

Level 3 Groups

The guiding principles in choosing appropriate activities for Level 3 are repetition and manipulation. People at this cognitive level are not goal directed. The process must interest them in order for them to be drawn to participate in an activity. Therapists should think of activities that focus on these attributes as strengths.

Many of our daily activities have the attributes of manipulation and repetition. Washing the dishes, sewing a button, clipping fingernails, and eating a bowl of cereal are examples. It is timing that is difficult for Level 3s, knowing when to begin and when to end. For example, in doing a woodworking project, clients at Level 3 may keep on sanding long after the wood is smooth. They will apply much more glue than is necessary. They will string beads until they get to the end or all the beads are used up. They may place tiles in a row along the edge of a frame, without regard for color or spacing. The therapist must be responsible for structuring the activity into steps and keeping track of time to move the group along.

The ADM identifies a variety of craft projects that are appropriate for Level 3 groups. Some of them are tile trivets, ribbon mugs, sticker cards, canvas placemats, bargello bookmarks, whale note holders, and recessed tile boxes. (All of these projects have standardized materials, which are available from S&S Healthcare, and a free catalog may be obtained by calling them at 1-800-243-9232.) Standardized materials are desirable to increase reliability of the therapist's observations in assessing the mode of performance within each cognitive level. The ADM is recommended for groups in acute-care or other settings in which the accuracy of assessment is important in planning for discharge.

However, in chronic-care settings, such as group homes or skilled nursing facilities, where functional maintenance programs are needed, more interactive group activities can be planned using Allen's guidelines. When selecting activities for Level 3 groups, repetition and manipulation should be the guiding principles. For example, one therapist who works with clients at Level 3 with dementia may have them make long chains with yarn with crochet hooks and attach balloons to decorate for a party or string popcorn and cranberries for a Christmas tree. An occupational therapy aide or recreation aide may be taught to use Allen principles in executing such activities.

The timing of a Level 3 group should not exceed 30 minutes, as that is the limit of their attention according to Allen. Many work tasks are ideal for Level 3, for example, stuffing envelopes, attaching labels and stamps, or collating multiple-page documents. Such tasks have successfully been assigned to sheltered workshops. The workshop might be contracted to assemble packets of plastic utensils, napkins, salt, pepper, sugar, and powdered creamer in plastic bags for serving meals on airlines. In a hospital or day treatment setting, a

Level 3 group might be assigned the task of copying and distributing an in-house newsletter or invitations to an event. Again, the principles of repetition and manipulation should guide selection of appropriate work tasks. All materials should be within arm's reach for each Level 3 participant, and the task should be structured so that one step at a time can be performed repeatedly.

Two examples of activities are included here. First, the "Recessed Tile Box" (Activity Example 7-2), a standardized craft activity selected from the ADM (Earhart, Allen, & Blue, 1993), is described. Although this craft is also used to assess clients at Level 4, only instructions for Level 3 have been given here. An ADM craft activity should be used for groups when assessment of the level and mode of functioning is desired. Activity Example 7-3 is an interactive skill maintenance activity called "Summer Salad," which uses the same Allen Level 3 principles, but is not set up as a standardized assessment.

Level 4 Groups

At Level 4, activities are goal directed. Sequences of steps toward a goal are now possible. Having a goal in mind represents an important step toward problem solving. However, attention is still limited, and group activities should not be planned to last for more than 1 hour. Projects are either completed in one session, or separate steps may be done in two sessions. For example, the wooden tile trivet may be sanded and painted in the first session, and tiles selected and glued in a second session.

Craft projects are ideal experiments in problem solving. A woodworking kit with three pieces, such as a napkin holder, can be structured into a simple sequence: 1) sanding, 2) painting, and 3) gluing. A finished sample must be available to represent the goal. This takes advantage of Level 4 patients' tendency to attend to visual cues. Some ADM crafts suggested for Level 4 are tile trivets, Indian key fobs, ribbon cards, Hug-a-bear, and various bear clothes. Many other crafts may be structured in a more group interactive way, using similar Allen Level 4 principles of goal orientation, several step sequences, and visually stimulating colors and contrasts.

The environment is of special concern to Level 4 groups because their usable task environment now extends beyond arm's reach to the entire visual field. Items necessary for the task to be accomplished should now be placed in plain view. But more importantly, all irrelevant items should be placed out of sight or they will cause major distraction. If a workroom is small, lacking in storage space, and/or has multiple uses, getting rid of visual "clutter" is easier said than done. Considerable preparation time must be spent setting up the room before a Level 4 group begins. Likewise, the storage of objects is guided by the principle of visibility. What cannot be seen, for all intents and purposes, does not exist. Once this is understood by the therapist, it is clear what must be done. Clients at Level 4 will not go searching in cabinets and drawers. The same principle holds true for the home environment.

Assistance needed at Level 4 will be with processes that are not visible, such as the drying of paint or the changing of color or glaze as it dries. Although many food preparation tasks are ideal for this level, processes that involve heating or cooling are not understood or considered. Verbal direction alone is not enough when giving instructions for a task; demonstration should accompany verbal instruction. Written instruction is not at all useful, but sometimes pictures or diagrams can assist the client in progressing through the steps of a task that is familiar. Clients at Level 4 have a tendency to come to the end of a step and then ask, "What do I do now?" They know there is a goal they are working on, a completed project, or a meal on the table, but they are not sure how to get there. Probing or asking leading questions can encourage the client to think about the sequence and use available cues, such as the sample or the work of other members, to learn to problem-solve at a higher level. If the task is too difficult or the client's cognitive abilities are lower than what is required, the therapist may need to "rescue" by correcting an error or completing a step for the client. The information gathered from client-therapist interactions is then used for selecting a more appropriate activity for the next session.

Level 5 Groups

At this level, the focus is on safety. The difficulties requiring intervention usually involve impulsivity and a lack of planning or anticipation. For this reason, clients at Level 5 are introduced to more complex tasks in groups. Some activities suggested are clay and mosaics, cooking, and advanced crafts. While one-step, demonstrated directions are not necessary, the safe use of tools and procedures must still be demonstrated at Level 5. Several steps can be taught at one time, and clients are capable of selecting projects and varying colors and designs. Planning is involved, and projects may continue for more than one session. The occupational therapist still needs to monitor safety and check understanding of directions, especially with regard to the intangible variables of time and temperature.

The ADM includes the following activities for Level 5: sewing Raggedy Ann and Andy dolls and doll clothes, constructing and stenciling multiple-piece woodworking projects, and an assortment of projects using stenciled designs or iron-on decals. The cautious use of hot irons, power tools, ovens, or hot plates under supervision is suggested so that the occupational therapist might observe the client's knowledge and use of caution when handling these items. Group projects involving cooking, grilling outdoors, or participating in recreational activities, such as hiking, swimming, boating, or fishing, can also be used therapeutically to learn/evaluate safety in Level 5 groups.

People functioning at Allen's Level 6 may be placed in craft groups for assessment purposes or included in Level 5 groups if possible decline is suspected.

Cognitive Disabilities Group Leadership

Introduction

Names are mentioned around the table for acknowledgment, and the therapists introduce themselves. The leader explains the purpose of the project in concrete terms. Each member has materials for the activity set up at his or her place in advance. The purpose of the group is different from its goals. Because each member's mode of functioning is different, the goals for each member are individual. But the goal of the group is to provide a practical example in problem-solving, which serves as both practice for the members and ongoing assessment for the therapist.

The purpose should be stated so as to elicit each member's best effort. The therapist should use concrete terms in explaining the purpose, the structure, and the procedure, in language known to be understood by the members at their cognitive level. Projects are to be kept by the clients once completed. The usefulness and desirability of the project should be emphasized, and this can be individualized. Social recognition is an important component when motivating clients to select and begin to work on a project. For example, the tile box may be a gift for someone special, so "you should do your best to make it look nice." Timing is mentioned for Level 4 and higher, and it should be stressed that anyone needing assistance may signal one of the therapists at any time during the group.

Activity

The structure of groups described by Allen resemble Mosey's "Project Groups" (see Appendix A). Interaction occurs mainly between the therapist and each member. Doing the activity really takes the entire session. Demonstration will be given according to the cognitive level, and the project sample can be referred to as the goal. Even for those not yet goal oriented (Level 3s), the sample is an important learning tool to use for error recognition and correction, imitation, and encouragement of higher-level thinking. Cleaning up, as appropriate to the task, may take up the last 5 or 10 minutes of the session. Assistance given by the occupational therapist enables engagement in the activity, and this assistance changes with each cognitive level.

Sharing

No formal sharing takes place in Allen groups. However, informal comments about the projects of others by group members can provide needed social recognition for members.

Processing

A brief discussion at the end may focus on processing. People at all levels should have an opportunity to express their feelings about doing the task. The concrete end product is usually the focus of this discussion. Leaders should be careful not to give false praise, but limit comments to appropriate, reality-based feedback.

Generalization

Generalization by clients is really not possible until Level 5. For lower levels, therapist comments reflecting the purpose and the goal can be made when appropriate. Level 5 groups should be encouraged to find meaning in the activity at hand, and appropriate discussion questions by the leader will elicit this response.

Application

Applying new learning to everyday life can be reviewed at the end of the session. The therapist is directive in individualizing applications. However, no individual feedback is given during the session regarding problem behaviors. The occupational therapist may choose to give feedback to clients individually after having an opportunity to score the activity (using ADM worksheets) or to determine the most useful response to specific situations.

At Level 5, application focuses on task equivalence and discussion of safety issues in the home or work environment. The use of peer discussion may help group members to accept critical feedback or the need for change. In terms of the *Occupational Therapy Practice Framework*, the occupational therapist facilitates an awareness of possible barriers to participation presented by safety issues of members.

Summary

The therapist ends with instructions about the project itself, that it may be taken (if completed) or that it may be picked up later (e.g., after paint is dry). Names should be put on projects if they are to be left. More interpersonal issues are mentioned as the level of the group increases.

Caregiver Education Groups

A new focus area on the Allen-related Web sites is caregiver education. This is an area for community-based intervention, where OTs have much to offer as Allen advisors. Web sites offer training in becoming an Allen advisor, as well as announcing locally held workshops for OTs wishing to take on this role in home care and communities. Using the cognitive disabilities approach, Tina Champagne (2003) has created a Web site for caregiver education, which includes guidelines for family or informal caregivers of people with cognitive dysfunction. Champagne also emphasizes the sensory modulation approach, which will be covered in Chapter 9. Levy and Burns (2005) apply Allen principles in the treatment of older adults with dementia, focusing on how the six levels and 52 modes can guide caregivers in adapting the physical context of tasks, simplifying the tasks of everyday living, and offering needed assistance in order to maximize the client's best ability to function. Each cognitive level requires specific environmental adaptations to ensure the safety of people with dementia, allowing them to function longer in their home environments. For caregiver guidelines visit http://www.caregiversupport-network.com/aclscreen.htm. The occupational therapist should include the client's Allen's Cognitive Level range (i.e., 4.0 to 4.4) to obtain correct guidelines. For current updates on Allen's Cognitive Levels, visit http://www.allen-cognitive-network.org.

Allen-Related Web Sites

- For selected topics:

  http://www.allen-cognitive-network.org

- Assessment tools:

  http://www.allen-cognitive-levels.com/acls.htm

- For applications to client groups:

  http://www.allencogadvisor.com

- For test kits or materials and instructions:

  http://www.ssww.com

REFERENCES

Allen, C. K. (1982). Independence through activity: The practice of occupational therapy (psychiatry). *American Journal of Occupational Therapy, 36,* 731-739.

Allen, C. K (1985). *Occupational therapy for psychiatric diseases: Measurement and management of cognitive disabilities.* Boston, MA: Little, Brown & Co.

Allen, C. K. (1987a). Measuring the severity of mental disorders. *Hospital & Community Psychiatry, 38,* 140-142.

Allen, C. K. (1987b). Eleanor Clarke Slagle lectureship-1987: Activity, occupational therapy's treatment method. *American Journal of Occupational Therapy, 41,* 563-575.

Allen, C. K. (1988). Cognitive disabilities. In S. C. Robertson (Ed.), *Focus: Skills for assessment and treatment.* Rockville, MD: American Occupational Therapy Association.

Allen, C. K. (1991). Cognitive disability and reimbursement for rehabilitation and psychiatry. *Journal of Insurance Medicine, 23,* 245-247.

Allen, C. K. (1994). Creating a need-satisfying, safe environment: Management and maintenance approaches. In C. B. Royeen (Ed.), *AOTA self-study series: Cognitive rehabilitation.* Bethesda, MD: American Occupational Therapy Association.

Allen, C. K. (1997). Cognitive disabilities: How to make clinical judgments. In N. Katz (Ed.), *Cognitive rehabilitation: Models for intervention in occupational therapy.* Rockville, MD: American Occupational Therapy Association.

Allen, C. K. (1999). *Structures of the cognitive performance modes.* Ormond Beach, FL: Allen Conferences, Inc.

Allen, C. K., & Allen, R. (1987). Cognitive disabilities: Measuring the social consequences of mental disorders. *Journal of Clinical Psychiatry, 48*(5), 185-190.

Allen, C. K., Blue, T., & Earhart, C. A. (1995). *Understanding cognitive performance modes.* Ormond Beach, FL: Allen Conferences, Inc.

Allen, C. K., & Earhart, C. (1992). *Occupational therapy treatment goals for the physically and cognitively disabled.* Bethesda, MD: American Occupational Therapy Association.

American Occupational Therapy Association. (2008). *Occupational therapy practice framework: Domain and process.* Bethesda, MD: Author.

Burns, T. (2003). *Cognitive performance update.* http://CPT. Update.htm. Retrieved 10-10-2010.

Champagne, T. (2003). *Occupational therapy levels (2.4-5.8) caregiver guides.* http://www.ot-innovations.com/index2. php?option=com_content&task=view&id=21&po. Retrieved 10-20-2010.

Earhart, C. A., Allen, C. K., & Blue, T. (1993). *Allen diagnostic module instruction manual.* Colchester, CT: S & S Worldwide.

Heinmann, N. E., Allen, C. K., & Yerxa, E. J. (1989). The routine task inventory: A tool for describing the functional behavior of the cognitively disabled. *Occupational Therapy Practice, 1,* 67-74.

Ikiugu, M. N. (2007). *Psychosocial conceptual practice models in occupational therapy.* St. Louis, MO: Mosby.

Josman, N., & Katz, N. (1991). Problem-solving version of the Allen Cognitive Level (ACL) test. *American Journal of Occupational Therapy, 45,* 331-338.

Katz, N. (2008). *Routine task inventory-expanded (RTI-E) manual.* Retrieved from http://www.allen-cognitive-network. org/index.php/allen-model/routine-task-inventory-ex

Levy, L. L., & Burns, T. (2005). Cognitive disabilities reconsidered: Rehabilitation of older adults with dementia. In N. Katz (Ed.), *Cognitive rehabilitation: Models for intervention in occupational therapy* (2nd ed., pp. 347-385). Bethesda, MD: American Occupational Therapy Association.

Levy, L. L. (1997). The use of the cognitive disability frame of reference in rehabilitation of cognitively disabled older adults. In N. Katz (Ed.), *Cognitive rehabilitation: Models for intervention in occupational therapy.* Bethesda, MD: American Occupational Therapy Association.

Reisberg, B., Franssen, E., Souren, L., Auer, S., & Kenowskky, S. (1998). Progression of Alzheimer's disease: Variability and consistency: Ontogenic models, their applicability and relevance. *Journal of Neural Transmission, 54,* 9-20.

Toglia, J., Golisz, K., & Coverover, Y. (2009). Multicontext treatment approach. In E. Crepeau, E. Cohn, & B. Schell (Eds.), *Willard & Spackman's occupational therapy* (11th ed., pp. 739-776). Philadelphia, PA: Lippincott, Williams, & Wilkins.

World Health Organization. (2001). *International classification of functioning, disability, and health.* Geneva, Switzerland: Author.

Cognitive Disabilities Activity Example 7-1
Rope Dancing (Level 2)

Materials: 12-foot-long piece of white nylon rope, 1-inch thick, with ends tied in a overhand knot, and a cassette player with instrumental music in a variety of rhythms (e.g., John Philip Sousa marches, Strauss waltzes, the overture from "The King & I").

Participants: Six maximum.

Directions: Start the music to alert members and get their attention. Therapist stands inside the rope circle and motions members to come toward him or her. Therapist greets each member and places each member's hand or elbow around the rope, approximately 2 feet apart. Begin by walking in a circle to the right, marching to the rhythm of the music. Turn to face the rope, and hold with both hands or elbows. Therapist leads group in raising rope up high, then down low, to the rhythm of the music. Group imitates the therapist in doing a variety of in/out motions with arms and legs, while holding the rope. Have members take turns ducking under the rope and standing inside the circle. Two members can hold the rope bending over so that rope is 1' high, while therapist leads other members in stepping over it. Teams of three then take each end and pull each other back and forth slowly, changing their force when pulled or pushed gently by the therapist. Action ceases when the music ends (approximately 20 minutes). Therapist says "goodbye" to each member by shaking hands, saluting, or other gesture of recognition and farewell.

No verbalizations are needed to direct this group. However, proprioceptive cues are used as needed to direct the actions of the group and to recapture attention of straying members.

Cognitive Disabilities Activity Example 7-2
Recessed Tile Box (Levels 3 and 4)

Materials: Box with lid; 3/8-inch tiles, two colors separated into bins; sandpaper; brown wood stain; brush; rag; glue; and one completed sample for every two patients (checkerboard pattern in two contrasting colors). See Figures 7-3A and 7-3B. Access to a sink and water for clean-up is preferred. Glue bottles should be opened, and stain uncovered and stirred.

Participants: Six to eight members. Seat people at table, each with individual set of supplies. Figures 7-3C and 7-3D depict the standardized set-up for evaluation.

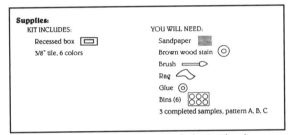

Figure 7-3A. Key for supplies needed. (© Claudia Allen, Allen Diagnostic Model. Reprinted with permission.)

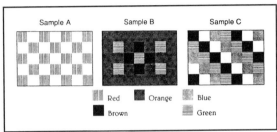

Figure 7-3B. Sample designs. (© Claudia Allen, Allen Diagnostic Model. Reprinted with permission.)

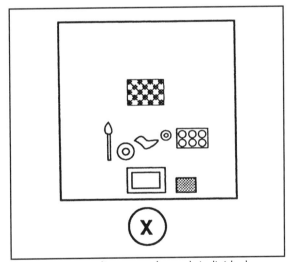

Figure 7-3C. Supplies set-up for each individual. (© Claudia Allen, Allen Diagnostic Model. Reprinted with permission.)

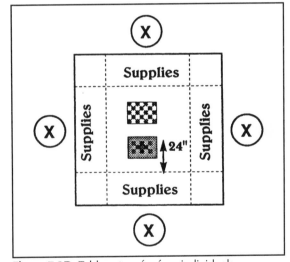

Figure 7-3D. Table set-up for four individuals. (© Claudia Allen, Allen Diagnostic Model. Reprinted with permission.)

Recessed Tile Box (Levels 3 and 4) (Continued)

Timing: Introduction and purpose—5 minutes

Sanding, staining, and gluing tiles—20 to 30 minutes

Processing and summary—5 minutes (does not include clean-up)

Because the maximum attention span for Level 3 is 30 minutes, progress must be monitored and timing adjusted accordingly. If more than half the group has not finished staining at the end of 15 minutes, it is recommended that gluing the tiles be done in a second session.

Directions: Introduce group and explain purpose of the activity. Instructions are taken from the ADM (1993, pp. B2-B5). "This is a tiled box [that] can be used to store jewelry, medicine, change, or other small items. All the supplies needed to complete it are in front of you. In order for me to see how you are doing today, it is important for you to try to make your box look as much like... the sample as possible."

Provide steps as indicated below as needed. Observe performance, provide appropriate prompts or assistance, and rate behavior for each step (see rating criteria). Move to the next step when the last one has been abandoned or when a person says "I'm done" or requests next step.

Step 1: Sanding—"The first step is to sand the wood on all sides until it is smooth." Pick up sandpaper and demonstrate sanding with the grain and feeling for smoothness.

Step 2: Staining—"This is stain. It may need to be stirred. It is painted on with the brush and then wiped off with the rag like this." Demonstrate painting and wiping one side. "Do all the sides."

Step 3: Gluing—"The tiles are glued on in rows like this." Demonstrate placing glue on the back of a red tile and placing it in the corner of the recess in the lid. Repeat with a white tile along the short side. Space the tile but do not comment on this. "Try to make a pattern like...this sample." Critical observations of each member's sanding, staining, wiping, gluing, and placing tiles are given, and rating is done by the therapist to assess the mode of functioning for each member according to the rating criteria. The critical observations for sanding are feeling/looking for smoothness, altering pressure and direction, turning box to access all surfaces, altering the shape of the sandpaper, and noting effects.

Rating Criteria: The ADM specifies detailed rating criteria for each step: sanding, staining, and gluing tiles. Table 7-7 shows behaviors expected at each cognitive mode (3.0 through 4.8) for the first step (sanding). Refer to Allen (1993) for ADM criteria for this and other steps of the craft.

Table 7-7

Sanding

3.0	Reaches for and grasps object; holds, feels, may name object
3.2	Sands randomly; may not look at box while working; stops and starts on command; may comment wtih short phrases.
3.4	May begin before instructions are given, fail to stop when asked; actions sustained 1 minute or longer, may change suddenly; looks at object inconsistently, does not note effects
3.6	Begins before instructions are given, stops when told; copies demonstration one step at a time; notes effects, moves location; may miss all/part of visible surface.
3.8	Stops between steps after visible surfaces are sanded and says "I'm done"; sands all visible surfaces but misses inside surfaces
4.0	Does not spontaneously refer to sample within 24 inches; sands all large visible surfaces; may miss or refuse to sand small or hidden surfaces
4.2	Refers to sample only when cued; may miss hidden surfaces or ask if inside/bottom should be done
4.4	Refers to and compares work to sample; may ask for verification before going on to next step; bends over box to reach back, still misses small edges
4.6	Scans environment to locate sample or supplies in plain sight; varies pressure/force/duration for better effects; may attempt to fold/tear sandpaper to do inside of box; rotates/examines all surfaces after sanding is completed; may not note grain of wood; may ask for help for best way to access small edges

© Claudia Allen, conference materials, 1997. Adapted with permission.

Processing and Summary: A brief discussion about how members liked the activity follows. All generalizations must be done by the therapist. Members may be asked questions about possible uses for their box—a gift, to keep jewelry, to store coins, etc. In summarizing, feedback from the therapist about the strengths of each member in following directions, responding to cues, and general workmanship is often helpful and appreciated, and ends the session on a positive note.

Cognitive Disabilities Activity Example 7-3
Summer Salad (Level 3)

This Level 3 group activity represents a functional maintenance activity that uses the same Allen guidelines as the standardized craft previously described but is more interactive. Up to eight members whose functioning has stabilized at Allen's Level 3 may be placed in groups like this, which are designed by a registered occupational therapist or certified occupational therapist assistant using the principles of repetition and manipulation. Other staff members may be instructed by the registered occupational therapist or certified occupational therapist assistant in leading these groups. The activity should not exceed 30 minutes, and sharing of tools and materials should not be required at this level.

Materials: One serrated plastic knife, one heavy plastic fork, and one cutting board or thick paper plate for each member. One big bowl in the center of the table is filled with as many pieces of fruit as there are members. Good choices are apples, pears, bananas, oranges, peaches, cantaloupe halves (wrapped in plastic), and pineapple slices (wrapped in plastic).

Participants: Six to eight members are ideal, with a co-therapist. Members should wash their hands before starting this group.

Directions: The therapist explains that the group will make a delicious fruit salad. The ground rules are that no one eats anything until all the fruit is cut, put back in the bowl, and mixed with a coconut-and-yogurt dressing. Each member introduces self and selects a piece of fruit from the bowl. Covering eyes and identifying fruit by touch may be an interesting variation. Members should be reminded not to eat the fruit, but to wait for a therapist to demonstrate to each member how their specific fruit should be prepared and cut into bite-size pieces. Approximately 15 minutes are spent cutting and trimming. A plastic-lined trashcan is passed around to throw away cores, pits, and peels with the help of the therapist. A volunteer mixes one pint of plain yogurt, one scoop of brown sugar, and half a cup of coconut flakes. Other volunteers take turns stirring the dressing into the fruit. Other volunteers scoop the fruit salad into bowls and pass them out to the members. Eating the fruit is a well-deserved reward for their hard work.

From Cole, M. B. *Group dynamics in occupational therapy: The theoretical basis and practice application of group intervention* (4th ed.). Thorofare, NJ: SLACK Incorporated. © 2012 SLACK Incorporated.

Cognitive Disabilities Activity Example 7-4
Falling Leaves (Level 4)

This is a basic craft group for Level 4 patients. It is a group project following the guidelines of goal orientation, visual cues (colors and shapes), and short sequences of steps, in this case, leading to a common end product.

Materials: The table is set up by the therapist for six to 10 patients. Half of the patients have a sheet of colored paper, a pencil, a pair of paper scissors, and a cardboard pattern of a leaf. Leaf shapes used are maple, elm, oak, ash, tulip, and birch. Real leaves can be traced to produce these patterns; however, this is done by the therapist. The other half of the patients have a piece of white poster board with a tree trunk and branches traced in black magic marker and the name of the tree outlined in black. Chunky capital letters are best, saying OAK, MAPLE, etc., with the centers to be colored in. Patients with the tree trunks also have two wide-tip markers, brown or gray and another color, and a small bottle of glue.

Directions: The therapist should demonstrate the processes.
1. Leaves. Place the leaf pattern on the colored paper, and trace around it with the pencil. Fit as many as you can on the paper without overlapping any lines. When finished, cut out each leaf along the lines you have traced.
2. Tree trunks. Color in the tree trunk with the appropriate color. Then, color in the letters with another color.

When finished, glue the appropriate leaves on the tree branches. Patients may work in pairs, so that maple leaves are glued to the maple tree trunk, etc. Colors of the leaves should be appropriate for autumn. For variation, two autumn shades may be used for each leaf to create a more interesting pattern.

Processing and Summary: Feelings about the craft activity and its end result are then elicited. Generalization discussion will center around the autumn season, what happens in the fall, and what kinds of tasks must be done to prepare for the autumn/winter season. Application can concretely be interpreted in discussing where to display the posters and what other decorations might be desired. Therapist feedback may be given in summary. The tree posters make a good decoration for the ward.

From Cole, M. B. *Group dynamics in occupational therapy: The theoretical basis and practice application of group intervention* (4th ed.). Thorofare, NJ: SLACK Incorporated. © 2012 SLACK Incorporated.

Cognitive Disabilities Activity Example 7-5
Straw Hats With Potpourri (Level 5)

This is an appropriate activity for spring and uses the strengths of Level 5, trial and error exploration in creating a pleasing result with the materials provided, using more than one sensory system (visual and olfactory). It also includes a safety check, as members are supervised in the use of the hot glue gun and are advised of the need for caution as needed.

Materials: 6-inch straw hats for each member, four rolls of thin satin ribbon (one each in pink, baby blue, red, and white), a variety of ½" silk flowers (daisies, roses, etc.), scissors, a glue gun with glue sticks, bags of potpourri in floral and herbal scents, nylon netting, spool of thread, and several colorful samples of finished hats.

Timing: Introduction—5 minutes
           Activity—30 minutes
           Processing/summary—20 minutes
           Clean-up—5 minutes

Directions: The leader introduces members and explains the project and its purpose. It could be a door decoration, a gift, or a preparation for the Easter holiday. Doing the craft will be a way to monitor the skill level of members and to observe how they deal with limited choices, verbal instructions, and safety precautions. The goal is for each member to design and decorate one straw hat.

Step 1: Potpourri—Cut a circle of nylon netting about 6 inches in diameter. Fill this with enough potpourri to fill the interior portion of the straw hat. Gather in the edges of the netting and tie it with a piece of string. Set this aside to be glued in later.

Step 2: Decoration—Choose ribbons to tie around the center portion of the hat. Ribbons may be tied with bows or knotted with streamers hanging down. Each member may choose two to four flowers to glue around the ribbon cluster. One piece of ribbon should be cut about 10" long, with the ends tied in an overhand knot to serve as a hanger.

Step 3: Gluing—The therapist should have the glue gun plugged in and heated to the correct temperature. A separated area with a fireproof surface and nothing flammable nearby should be maintained for gluing. Members can approach the gluing area several times during the session. First, the ribbons should be stabilized with a blob of glue right under the bow or knot. Next, the silk flowers are attached with glue. The nylon packet of potpourri is glued with the "tail" tucked inside the hat. Finally, the ribbon hanger loop is glued on the back, so that the hat may be hung from a hook on the door or wall.

Discussion and Summary: Feelings about the craft are elicited, followed by generalization of what other spring tasks around the house have similar attributes (i.e., getting out spring clothes, fixing up the house, making it smell nice). Discussing the use of the glue gun may be a good lead-in for reinforcing safety precautions around their homes. Other tasks involving heat and electricity (e.g., cooking, ironing, or using hair dryers, curling irons, or electric razors) should be discussed with each individual member with regard to safety. The straw hat activity may also trigger discussion of planning ahead for spring, the importance of spring cleaning, storage of winter clothes, care of lawns and gardens, or other tasks requiring anticipation, a typical problem area for Level 5. Summary should include feedback from the therapist. Hats are kept by the members to use however they like.

Chapter 8

DEVELOPMENTAL APPROACHES

In the temporal context, a client's developmental stage gives OTs important guidelines for exploring client occupational concerns. For example, social interactions and dating might be primary concerns for young adults, while productivity and caregiving might be more central concerns for the middle adult. Clients at midlife may have little interest in leisure occupations, while retired older clients may struggle with filling their leisure time with meaningful activities. The guiding principle of all developmental theories is that people develop in a more or less predictable sequence from birth to maturity and throughout life. This sequence is determined by both biological and environmental forces. Developmental stages are specific, progressive, and hierarchical. Development is divided into stages for the benefit of our understanding. In reality, the transition from one stage to the next is gradual and may involve cycles of regression and progression (backward and forward movement toward maturity). Each stage is subdivided into specific skills, issues, or conflicts, and each has characteristics that distinguish it from other stages.

Progressive refers to the idea that each stage increases in complexity and represents, in some way, progress toward maturity. It is assumed that maturity is the highest stage and, therefore, the goal. Bigsby (2003) discusses some current challenges to theories of ages and stages. She points out the importance of both environment and experience in explaining the variability of skills and behaviors in the development of children. Hierarchical means that each stage builds on the previous one. It reinforces the idea that there are foundation skills upon which higher-level skills are built. In applying developmental theory to rehabilitation, skills that are deficient must be relearned in the same sequence in which they normally develop. While this idea is common to most traditional developmental theorists, newer theorists incorporate a dynamic systems perspective, suggesting that the pathways to maturity are many and diverse, that stages may not always occur sequentially, and that maturity itself may be a work in progress.

FRAMEWORK FOCUS

Developmental stage is a part of each client's "personal context" as implied by the *Occupational Therapy Practice Framework* (American Occupational Therapy Association [AOTA], 2008). Developmental tasks at different stages of development are defined according to each theorist's unique focus. As one progresses developmentally, one's priorities in life will change, and one's occupational "performance patterns" are likely to reflect this. Illness and disability can disrupt the normal developmental progression, requiring a restructuring of the client's lifestyle. OTs may need to assist clients in exploring their priorities with regard to occupation and in changing or developing new habits, routines, and roles (AOTA, 2008).

The developmental frames of reference are best used as a guidepost by which to measure the effects of illness and thereby set realistic goals for recovery. Age is never a true measure of development. However, by viewing people with disability through the perspective of normal

Cole M.B. *Group Dynamics in Occupational Therapy:*
The Theoretical Basis and Practice Application
of Group Intervention (pp 217-248).
© 2012 SLACK Incorporated.

Table 8-1

Jung's Stages of Development (Spiritual)

Age	Stage
Birth to puberty (childhood)	Blissful ignorance, inherited predispositions
Puberty to age 35 (youth)	Conscious and doubting, taking on responsibility
Age 35 to old age (mid-life)	Change in direction to express laten parts of self-individuation and integration
Infirmity and death (old age)	Infirmity, acceptance of death, afterlife, and collective unconscious

development, discrepancies between developmental and chronological age can help the therapist to appreciate the true impact of disability on a person's life.

Most developmental theories define points of change, crises, or conflicts to be resolved before the person moves up to the next stage or level. These points of stress may be instrumental in bringing about the onset or exacerbation of illness. If the OT pays attention to developmental theory, he or she can take advantage of the knowledge that specific tasks need to be mastered in order to resolve the conflict or crisis that is really a normal part of development. These life tasks can serve as starting points for therapeutic groups in OT, offering clients the opportunity to discuss and find ways to progress developmentally by redesigning their own occupational life structure.

BASIC ASSUMPTIONS

There are many different theories of human development, some ending with adolescence (Freud) and others continuing right through old age (Erikson, Jung). Those discussed here are chosen because they help clarify our thinking about OT groups. Levinson borrows from Jung and Erikson among others in his theory of adult life transitions. Some theories of development map physical milestones (Gessell) while others address cognitive (Piaget) and moral reasoning (Kohlberg, Wilcox, Gilligan). Newer theories contribute to our understanding of older adult development, including Laslett, Baltes and Baltes, and Atchley, and the theories of socioemotional selectivity and gerotranscendence, which support, in part, Cumming and Henry's earlier theory of disengagement. Some of these depart from the concept of developmental stages and represent a complex systems approach. Finally, theories of physical aging and the contributions of social support theory are briefly summarized.

Jung

Jung, who wrote as early as 1914, might be considered the father of adult development theory. He differed from Freud in extending the developmental process throughout life and in acknowledging the contribution of external factors to growth and adaptation. Jung (1914) divided life into four basic stages:

1. Childhood
2. Youth
3. Mid-life
4. Old age

In Jung's view, childhood is spent in blissful ignorance. Although influenced by many inherited predispositions, children develop with no doubts, unaware of their own growth processes. Youth is marked by the onset of consciousness, doubts, problems, contradictions, and responsibilities. Jung described the second half of life as beginning between ages 35 and 40, when the essential character of life changes and energy becomes rechanneled. Before age 40, the individual has put his or her energy into external events such as establishing occupation, community position, marriage, and family. After age 40, Jung believes the individual turns inward, focusing more on the spiritual (Schultz, 1976).

Middle age is described by Jung as the "afternoon of life." Polarities are opposite tendencies of the self present in an individual, such as introversion versus extroversion, rationality versus intuitiveness, aggressiveness versus sensitivity, and action versus contemplation. At mid-life, Jung contends that whatever sides of the self were expressed in the person's youth, the opposite sides will prevail in mid-life. It was Jung who identified individuation as the true goal of life, a concept much in question in the 1980s. Individuation is a kind of enhancement of identity that involves further definition of the self. Individuation continues through each of the stages in greater depths and in different ways. The end result of individuation was thought to be integration, a uniting of all parts of the self into a qualified whole.

Old age is the final stage. As people age, they experience physical decline, remove themselves from positions of authority and responsibility, and face the inevitability of death. Jung assumed a belief in the presence of an afterlife and began the idea that all individuals ultimately contribute to a "collective unconscious," and so live on through others (Table 8-1). A recent application

Table 8-2

Erikson's Eight Stages of Development (Psychosocial)

Age	Stage
Birth to infancy	Trust versus mistrust
2 to 4 Toddlerhood	Autonomy versus shame and doubt
5 to 7 Early childhood	Initiative versus guilt
8 to 12 Middle childhood	Industry versus inferiority
13 to 22 Adolescence	Identity versus role confusion
23 to 35 Young adult	Intimacy verus isolation
35 to 50 Adulthood	Generativity versus stagnation
50 to death	Integrity versus despair

of Jung's theory is the Meyers Briggs personality assessment, which provides an effective tool for understanding and overcoming barriers to communication and learning and can serve as a guide for mending strained relationships or choosing appropriate occupational roles.

Erikson

Erikson (1978) also built on Freud's psychosexual stages and extended his theory to include adolescence and adulthood. His ideas are compatible with Jung's, but more social in nature and based on the central issues of each stage. Conflicts with Erikson's stages (described in Table 8-2) are well-known and often cited in OT literature. The conflict areas can guide our choice of activities in OT and can serve as a basis for setting goals at the various age levels. For example, trust issues can be worked on through movement activities, such as "falling" and "being caught," or through verbal activities, such as giving and receiving emotional support. Many social aspects of childhood and adolescence have implications for successful occupational performance and can therefore guide OT group interventions for those children or youth who struggle with the achievement of autonomy, initiative, industry, or identity, all of which must be learned through participation in occupational roles.

Adult Stages and Evidence

In the adult stages, intimacy in young adulthood includes the ability to make commitments to ongoing social relationships, and, in order to do so, the individual must have achieved a stable identity or sense of self. Intimacy and fidelity in relationships applies not only to marriages and partnerships, but also to long-term friendships and ongoing interactions with one's family members as they change and grow. Generativity, Erikson's middle adult stage, has been identified as continuing well into older adulthood and includes imparting wisdom to future generations (McAdams, Hart, & Maruna, 1998).

In a longitudinal study, Westermeyer (2004) found that generativity was significantly associated with successful marriage, close friendships, altruistic behaviors, and overall mental health. The achievement of Erikson's generativity stage in middle and older adulthood was found by researchers to have significant benefits for health and well-being later in life, such as maintaining a positive attitude toward oneself, having trusting and satisfying social relationships, continuing one's goals in life and a sense of direction, and independence and self-determination in resisting social pressure (McAdams, de St. Aubin, & Logan, 1993). Research has also supported that continuation of generativity, through volunteering in one's community, can greatly reduce the risk of mortality for older adults (Shmotkin, Blumstein, & Modan, 2003).

The final stage, integrity versus despair, is believed to occur at much later ages than originally thought. Occupations that promote integrity include taking steps to repair past unresolved problems and relationships through a variety of rituals such as gift giving, holiday or religious celebrations, or revisiting important places from one's past. Reminiscence and memoir writing can help older adults to reflect on the issues they need to resolve. A possible ninth stage was identified by Erikson and his wife Joan. They write about a "deliberate retreat from the usual engagements of daily activity... a paradoxical state that does seem to exhibit a transcendent quality" (Erikson & Erikson, 1997, p. 25).

Loss is a predominant theme in the lives of older people. Erikson's view of the final conflict to be resolved may be helpful in understanding how loss can be accepted. His eighth stage, integrity versus despair, suggests that contentment in old age results from the view of a life productively lived (Kaplan & Sadock, 2003). In later life, grandparents enjoy spoiling their grandchildren, and retired workers enjoy knowing that the younger generations will benefit from their life's work. Teachers may enjoy watching the success of their students, for example. According to Erikson, peace and contentment in old age occurs only if one has previously achieved intimacy and generativity. An older person needs to know that his or her life has been productive and that he or she has passed on his or her wisdom to others in some way. Without this belief, there is only despair. Despair, according to Erikson, is indicated by a fear of death and the realization that it is too late to start over.

Preparation for death is another necessary prerequisite for integrity in old age. As life is reappraised, old conflicts and unfinished business may be recalled. It is not unusual to wish for reconciliations with estranged friends or relatives. Often, there are old wrongs to forgive, apologies to make, and unkept promises to reconsider. These are important emotional concerns of the elderly and should not be prematurely dismissed. Those who are physically or cognitively impaired may need help in dealing with these issues. Even when actual reconciliations are not feasible, a great deal can be done through group experiences incorporating role-play and other creative activities. Developing a point of view about death is a spiritual and philosophical concern. Carl Rogers, psychotherapist and major spokesman for humanistic psychology, described a new interest in his 70s as he explored the world of the paranormal with his wife. His experiences changed his understanding of death. Whereas in his 50s and 60s he regarded death to be the end of the individual, he now considers it possible that the spiritual essence of man continues to live after death. He mentions the views of Arthur Koestler about each individual's consciousness being a part of the "cosmic consciousness" (Rogers, 1980, p. 88), a view that echoes Jung's ideas regarding the collective unconscious. Zemke and Gratz (1982) point out that, for the aged, illness and disability tend to renew earlier crises:

> The (occupational) therapist must acknowledge and work toward resolution of these just as she would with any other disabled adult. Only then can the ego integrity crisis be faced. Techniques such as remotivation or life review provide a basis for the thoughtful review and acceptance of life experience necessary for resolution at this final stage of life (p. 61).

Levinson

Levinson (1978) has published the most extensive (although admittedly controversial) research study to date on the developmental stages of adulthood. He based his findings on a longevity study of 40 men. Levinson presents adulthood as periods of stability alternating with periods of transition. The three life transitions he identifies are

1. Early adult—Ages 17 to 22
2. Mid-life—Ages 40 to 45
3. Late adult—Age 60 to 65

These periods of conflict are interspersed with periods of relative stability in which the individual lives within an established life structure and stays more or less on course. Sheehy (1981) popularized this theory with her best-selling book *Passages*.

Levinson contends that each transition period occurs during specific age ranges, and each transition has its own developmental tasks. Like Erikson, he saw each transition as requiring the resolution of conflicts before the person can move on to the next stage.

Primarily, the tasks of each transition period are to re-evaluate the existing life structure, explore the possibilities of change, and make choices that will restructure life in the next era. Eras are between stages of stability described as young, middle, and late adulthood. In the Levinson study of 40 men, work was considered to be a "base for life in society," giving the man his life structure in a cultural, class, and social sense as well as occupational sense (Levinson, 1978, p. 9). Since the thrust of the study was to examine the mid-life transition, subjects selected were age 35, from four different occupational groups, and were followed to age 45. Biographical information collected from these subjects forms the basis of the young adult transition. The late adult transition is only briefly covered by Levinson and is considered to parallel the preceding transition.

Levinson's theory has been selected for focus because it presents a good structure around which to understand life problems of clients and to plan OT groups.

The Early Adult Transition

The essence of this transition is the separation from the family of origin in order to establish a new home base. The separation is both geographical and emotional and generally creates a sense of loss. Yet, the excitement involved in establishing oneself in the adult world provides a sense of satisfaction. Exploration in the early adult transition quickly pushes toward commitment as the young man is required to take on adult responsibilities. Balancing exploration with the need for structure is an ongoing struggle. The major tasks of the early adult transition are forming the dream, finding a mentor, forming an occupation, and starting a marriage and family.

Forming the Dream

The first task that plays a powerful role in early adulthood is called forming a dream. Levinson states that the dream emerges during the early adult transition where the boy/man imagines himself settled in the adult world. This may be connected with concrete reality or far removed from his actual world. The ability to play make-believe in early childhood is the forerunner of this imagining in early adulthood. The dream is a vehicle for exploring his image and "provides a source of hope, self-esteem, and personal integrity" (Levinson, 1978, p. 93). The young adult's task includes forming relationships with others who can facilitate his work on the dream and finding ways of living it out in his life.

The Mentor Relationship

According to Levinson, the mentor relationship is very complex and extremely significant for a man during early adulthood. The mentor is a transitional figure in a person's life, serving as a teacher, sponsor, guide, and adviser. The most important function of the mentor is "to support and facilitate the realization of the dream" (Levinson, 1978, p. 98). Offering expertise and counseling to a young man, yet not being parental, the mentor is usually older than his protégé by a half-generation. All men in the study had male mentors, although Levinson's own mentor was a female, and it is expected that as more women enter currently male-dominated fields, they too will serve as mentors to both men and women.

In a study conducted by Margaret Hennig using 25 high-level women executives, it was shown that all had found male mentors early in their careers (Sheehy, 1976). Interestingly, these successful women chose careers rather than marriage in their 20s, yet realized around age 35 that something was missing and began to explore their feminine sides. Levinson reports a similar happenstance for men who become less involved with their mentors by age 40 and face the task of reintegrating the feminine side of their personality.

Choosing an Occupation

The process of choosing an occupation extends throughout the entire life cycle, beginning in childhood with make-believe games like "doctor" or "teacher." As Levinson remarks about other important life choices, "The great paradox of human development is that we are required to make crucial choices before we have the knowledge, judgment, and self-understanding to choose wisely" (1978, p. 162). Transforming one's early interests into an occupational choice during young adulthood is a complex psychosocial process, and a pattern usually emerges with some definition by the early 30s. An occupation often serves as an index of an individual's worth in society, both economically and socially, and defines his or her role in the community. For many of the men in Levinson's study, establishing an occupational identity is often tied up with parental expectations and the nurturing given to the dream concept with or without the presence of a mentor. There are enormous differences between individuals regarding the meaning of success and failure, and concepts around these values change as growth occurs throughout their lifespan.

This stage has important implications for OT. Because illness almost always interrupts the work role of the client, values around self and work need to be reconsidered. Group activities dealing with values around the work role and the exploration of alternate roles in the home and community are appropriate for a wide variety of client populations.

Marriage and Family

Undertaking the obligation to marry and have children does not necessarily mean one is prepared for the responsibilities and commitments. Often, this step is intricately bound up with the other tasks of early adulthood, such as separating from parents and finding support for the dream pursuit. Levinson describes a "special woman" (1978, p. 109) who facilitates a man's entry into the adult world by providing boundaries within which his aspirations can be realized and giving nourishment to his occupational journey. If the marital choice is made in such a way as to be antithetical to the dream, the relationship may suffer conflicts at a later date. Obviously, the relationship will be modified over time to accommodate the dreams of both the man and woman, and there are endless possibilities for creating a family pattern that is suitable for both. The importance of fatherhood and motherhood may not emerge until the individual has outgrown his or her occupational mentor and is prepared to provide those types of functions to his or her younger associates and to his or her own offspring.

The Mid-Life Transition

This period is said to provide the bridge from early to middle adulthood. It brings a man to question, search, and re-examine his life and his values. For the great majority of men in the Levinson study (80% of subjects), this great struggle within the self and the external world may reach crisis proportions. Often, several years are needed to go through the process and come to some resolution. A culminating event often signifies success or failure in the man's fantasy, and this self-judgment may be all-encompassing. If he fails to get a promotion, he may regard himself as a failure in other aspects of his life as well. This transition period begins when a man realizes that he cannot go on as before, that he cannot "become his own man" under his existing life structure, and that changes will be necessary in order to advance sufficiently in any chosen direction. Three main tasks are defined by Levinson for this stage of development:

1. To terminate the era of early adulthood (reappraising the past)

2. To take the first steps toward middle adulthood (modifying the life structure)

3. To deal with the polarities that are the sources of deep division in his or her life (individuation at mid-life)

Each of these broadly defined tasks has many specific aspects to consider.

Reappraising the Past

Recognition of his own mortality gives a man a renewed sense of urgency about the use of his remaining time. He examines his accomplishments in relation to earlier hopes, values, and expectations, asking "Have I accomplished all that I set out to do?" Because of the nature of a dream, which is essentially fantasy, many ideas, assumptions, and beliefs associated with the dream do not withstand the comparison with actual experience. Levinson defines "de-illusionment" as "a recognition that long-held assumptions and beliefs about self and the world are not true" (1978, p. 192). The process of de-illusionment is accompanied by emotions of disappointment, joy, relief, bitterness, grief, wonder, freedom, and pain. At this stage, a man may ask, "What have I done with my life? Is what I'm doing now what I want to be doing in the future? Have I reached success at my job? Am I fulfilled by my marital relationship? What are my present values and priorities? Am I spending my time on the things I really value? Is what I have done really meaningful? How have I been fooling myself? (and/or) What is my true worth in my eyes and society's?" OT groups can focus on some of these issues to help clients who are facing a mid-life transition to answer some of these questions.

Modifying the Life Structure

Having taken stock of the past, man now begins to plan for the next phase: exploration of new patterns for living occurs. Some changes are externally motivated. The realities of growing families, aging parents, and changes in spouse and the marriage require certain changes in role and point of view. Experience of world politics, economy, and cultural and social values also influence the planning of man's new life structure. But whether or not visible change occurs, one's outlook, values, and expectations of life are essentially different as a result of the developmental tasks of the mid-life transition. Questions to be asked are, "What do I want to change in my life? What are my options for change in occupation, marriage and family roles, roles in the community? What are the external changes in my life that put pressure on me to change? What pressures do I feel from society, friends, associates, and family, either to change or to remain the same? How can I feel more fulfilled? What parts of myself have gone undeveloped that I would now like to give expression? What faults do I see that I would like to eliminate? What new character traits can I work on developing? How can I set a more realistic goal for the future? What new beliefs can be adopted to replace the delusions of the past?" The possibilities of OT activities to help with the planning process are endless. Furthermore, the potential for self-discovery and exploration of options are maximized in group intervention.

Individuation at Mid-Life

At mid-life, individuation is a continuation of past separation and self-definition. Separation evolves from birth, gradually forming clearer boundaries between the self and the outside world. This individuation plays a part at each transition. Levinson takes his cue from Jung in describing the mid-life individuation tasks as resolving four polarities:

1. Young/old
2. Destruction/creation
3. Masculine/feminine
4. Attachment/separateness

Every life structure necessitates giving high priority to certain aspects of the self while minimizing others. In young adulthood, youth, creativity, masculinity, and attachment often outweigh their counterparts. At mid-life, neglected parts urgently seek expression.

1. *The Young/Old Polarity:* Young and old are viewed as relative terms, not specifically tied with any age. Young takes on such meanings as birth, growth, possibility, initiation, openness, energy, potential, promise of spring, fertility, and vision of things to come. Conversely, old represents termination, fruition, stability, rigidity, completion, impotence, senility, and death.

   The issues of the young/old dichotomy at mid-life are realization of one's own death, fear of loss of youth, decline in bodily and psychological powers, realization that one's time is limited, wish for immortality and fear that man is not immortal, loss of omnipotence, and acceptance of limitation. Out of the recognition of one's own mortality comes the imagery of the legacy, or what a man will pass on to future generations. Among possible legacies are children, teachings or discoveries, concrete and social structures, objects of lasting value, written documents, and artistic works.

2. *The Destruction/Creation Polarity:* A new awareness of the destruction as a universal process takes on several forms in the mid-life transition. A man must come to an understanding of his grievances toward others for their destructiveness toward him. This typically results in anger toward loved ones: parents, wife, mentors, and friends whom he sees as having hurt him. He must also look at his own destructiveness in terms of how he has hurt others. It is necessary for him to accept destructiveness as a natural part of life and to take responsibility for it. Taking action in any direction always has consequences, some creative and some destructive. "If he is forced to maintain the illusion that destructiveness does not exist, he will also be impaired in his capacity for creating, loving, and affirming life" (Levinson, 1978, p. 224).

3. *The Masculine/Feminine Polarity:* Levinson refers to the terms *masculine* and *feminine* as going beyond the biological and social differentiation. Masculinity refers to bodily prowess and toughness, homosexuality, rationality, achievement and ambition, and an intolerance of weakness. Femininity refers to

motherhood, caring and emotionality, artistic creativity, softness, and lack of strength and stamina. The masculine and feminine are really both aspects of the same person and are seen as poorly integrated in early adulthood, due to immaturity, cultural tradition, and the necessity for aggressive pursuit of one's occupation and social position. In middle adulthood, however, man comes to new terms with this polarity, seeing masculine and feminine as less rigidly divided within the self and combining them more creatively in work, personal relationships, and acceptance of self. Aggressiveness may give way to a more nurturing and sensitive side of the personality without really injuring the masculine role identity. The resolution of the masculine/feminine dichotomy opens new possibilities for the man in both love relationships with peer women and mentor relationships.

In OT, we are constantly faced with the masculine and feminine identities of our clients. In doing activity groups with male and female clients, it is important to consider their values and expectations. For example, male clients may refuse to do activities like cooking or sewing, which they consider to be "women's work." Female clients may have negative feelings about doing money management or using power tools. In using developmental theory, the age and gender of our clients as well as their disability will determine what activities they are willing to try.

4. *The Attachment/Separateness Polarity:* Attachment is defined by Levinson as "to be engaged, involved, needy, plugged in, seeking, and rooted" (1978, p. 239). Separateness is distinguished from isolation and loneliness in that it refers to a person's involvement in his or her inner world, his or her fantasies. In early adulthood, with marriage and mentor relationships, typically, attachment takes precedence at the expense of separateness. At mid-life, developmentally, a more equal balance between the two must be achieved. This generally means the man at mid-life moves further into himself and, through this process, is able to examine his own feelings, values, and goals apart from external and social expectations.

The Late Life Transition

Levinson (1978) positions the late adult transition at ages 60 to 65. The tasks of this period are to reappraise the past, create a new life structure, and make choices that are relevant to the final stage of life. Levinson's study does not extend beyond mid-life and must be viewed as speculation. The issues facing the older adult are physical decline, loss of a productive role, and coming to terms with death, both of self and loved ones. According to some theorists, changes in perception of

time begin at mid-life from "time since birth" to "time left to live." In the late adult transition, the approach of death can no longer be ignored. The limited time remaining must be devoted to resolving old conflicts, finishing unfinished business, deepening important relationships, and arranging to leave one's legacy. These life tasks lend themselves very nicely to group activities in OT. Life review groups are one example of how OT can address these issues. The late adult transition necessarily includes reviewing one's life experiences and reappraising them to sum up their worth. The results of this reappraisal may determine how an individual copes with the later years.

Piaget's Intellectual Development

Piaget (1972) studied the perceptions and problem-solving behaviors of young children to create his well-known stages of intellect or cognition. The sensorimotor stage, occurring from birth to age 2, provides a foundation for perception in the next stage, pre-operational (ages 2 to 7), which is characterized by egocentrism, problem-solving, and symbolic play. In the concrete operations stage (ages 7 to 11), logical mental processes are learned through games with rules and the influence of social demand. Formal operations (ages 11 to 15) include the ability to think abstractly; to consider past, present, and future within the context of problem solving; and to apply flexibility in solving problems. Piaget's developmental theory remains foundational to OT's work with children and families (Dunbar, 2007). Many OT theories incorporate the work of Piaget, including motor learning theory, Allen's cognitive disabilities frame of reference, Toglia's multicontextual approach, and the occupation-based model of Occupational Adaptation (Schkade & Schultz, 2003).

Many OTs are not aware that recent studies in adult cognitive development have expanded Piaget's theory beyond the formal operations stage. Piaget (1972) identified formal thought as the highest cognitive level, which he perceived to be applied throughout adulthood in order to adapt to changing life circumstances through the processes of assimilation (fitting new information into existing concepts) and accommodation (changing existing knowledge structures to account for new information), in order to balance internal needs with demands of the environment. However, several new theories have been proposed, which have been called "postformal stages" (Birney & Sternberg, 2006; Sinnott, 1993). Adults apply the newly identified stages in problem-solving and decision-making strategies within social, interpersonal, moral, political, and scientific domains, in ways that cannot be explained by Piaget's construct of formal operations. Adult developmental theorists have proposed that postformal reasoning is more complex and involves multiple ways of knowing. Using mathematical axioms, Commons and Richards (1999) identified four postformal stages:

Table 8-3

Kohlberg and Wilcox's Development of Moral Reasoning

Age	Stage
2 to 4 years	Preconventional level: Decisions made on the basis of punishment and reward Stage 1: Person is egocentric; no ability to empathize Stage 2: Reciprocity; makes deals with authority
6+	Conventional level: Decisions based on pleasing others Stage 3: Confirms identity as good; authority is fair; good people get best treatment Stage 4: Law and order orientation; rules necessary to maintain social structure; only one system is "right"
11 to 12 years	Post-conventional level: Fairness is free-standing logic Stage 5: Individual rights and human dignity can override rules; empathy influences decisions; right and wrong are separate from rules Stage 6: Ideal stage, rarely encountered in reality; unconditional value of rights of humanity; empathizes with all participants in a moral dilemma; creatively resolves polarities and contradictions

1. *Systematic order*—Defining relationships between various parts of a system, including multivariate causes, and building matrixes or models to describe complex inter-relationships. They estimate about 20% of the adult population is capable of thinking on this level.

2. *Metasystematic order*—Able to conceptualize entire systems interacting with each other and can identify metasystematic actions that can compare, contrast, transform, and synthesize systems into metasystems. Professors at top research universities might function at the metasystematic level.

3. *Paradigmatic order*—Create new fields from multiple metasystems by comparing, combining, re-organizing, or coordinating very large and seemingly unrelated fields of knowledge. When facing problems unexplainable through existing paradigms, these thinkers create new paradigms that account for previously unexplained phenomenon. Authors give the examples of Einstein (physics) and Euclid (mathematics) from scientific disciplines.

4. *Cross-paradigmatic order*—Paradigms applied in fields for which they were not created can profoundly transform large areas of knowledge. Authors state that interdisciplinary studies do not qualify for this level of thought and are mostly at the paradigmatic order level. Very few people have achieved this level of intellect. The example given is Charles Darwin, who intertwined the fields of biology, paleontology, geology, and ecology to form theory of evolution, an entirely new relationship among paradigms.

These complex levels of thinking seem consistent with complexity theory, chaos theory, and complex (dynamic) systems theory described in Chapter 3. Clearly, these stages apply more to ourselves as OT practitioners, educators, and scholars than to our clients. For example, the new discipline of occupational science, or the concept of OT in "high definition" might be represented by one of these higher levels of thought.

Practically speaking, OTs can apply these in two ways: as a way to help clients to understand that adults do not stop developing when they reach physical maturity around age 18, as Piaget once thought. Rather, intelligence continues to develop throughout adulthood. Some theories of aging have linked this fact with the need to encourage lifelong learning through adult education or "Third Age Universities (U3A's)" (Baltes & Smith, 2001). The second use of postformal theories for OT is to help us understand that people have multiple ways of thinking, learning, and communicating and that we as OTs need to consider this when trying to understand their problem-solving strategies, judgments, and life decisions.

Kohlberg and Wilcox

Kohlberg and Wilcox built on the work of Piaget, who developed stages of intellectual development. They looked at the way logic was used in the development of moral reasoning (Wilcox, 1979). How people get along in society, their view of themselves, and the social structure depend on how they make decisions about right and wrong. Kohlberg and Wilcox suggest three levels and six stages of moral development (Table 8-3). This perspective is useful in planning groups with clients who are not psychotic but have problems with society or in dealing with authority figures or rules. Motivation to move up to the next level comes from having experiences that contradict one's former beliefs and cause one to question his or her own reasoning. According to Kohlberg, all of the stages can be brought into adulthood. Many adults have been found to operate at the preconventional and conventional levels. Therapists should look for lags in moral reasoning as a possible explanation of behavior in clients.

Bruce and Borg (1993) suggest that OT group leaders encourage growth in moral reasoning by creating dissonance. Therapists do this by exposing the group members to reasoning at a slightly higher level and encouraging role taking and role reversal. Introducing moral dilemmas for a group to discuss and solve might provide an appropriate setting for this kind of developmental learning.

Gilligan—"A Different Voice"

Gilligan (1982) challenges previous theories of development in two respects. She sheds doubt on the "age and stage" concept of development, and she suggests that women have a different way of thinking about life than men do and that their developmental stages may also be fundamentally different. Gilligan points out that prior theorists, including Erikson, Kohlberg, and Levinson, have based their beliefs primarily on observations of men. A professor at Harvard, Gilligan performed her own research regarding men and women from childhood through maturity, regarding their identity and moral development, rights and responsibilities, and the role of conflict in development.

In relation to Kohlberg, Gilligan (1982) suggests that these stages relate more to men than women and do not consider the variables of culture, time, occasion, and gender. She observes that events of women's lives and of history promote the view that concern with individual survival is "selfish" or "bad," as opposed to the "responsibility" of a life lived in relationships. For women, life is caring in relationships. When the focus on individuation and individual achievement extends into adulthood and maturity is equated with personal autonomy, concern with relationships appears as a weakness of women rather than a human strength.

The stereotypes of adulthood or maturity suggested by Levinson and Erikson favor separateness or self-sufficiency over connection to others. This is primarily a "male" point of view, according to Gilligan (1982). According to these theorists, young adulthood is characterized by a conflict of commitment in which either identity or intimacy wins out. The male believes that separation empowers the self and permits full self-expression and intimacy, the choice of women, represents immaturity and impedes expression of the self. Gilligan states that "the silence of women in the narrative of adult development distorts the conception of its stages and sequence" (Gilligan, 1982, p. 156).

Gilligan does not suggest an alternative sequence of developmental stages, nor does she describe how pre-established stages are different for women. Yet, her points are well-taken and encourage us, in using this frame of reference, not to accept the proposed ages and stages as absolute reality.

In considering Gilligan's message for OT groups, we need to consider more carefully the role of relationships for our clients. There is no better place than a group to explore and work on the skills that affect relationships.

Baltes and Baltes Selective Optimization With Compensation Theory

Baltes began developing the selective optimization with compensation (SOC) theory in the 1980s as an attempt to unify previous theories of physical, biological, and spiritual aging (Baltes, Reese, & Lipsitt, 1980). He reviewed age and stage theories and determined that they did not account for the impact of social contexts and life experiences. In this view of the lifespan development, aging begins at birth and proceeds through biologically determined milestones within the context of selected life tasks aimed at growth and development until the child reaches reproductive maturity. Tasks (or occupations) are selected by the person and optimized by the physical, social, and cultural environment, while tasks or functions not relevant to the current goal are set aside through compensation. Through childhood and young adulthood, reproduction is the biological goal through which systems within the body self-organize. Culture and social contexts shape the way this goal is manifested for the individual. Young adults may or may not select tasks that help to optimize the goal of reproduction, such as dating, forming relationships, engaging in sports or other activities to maintain physical fitness, or obtaining an education or career training to prepare for financial independence from parents.

Throughout life, selection, optimization, and compensation constantly rebalance each other as people's life goals and priorities change over time. Social relationships play a large role in the SOC balancing process. For example, in middle adulthood, a married couple might divide the work of maintaining a home, earning a living, and raising children. For each partner, the goal represents the specific roles and occupations chosen as priorities, and in doing so, one partner compensates for the other. The wife may maintain a high-paying job outside the home. She selects career success as her goal and optimizes her opportunities by focusing all her energy to work-related activities. To compensate, she may delegate home management and meal preparation to the husband, whose work schedule may be more flexible. As parents, they may divide child-rearing activities so that each contributes what is most important to them.

Table 8-4

Laslett's Four Ages

Age	Description
First	Childhood, dependency, socialization, education, little responsibility
Second	Maturity, independence, familial and social responsibility, earning a living
Third	Retirement, crown of life, self-fulfillment, enjoying life for its own sake
Fourth	Dependency, disengagement, physical frailty, spirituality, preparing for death

Baltes' SOC theory is best known in connection with successful aging in older adulthood (Baltes & Baltes, 1990; Baltes & Smith, 2001). When people begin to lose energy, physical, or mental capacities, whether due to injury, illness, or the aging process itself, they find it most important to focus their limited energy and abilities on occupations that have the highest priority for them. Older adults select personally meaningful roles and occupations from among those afforded by the resources available to them. They also select environmental contexts in order to optimize their ability to accomplish their goals. As people age, they need more assistance to compensate for the abilities they have lost, and they need the support of others in order to compensate for the tasks they no longer can or wish to do.

The dynamic SOC balancing throughout life incorporates many of OT's concepts and constructs of occupational adaptation. This theory has inspired many research studies that support OT's role in helping clients adapt to changing life circumstances, especially for older adults.

Laslett's Fresh Map of Life

Peter Laslett (1989) also developed his theory in response to emerging information that previous theories failed to explain. He noted the demographics of the population had changed dramatically during the last quarter of the 20th century; that the population in Western countries got increasingly older; and that older adults over 65 continued to live active, productive, and healthy lives well into their 70s, 80s, and even 90s. Compare this with Levinson's theory, for example, that the older adult transition occurring from ages 60 to 65 included coping with physical decline and coming to terms with death. Laslett noted that for those with continued good health, these life tasks did not typically occur until much older ages. Of particular interest to Laslett was the lifestyles and occupations of older adults between the time they retired and the onset of disability. He identified four stages of life, but did not connect them with chronological ages (Table 8-4). Rather, the stages are defined by the life goals and occupations within them, which can occur in a different sequence depending on life circumstances.

Laslett's First and Second Ages

The first stage includes childhood and preparation for work. While childhood must come before adulthood, many people find themselves revisiting this stage as adults, for example if they become unemployed or decide to change their career in middle or older adulthood. The Second Age is defined by employment and raising one's family. Within a range of socioeconomic levels, people identify themselves by the occupations they perform as adults. However, the key concept defining this life stage is the need to earn a living by working. Productive occupations have different meanings in retirement than they do in the Second Age, as described in the next section.

Laslett's Third Age

Defining the Third Age represents Laslett's unique contribution to adult development because he is the first to recognize the distinctive life goals and tasks that characterize the time period (often 20 to 30 years) between retirement and the onset of disability. Any OT practicing in the field of gerontology cannot ignore the global phenomenon of the Third Age model (Christiansen, 2008), which Laslett has called "the age of active retirement" (1989). Entering the Third Age, older adults are no longer constrained by the economic necessity of working, a phenomenon that in many countries is facilitated by the bestowal of government subsidies like social security or public or private pensions. Third Agers have a whole new set of life tasks, that are different from any previously identified stage of older adulthood: self-fulfillment, life-long learning, creative expression, civic engagement, and making a contribution to society (advocacy). The Third Age has generated thousands of "Third Age Universities (U3As)" throughout the world, with the mission of offering continuing education and/or career development to retirees while also conducting research about the process of successful aging. Laslett (1997) points out that, while governments continue to subsidize Third Agers, these individuals have a responsibility to use their productive energy in the service of humanity. The current situation may provide a window of opportunity for Third Agers to change the culture of retirement to include valued social roles that simultaneously offer self-fulfillment while promoting social (and occupational) justice and addressing the unmet needs of society.

While most people enter the Third Age as older adults, some do so at younger ages for a variety of reasons. For example, young artists or composers of music may pursue these creative, self-fulfilling endeavors despite their inability to earn a living by doing so. People who acquire serious injury or illness at younger ages may be forced to retire from competitive employment and to redefine their life roles based on limited abilities and resources. Many people in this category could become OT clients, and this theory may guide our professional reasoning when collaborating with them to create a new vision for their future occupational roles.

Laslett's Fourth Age

The Fourth Age begins when people become dependent on others to meet their basic needs. It includes some of the life tasks described by previous theories of aging, such as adjusting to physical decline and preparation for death. Several theories have confirmed the transition from Third to Fourth Ages by identifying changes in life goals, structure, and social relationships as well as a shift in occupational priorities. Baltes and Smith (2001) discuss how the onset of disability creates a need to shift the balance of optimization (environmental supports) and compensation (services from others) in order to continue to engage in the occupations older adults select as priorities. Two other theories address the change in activity and lifestyle priorities that seems to occur in very old age: socioemotional selectivity theory and gerotranscendence.

Socioemotional Selectivity Theory

Selectivity involves a voluntary narrowing of one's social networks and a disengagement from certain types of activities that once held meaning. Researchers have found that, in those older than 80 years, present-oriented goals have a higher priority than future-oriented goals (Carstensen, 1992; Lockenhoff & Carstensen, 2004). Social relationships are limited to significant family members and longtime friendships, and Fourth Agers no longer have interest in activities involving meeting new people or making new friends (Adams, Roberts, & Cole, 2011). The narrower social circle helps elders conserve emotional energy, only worrying about the people who matter most. Additionally, emotional intensity seems to diminish as Fourth Agers accept their own mortality. Those older than 85 years feel comfortable spending more time sleeping or engaging in solitary activities (Adams et al., 2011; Larson, Czikszentmihalyi, & Graef, 1982).

Gerotranscendance

This theory views the shift from a lifestyle of continued activity to one of disengagement as a positive adaptation to changing life circumstances. Researchers denote a shift in occupational priorities away from pragmatic and performance-oriented activities toward more spiritual and transcendent occupational interests.

Atchley's Continuity Theory

Continuity theory acknowledges that many established patterns of thinking, doing activities, and maintaining social relationships continue throughout life despite changing circumstances. As people age, they make adaptive choices that seek to maintain their self-identity and basic world view (Atchley, 1999). In other words, internal patterns (such as personal goals, beliefs, and values) and external patterns (such as lifestyle, social networks, and daily routines) continue through each transition or adaptation, helping the person to maintain a sense of well-being and personhood. Continuity does not discredit the likelihood that predictable life changes occur for everyone as they move through adulthood, but it looks at each adaptation as building upon prior life experiences. In this view, people become better at solving life problems and adapting as they grow older, counterbalancing the alternate view that people lose cognitive abilities as they age. Adults who have learned to use environmental feedback to increase the efficiency, effectiveness, and satisfaction of their responses have the potential to achieve exceptional adaptive ability and resilience (Baltes & Smith, 1990). Atchley's continuity theory is congruent with many OT occupation-based models that view occupational adaptation as an upward spiral of ongoing development.

FUNCTION AND DYSFUNCTION

If one uses an age-and-stage theory, then healthy functioning is having achieved age-appropriate developmental tasks. For example, a 23 year old will have separated from his or her parents, chosen a career, and, if not married, at least developed a support system of peers with whom to identify. Conversely, dysfunction may be looked at as failure to develop age-appropriate skills or failure to achieve the tasks of one's developmental stage. The stages of childhood and adolescence have been studied historically in much greater detail than those of adulthood. However, even these age-stage matches have been challenged. OT practitioners are advised to regard the ages given for developmental tasks as only approximate guidelines. Furthermore, as illness interferes with normal development, the discrepancy between age and developmental level may become so great that the term *age-appropriate* becomes meaningless. It is the developmental stage that we as OTs are concerned with because that is what determines the level of function and adaptation to the environment.

Dysfunction can be seen as a lack of adaptive skills necessary for effective and satisfying interaction with one's environment. It can be caused by a failure to develop these skills (developmental delay), a loss of these skills (e.g., due to brain trauma), or a regression to an earlier stage of development (such as that caused by depression or schizophrenia).

In adult development theory, just the normal tasks at each transitional stage may be enough to cause a crisis situation. If Levinson (1978) speaks of the mid-life transition as a potential crisis for 80% of the population, think of the impact it must have on those with physical or mental disability. If Levinson is right, the stress produced by this kind of crisis is likely to contribute to physical and mental breakdown, even in those without previous illness.

Development is almost always affected by illness. As clients with disability are referred to OT, the assessment process is likely to uncover missing skills that clients have failed to learn in earlier stages of development. The difficulty in coping with illness in the present is often due to the inadequacy of earlier skill development. Because the stages of development are hierarchical, OT cannot address issues of the client's current age until earlier skills are learned. For example, a 20-year-old may not be expected to work on career choice and separation from parents if his or her illness has resulted in a lack of ability to form peer relationships and his or her own identity is not developed. Because of discrepancies between chronological and developmental age in people with illness and disability, groups in OT often include clients of varying ages. OTs organize group interventions by developmental levels (not age levels) so that members can work together on similar skills.

CHANGE AND MOTIVATION

Motivation comes from an individual's natural desire for mastery of age-appropriate skills. The drive toward mastery is, at least in part, biologically determined. However, as a person matures, the environment plays a greater part in motivation. If a person's attempts to progress developmentally are met with success, motivation will likely remain intact. Repeated failures to keep up with peers, on the other hand, may discourage a person from continuing to try. OT may encourage the rediscovery of the drive toward mastery by creating a "just-right challenge." This is a task or situation that encourages a client to use higher-level skills, but one that is not beyond his or her reach.

When there is a developmental lag or loss of skills, they must be learned or relearned in the correct developmental sequence. Mosey (1970) called this "recapitulation of ontogeny." If the client is more than one level behind, the change process may be slow, but it follows a more or less predictable pattern. Because developmental stages are hierarchical, the earlier skills must be mastered before the learning of later-developing skills is possible.

Consider a group of individuals with persistent mental illness. The age of onset for several chronic mental illnesses is the early 20s. Often, clients have achieved at least some of the developmental tasks of the young adult transition before becoming ill. Many have vocational or educational training in a chosen career, some have begun working and have moved out of their parents' homes, and some have married and had one or two children. These are accomplishments beyond the capacity of most clients with chronic mental illness. One might see these clients as regressed. Because of their illness, they have gone backward to an earlier, less mature stage of development. In treating these clients, the OT needs to determine the correct level at which to begin. This will be the level at which mastery is possible and growth and change can be motivated.

Mosey's concept of the six adaptive skills is helpful in identifying a client's correct developmental level, as well as determining which skills need work. These skills are as follows:

1. Perceptual motor
2. Cognitive
3. Dyadic interaction
4. Group interaction
5. Self-identity
6. Sexual identity

Each adaptive skill has several subskills whose typical ages of development are identified. These are described fully in Appendix C (Mosey, 1986).

Change occurs through the learning of new skills. This can be encouraged by setting up a growth-facilitating environment. The OT looks carefully at the physical environment in terms of safety. The emotional environment may best be set through the client-therapist relationship and through the use of groups. Mosey's (1970) concept of developmental groups is useful here. The hierarchy of group structure and leadership requirements in these groups can help OTs to plan group interventions for clients that are appropriate to their level of development (see Appendix B).

However, the benefits of group intervention go beyond the learning or relearning of group interaction skills. All six adaptive skills identified by Mosey may be effectively learned in a group context through engaging in an OT activity. At the higher developmental levels, the tasks of adult development may be facilitated through group activities in OT.

GROUP INTERVENTION

As implied in this frame of reference, groups are best organized along the lines of developmental level rather than age. OT groups would be primarily homogeneous. At earlier levels of development, clients in a parallel group may be participating in activities that promote sensorimotor or cognitive skill development. At higher levels, groups may use interaction skills to work on career choice in the young adult transition, re-examine their values in the mid-life transition, or participate in retirement planning in the late-life transition. The structure of OT group intervention is organized according to the developmental level, and this guides the OTs' choice of activity as well.

The limitations for use of this frame of reference are minimal. Clients of every age and almost any type of disability are appropriately treated within its bounds. The theories of adult development described in this chapter, however, are most helpful in planning groups for the later stages of development. Guidelines for the earlier stages, dealing with sensorimotor and cognitive development, are described in Chapters 6 and 9.

Role of the Leader

In developmental groups, the OT takes a directive role. Knowledge of the predictable conflicts and skills in each developmental stage guides the use of activities and setting of group goals. He or she evaluates clients' skills to determine their developmental levels and attempts to predict their potential for further development. When placed in appropriate groups, clients can work together on their mutual tasks with the leader's guidance. Because the sequence of learned tasks is hierarchical, the OT cannot give too many choices to the group. If the groups are planned appropriately, their area of interest should coincide with the developmental tasks of their level. OTs need to challenge their groups to develop further by consistently introducing higher-level activities at appropriate times.

It is also the responsibility of the leader to create and maintain a growth-facilitating environment (Mosey, 1970). In the intervention setting, clients should be supported and rewarded for growth, not discouraged. If a group is ready to take on more responsibility, this should be allowed. If growing requires a stage of upset and turmoil, and it has to get worse before it gets better, this should also be met with patience and support.

The OT should be on the lookout for signs of developmental transitions in clients with physical disability as well as mental illness. Even when the illness is physical, addressing developmental issues can be the most beneficial in helping the client to cope. Coping with illness or developmental crises often requires the learning of enabling skills. These are specific cognitive, psychosocial, or sensorimotor learned behaviors that make it possible for the individual to meet his or her developmental needs (Bruce & Borg, 1993). Examples are reading and writing, communication skills, or the ability to empathize with others. Mosey's adaptive skills might be used as a guide.

Examples of Activities

The chosen activities should address issues to be resolved or specific skills appropriate to the developmental level of the client group. The theorist, the specific stage to be addressed, and the specific task or skill within that stage should be identified. Because most of the theorists have an identified hierarchy of issues, tasks, or skills to be learned at each level, these can easily serve as guidelines for activity choice. See Activity Examples 8-1 through 8-10. Most of the group activities at the end of this chapter originally appeared in Cole and Gross (1982).

GROUP LEADERSHIP

The seven steps of group leadership can remain intact when working with most adult groups in this frame of reference. The introduction is done according to the guidelines offered in Chapter 1.

Activity

Activities and goals are chosen using specific guidelines from the ages and stages of development. The learning exercise in Worksheet 8-1 may be helpful in identifying the theory and stage that is appropriate for a particular group of clients. Fill in the chart by writing under the various chronological ages the appropriate information from the theories reviewed at the beginning of this chapter. However, Ikiuku (2007) warns that client input should also guide activity choice, rather than just strict adherence to developmental models.

Transitions have been highlighted recently as times when people may need OT services. For young adults, the transition from school to work can be full of stumbling blocks. OTs can apply knowledge of the theories of young adult transitions to help young clients to better prepare for the new work and social roles in which they seek to participate. Gibson and colleagues identify three transitions for which OTs are well prepared to assist clients (Gibson et al., 2010):

- *Children entering school*—Whether preschool or kindergarten, children face many challenges when first entering an unfamiliar environment and taking on the uncertain role of student in a classroom setting.

- *High school graduates transitioning to work settings*—Have many challenges as outlined by developmental theorists, when taking on new work roles and responsibilities and establishing independence from parents.

- *Older adults transitioning to new environments later in life*—For example, when parents of a child with disabilities grow older, difficult decisions must be made for parents and for the adult child who needs ongoing care.

Worksheet 8-1
Developmental Theories Comparative Chart

Directions: Using information from this text and others, fill in the developmental stages for each of the theorists. Estimate the chronological age range for each stage and fill in on the chart below.

Chronological Age	Childhood	Adolescence	Young Adulthood
Jung (Spiritual stages)			
Erikson (Psychosocial stages)			
Levinson (Life transitions)			
Kohlberg (Moral development)			
Piaget and Postformal			
Mosey (Appendix C) (Adaptive skills)			
Baltes and Baltes			
Laslett			
Socioemotional selectivity			
Gerotranscendence			
Atchley's continuity			
Physical milestones/ attributes typical of age			

From Cole, M. B. *Group dynamics in occupational therapy: The theoretical basis and practice application of group intervention* (4th ed.). Thorofare, NJ: SLACK Incorporated. © 2012 SLACK Incorporated.

Developmental Theories Comparative Chart (Continued)

Chronological Age	Middle Adulthood	Third Age	Fourth Age
Jung (Spiritual stages)			
Erikson (Psychosocial stages)			
Levinson (Life transitions)			
Kohlberg (Moral development)			
Piaget and Postformal			
Mosey (Appendix C) (Adaptive skills)			
Baltes and Baltes			
Laslett			
Socioemotional selectivity			
Gerotranscendence			
Atchley's continuity			
Physical milestones/ attributes typical of age			

From Cole, M. B. *Group dynamics in occupational therapy: The theoretical basis and practice application of group intervention* (4th ed.). Thorofare, NJ: SLACK Incorporated. © 2012 SLACK Incorporated.

Knotts (2008) reviews the typical transitions of older adulthood, including 1) work to retirement, 2) changes in health status, 3) relocation or place transitions, 4) transitions in social relationships, and 5) adaptation to loss of significant others. Because transitions can be highly stressful, many people need help in coping with the complex and dynamic consequences of difficult transitions in their lives. Knotts (2008) suggests that occupations can serve as a bridge; OT can facilitate the continuation of familiar occupational patterns and routines to help maintain a sense of competence and well-being through many changing circumstances.

It is especially important to plan an environment that incorporates safety, support, and challenge. The goals for these groups are to help members progress to higher levels of development. The timing of groups may be altered to suit the group, the activity, and the goal. Many of the tasks of adult development are quite complex, and there are many aspects to be explored. Activities such as those listed above may take several sessions, depending on how they are planned and how much discussion seems appropriate. If clients are motivated by a particular activity, it may be desirable to give homework. Clients may be asked to think about the issues discussed between sessions, to explore options for change, or to try out new behaviors with family and friends.

A good resource for the late-life developmental tasks is the AOTA publication, Lifestyle Redesign: Implementing the Well Elderly Program (Mandel, Jackson, Zemke, Nelson, & Clark, 1999). This manual provides many prevention activities dealing with transitions of older adulthood.

Sharing and Processing

Sharing, including self-expression and feedback, is an important part of the developmental group. However, while members are working on similar tasks, there is no expectation that they will produce similar results, because each person must complete a developmental task in his or her own way. This expectation is consistent with the concepts of client-centered practice (AOTA, 2008). Processing the group may uncover many feelings about both past and present experiences. This is one frame of reference in which talking about past events is not discouraged. Relationships among members evidenced during processing can be helpful in supporting clients through many traumatic memories as well as stressful present-day realities. Group cohesiveness in this frame is desirable and encouraged.

Generalizing and Application

Generalizing an experience should be somewhat predictable, because most of the activities will address specific developmental issues. The therapist really has to take the lead to guide the discussion of general principles along developmental lines.

Application is a particularly important aspect of developmental groups, because the group experiences are designed to have a specific impact on development. If there is a focus to the discussion of developmental groups, it should be the application of learning to each individual's everyday life. The summary can be shared by members and the leader, depending on the ability of the group, and this should also stress application of learning.

There are quite a few theories added to this edition, so, as a preparation for group planning, students can use Worksheet 8-1 to compare the different theories and approximate age groups to which they apply. Because chronological ages rarely coincide with developmental life stages of the various theorists, using childhood, adolescence, young, middle, and older adulthood as groupings might be more contemporary. Put the entire chart on a word processor to accommodate the many new criteria and conditions, and add your own subtitles.

REFERENCES

Adams, K. B., Roberts, A. R., & Cole, M. B. (2011). Changes in activity and interest in the Third and Fourth Age: Associations with health, functioning, and depressive symptoms. *Occupational Therapy International, 18,* 4-17.

American Occupational Therapy Association. (2008). Occupational therapy practice framework: Domain and process. *American Journal of Occupational Therapy, 62,* 625-683.

Atchley, R. C. (1999). *Continuity and adaptation in aging: Creating positive experiences.* Baltimore, MD: Johns Hopkins University Press.

Baltes, P., & Baltes, M. M. (Eds.) (1990). *Successful aging: Perspectives from the behavioral sciences.* New York, NY: Cambridge University Press.

Baltes, P., Reese, H. W., & Lipsitt, L. (1980). Lifespan developmental psychology. *Annual Review Psychology, 31,* 65-110.

Baltes, P., & Smith, J. (1990). The psychology of wisdom and its ontogenesis. In Sternberg, E., *Wisdom: Its nature, origins, and development.* New York, NY: Cambridge University Press.

Baltes, P., & Smith, J. (2001). *New frontiers in the future of aging: From successful aging of the young old to the dilemmas of the Fourth Age.* Retrieved from www.valenciaforum.com/Keynotes/pb.html.

Bigsby, R. (2003). Developmental and neurological perspectives. In E. Crepeau, E. Cohn, & B. Boyt Schell (Eds.), *Willard & Spackman's occupational therapy* (10th ed., pp. 243-245). Philadelphia, PA: Lippincott, Williams & Wilkins.

Birney, D., & Sternberg, R. (2006). Intelligence and cognitive abilities as competencies in development. In Bialystok & F. Craik (Eds.), *Lifespan cognition* (pp. 315-330). New York, NY: Oxford University Press.

Bruce, M. A., & Borg, B. (1993). *Frames of reference in psychosocial occupational therapy* (2nd ed.). Thorofare, NJ: SLACK Incorporated.

Carstensen, L. L. (1992). Social and emotional patterns in adulthood: Support for socioemotional selectivity theory. *Psychology and Aging, 7,* 331-338.

Christiansen, C. (2008). Envisioning a key role for occupational therapy to support healthy aging in the 21st century. In S. Coppola, S. Elliot, & P. Toto (Eds.), *Strategies to advance gerontology excellence: Promoting best practice in occupational therapy* (pp. 501-512). Bethesda, MD: American Occupational Therapy Association.

Cole, M., & Gross, M. (1982). *Structured group experiences for life's adult transitions.* Unpublished manuscript.

Commons, M. L., & Richards, F. A. (1999). Four postformal stages. In J. Demick (Ed.), *Handbook of adult development.* New York, NY: Plenum (Elsevier).

Dunbar, S. B. (2007). Theory, frame of reference, and model: A differentiation for practice considerations. In S. Dunbar, (Ed.), *Occupational therapy models for intervention with children and families* (pp. 1-9). Thorofare, NJ: SLACK Incorporated.

Erikson, E. H. (1978). *Adulthood.* New York, NY: Norton.

Erikson, E. H., & Erikson, J. M. (1997). *The life cycle completed.* New York, NY: Norton.

Gibson, R. W., Nochajski, S., Schefkind, S., Myers, C., Sage, J., & Marshall, A. (2010). The role of occupational therapy in transitions throughout the lifespan. *OT Practice, June 28,* 11-14.

Gilligan, C. (1982). *A different voice.* Cambridge, MA: Harvard University Press.

Ikiuku, M. (2007). *Psychosocial conceptual practice models in occupational therapy: Building adaptive capability.* St. Louis, MO: Mosby.

Jung, C. G. (1914). *On psychological understanding. In Collected Works 3.* Princeton, NJ: Princeton University Press (1960).

Kaplan, H., & Sadock, B. (2003). *Synopsis of psychiatry* (9th ed.). Baltimore, MD: Williams & Wilkins.

Knotts, V. J. (2008). Transitions for older adults. In S. Coppola, S. Elliott, & P. Toto (Eds.), *Strategies to advance gerontology excellence: Promoting best practice for occupational therapy.* Bethesda, MD: American Occupational Therapy Association.

Larson, R., Csikszentmihalyi, M., Graef, R. (1982). Time alone in daily experience: Loneliness or renewal? In L. A. Peplau, & D. Perlman (Ed.), *Loneliness: A sourcebook of current theory* (pp. 40-53). New York, NY: John Wiley & Sons, Inc.

Laslett, P. (1989). *A fresh map of life: The emergence of the Third Age.* Cambridge, MA: Harvard University Press.

Laslett, P. (1997). Interpreting the demographic changes. *Philosophical Transactions of the Royal Society of London. Series B, Biological Sciences, 352*(1363), 1805-1809.

Levinson, D. (1978). *The seasons of a man's life.* New York, NY: Ballantine Books.

Lockenhoff, C. E., & Carstensen, L. L. (2004). Socioemotional selectivity theory: aging, and health: The increasingly delicate balance between regulating emotions and making tough choices. *Journal of Personality, 72,* 1395-1424.

McAdams, D. P., Hart, H. M., & Maruna, A. S. (1998). The anatomy of generativity. In D. P. McAdams & E. de St. Aubin (Eds.), *Generativity and adult development* (pp. 7-43). Washington, DC: American Psychological Association.

McAdams, D. P., de St. Aubin, E., & Logan, R. (1993). Generativity among young, midlife, and older adults. *Psychology and Aging, 8,* 678-694.

Mandel, D., Jackson, J., Zemke, R., Nelson, L., & Clark, F. (1999). *Lifestyle redesign: Implementing the well elderly program.* Bethesda, MD: American Occupational Therapy Association.

Mosey, A. C. (1970). *Three frames of reference for mental health.* Thorofare, NJ: SLACK Incorporated.

Mosey, A. C. (1986). *Psychosocial components of occupational therapy.* New York, NY: Raven.

Piaget, J. (1972). Intellectual evolution from adolescence to adulthood. *Human Development, 16,* 346-370.

Rogers, C. (1980). *A way of being.* Boston, MA: Houghton Mifflin.

Schultz, D. (1976). *Theories of personality.* Monterrey, CA: Brooks/Cole.

Schkade, J., & Schultz, J. (2003). Occupational adaptation. In E. Crepeau, E. Cohn, & B. Schell (Eds.), *Willard & Spackman's occupational therapy.* Philadelphia, PA: Lippincott, Williams, & Wilkins.

Sheehy, G. (1976). *Passages: Predictable crises of adult life.* New York, NY: E. P. Dutton.

Sheehy, G. (1981). *Pathfinders: Overcoming the crises of adult life.* New York, NY: E. P. Dutton.

Shmotkin, D., Blumstein, T., & Modan, B. (2003). Beyond keeping active: concomitants of being a volunteer in old-old age. *Psychological Aging, 18,* 602-607.

Sinnott, J. D. (1993). Yes, it's worth the trouble! Unique contributions from everyday cognition studies. In J. M. Puckett & H. Reese (Eds.), *Mechanisms of everyday cognition* (pp. 73-95). NJ: Lawrence Erlbaum Association.

Westermeyer, J. (2004). Predictors and characteristics of Erikson's life cycle model among men: A 32 year longitudinal study. *International Journal of Aging and Human Development, 58,* 29-48.

Wilcox, M. (1979). *Developmental journey.* Nashville, TN: Abington Press.

Zemke, R., & Gratz, R. R. (1982). The role of theory: Erikson and occupational therapy. *Occupational Therapy in Mental Health, II*(3), 45-63.

Developmental Activity Example 8-1
Ideal Man/Ideal Woman

This activity addresses Levinson's early adult transition, specifically the tasks of finding a special woman or man and finding a mentor.

Materials: 12- x 18-inch sheets of white drawing paper, pastels, pencils, erasers, and tissues.

Directions: First, look into your fantasy, and envision a person of the opposite gender who you consider to be ideal, having all the qualities you would wish for in a mate, companion, and friend. What does that person look like? Notice hair, eyes, facial expression, stature, clothing, style of movement. What is that person doing? Perhaps he or she is sitting across from you at dinner, participating with you in an active sport, sitting by the fireside planning a new project with you, having lively interactions with others at a party, seriously engaging in a business venture, or walking alone on a deserted beach. When an image has come to mind, try to capture its essential qualities by drawing them.

Fold the paper in half, and draw your first picture on the left half of the page. Never mind if your drawing does not look exactly like your mental image—just do the best that you can. You have 15 minutes for the drawing. After 10 minutes, next to your drawing, make note of any particular personality traits, habits, attitudes, values, and other internal attributes possessed by the person you drew. Is this person sensitive, strong, energetic, intellectual, responsible, gentle? What talents and abilities does the person possess?

Now, imagine a person of the same gender, who you consider to be ideal. Maybe the person is someone whose accomplishments you admire or whose lifestyle seems appealing. Perhaps the person holds a position in life you aspire to or has talents you desire to develop in yourself. Do not think too much about this, but allow images to enter your mind, remembering that this will be a person you create, not necessarily someone you know. You may combine attributes of several people or just make up new ones. Keep in mind the images you consider most ideal, and when the image crystallizes, begin to draw it on the second side of your paper. Do the same as you did for the first part, considering physical appearance, activity or situation, and both external and internal traits. Write down those elements that cannot be defined by drawing (15 minutes).

Developmental Activity Example 8-2
Times of Your Life Collage

This activity addresses Levinson's mid-life transition in providing an opportunity to review past accomplishments as well as unrealized expectations. It will assist clients in re-evaluating the past and present life structures in preparation for making changes in middle adulthood (Figure 8-1).

Materials: Variety of magazines suitable to patients, large poster board, glue, scissors, and marker for each patient. If patients in the group are of similar or known ages, the poster board may be set up ahead of time to provide a space for every 5 years of their lives up to their present ages.

0 to 5	5 to 10	10 to 15	15 to 20
20 to 25	25 to 30	30 to 35	35 to 40

Figure 8-1. Times of your life collage. Draw format on larger posterboard. Adapt ages for each member.

Directions: The object of this exercise is to get a temporal perspective on our lives and to see how the parts fit into the whole to make us the people we are today. The poster board will represent the whole. Our life will begin on the upper left and proceed to the lower right, divided into time intervals of 5 years. Leave one space for the present. (Show example.) Now, think about the events that occurred in each segment of your life, what you were like then, people who were in your life, places where you lived or traveled, accomplishments you achieved, and decisions you made. Then, look through the magazines and find pictures, words, and phrases that best describe the major event or aspect of each segment of your life up to and including the present.

This activity can take up to 2 hours. Depending on patient group, the project can be done on one day and discussed the next, or it can carry over several group sessions. Discussion should center around evaluation of events and account for spaces left blank. High and low points may be identified. Emotional responses to events or patterns may be identified. Are there patterns? Were there changes? How were the changes made? Markers may be used to identify highs, lows, and emotions surrounding events.

Change options should then be explored. What accounts for the decisions in your life? Were they made impulsively? Influenced by others? Done with careful planning? If you could go back and change parts of your life, what would you change? What do you wish you could add or delete? What was missing in your life development that you wish had been there?

A follow-up drawing can be added to this exercise, entitled "The Future." Planning the next 5 or 10 years can be done using the same collage techniques.

From Cole, M. B. *Group dynamics in occupational therapy: The theoretical basis and practice application of group intervention* (4th ed.). Thorofare, NJ: SLACK Incorporated. © 2012 SLACK Incorporated.

Developmental Activity Example 8-3
Fabric of Life

This simple weaving activity addresses the life review task of Levinson's late-adult transition. It is in keeping with the views of Erikson and Jung as well. The use of colors, patterns, and materials encourage the incorporation of emotional and substantive memories or essences, as well as marker events (Figure 8-2). This exercise requires two or three 1-hour sessions for most groups.

Materials: Pencils, paper, and a medium paper bag for each group member to plan his or her project. A heavy wire circle (loom) 12- to 18-inches in diameter (warped with strong yarn dividing the circle into 16 equal parts, tied together in the center) and one pair of sharp scissors should be provided for each person. A large variety of fabric remnants (can be scraps from a seamstress or cut from old, donated clothes, curtains, sheets, tablecloths, etc.), trimmings, ribbons, and several colored balls of yarn. Fabrics should be cut into long 1-inch strips.

Directions: Fabrics are, for most of us, associated with clothing, home furnishings, draperies, bed sheets, and the like. They are adorning and surrounding us constantly, and although often not the focus of our attention, they influence our sensory experiences and our mood and color our lives in ways of which we may be unaware. In this exercise, we will associate key events, places, and people in our lives with a sensory awareness of the fabrics that may symbolize them. We will choose fabrics, trimmings, or ribbons to represent both events and significant others in our lives. In addition, each of us will choose one special yarn or fabric to represent ourselves. Begin by writing down any of the following that apply most to you. As you choose fabrics, trimmings, and ribbons for each memory, cut an arm's length of it and place it in your paper bag.

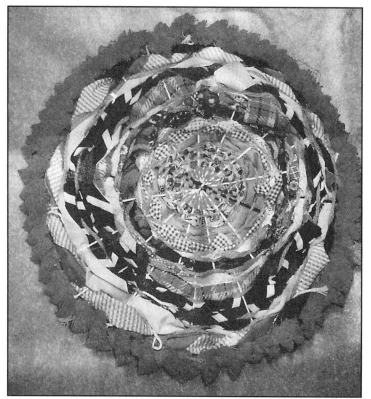

Figure 8-2. Fabric of life.

Developmental Activity Example 8-3
Fabric of Life (Continued)

1. Birth and young childhood—Envision your room or most memorable environment as a child. What do you see? What can you feel? Is there a favorite blanket or stuffed toy? What color is there? How does the texture of the fabric feel to your touch? Choose a fabric or material from the collection to represent this association as closely as possible.

2. Parents—Envision each of your parents, either separately or together, doing whatever they ordinarily were doing when you were a child. How were they dressed? What was their favorite color? Style? Summon an image of each of your parents as you would like to remember them from childhood. Then, choose a fabric to represent that image. Take a few minutes to re-experience visual, tactile, auditory, or olfactory memories (sights, sounds, textures, and smells) associated with each of the items to follow, and continue to select fabrics and place them in your bag.

3. Friends from childhood

4. Relatives and siblings

5. A childhood home (imagine your room)

6. First day of school (what did you wear?)

7. Communion, bar mitzvah, or joining a church

8. First date

9. First school dance

10. First boyfriend or girlfriend

11. Graduation

12. First job (or significant ones)

13. Marriage

14. First house or apartment

15. Death of loved one(s)

16. Important travels

17. Awards or promotions at work

18. Adult friends

19. Birth of children and their significant others

20. Marriage, graduation, or jobs of children

21. Birth of grandchildren

22. Organizations or committees

23. Adult hobbies or leisure activities

24. Other important events or milestones

Planning takes at least a 1-hour session and should be discussed before the session ends. Memories can be verbalized and elaborated. If desired, a small scrap of fabric can be taped to the paper and labeled after each item is planned, so the group member will not forget what was chosen for which at the next session. Be sure to put names on paper bags. Planning paper can be folded and placed inside.

From Cole, M. B. *Group dynamics in occupational therapy: The theoretical basis and practice application of group intervention* (4th ed.). Thorofare, NJ: SLACK Incorporated. © 2012 SLACK Incorporated.

Developmental Activity Example 8-3
Fabric of Life (Continued)

Procedure for Weaving: Begin with the ball of yarn that represents you. Tie the end to the center and weave it under and over each warp thread, clockwise around the circle for five or six rows. This yarn will touch and become a part of all the other materials you have chosen. How much of each other material you use depends on how large a part its associated element played in your life. Begin with childhood and work chronologically, adding chosen materials and weaving them over and under with the yarn, around and around the circle. From time to time, rake the yarn toward the center with your fingers to push it together. End when you have used up all the materials selected. Wind the yarn (or add ribbon or trim) around and around the wire circle to cover it, and tie in a loop knot at the end to hang it on the wall. (See Figure 8-2 for example.)

Discussion should be encouraged during the weaving process, and the therapist will help patients as needed. Feelings about the project at the end are especially important. The doing process often evokes many hidden feelings that need to be expressed and explored. Is the review of life positive or negative? Which parts are positive or negative? What is missing? Patients should be encouraged to keep their own projects and to reflect on the significance of them, and not to use them as gifts, at least for a while. Remember, a life review is only the beginning of the task of evaluation and integration, which Jung and Erikson have suggested is necessary for contentment in old age.

From Cole, M. B. *Group dynamics in occupational therapy: The theoretical basis and practice application of group intervention* (4th ed.). Thorofare, NJ: SLACK Incorporated. © 2012 SLACK Incorporated.

Developmental Activity Example 8-4
The Doctor's Dilemma

This activity refers to Kohlberg's fourth and fifth stages of moral development. The group's discussion is intended to cast doubt upon a strict "law and order" kind of reasoning about morality and to encourage empathy with more than one participant in a given situation.

Directions: First, I will read you a story that has several characters who do not agree with one another. Listen carefully to the story, and then, as a group, decide who is right, who is wrong, and what should be done about the situation.

Story: Jenny was a healthy 24-year-old woman who went into the hospital unexpectedly to have her appendix removed. It was 8 p.m. and Dr. Struthers had just completed a long, tiring day of surgery. Jenny's sister Carol brought her to the hospital in terrible pain; it was evident that she needed to be operated on at once. The emergency room nurse, Eva, interviewed Jenny and prepared her for surgery. Eva wrote down on her report that Jenny had her last meal 1 hour ago, which put her at considerable risk of choking when given general anesthesia. However, the doctor did not read the report carefully. He operated anyway, and the patient choked to death on the table.

Carol was in shock; she suspected negligence and sued the doctor for $1 million. Although Jenny was not married and had no children, Carol missed her sister and felt that those who mistreated her sister should pay. But mostly, she could really use the money. She and her husband had just bought a house and had defaulted on the past few payments. A settlement of $500,000 would just about pay off their mortgage, and prevent them from losing their home.

Eva, the nurse who prepared the report, was secretly in love with the doctor. Out of love, she offered to alter the report, changing the "1" hour since last meal to a "9." This would clear Dr. Strothers of any blame for Jenny's death. Eva saw that Dr. Struthers was a caring and brilliant young doctor, capable of saving many more lives if allowed to continue his practice. Of course, a verdict of guilty in the lawsuit would prevent him from ever practicing again. Eva was willing to give up nursing and take the blame for the man she loved. She hoped perhaps he would marry her if she did this, and after a brief jail sentence, they could live happily ever after.

Dr. Struthers was faced with a dilemma. Should he take the blame, plead guilty in the lawsuit, and give up his life's work? Should he accept Eva's offer to take the blame? Should he meet with Carol and offer to pay her $500,000 to withdraw the lawsuit? How should the story end? It is up to you.

Developmental Activity Example 8-5
Families of Clay

Margo Gross, MS, OTR/L, is acknowledged as the creator of this activity, which relates to Levinson's individuation in both the early-adult and middle-adult transitions.

Materials: A ball of soft clay, approximately 4 inches in diameter, a piece of cardboard or poster board (18 x 24 inches) for each member, clay modeling tools, water and paper towels for clean-up, markers, and small post-it notepads.

Directions: Divide your clay into sections for each member of your family, including yourself. Sculpt an abstract figure that represents how you feel about each person. Try to use non-concrete representations. Arrange the people on the board in such a way as to describe the relationships in your family. Label each member.

Discussion: Discuss how you saw your family system at ages 5, 15, 25, 35, etc. How would you like to see the relationships in your family placed, ideally? What happened to the structure when new members were introduced? Geographical moves? Marriage or divorce? Death?

Individuals beginning to separate from their family of origin can look at the structure and their place in it from a distance. Assessing the aspects of learning derived from each parent, hidden messages, and alliances and conflicts between members is an important step in the individuation process. At mid-life, individuation takes on a qualitatively different process, as the role of parent to offspring ends and becoming caretaker for one's own aging parents is more of a reality. Whether or not family ties remain close, individuation continues psychologically as one ages. One's perception of each family member is altered as the individual becomes more fully integrated.

From Cole, M. B. *Group dynamics in occupational therapy: The theoretical basis and practice application of group intervention* (4th ed.). Thorofare, NJ: SLACK Incorporated. © 2012 SLACK Incorporated.

Developmental Activity Example 8-6
Eulogy for Yourself

Margo Gross, MS, OTR/L, is acknowledged as the creator of this activity, which addresses Levinson's middle and late life transitions.

Materials: Pencil and paper for each member.

Directions: This exercise will help you see your life more clearly from the perspective of your imagined death. Write the eulogy that your best friend might read at your funeral. Include any major accomplishments, special family relationships, contributions to the community, and values or morals that you strongly uphold. What has been the significance of your life, and how might you be leaving the world a better place?

Within the group format, pass your eulogy to the person at your right, and take turns reading them out loud. Record your response as you hear about your life in retrospect.

Discussion: What periods of your life were the most/least fulfilling in terms of career, family relationships, involvement in community life? Where were the major turning points? What values did you act on consistently? How can you plan to complete any unfinished business in the time left before your death?

This exercise has direct implications for those individuals approaching mid-life, where the sense of aging becomes more acute due to the beginning of the physical and cognitive decline. Their sense of mortality is accentuated by the change in generational status, by the aging of parental figures, and by the death or illness of friends or contemporaries.

Assessing the climb up the ladder of success and deciding whether earlier goals were attained or new goals need to be defined are aspects of this developmental period. The activity will reinforce the fact that each individual still has a period of life ahead to restructure a change to reach different or new goals.

For individuals in the late adult transition, the activity serves to assist in life review. It is a concrete way of seeing and hearing how the major themes and events in a life come together to unify the self.

Developmental Activity Example 8-7
Major Accomplishments

Margo Gross, MS, OTR/L, is acknowledged as the creator of this activity, which addresses Levinson's middle and late life transitions. Two 1-hour sessions are needed for this exercise.

Materials: 12- x 12-inch plywood boards for each member, sandpaper square, scissors, magazines, personal photographs if available, decoupage glue, water-based wood stain, rags, brushes, water and paper towels for clean-up, and permanent color markers.

Directions: Prepare the wood board by sanding the edges and corners and also both surfaces of the wood until smooth to the touch. Wipe away the sawdust. Brush the stain onto all sides of the wood in the color of your choice. Use a small rag to wipe off excess stain and set aside to dry. From the magazines, choose pictures and words that describe your major accomplishments up to the present time. Arrange them in front of you as you process the first session. Write your name on the back of your board with a marker, and place your clippings in a plain envelope with your name.

Bring any photographs, actual newspaper clippings, or mementos you have found at home to the second session. Arrange the clippings and photos on the board in a pleasing manner. You may wish to overlap the pictures, which means applying several coats of decoupage glue to adhere each layer of the design. Be sure to smooth the pictures well to eliminate air bubbles underneath, which can cause wrinkling of the pictures as the glue dries. Apply a final coat of glue to finish the plaque and give the project a glossy shine. Be sure to apply decoupage glue to the edges to seal and protect the plaque. When dry, a tooth hook may be applied to the center of the back for hanging.

Discussion: Depending on the transitional period in which members of the activity group are involved, the pictures chosen will represent feelings about their accomplishments to date. Individuals in the middle adult transition will use this activity to re-evaluate the past and take stock of their progress. For late adult transitions, the plaque serves as a life review. People facing retirement, changes in financial status, or widowhood may find the decoupage a concrete daily reminder of their self-worth, which may be shaky during such periods of adaptation. Categories of successes may be separated into family, career, or personal accomplishments. A discussion of how a future plaque might look will assist those in the process of designing a new life structure.

Developmental Activity Example 8-8
Exploring Sex Roles

Margo Gross, MS, OTR/L, is acknowledged as the creator of this activity, which addresses Levinson's early adult transition.

Materials: Worksheets and pens for each member, large newsprint pad with easel, and magic marker.

Directions: This activity is designed to explore and clarify sex roles in our lives. Using the headings provided, fill in the incomplete sentences, trying not to censor any ideas that come to mind, even if the statements seem to be contradictory. After 10 to 15 minutes, ask the group to stop writing and look over their answers. On the newsprint pad, write down the men's and women's responses as they are shared.

Discussion: Which items on your list seem the most powerful or important to you? Which items are self-imposed? Which show family influences? Which items are similar for the men? For the women? Which items from the opposite sex surprised you the most? How might your roles be the same or different from roles of your parents? Which did you neglect, which did you emphasize? Which items are age-specific for you right now?

Exploring Sex Roles (Continued)

Exploring Sex Roles Worksheet (Male)

If I were a woman, I could...

1.
2.
3.
4.
5.

Because I am a man, I must....

1.
2.
3.
4.
5.

Exploring Sex Roles Worksheet (Female)

If I were a man, I could...

1.
2.
3.
4.
5.

Because I am a woman, I must....

1.
2.
3.
4.
5.

Developmental Activity Example 8-9
Childhood Games and Occupational Choice

Margo Gross, MS, OTR/L, is acknowledged as the creator of this activity, which addresses one of the life tasks of Levinson's early and middle adult transitions.

Materials: Worksheets and pencils.

Directions: Children from a young age until they are well into adolescence spend much of their free time in some form of play. Make a list of 10 childhood games that you remember playing. Think about games you played alone and ones you played informally with peers. Include both indoor and outdoor games, fantasy and make-believe, as well as group games and sports.

After you complete the list, analyze each game by placing the symbols next to it that best apply. Then, apply these same symbols to your current occupation.

Discussion: What are the similarities and differences between your childhood play and current occupation? Consider whether your present occupation involves the characteristics of play that you enjoyed the most. Have you accepted or rejected aspects of yourself that you value and want to be a part of your life today?

From Cole, M. B. *Group dynamics in occupational therapy: The theoretical basis and practice application of group intervention* (4th ed.). Thorofare, NJ: SLACK Incorporated. © 2012 SLACK Incorporated.

Developmental Activity Example 8-9
Childhood Games and Occupational Choice (Continued)

Childhood Games and Current Occupation Worksheet

Name:

Job title of current or most recent occupation:

List 10 childhood games you remember playing (before the age of 15):

1.

2.

3.

4.

5.

6.

7.

8.

9.

10.

After you complete the list, analyze each game by placing the symbols next to it that best apply:
M—Male oriented
F—Female oriented
U—Unstructured
S—Structured
A—Played alone
G—Played with others/groups
Ab—Abstract, fantasy oriented
C—Concrete, reality oriented
O—Objects or props necessary
M—Imagined or mentally created

Now, apply these same symbols to your current occupation.

From Cole, M. B. *Group dynamics in occupational therapy: The theoretical basis and practice application of group intervention* (4th ed.). Thorofare, NJ: SLACK Incorporated. © 2012 SLACK Incorporated.

Developmental Activity Example 8-10
Reminiscence

Life review has a place in almost every developmental theory addressing the older adult. Erikson, Jung, and Levinson all define some form of re-evaluation of the meaning of one's life as its end draws nearer. Reminiscence is a review of past experiences, with a goal of establishing a sense of integrity and satisfaction with oneself through the process of remembering. Drawing, writing, and storytelling are creative ways to assist members in recalling their specific experiences. Once written or drawn, members should share through discussion. Some suggested themes include the following:

- Specific years or events: The Great Depression, World War II, the 50s, the 60s.
- What were you doing when... Pearl Harbor was bombed? Franklin D. Roosevelt died?
- What was the most difficult period in your life?
- When did you get your first car? First house?
- Describe your first date. First job. First child.
- Describe your first encounter with death (relative, close friend).
- What was your proudest moment?
- Whom do you admire most in your family?
- What values would you choose to leave to your children? To society?
- Bring in favorite music/songs from the past, and discuss their significance.

It should be noted that reminiscence does not restore memory for people who have cognitive deficits. However, people with mild or moderate dementia often retain remote memories, and discussing these in groups can help them re-establish a sense of normal social functioning.

From Cole, M. B. *Group dynamics in occupational therapy: The theoretical basis and practice application of group intervention* (4th ed.). Thorofare, NJ: SLACK Incorporated. © 2012 SLACK Incorporated.

Chapter 9

SENSORIMOTOR APPROACHES

The sensorimotor approaches include a range of frames of reference that address motor, sensorimotor, perceptual, and cognitive problems due to developmental or acquired conditions affecting the brain. The motor control approaches in particular have undergone some major theoretical changes in recent years (Trombly & Radomski, 2008). Earlier sensorimotor approaches arose from the principles of neuroscience and generally follow an ontological sequence of development, which might also be described as linear. Using complexity theory, OT theorists have transformed many of these approaches with a more holistic and occupation-oriented perspective. Yet, for specific types of sensorimotor dysfunction, earlier frames of reference and their techniques for assessment and intervention have much to contribute. Experienced OTs will be able to use specific techniques within the context of client-centered, occupation-based interventions that are compatible with today's OT paradigm. This chapter will briefly review Trombly's Occupational Functioning Model (OFM), the task-oriented approach, motor learning theory, and Carr and Shepherd's Motor Relearning (Sabari, 2002), as well as the more traditional approaches to motor control. The sensory integration (SI) theory of Ayres and subsequent sensory modulation approaches will also be briefly reviewed. Ayres' SI theory paved the way for the group approaches devised by King and Ross. Recently, sensory modulation has emerged as an effective intervention for many populations across the age span, including autism spectrum disorders, learning disabilities, persistent mental illness, addiction disorders, stroke, and dementia. Extensive literature exists by

and about all of these theories, and the reader is referred to other books and articles for a more in-depth understanding of each specific theory.

FRAMEWORK FOCUS

Traditionally, this approach has been used to facilitate learning or relearning of motor skills by applying controlled sensory input to specific body structures as defined in the *Occupational Therapy Practice Framework* (American Occupational Therapy Association [AOTA], 2008). Body functions such as learning, memory, and motor planning interact with body structures and environmental contexts to produce optimal occupational performance. SI moves beyond motor responses and addresses process skills, such as attending and listening, emotion modulation, eye-hand coordination, and academic learning ability. Current evidence suggests that using motor facilitation techniques is most effective when practiced within specific "contexts" and "activity demands."

For OT, the primary use of this approach has been with developmental disabilities affecting the central nervous system (CNS) and those who have suffered trauma or disease to the CNS. However, recent studies of the brain have linked neurophysiological and CNS dysfunction to mental disorders as well. Applying SI principles of intervention with the geriatric population is increasing and shows promising results. OT groups using this frame of reference should use activities that stimulate the

Cole M.B. *Group Dynamics in Occupational Therapy:
The Theoretical Basis and Practice Application
of Group Intervention (pp 249-280).*
© 2012 SLACK Incorporated.

senses, produce purposeful movement, promote cognition and affect, and use real-life tasks to approach the CNS in a systematic way.

BASIC ASSUMPTIONS

This group of approaches encompasses many theorists (and techniques), among them Trombly, Carr and Shepherd, Rood, the Bobaths (neurodevelopmental treatment [NDT]), Brunnstrom, Ayres' sensory integration, and Dunn's sensory processing frames of reference. These frames are not necessarily intended to be used with groups; however, the principles of intervention can be applied when planning group activities. Examples of OT group intervention approaches using these theories are reviewed, including the writings of King and Ross. Some of these approaches make the assumption that brain function is hierarchical and rehabilitation follows a developmental sequence, while others view brain function as parallel and simultaneous and organize interventions around specific tasks. All of the theorists agree on the importance of sensation in this process and the importance of practice and feedback in motor learning.

Holistic Systems Approaches

The newer sensorimotor approaches incorporate varying degrees of dynamic systems theory, which is closely associated with complexity theory described in Chapter 3. When applied to physical disabilities, this theory defines motor control as a blend of reflexes and voluntary control that is dependent on the demands of both task and environment. The CNS interprets cues from the environment and involves multiple subsystems when planning to reach desired goals. In contrast to hierarchical models, this is seen as "parallel distributed processing" in which many signals may be processed simultaneously among many brain structures. Movement is then generated by an open-loop feed-forward system with emphasis on anticipatory postural adjustments made as part of the total movement pattern. Behavior, therefore, is a product of the interaction between the individual, the task, and multiple environmental factors (Bowler, 1999).

Trombly's Occupational Functioning Model

The occupational functioning model (OFM) was primarily developed for people with physical disabilities. This model adds a holistic perspective in the application of more traditional biomedically based frames of reference. In 1995, Catherine Trombly introduced her OFM in her Eleanor Clarke Slagle Lecture. She pointed out that when a client "got to choose an activity...the chosen activity was meaningful and kept the person interested and working" (Trombly, 1995, p. 960). Her model incorporates this idea in a "descending hierarchy of roles, tasks, activities, abilities, and capacities." The goal of her model is to "develop a sense of competency and self-esteem" (p. 961). Evidence has demonstrated that a strong relationship exists between life satisfaction and one's roles related to social integration and work (Dijkers, 1999; Trombly, 2008). This supports the model's use of occupation as both "means" (to build foundation skills) and as "end" (to improve performance). A basic assumption of the OFM is that "ability to carry out one's roles and activities depends on basic abilities and capacities. However, acknowledging the complex nature of human occupation, Trombly interprets current research to suggest that the relationship between low level capacities and abilities and higher level tasks and roles is not direct" (Trombly & Radomski, 2008, p. 4). Developing stronger muscles does not guarantee that a person can carry luggage or bring in the groceries. Many abilities and capacities work together to produce occupational performance (Dagfinrud et al., 2005).

Trombly (2008) acknowledges that environment plays a much larger role in physical rehabilitation than was previously thought. Evidence shows that clients best perform occupations related to valued roles when practiced in the environments and contexts particular to that individual. However, after injury, physical deficits often present barriers to successful occupational performance in natural contexts (home or work settings). When faced with physical obstacles, clients need to work on foundational capacities (such as motor control or postural endurance) in order to develop or restore confidence in their ability to perform valued occupations, otherwise known as self-efficacy. Self-efficacy (Bandura, 1977, 1997), a cornerstone of the OFM, requires clients to build a history of successful occupational performance. In the absence of natural settings during the acute stages of recovery, the OT can facilitate small groups to provide one another the social and emotional support needed to develop or restore self-efficacy. The OT group leader can guide members working on foundational abilities in choosing which occupations they prefer to engage in as a means of recovering lost abilities, for example, playing board games or baking cookies as a means to practice postural and upper extremity motor control. This suggests that clients who have mastered the foundational capacities, abilities, and skills may be more appropriately treated in groups. For example, OTs can compose groups of clients to work on valued roles in self-maintenance, self-advancement, or self-enhancement using a task-oriented approach. The group provides a social and cultural context within which each member is motivated to meet the task demand. Trombly calls this method of using tasks as intervention "occupation-as-end" (p. 6). See Table 9-1 for an overview of the OFM.

Table 9-1

Trombly's Occupational Functioning Model Hierarchy

- Sense of self-efficacy and self-esteem
- Satisfaction with life roles
- Competence in tasks of life roles
- Activities and habits

- Abilities and skills
- Developed capacities
- First-level capacities
- Organic substrate

Task-Oriented Approach

This approach is based on the theories of motor learning and dynamical systems theory (described earlier). Functional tasks, chosen collaboratively by client and OT, are believed to help organize motor behavior. Principles from learning theory are applied to the doing of meaningful tasks, which are graded and sequenced according to each client's needs and abilities. The client's occupational performance results from the interaction of multiple systems, both internal and external. From the *Occupational Therapy Practice Framework* perspective, "client factors," such as anatomy, physiology, and physical and mental functioning, are influenced by multiple "contexts" and "activity demands" in producing occupational performance. After CNS damage, a client's behavior may seem purposeless, but, in this approach, all behavior is interpreted as a client's attempt to achieve functional goals. Each task requires practice and experimentation with a variety of strategies in multiple contexts in order for motor skills to be learned.

Bass-Haugen, Mathiowetz, and Flinn (2008) list the following five principles of the task-oriented approach:

1. Client-centered focus
2. Occupation-based focus
3. Person and environment
4. Practice and feedback
5. General treatment goals

Each will be reviewed briefly here.

Client-Centered Focus

Research shows that "clients who are actively engaged in their treatment show achievement in self-identified goals, increased functional independence at discharge, and (are) discharged to less restrictive environments (Gibson & Schkade, 1997)" (Trombly & Radomski, 2002, p. 484). Client priorities can be very task focused, and clients are often motivated by the wish to perform valued life roles. OTs form therapeutic relationships with clients during evaluation that involve a discussion of personal interests, values, and preferences; identification of meaningful life roles; and collaboration on goals and priorities. Choices of intervention tasks and decisions about group membership are a natural consequence of this continued collaboration. Clients with common goals can benefit from engaging in group tasks in which members participate in planning, implementing, group problem-solving, outcome evaluation, and mutual feedback. The OT who facilitates a task-oriented group will contribute professional expertise and resources as needed or requested by client members. Some such groups will require more direction than others.

Occupation-Based Focus

This approach uses actual functional tasks as opposed to exercise to achieve movement goals. Tasks that are selected should be both meaningful and important to the client's life roles. "Life satisfaction is not determined by successful completion of a random set of functional tasks (changing a diaper...). Satisfaction or reward comes from the feeling that roles are fulfilled (parent...)" (Bass-Haugen, Mathiowetz, & Flinn, 2008, p. 602). Selecting tasks collaboratively with clients and reinforcing their relevance to life roles is likely to enhance client motivation. However, clients need our assistance to avoid early failure with tasks that are initially too difficult. The OT must also carefully analyze the selected tasks and adapt or grade the task demand to match client abilities and learning needs.

Person and Environment

It is important for the OT to observe the performance of tasks that are difficult for the client. Many systems interact to influence occupational performance. Part of the OT intervention will be to identify both personal and environmental factors that facilitate or inhibit task performance so that adaptation of these factors can be explored. Client and OT can collaborate to develop strategies to prevent interfering variables and to adapt the task and environment to promote optimal functioning.

Practice and Feedback

Skill practice in a variety of settings is necessary for learning to occur. This reflects an important principle of motor learning, the principle of encoding specificity. According to this principle, events stored in memory are embedded in specific contexts, which limit the transfer or generalization of learning in a different context. Flinn and Radomski (2008) suggest using contextual interference by varying the context and the task for which a skill is practiced. This encourages more complex processing strategies, which include problem-solving and adapting the skill in different situations. Motor learning theory also stresses the importance of feedback, both intrinsic and extrinsic. Intrinsic feedback is usually somatosensory or visual, experiencing the sensation of the movement. Extrinsic feedback comes from others. The OT may give feedback concurrently, coaching the client during task performance. This type of feedback is called knowledge of performance (KP). The outcome of task performance is called knowledge of result (KR). Research shows giving feedback on performance is more productive at the beginning stages of rehabilitation and giving feedback on outcome or result is better if given intermittently. A decision needs to be made about whether to practice one part of a task (part learning) or the whole task (whole learning). A whole task is more readily stored in long-term memory than parts of a task. Storage and retrieval are both necessary for motor learning to occur.

General Goals

The overall goals of the client learning process are to discover the optimal movement patterns for task performance. Flexibility, efficiency, and effectiveness are important for any task, and these may develop as clients continue to practice skills in varying natural environments. Ultimately, clients need to develop problem-solving skills so that they can continue to identify their own solutions in both home and community environments.

Motor Learning Theory

Motor learning has been defined as a "set of processes associated with practice or experience leading to relatively permanent changes in the capacity for responding" or producing skilled motor action (Schmidt, 1988, p. 346). Central to this theory is the growing body of knowledge on neural plasticity. Organisms demonstrate an inherent capacity to self-organize throughout life. Neural plasticity is the ability of the nervous system to become more efficient at the cellular level and to change the way the whole system works by modifying neural connections. Short-term learning depends on short-term, or working, memory, which allows us to attend to a phone number long enough to dial it. This may be equated with the random access memory on a computer. Only when we "save" information to a hard drive on a computer can we then retrieve the information and use it later. Long-term memory acts in much the same way, as a necessary step in making permanent and lasting change. OTs are most interested in long-term modulation of synapses that results from experience. Using these principles, therapeutic activities can be devised by OTs to effect lasting changes in motor functioning for clients.

Schmidt (1988) identified four basic concepts for motor learning:

1. Learning is a process of acquiring the capability for skilled action.
2. Learning results from experience or practice.
3. Learning cannot be measured directly, rather it is inferred from behavior.
4. Learning produces relatively permanent changes in behavior.

Motor learning during rehabilitation occurs in three stages, according to Fitts and Posner (1967). At first, the client attempts to understand the nature of the task. The OT discusses various strategies for doing the task and evaluating performance. This is the cognitive stage. The second, associative stage, involves refining and perfecting the skill through practice. The third stage occurs when the skill becomes habitual, and a low degree of attention is required for optimal performance. This is called the autonomous stage. Shumway-Cook and Woollacott (2006) review a multitude of evidence supporting motor learning theory. Within this approach, the OT facilitates motor relearning using teaching-learning strategies and incorporates them into meaningful occupations using many of the task-oriented approaches described earlier.

Carr and Shepherd

Carr and Shepherd (1987, 1998) developed a Motor Relearning Program (MRP), which focuses on teaching clients how to use feedback to modify their performance. These theorists use dynamical systems theory, which views changes in neural connections as initiated by environmental opportunities. In other words, they assume that voluntary movements are initiated by functional task goals instead of exercise. An important principle of dynamical systems theory is attraction states, or preferred patterns of movement. A deeply entrenched movement pattern can become a barrier to lasting change. For example, if a person develops a faulty golf swing and uses it many times, it is very difficult to unlearn. It is the same with maladaptive movement patterns following brain damage. If the pattern is new and unpracticed (shallow), it is much easier to change. Control parameters are those factors that influence preferred patterns of movement. For example, a wet floor or an icy sidewalk will alter one's movement patterns while walking. Some control parameters are external, while others are internal. For example, fatigue might be an internal factor that alters one's pattern of walking.

Carr and Shepherd use four principles of intervention to shape long-term learning:

1. Oral instruction: The most important aspects of movement are used to create an objective goal (e.g., "touch the spoon handle").
2. Visual demonstration: The therapist models the movement for the client. Photographs and drawings can also be used. The demonstration focuses on the most essential task components.

Table 9-2

Carr and Shepherd's Motor Assessment Scale Categories

- Supine to side lying on intact side
- Supine to sitting on edge of bed
- Balanced sitting
- Sitting to standing

- Upper arm functions
- Hand movements
- Advanced hand activities

3. Manual guidance: The OT moves the client through a sequence, attending to inhibition of constraining components.

4. Accurate and timely feedback: Feedback is offered to reinforce actual improvements in performance. While effort can be acknowledged, it should not be treated in the same way as actual improvement.

In dealing with motor abnormalities, four general categories of motor performance are addressed:

1. Standing up and sitting down

2. Walking

3. Reaching and manipulation

4. Balance

Carr and Shepherd (1998) have devised an assessment tool, the Motor Assessment Scale (MAS), using a seven-point scale to evaluate seven specific movements related to the above categories. These movements are listed in Table 9-2. For the full assessment scale, see Carr and Shepherd (1987).

An important aspect of the Carr and Shepherd intervention technique is grading the activity demand. The following are guidelines for grading an activity to elicit specific motor response patterns:

- Change the position of the person, the seating, the support, or the alignment.

- Change object placement, position relative to body, or distance.

- Change the object characteristics, weight, size, one- versus two-handed lifting.

- Change temporal demands, such as using stationary versus moving objects.

Carr and Shepherd (1998) go on to define the essential features of each movement category addressed by their theory. Potentially, the most interesting category to be addressed by group intervention is the fourth: reach and manipulation. This category is said to have the greatest number of degrees of freedom or potential variations in complexity of movement. This is addressed by combining several movements into synergistic combinations. Relearning of reach and grasp requires initial passive stretch of the shoulder muscles to maintain range of

motion. This passive stretching using the unaffected arm might be one example of an activity that can be learned in a group format, perhaps while moving to music or incorporating visualization. Client members might learn to observe one another and offer feedback using guidelines modeled by the OT facilitator.

Traditional Neurophysiological Approaches

The following group of theories has come to be known as the reflex-hierarchical models of motor control. The reflexive basis of human movement has been challenged in recent years by research that suggests that motor behavior is not primarily controlled by the CNS in a top-down hierarchy. The dynamical systems theory and the motor learning theory have cast doubt as to the legitimacy of some of these earlier theories, which discouraged the use of functional tasks for fear of developing "splinter skills" or skills learned by rote, which skipped ahead of the normal developmental sequence. Thus, doubt is cast upon approaches that emphasize adherence to a developmental sequence at the expense of functional performance (Trombly & Radomski, 2008). However, these theorists continue to influence practice, and some, such as NDT, are being researched and updated.

Rood

Margaret Rood's work preceded most of the other theorists covered in this chapter, and her ideas seem to have inspired many of the concepts of SI developed later. Rood was the first to focus on the importance of reflexes. Rood (1954) states:

...motor patterns are developed from fundamental reflex patterns present at birth which are utilized and gradually modified through sensory stimuli until the highest control is gained on the conscious cortical level. It seemed to me then, that if it were possible to apply the proper sensory stimuli to the appropriate sensory receptor as it is utilized in normal sequential development, it might be possible to elicit motor responses reflexively and by following neurophysiological principles, and establish proper motor engrams.

Table 9-3

Rood's Eight Ontogenetic Motor Patterns

1. Supine withdrawal
2. Segmental rolling
3. Pivot prone (prone extension)
4. Neck co-contraction Supporting self on elbows

5. Supporting self on elbows
6. All-fours movement patterns
7. Standing
8. Walking

Rood's (1954) theory has four basic components:

1. Sensory input is required for normalization of tone and evocation of desired muscular responses.
2. Sensorimotor control is developmentally based.
3. Movement is purposeful.
4. Repetition of movement is necessary for learning.

Most OTs recognize Rood's techniques of facilitation and inhibition. Light stroking, brushing, icing, and joint compression are used to facilitate movement. Joint approximation (light compression), neutral warmth, pressure on tendon insertion, and slow rhythmical movement are used to inhibit unwanted movement. Many of Rood's facilitation and inhabitation strategies have been adapted by later theorists, and the basic principles have been applied in activity selection for group programming for many different populations, such as the sensory trauma-informed approach to restraint reduction described later in this chapter.

Rood recommended the facilitation of normal movement in a developmental sequence. First, phasic reciprocal contraction, such as flexion to extension and back, is practiced repeatedly until learned. Next, stabilization through co-contraction of major muscle groups is facilitated. A third phase combines these, practicing movement imposed on stabilization, and a final phase incorporates the development of skilled movement. Table 9-3 states Rood's eight ontogenetic motor patterns.

This sequence gives OTs some very specific guidelines for planning movement activities for clients with neurodevelopmental disorders. When planning group intervention, each client's unique developmental level with respect to movement needs to be carefully considered. Movement groups can be set up at many levels but should progress from earlier to later stages in the ontogenetic sequence. Clients should not be asked to perform movements at higher levels than they are capable. Positioning is a primary concern, especially at the lower levels. It may involve the extensive use of mats, bolsters, beach balls, or other specialized equipment.

Many games can be devised that involve pushing and pulling, throwing and catching, and rolling and creeping to move the body from one place to another. These activities should be set up to incorporate the correct therapeutic movement sequences for each client, while the clients are participating in goal-directed activities.

The Bobaths' Neurodevelopmental Therapy

Dr. and Mrs. Bobath are a neurologist and a physiotherapist from England who originated the therapeutic technique best known as neurodevelopmental therapy (NDT; Bobath, 1972). One of their most important contributions to theory is their focus on sensorimotor learning. It is not movement itself but the sensation of movement that is learned and remembered. Much of the Bobaths' work was done on children with cerebral palsy and adult hemiplegia post-stroke (Bobath, 1990). The techniques are widely known and used but little researched prior to 1990, according to Levit (2008). Since the Bobaths' deaths in 1990, the Neurodevelopmental Treatment Association in the United States, as well as similar groups in other countries, have been working to update the theoretical basis and practice techniques for NDT. Although it addresses mainly the motor and sensory components of performance, NDT intervention is individualized to meet specific client goals and represents an interactive process among the individual, caregivers, and members of the interdisciplinary team (Levit, 2008). The approach works best when all helpers, including family members, use the same approach.

Following the Bobaths' focus on sensation, their handling of children with cerebral palsy, and subsequently of adults with hemiplegia, concentrated on repetition of correct motor responses. The assumption is that when clients experience normal movement, this results in correct sensory feedback to the CNS. NDT involves teaching the client how correct movement feels. To this end, great effort is made to inhibit primitive reflexes through "reflex inhibiting patterns" (RIPs) (Levit, 2008, p. 651) and to elicit righting and equilibrium responses.

In NDT, sensory stimulation is regulated with great care. Weight bearing, placing and holding, tapping, and joint compression are used to activate normal movement and posture. However, these stimuli are withdrawn as soon as an abnormal response occurs. In hemiplegia, sensory deficits are interpreted as an indication of poor prognosis for regaining normal control of movement. Stress is avoided because it is thought to promote abnormal tone and movement.

After stroke or head trauma, the sequence of relearning movement approximates normal development. While

Table 9-4

Brunnstrom's Six Stages of Recovery

1. Flaccidity, no voluntary movement
2. Synergies or minimal voluntary movement
3. Synergies performed voluntarily
4. Some deviation from synergy
5. Independent or isolated movement
6. Individual joint movement nearly normal with minimal spasticity

compensatory movement that uses one-handed techniques is discouraged, tasks that are client priorities may be practiced using bilateral movements and key points of control. Some researchers have demonstrated that an approach that combines traditional NDT with instruction in home exercise showed greater improvement in functional control than NDT alone (Sunderlund et al., 1992). Therapist assistance is needed initially to inhibit abnormal movement patterns during task performance. Recovery from stroke and trauma generally involves a flaccid stage followed by a spastic stage. Many specific exercises and handling are suggested in each of these stages following the developmental process. These involve positioning, weight bearing, holding and placing, balance reactions, and protective extension, among others. Levit (2008) suggests a good source of both individual and group activities based on the Bobaths' NDT approach is Eggers' *Occupational Therapy in the Treatment of Adult Hemiplegia* (1983).

Brunnstrom

Unlike the other theorists so far, Signe Brunnstrom took an opposite view of the use of reflexes. Her basic assumption was that as normal development progresses, spinal cord and brainstem reflexes become modified and their components rearranged into purposeful movement through the CNS. Therefore, reflexes can and should be used to elicit movement where none exists as part of a normal sequence (Trombly & Radomski, 2002). Both proprioceptive (resistive) and exteroceptive (tactile) stimuli are used to elicit reflexes, and the client is encouraged to think about the movement that results and try to gain control of that movement.

The Brunnstrom approach seeks to elicit associated reactions and synergies. For example, resistive stimuli are believed to achieve both reflexive movement on the noninvolved side and similar synergistic movement on the involved side. A synergy is defined as the total flexion or extension movement of a joint or limb. Six stages of recovery are defined by Brunnstrom for the upper and lower extremity as listed in Table 9-4.

These are specifically defined, and interested students are encouraged to read about specific assessment and treatment techniques in Brunnstrom's *Movement Therapy in Hemiplegia* (1970).

Groups using the principles of NDT, as well as other neurodevelopmental theories, may be designed with clients who have achieved a fair degree of voluntary movement. Exercise groups, movement to music, and simple games are best suited to these clients, many of whom are likely to have language and cognitive problems as well.

Ayres' Sensory Integration

Sensory integration (SI) is "one of the most cited and applied of all theories within occupational therapy" (Mulligan, 2002). The term, sometimes used interchangeably with sensory processing in the interdisciplinary literature, refers to a theory of normal sensory development, a group of disorders, and a specific OT evaluation and intervention. A. Jean Ayres, an OT and educational psychologist, is credited with developing the theory of sensory integration (Ayres, 1961, 1974, 1979; Bundy, Lane, & Murray, 2002). Ayres maintained an active private practice with children in Southern California. Her research focused on sensory processing in an attempt to explain the underlying causes of learning disabilities and behavioral and motor difficulties in children. As a neurodevelopmental approach, SI assumes that remediating underlying neurological processes will improve a child's motor coordination and ability to attend and learn in the classroom. Ayres proposed that sensory systems build upon one another from birth and that the visual and auditory systems depend on more foundational body-centered senses (tactile, proprioceptive, and vestibular systems). Therapeutic interventions using sensory input affect multisensory systems and therefore influence both learning and behavior. Applying Ayres' principles in today's practice, sensory processing must connect with occupation, so that effectiveness of SI interventions can be seen through the client's successful engagement in occupations and participation in life roles (Roley, Mailloux, Miller-Kubaneck, & Glennon, 2009). Two basic assumptions currently dominate SI theory: neuroplasticity and a hierarchical view of the CNS. Neuroplasticity of the brain refers to its ability to adapt and change. According to Mulligan (2002), an abundance of evidence exists to support the concept of neuroplasticity. While concept of CNS hierarchy has been challenged in recent years, its usefulness as a central concept in the SI frame of reference for OT lies in its many specialized intervention techniques that are firmly rooted in the occupation of play. SI largely focuses on the remediation of brainstem functions as a way to improve functional skills within the context of play, learning, and social interaction (Blanche & Kiefer, 2007). Ayres refers to the normal developmental sequence in her study of the use of sensory input. She suggests four levels of the sensory integrative process. Her concept of foundation skills implies that lower level (brainstem) functions precede higher levels in Stages 1 through 4. These stage descriptions are adapted from Ayres' flowchart for the senses, integration of their input, and end products, which was copyrighted by Western Psychological Services in 1979.

Primary Level

At this level, Ayres (1974) identifies the three basic sensory systems as vestibular, proprioceptive, and tactile. Visual and auditory are acknowledged but not thought to play a major integrative role in the earliest stages of development. Touch is cited as the basis for the infant's first emotional bond with mother. The processing of these initial touch sensations is seen to be responsible for establishing a basic sense of security.

The proprioceptive and vestibular senses offer another kind of basic security—gravitational security. These help the child develop balance for standing and walking and prevent the fear of falling. This level includes the eye movements, posture, balance, muscle tone, and gravitational security all resulting from the vestibular and proprioceptive integration. Sucking, eating, the mother-child bond, and tactile comfort are seen as the result of integration of tactile sensations.

Second Level

At this level, the three basic senses are integrated into a body precept, coordination of the two sides of the body, motor planning, attention span, activity level, and emotional stability. Sensory information from vestibular, proprioceptive, and tactile receptors are used to form precepts, or maps, of the body that are stored in the brain. With this mechanism, one is constantly aware of where his or her body is and what it is doing. This precept has information about right and left sides of the body, which allows the two sides to work bilaterally to accomplish tasks. The precept also allows a person to plan motor actions (e.g., catching a ball or feeding him- or herself). The organization of sensory input by the brain is also reflected in the ability to focus attention and adjust the level or pace of activity. Hyperactivity, hypoactivity, and the inability to attend are thus explained by poor integration at the secondary level of SI.

Third Level

Speech and language, eye-hand coordination, visual perception, and purposeful activity are possible at this level due to the impact of auditory and visual sensations.

According to Ayres (1974), the vestibular and auditory systems are intimately related. The vestibular system, as stated above, is responsible for the ability to attend to what is heard. Language comprehension likewise begins with the child's touching, moving, lifting, and otherwise interacting with the objects in his or her environment. Only through this experience can he or she begin to appreciate the unique properties of an object and know its name. Visual perception is also seen as an end product of earlier SI: how big something is, how far away it is, and what its relationship is to other parts of the environment are all experienced first by reaching and touching. The visual experience is thus intimately related to the tactile and vestibular systems as well. With an understanding of what he or she hears and what he or she sees, the child's actions with respect to the environment can be purposeful. Visual sensation directs the child's hand to reach out to pet the kitten. He or she alters his or her posture to keep his or her balance as the kitten moves under his or her touch. The child hears the kitten purr and repeats the action. Visual, auditory, tactile, and vestibular systems all work together to help the child explore and learn about his or her environment.

Fourth Level

The fourth and final level of SI includes the following end products: the ability to organize and concentrate, self-esteem, control and confidence, academic learning ability, capacity for abstract thought and reasoning, and development of dominance and hemispheric specialization. From Ayres' (1974) point of view, it does little good for OTs to attempt to directly teach these skills when the earlier stages of integration are not adequately developed. This point of view has been challenged in recent years.

Skilled voluntary fine motor hand movement, for example, cannot be taught to the disabled child by giving practice exercises. Ayres describes the development of hand movement as a sequence of many steps:

- Control of neck and eye movements
- Trunk stability and balance
- Scapular and shoulder stability and movement
- Elbow motion
- Gross grasp
- Wrist positioning and movement
- Release of grasp
- Forearm supination and pronation
- Individual finger manipulation.

Overlapping this sequence is the coordination of visual and sensorimotor mechanisms. Movements begin as spinal reflexes and are modified and refined to achieve a behavioral goal. In this way, reflex movement becomes voluntary. Regarding the role of sensation in this process, Ayres states two basic assumptions:

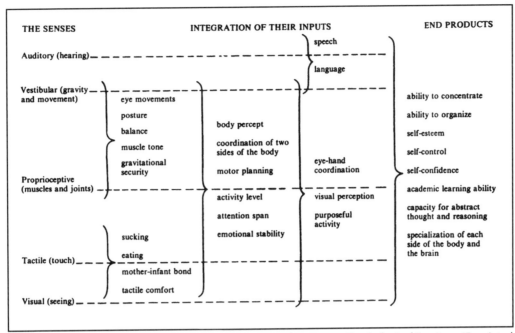

THE SENSES   INTEGRATION OF THEIR INPUTS   END PRODUCTS

Figure 9-1. A. Jean Ayres sensory integration theory. 1979 by Western Psychological Services. (Reprinted from *Sensory Integration and the Child* by permission of the publisher, Western Psychological Services, 12031 Wilshire Blvd., Los Angeles, CA 90025.)

1) therapeutic activities to address identified deficits are designed with specific attention to the contribution of tactile, proprioceptive, and vestibular sensations to function and 2) "ongoing motor learning and behavior are strongly influenced by if not dependent on incoming sensation" (Ayres, 1979). She proposed "playful" interventions to engage the child's "inner drive" to learn and develop. In this way, OT facilitates enhanced neuronal growth and development (brain plasticity) that leads to increased skill, self-confidence, and independence in daily life activities (Ayres, 1974). A great deal has been written about sensory integrative function and intervention, and the reader is referred to Ayres' *The Development of Sensory Integrative Theory and Practice* (1974) and *Sensory Integration and the Child* (1979) for a more in-depth discussion of Ayres original theory and research (Figure 9-1).

Theoretical Updates

Volumes of evidence for various aspects of SI have been reviewed and summarized (Miller, 2003; Mulligan, 2002, 2003). The results remain inconclusive because most studies had deficiencies in methodology. Stronger evidence exists for SI applications for specific disabilities such as autism, Asperger's syndrome, or attention deficit disorders (Miller, Coll, & Schoen, 2007; Roberts, King, Thomas, & Boccia, 2007; Schilling & Schwartz, 2004; Smith, Press, Koenig, & Kinnealey, 2005), for which SI interventions produced enhanced occupational performance and raised scores on cognitive, behavioral, and psychological measures.

Recently, Ayres' family members, the Baker/Ayres Trust, have trademarked the name "Ayres Sensory Integration." They did so in response to concerns by many OT professionals that a large number of research studies and publications today do not include the basic OT principles of adaptive responses and engagement in occupation that Ayres intended. Non-OTs have used the term sensory integration referring to passive sensory input or have promoted the interventions indiscriminately as a form of early learning. While some other professions have questioned the research evidence for SI interventions, others have published research based on techniques that widely deviate from Ayres original concepts (Glennon & Smith Roley, 2006). The move to trademark Ayres SI is intended to preserve the original body of work and promote research and practice that correctly represents it. Another safeguard for Ayres SI is the establishment of a global network Web site (www.siglobalnetwork.org), which was created by OTs worldwide to preserve the original Ayres SI theory and research (Stzelecki, 2008). Miller's sensory processing disorders (SPD) Web site also makes Ayres theory more accessible to both parents and OTs and reviews the latest research linking sensory integration disorders with autism, Asperger syndrome, and other learning disabilities (www.spdfoundation.net) (Miller, in Strzelecki, 2008). Parham and colleagues (Parham et al., 2007) added another safeguard, a fidelity tool to ensure correct adherence to Ayres principles in the theory and practice of SI. The fidelity measure requires systematic ongoing documentation of the delivery of intervention, including not only observed behaviors but also process elements, such as the quality of the therapeutic relationship, interactions with peers, and other critical treatment events (Strzelecki, 2008).

One of the major advantages of the sensory integration frame of reference is its highly standardized assessment tools. Ayres Sensory Integration and Praxis Tests (SIPT) were standardized on thousands of children nationwide, and these tools along with others, such as the Postrotary Nystagmus Test (PNT), and, more recently, the Sensory Processing Measure (SPM) provide reliable, quantifiable descriptions of a child's sensory processing issues. Such measures, which OTs are trained to administer, clearly demonstrate the need for OT SI interventions and also facilitate a team approach in school-based OT practice (Ayers, 1972; Henry, Ecker, Glennon, & Herzberg, 2009).

A systems view of brain function has largely replaced the hierarchical view. According to systems theory, the brain works as an integrated, holistic system. As early as 1991, Fisher and Murray proposed the updated view that SI dysfunction results from a number of inter-related systems that are not functioning optimally. Recent practice tends to combine SI techniques with other approaches that incorporate research evidence from multiple sources.

The spiral of development, a newly developed addition, combines Ayres' original theory with studies of normal development, systems theory, and humanistic psychology. As children spiral upward toward maturity, their development includes the adaptive use of sensory information in the context of sensorimotor activities to further develop the sensory integrative capacity of the brain. Children's natural tendencies to explore and master their environment move them ever closer to self-actualization (Bundy, Lane, & Murray, 2002).

Dunn's Sensory Processing Model

Some researchers note that, in OT literature, the terms sensory integration and sensory processing are used interchangeably. However, in respect for Ayres SI, other models that address sensation are more appropriately called sensory processing, modulation, or otherwise (Davies & Gavin, 2009). One such model is Dunn's (2009) sensory processing, which looks at a wider range of sensory systems in her model than Ayres, including the following three categories of sensation:

1. Chemical senses including olfactory (smell) and gustatory (taste) sensations.
2. Body senses include somatosensory (tactile), proprioceptive (body position), vestibular (balance and movement).
3. Environmental senses include auditory (hearing) and visual systems.

Although each of these sensory systems has discrete properties, they all have common processing features and mechanisms. The first is centrifugal control, defined as the ability of the brain to regulate its own input. It does so in three ways: 1) suppression—tuning out some stimuli so that others become easier to attend to, 2) divergence—sending a single sensation to multiple parts of the brain, and 3) convergence—bringing together input from multiple sensory systems.

Another assumption of this model is the balance of excitation and inhibition. Through feed forward and feedback mechanisms, the brain is constantly balancing the effects of sensory stimuli, so that only when something tips the balance toward excitation does an action response occur. Sensory feedback allows the brain to fine-tune response patterns, making it possible for movements and other responses to become more skilled or accurate with practice.

Once sensory input is received, the brain processes it by organizing various inputs, comparing them with past sensory experiences and assigning meaning or interpretation. People use sensory processing to guide and regulate daily behavior as well as alerting them of potential threats from the environment.

Dunn's model consists of four sensory processing patterns that occur normally in all people. These are derived from the continua of nervous system thresholds and self-regulation strategies. Some individuals have a lower threshold; that is, they need less sensory input in order to activate their neurons, while others have a higher threshold, more resistant to response activation. Self-regulation of sensory input can also differ: some people tend to actively seek or avoid sensory experiences, while others remain more passive. These tendencies result in the following four patterns:

1. *Sensation seeking:* High thresholds and active self-regulation.
2. *Sensation avoiding:* Low thresholds and active self-regulation.
3. *Sensory sensitivity:* Low thresholds and passive self-regulation.
4. *Low registration:* High thresholds and passive self-regulation.

To determine a person's typical sensory-processing patterns, Dunn designed an evaluation tool, the Sensory Profile. This is a standardized observation and self-report instrument with separate versions for children and adults (Brown & Dunn, 2002; Dunn, 1999). Most of the evidence for this approach comes from the neurosciences; however, evidence for the specific patterns identified in Dunn's model are also substantial (Dunn, 2009). Research supports the use of specific SI strategies for children with sensory-processing dysfunctions, such as the use of weighted vests or blankets (Smith et al., 2005) or the use of chair ball seating (Schilling et al., 2003).

Sensory Processing Disorders in Adulthood

Most of the literature about SI addresses children. However, many adults demonstrate the same sensory-processing disorders. When children with undiagnosed and untreated conditions such as autism and attention deficit disorders grow up, they have learned to cope with sensory defensiveness or sensitivity, so that they don't seek treatment until either they are overwhelmed or they encounter children who are receiving OT SI interventions. Kinnealey notes that adults with sensory modulation or processing disorders often have issues related to anxiety, depression, and social-emotional functioning (Kinnealey & Oliver, 2002). Wilbarger first described sensory defensiveness (now called sensory modulation disorder) as "a constellation of symptoms related to aversive or defensive reactions to non-noxious stimuli across one or more sensory systems" (Wilbarger & Wilbarger, 1991, in DiMatties & Sammons, 2009, p. 16). Defensive reactions affect one's state of alertness, emotional tone, stress level, and ability to attend. Tactile defensiveness, for example, makes a woman unable to advance in her career because she is unable to tolerate wearing classic business clothing. Wilbarger developed the use of "sensory diets," using sensory input in controlled increments aimed at desensitizing clients to the offending sensation. The Wilbarger protocol, which uses brushing, deep pressure, and selected joint compression strategies, requires special training (DiMatties & Sammons, 2009).

May-Benson (2009) summarizes adult sensory modulation (defensive) dysfunctions as the following:

- *Tactile*—Sensitivity to clothing textures, aggressive responses to light touch interferes with friendship and intimacy, tend to avoid crowds, parties, or other social gatherings.
- *Auditory*—Sensitive to/irritated by certain sounds, interfering with work or social participation outside home.
- *Vestibular*—Frequent motion sickness, balance issues, especially when walking on uneven surfaces, avoid elevators, fear/avoid flying.
- *Motor/dyspraxia*—Feel clumsy or awkward when moving, problems with driving, parking, operating machinery, often fail at work because of inability to organize or complete projects or multitask.

Because few standardized tests exist for adult sensory processing, clients are usually evaluated by interview, clinical observations, or adaptation of one of the tests intended for children, such as Ayres Sensory Integration and Praxis Tests, Postrotary Nystagmus Test (for vestibular deficits), the Sensory Processing Measure (Glennon et al., 2007), or Dunn's sensory profile for Adults (Brown & Dunn, 2002). The overarching goals of OT using the SI frame of reference apply equally well to both children and adults. A typical program for adult sensory modulation involves several stages (adapted from May-Benson, 2009):

1. *Preparation:* Education about the mechanisms of dysfunction and sharing evidence about sensory input as remediation, leading to development of insight through OT therapeutic use of self. OT demonstrates using SI activities to establish and maintain an appropriate level of arousal. Some typical techniques used for this are use of deep pressure (such as weighted blankets) or myofascial or craniosacral therapy techniques.

2. *Sensory activity aimed at the unregulated sensation:* For example, strong vestibular input (such as spinning followed by visuomotor exercises) or use of the Wilbarger protocol for tactile input.

3. *Integrating activity:* Using multisensory systems, such as the infinity walk (walking in figure 8s while performing visual tracking) to elicit adaptive responses, log rolling (rolling across varied surfaces), or using a swinging balance board. OT provides increasing challenge as activities are mastered.

4. *Organizing wrap-up activity:* Such as heavy work activities aimed at self-regulation to decrease defensive responses. Clients identify occupations within their daily routine that can meet sensory needs and collaboratively design strategies to cope with and/or prevent sensory overload during occupational engagement.

Home programs often include heavy exertion activities (such as running or workouts) early in the day to prepare for work and social occupations and to avoid overload. Adults need to learn self-advocacy in daily situations in order to prevent adversely affecting social participation and relationships. Self-regulation for adults is parallel to the well-known "How does your engine run" program (Williams & Shellenberger, 1994), which teaches children simple changes to their daily routine (breaks of brisk walking before doing homework) to help them keep their brain working "just right" (DeMatties & Sammons, 2009, p. 17). Sensory modulation issues often affect mental health, a fact that supports the use of sensory modulation training as a prevention strategy (Strzelecki, 2008, citing Kinnealey & Oliver, 2002). In this regard, OTs might design group interventions for people with sensory modulation issues secondary to trauma, post-traumatic stress disorder (PTSD), depression, or anxiety disorders, using education and self-regulation activities based on sensory integration or sensory processing theory. For example, of veterans returning from overseas, a recent study reported that 19% show signs of PTSD, and an additional 7% have a traumatic brain injury or depression in addition to PTSD (Hofmann, 2008). This is a population that could be assessed and treated using a sensory processing frame of reference to enable their transition to stateside or civilian employment. Most of the evidence in support of these strategies is anecdotal, and additional research is needed to demonstrate OT's use of SI and sensory processing frames of reference with adults.

Group Approaches

King's Sensory Groups in Mental Health

While most of the research of Ayres and her associates applies to children, several OTs have written about the treatment of mentally ill adults using neurodevelopmental and sensory integrative techniques. The best known of these is Lorna Jean King, who pioneered the use of SI approaches with chronic schizophrenic adults.

Lorna Jean King has noted the lack of SI in both schizophrenic and autistic clients by observing the kinds of sensory stimulation they seek from the environment. For example, she evaluates a retarded and autistic adolescent by observing his or her preference for vibratory input (plays with a hand-held vibrator), proprioceptive input (constant self-hugging), and calming vestibular input (distractible and disruptive behavior is reduced by slow swinging and rocking) (Larrington, 1987).

Paul Schilder noted as early as the 1930s that schizophrenic clients are markedly under reactive to vestibular stimulation as measured by post-rotary nystagmus (rapid eye movements) (King, 1974). King linked the vestibular system abnormalities with the postural and movement limitations (pacing, adduction, and internal rotation) observed in the chronic process schizophrenic client, more currently called the negative symptom schizophrenic (Figure 9-2).

Process schizophrenia is a subtype of schizophrenia, a mental disorder that develops insidiously from childhood and is not the result of a severe or recognizable stress. Process schizophrenics do not respond readily to medical or behavioral intervention and so tend to be chronically institutionalized.

King refers to numerous studies of the neurological deficits in schizophrenia (and also autism) that link faulty vestibular and proprioceptive processing to schizophrenic symptoms. Some of these symptoms include perceptual deficits, feelings of fatigue and slow movement, postural insecurity (fear of falling), concrete thinking, and lack of emotional response. King's hypothesis is that some schizophrenic clients have "defective proprioceptive feedback mechanisms, the vestibular component in particular being under reactive in its role in the sensorimotor integration" (King, 1974, p. 534).

Considering today's emphasis on the biochemical etiology of all mental illness (including schizophrenia), King's theory of the central role of movement in

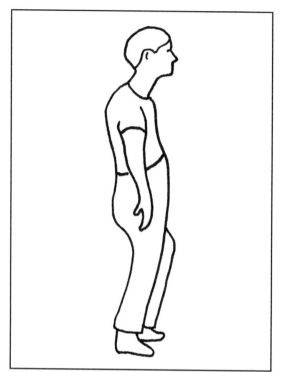

Figure 9-2. Postural abnormalities due to faulty proprioceptive feedback in the person with process schizophrenia (flexion, adduction, internal rotation).

altering biochemical states, as well as biochemistry affecting movement, remains timely. Movement and sensation are known to produce chemical changes just as taking medication produces changes in brain chemistry. Furthermore, King (1974) states "...this model...applies not only to etiology but also to treatment. Although we cannot be sure which chemicals to alter, or in what direction, we can intervene in the motor behavior of the individual with the knowledge that there will be effects upon the thought processes and upon biochemistry" (p. 534).

In later publications, King notes the role of activities in coping with stress. A strenuous action, or "fight or flight" response to stress (Gal & Lazarus, 1975), was found to be responsible for the rapid metabolism of stress hormones, thus preventing secondary damage to the system. This suggests that strenuous or heavy work activity can serve to normalize the neurotransmitter balance that has been deranged by stress (King, 1978, 1988).

The intervention techniques King used with groups of chronic schizophrenic clients are adaptations of the techniques Ayres used with children. They are gross motor activities aimed at normalizing patterns of excessive flexion, adduction, and internal rotation and increasing range of motion. Vestibular and tactile stimulation are provided through the use of the standard props—hammocks, scooter boards, balls, and blankets. Heavy work patterns suggested by Rood in King (1974) resisted use of tonic muscle groups, and co-contraction patterns are also incorporated. King has also added parachutes, balloons, and beanbag chairs.

Table 9-5

Adapting Ross' Five-Stage Groups: Alerting Versus Calming Sensory Stimuli

	Alerting	**Calming**
Environment	Bright light, bright colors, high contrasts, loud sounds, rapid rhythms, uneven sounds	Low light, pastel colors, similar hues, soft melodic sounds, slow even rhythms, closing one's eyes
Smell/taste	Pungent odors; cold/hot foods/liquids; crunchy, strong flavors	Sweet or herbal smells, smooth textures, mild flavor, temperate foods
Touch/movement	Light touch, sudden touch, rapid movement, rotation or changing direction, jumping/hitting/clapping	Steady moderate pressure, slow rhythmic movement, vibration, slowly rotating movement, holding on, hugging

King suggests two criteria for the selection of activities: (1) attention must not be centered upon the motor process but rather on the object or outcome and (2) the activity must be pleasurable and evoke smiles, laughter, and feelings of fun. Clients should not have to think about what they are doing or how they move; the goal is to elicit spontaneous movement and affect. Vestibular and proprioceptive processing occurs at the brainstem level and produces automatic responses, not cortical (voluntary) responses. Therefore, if a ball is thrown to a client and his or her hands extend spontaneously to catch it, we can assume that this automatic action reflects adaptive vestibular processing at the brainstem level. The goal of group activities using this frame of reference is to stimulate the sensory-processing systems so that they will function more adaptively. As OTs, we see spontaneous and purposeful motor responses as evidence that we are reaching that goal.

Ross' Five-Stage Groups

Mildred Ross further developed the use of sensory integrative theory and techniques with chronic populations, including older adults with dementia, neurological impairment, or persistent mental illness. Ross provides mostly anecdotal evidence for the usefulness of these groups for facilitating occupational engagement in long-term care facilities. Improvement in adaptive responses was demonstrated with older adults in nursing homes (Corcoran & Barrett, 1987). Ross later applied SI principles in groups of younger clients with mental retardation and adapted the approach for clients of any age with disabilities that prevent adequate functioning in the community (Ross, 1997; Ross & Bachner, 2004). Ross developed her group techniques over more than 20 years of clinical experience. Her group sessions occur in five stages, which move developmentally from alerting activities involving tactile, kinesthetic, and proprioceptive input to graded opportunities for organized cognitive thought and behavior (Table 9-5). The following is a summary of Ross' five-stage groups.

Stage I

Stage I acknowledges the presence of each member to each other member of the group. Introductions or saying names can easily accomplish this. The purpose of the session is established by the therapist or group members in Stage I, and this orients members to the session. Explanations should be kept brief and on a level the members can understand. The attention of members should be captured in Stage I.

Stage II

Stage II provides maximum exertion in movement. A variety of gross motor movement is suggested here, incorporating all three planes—horizontal, vertical, and sagittal. Exercise, dance patterns, or games may be adapted for this stage. Pleasure, communication, and interaction or "cohesiveness" are possible goals. The effect of this stage is to stimulate, mobilize, and energize.

Stage III

Stage III emphasizes perceptual-motor skills. Activities may be chosen that require less vigorous movement and more judgment and focus action to accomplish a purposeful task. Making a fruit salad or drawing a picture are examples. The activities should be short-term and able to be finished in 30 minutes or less. This stage should have the effect of calming and focusing.

Stage IV

Stage IV is the time for cognitive stimulation. A discussion of the previous stages, memory games, or poetry reading is suggested by Ross. "This is the opportunity for cortical controls to be demonstrated through organized behavior such as impulse control or creative expression. It is the highest point for display of attentiveness and group cohesiveness" (Ross, 1997, p. 9). The length of this stage may be changed depending on the activity chosen and the level and interest of the group. Music or current events discussion may take a major portion of the time, while a short inspiring poem may take less than 5 minutes. Preparation for closure should be kept in mind in selecting activities for this stage.

Stage V

Stage V provides resolution and termination. A way to say goodbye, when to meet next, or suggestions of what to do next time might serve as endings. When the therapist feels that the group was good, it may be appropriate to verbalize this in summarizing. Statements of satisfaction with the group by the therapist and clients can achieve a sense of peacefulness at its end, as illustrated in Figure 9-3.

Role of the Therapist

Using Ross' stages, the therapist plans and leads the activity, guided by knowledge of the principles of sensorimotor integration and activity analysis but taking his or her cues from the group as well. The OT must be quite skilled to lead this kind of group effectively, keeping control while gently encouraging members to get involved. The stages provide a clear structure around which to plan appropriate activities. Ross, in *Integrative Group Therapy: Mobilizing Coping Abilities With the Five-Stage Group*, offers excellent guidelines for considering when an activity should be introduced and how it should be presented (1997). Application for adults with developmental disabilities is extensively outlined in Ross and Bachner (2004).

Sensory and Trauma Informed Interventions, A Population Approach

LeBel and Champagne (2010), researchers in Massachusetts, designed a sensory processing model to reduce the use of restraints in all publically funded programs and facilities, including mental health treatment settings, correctional facilities, veterans' treatment centers, and public schools. The authors note that exposure to trauma is a significant factor among populations of people with mental illness (90%), returning veterans with post-traumatic stress symptoms, inner city children and youth, and prisoners in correctional facilities. Many studies attest to trauma's profound effect on a person's response to everyday sensory experiences and their implications for emotional and physical safety (LeBel, Champagne, Stromberg, & Ryan, 2010). Trauma-informed sensory approaches use occupations to foster feelings of safety and support while offering opportunities for recognizing and regulating sensory experiences (Champagne & Stromberg, 2004; Fisher, 2006). There is an emerging evidence base in OT for identifying sensory disorders and designing sensory modulation/integration interventions (Moore & Henry, 2002; Smith, Press, Koenig, &

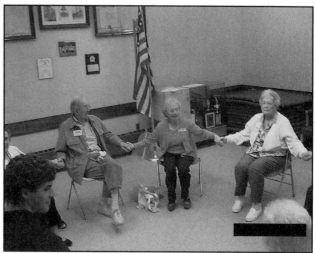

Figure 9-3. Mildred Ross (center) provides a warm and calming closure to her five-stage group. Baldwin Senior Center, Stratford, CT, reprinted with permission.

Kinnealey, 2005). For example, a youth crisis plan was developed that helps teens identify what upsets them, how it feels in their body, and what sensory-based activities help calm them down (Massachusetts Department of Mental Health, 2010). This recent Massachusetts initiative, while beginning as a restraint reduction effort, has evolved into a statewide and nationwide training effort, in which OTs are involved as educators and trainers in the use of sensory interventions for calming, self-soothing, and de-escalation. These interventions, based on the principles of sensory processing and sensory integration described earlier, form the basis of client group programming. Consulting OTs also design staff education groups, help publicly funded facilities to develop appropriate sensory evaluations, and provide training in the use of sensory interventions for calming, reducing anxiety, and addressing different types of sensory sensitivity.

This advocacy initiative on the part of Massachusetts-based OTs has provided a unique opportunity for OTs in other states to become involved in this large-scale public health initiative. However, because using SI with adults is an emerging practice area, OTs need to proceed with caution and to make sure the programs they design remain true to occupation-based theories and Ayres SI principles, methods, and outcomes.

FUNCTION AND DYSFUNCTION

In the sensorimotor frames of reference, functioning may be viewed as adequate when a person is able to learn and use all of the adaptive skills characteristic of his or her age. Because there is assumed to be a sequence of neurological and physiological development, dysfunction can be defined as a lag in development causing the client to function below his or her age level. An adult is dysfunctional when neurological or physiological malfunctioning interferes with normal daily activity and participation in life. This view of dysfunction in any illness encourages the identification of a physical cause. Even mental illness, as King has discussed, can respond to a neurodevelopmental intervention approach that follows the guidelines of early development. In using movement and games, the client's active participation is encouraged to produce an adaptive response in activities that are both functional and meaningful.

CHANGE AND MOTIVATION

Change in neurophysiological functioning is thought to be brought about through several methods. Physical activity can produce change through its effect on muscle tone, muscle strength, and range of motion. Physical activity has also been shown to produce chemical changes; this is how the "runner's high" has been explained. During OT activities, changes in brain and body function can be brought about through sensory stimulation and repetition of movement. Using the traditional theories, change occurs in a specific sequence and progresses stage by stage up the hierarchy toward maturity. In an illness that has left clients without normal movement patterns and sensory processing skills, a baseline level must be established through careful sensorimotor assessment. Then, through a repetition of the developmental sequence, sensory and motor components of activity can be used by the OT in such a way as to facilitate sub-cortical learning. Automatic movement and postural responses will precede more advanced cognitive responses. The changes we look for in the sensorimotor frames can often be seen as spontaneous self-corrections, such as an increased state of alertness or a more functional body posture. These normalized neurological states can then serve as building blocks for working on more skilled purposeful movements and the use of language in interactions within groups.

As Ross points out, activities we offer clients can have powerful effects on the CNS. These effects can be both positive and negative. Activities should be carefully planned to approach the CNS in a way that it can accept and handle and to do so in a way that facilitates positive change. The OT does this through control and limitation of sensory input (Ross, 1997).

Change from the motor learning perspective comes about through repetition of a sequence of actions in performing functional tasks. This repetition in varied contexts and environments encourages the formation of new or alternate neural pathways that circumvent damaged areas. When linked with self-directed goals, repetition of adaptive strategies, and environmental adaptation, practice, and feedback pave the way for habituation of adapted motor and process skills (Bass-Haugen et al., 2002).

Motivation comes in the form of accepting the challenge to be a more active participant in life. Clients, after illness or injury, may be motivated to go back to work and to do things the way they used to. The lack of motivation comes when they expect too much change too fast, and, therefore, they feel they have failed. With long-term physical dysfunction, clients may be unable to modify their goals or accept new methods for meeting their needs. Chronic illness may leave clients without hope. When cognitive impairment accompanies the physical or emotional dysfunction, long-term goals may no longer be understood. The spontaneous urge to advance one's development must often be rekindled after illness. Interventions such as sensory stimulation and movement play can encourage the client with chronic illness to pursue more active participation with others and the environment. Once success or pleasure is experienced, clients may be more motivated.

GROUP INTERVENTION

King and Ross have given some helpful guidelines on how to structure groups. Gross motor activities are the common element. While movement activities are used extensively with pediatrics and physical dysfunction populations, movement is too often overlooked as an effective media for psychosocial dysfunction and geriatrics. As OTs, we need to expand our repertoire of tools to include more activities involving movement. Much of our training in physiology, neuroanatomy, and sensorimotor integration prepares us well for doing so. Perhaps our level of comfort in using movement with our clients is not as high as it could be. Often, OTs need to be comfortable with their own ability to move and play before they are able to share this with clients.

Role of the Occupational Therapist

In the sensorimotor frames, the OT is a directive leader. The therapist needs a fairly thorough knowledge of neurodevelopment, neurophysiology, and SI in order to lead these groups competently. In most cases, clients with whom we are working are at low levels of functioning. Often, verbal communication is at a minimum, and it is through imitation and role modeling that our clients perform activities therapeutically. The OT plans movement, sensory, or cognitive activities that match their level and are relatively sure to succeed. The concept of the "just-right challenge" applies here. Activities should interest and challenge the clients but should not be so complex as to overwhelm them. In movement groups as described by King, Ross, and Levy, the OT is the undeniable leader. He or she comes prepared with equipment and ideas and guides the group from start to finish, taking cues from clients as needed along the way.

Neurodevelopmentally based movement groups can be effective with some higher cognitive level populations as well. When this is done, care should be taken to explain the purpose thoroughly so that clients understand how the exercises and movements will help them.

Goals

Some of the goals mentioned by the various theorists may be summarized as follows:

- Provide sensory stimulation and opportunities for adaptive response. The client will develop skill in sensorimotor performance and strengthen normal sensorimotor integration.

- Improve and maintain muscle tone, posture, and motor planning. The client will demonstrate these successfully during participation in activities.

- Motivate the client to participate. The client will respond to stimulation by imitating or initiating activity.

- Facilitate the development of higher-level cognitive skills through the integration and assimilation of lower-level skills. The client will demonstrate higher-level skills through participation in activity.

- Provide multiple opportunities for practice of functional and meaningful tasks. Group members can support one another, provide valuable feedback, and benefit from group problem-solving.

- Achieve a sense of mastery and well-being. The client will demonstrate positive affective responses during participation in activity.

Specific goals for individual clients may be easily set and measured. All of the goals may be worked on appropriately through the use of group activities.

Examples of Activities

Movement activities of all types may be adapted in this frame of reference, from simple calisthenics to dance and sports, to laying bricks and digging in the garden. When working with adult populations, the therapist must be careful not to make the activities seem too childish. The qualities of group activities are carefully chosen and graded according to the type and amount of sensory input they provide, as well as their implications for adaptive responses from members.

New Games

One particularly rich source of activities that are adaptable is the handbook of the New Games Foundation (Fluegelman, 1976). The New Games Foundation is an organization that originated at San Francisco State College in 1966 as a resistance to the Vietnam War. The group was against any type of competition, even in sports, so they designed games that provided opportunities for individuals to express aggressiveness without anyone winning or losing. The games were designed for all ages and levels of activity, and since 1974, every few years, they publish another book of newly invented games; see Activity Examples 9-1 and 9-2.

The New Games followers suggest what OTs already know: that all the games can be adapted by changing the rules or that new games can be invented to meet the special needs and goals of our clients.

Parachute Games

King suggests parachute play as effective for spontaneous range of motion and postural correction as well as vestibular-proprioceptive stimulation (Figure 9-4). A real parachute (with no strings) works best and can be obtained in surplus stores or sports equipment supply catalogs.

Parachute games (Activity Example 9-3) are rich in sensorimotor integration potential. The basic movement involved requires reaching high above the head, an extension of the shoulders, elbows, and wrists to the full range of motion. The head tends to roll back as the client looks at the effect of his or her movement, the parachute rising high in the air. Lowering the parachute to below the knee requires the client to flex the spine forward at the waist and to extend the head forward, again following the movement of the parachute. The motion of the head and joints provides both proprioceptive and vestibular stimulation. Other movements may also be analyzed in this manner to aid in intervention planning to meet specific goals.

Bioenergetics Groups

These are groups aimed at the expression of feelings through movement. The major spokesman for this approach to movement is Alexander Lowen. Lowen's bioenergetics exercises were developed from his bioenergetics theory of personality, which is understood in terms of the body and its energetic processes (Lowen & Lowen, 1977). More recently, Lowen's workshops have been offered as an extension of the myofascial release therapy workshops given by John Barnes, a physical therapist. Bioenergetics exercises can offer OTs guidelines in the use of breathing and movement exercises to heighten emotional awareness and expression. Some of the bioenergetics exercises can release very powerful feelings and should not be done without training. However, the basic concept is useful in planning expressive exercises in moderation. For further information about this approach, the reader is referred to Lowen and Lowen's book, *The Way to Vibrant Health* (1977).

The activity groups discussed in Activity Examples 9-4 and 9-5 are based on this concept and have been used with adult clients with mental illness who are inhibited in the expression of feelings. In doing these activities, the OT should be careful not to overstimulate potentially volatile clients. The exercises

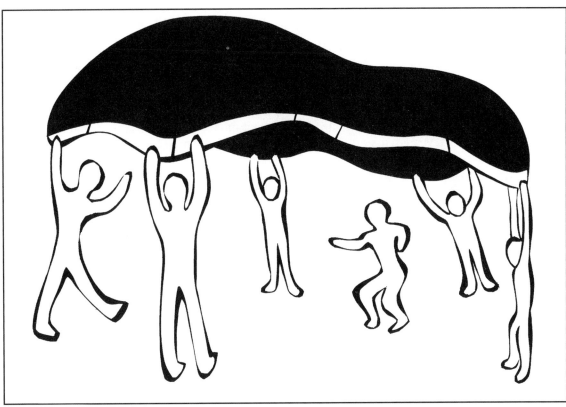

Figure 9-4. Parachute play.

should not be done with clients who are excitable or are at risk for violent behavior. These neurophysiological techniques are especially well-suited to intervention with depression.

Exercise Groups

Exercise to music or dance activities has good potential as a therapeutic tool. Circle or group dancing is usually best suited to our purpose in OT. In physical disability areas where goals involve maintaining and increasing strength and range of motion, group activities that accomplish these goals are more enjoyable and motivating than individual exercise programs. A good example of this type of group is the "Range of Motion Dance," an exercise program for clients with rheumatoid arthritis developed by Diane Harlowe and Patricia Yu at St. Mary's Hospital Medical Center in Madison, Wisconsin (Van Deusen & Harlowe, 1987). This is a guided fantasy done with groups of clients with arthritis seated in chairs. The exercises, while following the story, go systematically through the range of motion for nearly every joint in the body. Once the sequence of motions is learned, it can be repeated by the clients at home by listening to the story on an audiotape. Greenfield and Godinez have introduced a similar group for clients with stroke, called "Self Range of Motion Exercises" (Greenfield & Godinez, 1989). They have defined eight skill levels for these exercises, ranging from complete

dependence on the therapist leader to independence in performing the exercises.

In doing such groups, it is important to use the potential of the group to provide mutual support, encouragement, and feedback. Do not let the activity speak for itself; combine it with verbal reinforcement, progress checks, and education about how and why it is helping. It is generally the social and emotional aspects of a group that keep members coming back.

Sensorimotor Activity Groups Addressing Anxiety, Hostility, and Despair

Sensory and trauma-informed interventions have been used in mental health facilities, correctional facilities, and public schools, as alternatives to the use of seclusion and restraint (LeBel & Champagne, 2010). Some of the sensory techniques suggested for these uses are hugging or punching pillows, applications of heat or cold (showers, hot tubs, swimming pools), wrapping in blankets, moving to music, and walking, running, or other high-energy activities. For example, Bazyk and Bazyk (2009) used sensorimotor group activities to help low-income urban youth to express feelings appropriately and learn strategies for dealing with anger. For older adults in nursing homes, following Dunn's sensory processing model, Lape (2009) used multisensory environments to decrease negative behaviors such as agitation, wandering, fight and flight responses, social withdrawal, and lethargy in nursing home residents with dementia. She began with a group of three residents, facilitating their interaction with the sensory environment with each one individually in 30- to 45-minute sessions three times per week for 6 weeks. All three residents, while responding differently to the various stimuli, reduced or eliminated their negative behaviors for several hours after the sessions and demonstrated an ability to more fully engage in occupation-based activities, such as group dining or participation in "bingo" (Lape, 2009, p. 12). This program used sensory media derived from the "snoezelen" approach, such as a bubble tube with triple mirrors, beanbag chairs, a leaf swing, fiber-optic light, music systems, and an illuminated parachute ceiling cover (Burns, Cox, & Plant, 2000). During sessions, additional sensory input for smell, taste, and touch were also introduced. Before implementing such a group, it is recommended that each participant be evaluated for their sensory preferences, sensitivities, and typical sensory processing patterns, so that appropriate calming or alerting stimuli can be facilitated. Adult versions of Dunn's Sensory Profile might be adapted for use with older adults (Brown & Dunn, 2002).

Ross' Five-Stage Groups

Mildred Ross gives us a sequence of specific guidelines for the selection of activities. Because the five-stage group is designed for severely impaired and chronic populations, movement and sensory stimulation are key elements of activity. "A routine of organized sequences enhances the likelihood of an automatic habitual response" (Ross, 1997, p. 2). The purpose of the five separate organized sequences is to motivate interaction with the environment. Sensory stimulation produces the heightened arousal and alertness to one's surroundings that maximizes the potential for adaptive responses. The outcome must be calm alertness that makes adults ready to move on in an organized way to the next activity of the day.

Table 9-6 may be useful in creating and modifying activities to help accommodate and manage the behaviors that emerge during the five-stage group.

Activity Examples 9-6 and 9-7 suggest specific organized sequences. In Ross' book Integrative Group Therapy, many other activity sequences are suggested. Because different populations have differences in their abilities to integrate sensory information, the examples given cover medium (Activity Example 9-6) and low (Activity Example 9-7) levels of processing skill.

Movement Therapy Groups for Children With Disabilities

Sophie Levitt (1982) suggests therapeutic group work using a neurodevelopmental approach for children with cerebral palsy and motor delay. Both play groups and structured groups are seen as more effective than individual intervention for several reasons. The group often curtails rebellion and encourages cooperation. Children imitate other children and often instruct each other in doing what is required. Children seem to be able to concentrate more than twice as long with the stimulation of the group setting (1 to 1.5 hours as opposed to 20 minutes individually, Levitt reports). Levitt emphasizes the interdisciplinary nature of these groups. Occupational and physical therapists, nurses, speech therapists, and teachers all contribute to planning and implementing the activity.

In groups for children with disabilities, it is not useful to group by diagnosis. Children should be selected for the groups according to their functional problems. The basis of selection may be motor problems such as poor grasp and release, poor balance, or recurring abnormal movement patterns or postures. The developmental or cognitive level of group members should be similar. Some children who are too severely involved to be aware of the group may not be appropriate. The selected group should be capable of working together and establishing a degree of group spirit. The specific activities should be selected according to the deficits of the members (Levitt, 1982).

It is evident that adults as well as children should be treated in groups of similar developmental level and that the same principles for selection and planning apply. It would be encouraging to see more groups of physically disabled adults treated in a manner that encourages interaction and takes advantage of general group dynamics principles. Some more current resources for groups with children are Mannix's *Self-Esteem Activities for Secondary Students With Special Needs* (1996) and *Social Skills Activities for Special Children* (1993).

Task-Oriented Groups for Physical Disabilities

Client-centered interviews will determine which goals and tasks have priority for clients with acquired brain damage. Clients who have reached a level of voluntary control may benefit from groups that address similar goals. Activity Example 9-8 uses the materials for a cooking task as the basis for practice of reach and grasp. It uses the principle of variation of strategies by presenting objects of different shapes, sizes, and weights, which are placed at different shelf levels, to achieve optimal learning.

Table 9-6

Rood's Sensory Guidelines for Movement Facilitation and Inhibition

Facilitation or Alerting	Movement Response	Inhibition or Relaxation	Activity Examples
Light touch, brushing, stroking	Fast brushing produces strongest contraction	Neutral warmth	Warm bubble bath, hot tub, light fleece blanket covers
Icing—2 types: • A-icing—3 quick swipes of ice pack across muscle • C-icing—hold ice pack for 3 to 5 seconds	A-icing applied to palms or soles of feet produces reflex withdrawal C-icing produces postural tonic responses	Slow, rhythmic stroking	Light massage, feeling warm breezes, sifting sand, petting an animal, handling soft textures or materials
Quick stretch (proprioception)	Facilitates muscle contraction and inhibits antagonistic muscles	Sustained pressure	Wrapping in blanket, bandage wrapping, weighted clothing, hugs
Vibration to tendon (proprioception)	Releases tension, allows slow stretch	Prolonged stretch	Yoga, pulling or lifting heavy objects
Stretching hand muscles or forceful grasping	Co-contraction/stabilization of shoulder joint	Joint approximation (pushing together)	Pushing or supporting heavy objects
Movement of head position (vestibular)	Spinning, bending over, rapid forward movement	Tendon pressure	Heavy massage
Heavy joint compression (strong proprioceptive input)	Co-contraction around joints, righting response	Slow, rhythmic rocking or slow rolling	Rocking chair, slow dancing, swaying to music, walking, swinging in a hammock
Pungent smells and tastes	Arousal, alerting response	Pleasant smells and tastes	Relaxation response
Visual—Bright light, high-contrast, non-patterned movement	Avoidancem or stimulation-seeking/alerting behavior	Dim light, mid-range colors, low-contrast, slow-patterned movement	Promotes feeling of safety and well-being, or apathy
Sharp or loud nonrhythmic sounds	Alerting response	Soft, mellow, rhythmic sounds	Relaxation response

Music in Movement Groups

The use of music in therapy groups has been mentioned briefly. Music has qualities that can both relax and invigorate; it can energize a group, distract it, or put it to sleep. The choice of music should be made with care; instrumental rather than vocal may be less distracting. The clients' level of stimulation should be closely monitored, as Ross suggests. Music can change the mood of the group, but the key is to do it gradually; the music should match the mood of the clients to begin with, and then change little by little, accompanied by appropriate movement activities. It can arouse emotion easily because it has an effect on the body and the mind. Selection of music may depend to a great extent on what you want to accomplish with the client. With clients with depression, the therapist may want to energize them by playing music with a lively beat. Clients susceptible to anxiety might benefit more from slow, mellow rhythms and ballads that soothe the nerves. In any case, OTs usually use music in combination with movement activities, and it is the activity that should remain the focus with the music providing an appropriate background.

GROUP LEADERSHIP

Introduction

In neurodevelopmental groups, the explanation of purpose should match the clients' ability to understand it. The level of cognition is the most important factor, and this varies widely in groups using the neurodevelopmental approach.

The warm-up is essential and takes on a somewhat different emphasis here. The warm-up should prepare the members for the activity not only psychologically, but physiologically as well. As Ross has stressed, there is a systematic way to approach the CNS (1997). If members are unable to screen out nonessential sensory stimulation, they may be overloaded very quickly. With client populations that are at risk for this, such as those with stroke, head trauma, autism, developmental delay, or chronic mental illness, the warm-up can offer limited and gradually increasing stimuli to test the group for an acceptable level of sensory stimulation.

Likewise, with the physically ill, the warm-up may be used as a testing experience to determine what level of physical exercise can be tolerated. Naturally, the OT has evaluated the client members prior to the group planning, so he or she should already be aware of the limits of safety. However, clients' conditions will vary on a daily (or hourly) basis, and changes need to be taken into account. Based on the warm-up, the time frame or the activity itself may have to be modified.

Activity

The activities used will vary widely depending on the client population. Sensorimotor or cognitive-perceptual tasks are most common. Activities will generally address some aspect of neurological or physical functioning and will facilitate some kind of adaptive response. Unlike previously described frames of reference, there may be several short-term activities planned during each session. The activities are organized and sequenced according to neurophysiological theory, so that simpler sensorimotor activities can build up to advanced, more complex activities. Likewise, high stimulation activities are followed by slower, more calming ones, so that the CNS does not get over-stimulated. Materials that facilitate movement, like mats, balls, props, and pillows, are often used. Craft activities or work activities that incorporate gross motor actions are useful. Materials and environments may be set up to provide cues for functional tasks so that activity demand matches or challenges the performance capacities of clients. Timing depends on the endurance and attention span of members, and sessions can be relatively short, 30 to 50 minutes.

Sharing and Processing

Sharing in movement groups occurs within the bounds of the activity. Clients can observe each other's movements; the cognitive or symbolic meaning of the movement is really not the point and, therefore, is not necessary to share. Processing involves expressing feelings about the group and, when possible, should be done verbally. Verbal processing can reveal hidden resistances and bring out other notable problems clients have while participating in the activity.

Generalizing and Application

The principles learned are associated with the effects of activity or movement of various kinds on the body and the emotions. The knowledge of the therapist may be shared with the group, when appropriate, to facilitate this learning. For example, a group of clients with depression may notice that after the physical expression of anger and hostility, they feel more energy. The lesson in this is that expression of feeling is natural and healthy. The application is to find ways to express feeling without hurting others or otherwise getting into trouble.

Application, even with clients at a lower cognitive level, may involve learning to repeat a desired adaptive response. When movement activities result in spontaneous laughter, for example, the pleasure of this response may motivate the client to repeat the movement that produced it. The neurodevelopmental response to movement activities tends to be spontaneous and not planned. As clients integrate new movement patterns into their repertoire, they will use them spontaneously at times outside of the group. The goal is to stimulate the development of higher-level skills and more adaptive functioning in the client's everyday life.

Neither generalization nor application need to be separate phases of the sensorimotor group. The verbal summary is sufficient to reinforce this learning. However, discussion of learning and applications in life activities can be useful for those clients who are capable of such verbalization and insight.

REFERENCES

American Occupational Therapy Association. (2008). *Occupational therapy practice framework: Domain and process.* Bethesda, MD: Author.

Ayres, A. J. (1961). Development of the body scheme in children. *American Journal of Occupational Therapy, 15,* 99-102.

Ayers, A. J. (1972). *Southern California sensory integration tests.* Los Angeles, CA: Western Psychological Services.

Ayres, A. J. (1974). *The development of sensory integrative theory and practice.* Dubuque, IA: Kendall Hunt.

Ayres, A. J. (1979). *Sensory integration and the child.* Los Angeles, CA: Western Psychological Services.

Bandura, A. (1977). *Social learning theory.* Englewood Cliffs, NJ: Prentice Hall.

Bandura, A. (1997). *Self-efficacy: The exercise of control.* New York, NY: W. H. Freeman.

Bass-Haugen, J., Mathiowetz, V., & Flinn, N. (2008). Optimizing motor behavior using the occupational therapy task oriented approach. In M. V. Radomski & C. Trombly Latham (Eds.), *Occupational therapy for physical dysfunction* (6th ed., pp. 598-617). Philadelphia, PA: Lippincott, Williams and Wilkins.

Bazyk, S., & Bazyk, J. (2009). Meaning of occupation based groups for low income urban youth attending after school care. *American Journal of Occupational Therapy, 63,* 69-80.

Blanche, E. I., & Kiefer, D. B. (2007). Sensory integration and neurodevelopmental treatment as frame of reference in the context of occupational science. In S. B. Dunbar (Ed.), *Occupational therapy models for intervention with children and families.* Thorofare, NJ: SLACK, Incorporated.

Bobath, B. (1972). The neurodevelopmental approach to treatment. In P. Pearson (Ed.), *Physical therapy services in developmental disabilities.* Springfield, IL: Charles Thomas.

Bobath, B. (1990). *Adult hemiplegia: Evaluation and treatment* (3rd ed.). London, UK: Heinemann.

Bowler, D. (1999). *Functional improvement through motor learning.* Presentation handout given in White Plains, NY sponsored by Preventionworks, Nov. 14, 1999.

Brown, C., & Dunn, W. (2002). *Adolescent/Adult Sensory Profile.* San Antonio, TX: The Psychological Corp.

Brunnstrom, S. (1970). *Movement therapy in hemiplegia.* New York, NY: Harper & Row.

Bundy, A. C., Lane, S. J., & Murray, E. A. (2002). *Sensory integration: Theory and practice* (2nd ed.). Philadelphia, PA: F. A. Davis.

Burns, I., Cox, H., & Plant, H. (2000). Leisure or therapeutics? Snoezelen and the care of older persons with dementia. *International Journal of Nursing Practice, 6,* 118-126.

Carr, J. H., & Shepherd, R. B. (1987). *A motor learning program for stroke* (2nd ed.). Rockville, MD: Aspen.

Carr, J. H., & Shepherd, R. B. (1998). *Neurological rehabilitation: Optimizing motor performance.* Oxford: Butterworth-Heinemann.

Champagne, T., & Stromberg, N. (2004). Sensory approaches in inpatient psychiatric settings: Innovative alternatives to seclusion and restraint. *Journal of Psychosocial Nursing, 42,* 35-44.

Corcoran, M. A., & Barrett, D. (1987). Using sensory integration principles with regressed elderly patients. In Z. Mailloux (Ed.), *Sensory integrative approaches in occupational therapy* (pp. 119-128). New York, NY: Haworth Press.

Dagfinrud, H., Kjeken, I., Mowinckel, P., Hagen, K. B., & Kvien, T. K. (2005). Impact of functional impairment in ankylosing spondylitis: Impairment activity limitation and participation restrictions. *Journal of Rheumatology, 32,* 516-523.

Davies, P. L., & Gavin, W. J. (2009). Validating the diagnosis of sensory processing disorders using EEG technology. In Royeen & A. J. Luebben (Eds.), *Sensory integration: A compendium of leading scholarship* (pp. 58-77). Bethesda, MD: American OT Association.

Dijkers, M. P. (1999). Correlates of life satisfaction among persons with spinal cord injury. *Archives of Physical Medicine & Rehabilitation, 80,* 867-876.

DiMatties, M. E., & Sammons, J. H. (2009). Understanding sensory integration. In C. Royeen, & A. Luebben (Eds.), *Sensory integration: A compendium of leading scholarship.* Bethesda, MD: American Occupational Therapy Association.

Dunn, W. (1999). *The sensory profile manual.* San Antonio, TX: Western Psychological.

Eggers, O. (1983). *Occupational therapy in the treatment of adult hemiplegia.* London: William Heinemann Medical Books.

Fisher, A., & Murray, E. A. (1991). Introduction to sensory integration theory. In M. Fisher, E. A. Murray, & A. Bundy (Eds.), *Sensory integration: Theory and practice.* Philadelphia, PA: F. A. Davis.

Fisher, J. (2006). *Working with the neurobiological legacy of early trauma (lecture series presentation).* Boston, MA: The Trauma Center.

Fitts, P., & Posner, M. (1967). *Human performance.* Belmont, CA: Brooks/Cole.

Flinn, N., & Radomski, M. (2008). Learning. In M. Radomski & C. Trombly (Eds.), *Occupational therapy for physical dysfunction* (6th ed.). Philadelphia, PA: Lippincott, Williams & Wilkins.

Fluegelman, A. (1976). *The new games book.* Garden City, NY: Doubleday.

Gal, R., & Lazarus, R. S. (1975). The role of activity in anticipating and confronting stressful situations. *Journal of Human Stress, 4,* 4-20.

Glennon, T. J., & Smith Roley, (2006). *Sensory integration: Inside and outside of occupational therapy practice.* Paper presented at the 2006 American OT Association Annual Conference and Expo, Charlotte, NC on April 28, 2006.

Greenfield, J. M., & Godinez, M. (1989). Clients with stroke learn independence by leading their own therapy group. *OT Week, April 20.*

Henry, D., Ecker, C., Glennon, T., & Herzberg, D. (2009). Using the Sensory Processing Measure (SPM) in multiple practice areas. *OT Practice, June 19,* 9-13.

Hofmann, A. O. (2008). Veterans affairs. *OT Practice, Sept. 8,* 12-14.

Kinnealey, M., & Oliver, B. (2002). *Adult sensory questionnaire.* Unpublished document.

King, L. J. (1974). A sensory integrative approach to schizophrenia. *American Journal of Occupational Therapy, 28,* 529-536.

King, L. J. (1978). Toward a science of adaptive responses. Slagle lecture. *American Journal of Occupational Therapy, 32,* 429-437.

King, L. J. (1988). *Occupational therapy and neuropsychiatry in mental health focus.* Rockville, MD: American Occupational Therapy Association.

Lape, J. E. (2009). Using a multisensory environment to decrease negative behaviors in clients with dementia. *OT Practice, May 26,* 9-13.

Larrington, G. (1987). Sensory integration based program with a severely retarded autistic teenager: An occupational therapy case report. In Z. Mailloux (Ed.), *Sensory integrative approaches in occupational therapy.* New York, NY: Haworth Press.

LeBel, J., & Champagne, T. (2010). Integrating sensory and trauma-informed interventions: A Massachusetts state initiative, Part 2. *Mental Health Special Interest Section Quarterly, 23,* 1-4.

Levit, K. (2008). Optimizing motor behavior using the Bobath approach. In M. V. Radomski & C. Trombly (Eds.), *Occupational therapy for physical dysfunction* (5th ed.). Philadelphia, PA: Lippincott, Williams and Wilkins.

Levitt, S. (1982). *Treatment of cerebral palsy and motor delay.* Boston, MA: Blackwell Scientific Publications.

Lowen, A., & Lowen, L. (1977). *The way to vibrant health.* New York, NY: Harper and Row.

Mannix, D. (1993). *Social skills activities for special children.* New York, NY: Prentice Hall.

Mannix, D. (1996). *Self-esteem activities for secondary students with special needs.* New York, NY: Simon & Schuster.

Massachusetts Department of Mental Health. (2010). Restraint/seclusion reduction initiative (RSRI) Retrieved from http://www.mass.gov/?pageID=eohhs2modulechunk&L=4&L0=Home&L1=Government&L2=Departments+and+Divisions&L3=Department+of+Mental+Health&sid=Eeohhs2&b=terminalcontent&f=dmh_p_rsri&csid=Eeohhs2

May-Benson, T. (2009). Occupational therapy for adults with sensory processing disorder. *OT Practice, June 15,* 15-19.

Moore, K. M., & Henry, A. D. (2002). Treatment of adult psychiatric patients using the Wilbarger protocol. *Occupational Therapy in Mental Health, 18,* 43-63.

Mulligan, S. (2002). Advances in sensory integration research. In A. C. Bundy, S. J. Lane, & E. A. Murray (Eds.), *Sensory integration: Theory and practice* (2nd ed.). Philadelphia, PA: F. A. Davis.

Parham, D., Cohn, E., Spitzer, S., Koomer, J., Miller, A., Burke, J., et al. (2007). Fidelity in sensory integration intervention research. *American Journal of Occupational Therapy, 61,* 216-227.

Roley, S. S., Mailloux, Z., Miller-Kubaneck, H., & Glennon, T. (2009). Understanding Ayres Sensory Integration. In C. Royeen & A. J. Luebben (Eds.), *Sensory integration: A compendium of leading scholarship* (pp. 19-31). Bethesda, MD: American Occupational Therapy Association.

Rood, M. S. (1954). Neurophysiological reactions as a basis for physical therapy. *Phys Therapy Rev, 34,* 444-449.

Ross, M. (1997). *Integrative group therapy: Mobilizing coping abilities with the five stage group.* Bethesda, MD: American Occupational Therapy Association.

Ross, M., & Bachner, S. (Eds.). (2004). *Adults with developmental disabilities: Current approaches in occupational therapy.* Bethesda, MD: American Occupational Therapy Association.

Sabari, J. S. (2002). Optimizing motor control using the Carr and Shepherd approach. In C. Trombly & M. V. Radomski (Eds.), *Occupational therapy for physical dysfunction* (5th ed.). Philadelphia, PA: Lippincott, Williams & Wilkins.

Schilling, D., Washington, K., Bilingsley, E., & Deitz, J. (2003). Classroom seating for children with attention deficit hyperactivity disorder: Therapy balls vs. chairs. *American Journal of Occupational Therapy, 57,* 534-541.

Schmidt. (1988). *Motor control and learning: A behavioral emphasis* (2nd ed.). Champaign, IL: Human Kinetics.

Shumway-Cook, A., & Woollacott, M. (Eds.). (2006). *Motor control: Translating research into clinical practice* (3nd ed.). Philadelphia, PA: Lippincott, Williams & Wilkins.

Smith, S. A., Press, B., Koenig, K., & Kinnealey, M. (2005). Effects of sensory integration intervention on self-stimulating self-injurious behaviors. American *Journal of Occupational Therapy, 59,* 418-425.

Strzelecki, M. V. (2008). Moving forward: A look at sensory integration. *OT Practice, Sept. 8,* 17-21.

Sunderland, A., Tinson, D., Bradley, E., Fletcher, D., Langton Hewer, R., & Wade, D. (1992). Enhanced physical therapy improves recovery of arm function after stroke. *Journal of Neurology, Neurosurgery, & Psychiatry, 55,* 530-535.

Trombly, C. (1995). Occupation: Purposefulness and meaningfulness as therapeutic mechanisms. American *Journal of Occupational Therapy, 49,* 960-972.

Trombly, C. (2008). Conceptual foundations for practice. In C. Trombly, & M. V. Radomski, (Eds.), *Occupational therapy for physical dysfunction* (6th ed., pp. 1-20). Baltimore, MD: Williams and Wilkins.

Van Deusen, J., & Harlowe, D. (1987). The efficacy of the ROM dance program for adults with rheumatoid arthritis. *American Journal of Occupational Therapy, 41,* 90-95.

Wilbarger, P., & Wilbarger, J. L. (1991). *Sensory defensiveness in children aged 2-12: An intervention guide for parents and other caregivers.* Denver, CO: Avanti Educational Programs.

Sensorimotor Activity Example 9-1
Blob

The Blob begins as a game of tag. When the person who is "it" catches someone, that person joins hands and becomes part of the Blob. Only the outside hand on either end of the Blob can snatch runaway players. Thus, the insidious Blob keeps growing, cornering stray runners and forcing them to join up. In large groups, the Blob may split itself into parts and organize raiding parties to round up the last few strays. Boundaries must be set for this game, so eventually everyone is caught. "The thrilling climax occurs when there's only one player left to put up a heroic last ditch stand on behalf of humanity" (Fluegelman, 1976, p. 107). The last survivor can start the next Blob as the game continues.

This game is obviously for people who are ambulatory, have good balance and coordination, and have enough cognitive understanding to be able to follow simple rules. Blob is a simple concept that can be fun even for those who do not grasp its deeper implications. Done inside a room with the elderly, a therapist can talk the group through any difficulties, or he or she can begin by being the Blob. It may be done slowly or quickly to adapt to patient ability, and it provides light exercise with an element of fun and challenge.

Sensorimotor Activity Example 9-2
People to People

Here is a new game that is made for OT. It is especially good for integrating movement, motor planning, and cognition. Everyone chooses a partner, and the game begins with a rhythmic clapping and snapping in unison (clap-clap-right hand, snap-snap-left hand). The caller names two body parts, one on the right snap, the other on the left snap (e.g., "elbow to ear"). On the next snap-snap the whole group repeats "elbow to ear" while simultaneously one partner places his elbow on the other partner's ear. The caller continues to name body parts, trying to challenge the group by naming obscure anatomical structures (esophagus to gastrocnemius) or forcing them to take awkward positions. When the caller gets tired of this, he may call out "people to people." Then everyone must change partners, and in the confusion, the caller grabs a partner, leaving another member to become the new caller.

Adaptations for this game are endless. At the very least, it is a great socialization ice breaker, sure to get everyone laughing. It is also an excellent way for OT students to study their anatomy. Patients can practice bilateral coordination (clapping and snapping), motor planning (touching parts with partner), body awareness (identifying parts), and cognition (naming and recognizing body parts). A fair amount of balance, coordination, and visual-motor integration are required to perform this activity successfully. Care should be taken with this and other games requiring touch that patients are not threatened by the close proximity to others.

The New Games followers suggest what OTs already know—all the games can be adapted by changing the rules or new games can be invented to meet the special needs and goals of our patients.

From Cole, M. B. *Group dynamics in occupational therapy: The theoretical basis and practice application of group intervention* (4th ed.). Thorofare, NJ: SLACK Incorporated. © 2012 SLACK Incorporated.

Sensorimotor Activity Example 9-3
Parachute Games

All the games begin with group members holding an edge of the parachute at even intervals. It will take a few tries to move the parachute up over heads and down to the knees in unison to "catch the air." When the group has accomplished this, members can take turns running under the chute and exchanging places with one another across the circle. Other variations of parachute play are as follows:

- *Popcorn*—When the parachute is down, a few tennis balls can be tossed in the center. The group makes the balls "pop" into the air and catches them with the parachute.
- *Round the World*—One ball is placed in the center of the parachute. The group is instructed to work together to make the ball roll around the edge of the parachute by moving it in unison.
- *Down the Drain*—Two colored balls are placed in the parachute. One side (blue ball) tries to get the other side's ball (red ball) to drop through the hole in the middle of the parachute.
- *Secret Club*—Billow the parachute by the unified above the head, below the knees motion of the group. Then, on the count of three, group members bring the parachute edge down behind their backs and proceed to sit on the edge of the parachute. The air in the middle produces a "tent" in which the "secret club" can meet (but not for long or the air can get very stale!).
- *Shark*—The members gather up the edge of the chute at just about waist level until a "calm sea" is produced. Then, the "shark" ducks under and stalks the group with one finger pointing up touching the parachute from below, so that his or her movements may be observed from the top of the parachute. At an unexpected moment, the shark grabs the legs of an unsuspecting group member. The "victim" screams loudly as he or she is pulled under to become the next "shark." Two or three sharks at a time may be used in larger groups.

From Cole, M. B. *Group dynamics in occupational therapy: The theoretical basis and practice application of group intervention* (4th ed.). Thorofare, NJ: SLACK Incorporated. © 2012 SLACK Incorporated.

Sensorimotor Activity Example 9-4
Expressing Anger With Movement

Materials: Exercise mats or thick carpeting and pillows.

Directions: Give directions for each step of the sequence, and allow members to take the time they need for each step.
1. Lie down on your back on the mat, and extend both legs. Kick your legs rhythmically, and allow your energy to flow into this motion. Take a few minutes to do this, setting your own pace.
2. Stand up and form a circle. Kick alternately with the right, then the left leg into the center of the circle.
3. Clench your fists, and as you kick into the center of the circle, say "No!" Louder!
4. What other words can we say? As members make suggestions, have the whole group try them. Try punching into the center of the circle and saying words or making sounds.
5. Rest a few minutes, and concentrate on breathing. Walk slowly around the circle, then turn and walk the other way. The slow walking has a calming effect after the excitement of kicking and punching.
6. Lie down on your stomach with your pillow in front of you. Punch pillow with right and left fists in a rhythmic motion. Do this for a few minutes, and set your own pace.
7. As you punch the pillow, say "No!" If you feel like kicking also, allow yourself to do this.
8. If you would like, give the pillow a name. (Therapists should do this with caution, so as not to arouse too much anger.)
9. After a few minutes, wind down, and just breathe slowly, resting head on pillow.
10. Stand up again when rested. Shrug shoulders in a backward roll, and loosen tension in the neck area.
11. As patients shrug, say "Get off my back!" Louder!
12. Sit in a circle, and massage muscles in back of neck. Each person massages the back of the person in front of him or her.

This exercise must be processed so that clients are not left with unresolved angry feelings. One goal is awareness of anger so that its appropriate expression can be discussed. Another goal is eliciting normal movement patterns sub-cortically. The careful planning and adaptation of this type of activity can utilize the concepts of Rood, NDT, PNF, Brunnstrom, or sensory integration.

Sensorimotor Activity Example 9-5
Acting Out Feelings

Materials: Twenty index cards with feeling words, paper, pencils, and stopwatch. Words for cards are lonely, disgusted, excited, pleased, annoyed, infuriated, friendly, jealous, miserable, crabby, ecstatic, impatient, giddy, silly, moody, spacy, frightened, terrified, hopeless, hurt. Other feeling words may be added or substituted.

Directions: Each member draws a card and takes 30 seconds to act out the feeling on the card. Someone should be designated as timekeeper. Players may make sounds, but no words are allowed. Players can walk back and forth in front of the group, sit, stand, lie down, and make gestures and facial expressions. The entire 30 seconds should be used. Nonverbal interaction with other members may be allowed as long as no one is hurt.

Members do not shout out their guesses; this is not charades. When time is up, group members write down what they think the feeling is. As each "mini-drama" ends, members read out their feeling words and discuss why they thought so. After a brief discussion, the player shows the group the card. Members continue to draw cards and act out feelings until they are all used.

Sensorimotor Activity Example 9-6
Ross' Five-Stage Group for Medium/Verbal Members

Materials: Six to eight clients, blackboard and chalk (or newsprint pad and large marker), and a basketball. Arrange chairs in a circle.

Stage I (5 minutes)—The therapist introduces self and states, "We are all going to exercise our muscles and our brains so we can share ideas and learn from each other. To begin, I'd like each of you to take a turn coming up to the board and writing your name." The chalk is handed to the first volunteer, who sits back down when finished. The group will read each name aloud as it is written. Note that everyone is needed to complete the circle; gather any late or distracted members.

Stage II (10 to 15 minutes)—An agitated group is organized by asking members to pass the basketball from one to another with both hands while sitting. Members may then stand and bounce the ball to each other across the circle. Members take turns walking around the outside of the circle bouncing the basketball; then, the members stand in a circle, facing right, an arm's length apart from each other. They must pass the basketball between their legs to the person behind them. The whole group jogs around the outside of the circle of chairs for maximum exertion. Members face left, arm's length apart, and pass the basketball backwards over their heads to the person behind them. The group can create its own movement sequences by requiring the ball to be passed without hands or from member to member in a predetermined pattern.

Stage III (15 minutes)—Members move chairs back a few feet before sitting down, thus expanding the circle. A large, empty wastebasket is placed in the center. Members take turns bouncing the basketball once and trying to get it in the "basket." The group can be split into "teams," keeping score on the board. If teams are uneven, reshuffling should occur. Blocking may be done if skill permits for "offensive and defensive play." Members of teams sit alternately and attempt to block winning plays with arm movements. Different colored bandannas may be tied around the members' necks or heads to signify the different teams.

End group with a series of stretches (e.g., pantomime throwing a free point, reaching for the hoop, and blocking). Finally, pantomime congratulating each other on a winning game. Check level of excitement; use a calming strategy from Table 9-1 if needed.

Stage IV (15 minutes)—Discussion of favorite sports can follow. Each member takes a turn remembering an experience involving a sport. What athletics do members know? Admire? Dislike? What do they remember about Winter or Summer Olympics? What about leisure or solitary sports, such as swimming, fishing, or bicycling? The goal of the discussion is to learn about each other and from each other about different sports. Encourage members to ask each other questions or respond to one another's comments.

If discussion is somewhat beyond the group, substitute taking turns with the chalk and drawing a piece of sports equipment on the board. Have the group guess what it is or what sport uses the equipment. Examples include fishing line with hook, swimming pool, boxing glove, golf club, baseball bat, tennis racquet, pair of skis. Congratulate the group for sharing their knowledge and experience with each other.

Stage V—To summarize, the therapist asks members to remember parts of the session. "What things did we do today? Which did you like best? What did you learn about each other?" End with a firm handshake and say goodbye by name as each member leaves.

From Cole, M. B. *Group dynamics in occupational therapy: The theoretical basis and practice application of group intervention* (4th ed.). Thorofare, NJ: SLACK Incorporated. © 2012 SLACK Incorporated.

Sensorimotor Activity Example 9-7
Ross' Five-Stage Group for Low/Verbal Members

Materials: Hand lotion, candle, balloons, party favor blowers, card table, cards with different colors, 10 to 12 pairs of matching objects, tray, and bag.

Stage I—Clients sit in a circle. The therapist greets each member by name and asks everyone to hold out their hands. A dot of herbal-smelling hand lotion is squeezed into their palms; the therapist demonstrates rubbing it into the hands. Ask members to notice how it smells. A vanilla- or spice-scented candle is then passed from member to member, and sniffing is encouraged.

Stage II—Every member chooses a colored, blown-up, 6-inch diameter balloon to hold between their hands. "Don't let go… don't drop it… hold onto it." The therapist then asks members to imitate holding it out in front, above the head, swinging to the left and the right (shoulder height), gently throwing and catching it, and touching the balloon to knees, ankles, floor, lap, chin, and each shoulder.

Put on music, such as a waltz tempo (e.g., Strauss) or a song that suits the members' age group. Ask the group to stand and imitate movements to the music: swinging the balloon back and forth, up and down, and around in a circle.

Batting balloons in the air begins as another song is played. Members try to keep all the balloons in the air until the music ends. Observe behavior and modify as needed.

Stage III—All balloons are collected except one. The therapist passes this balloon with his or her elbows and asks a member to begin passing it around the circle with no hands. This can be done sitting or standing. If it is someone's birthday, ask the members to sing "Happy Birthday" (many people who no longer speak can still sing). Party blowers are passed out, and everyone practices blowing by imitating the therapist. A small table is set up, and balloons are placed on the table. Members attempt to knock all the balloons off the table using the party blowers (again, no hands). Pick them all up and do it again. Passing a single balloon from one side of the table to the other can follow.

Stage IV—Cards with different colors are passed to each member. Colored cards matching these are placed down on the table. Members take turns choosing a card from the table until they find one that matches.

The therapist makes a board or tray with 10 or 12 common objects. Matching objects are placed in a bag. Members draw an object, guessing what it is by touch if they can, and pointing to the matching object on the tray. They look at the object to see if they guessed correctly.

Stage V—Play a short waltz tape, and ask members to stand and join hands for a group sway.

From Cole, M. B. *Group dynamics in occupational therapy: The theoretical basis and practice application of group intervention* (4th ed.). Thorofare, NJ: SLACK Incorporated. © 2012 SLACK Incorporated.

Sensorimotor Activity Example 9-8
Grocery Game for Adults With Physical Disabilities

Goal: Upper extremity strengthening, grasp and release practice, and improvement in efficiency of movement using a variety of shapes, sizes, and weights.

Position: Six members, seated in wheelchairs in a circle, no table.
Timing: Warm up: 5 to 10 minutes
Activity: 10 to 15 minutes
Discussion: 20 to 30 minutes
Summary: 5 minutes

Materials: Six each of the following: 8 oz. can of beans, 16 oz. can of tomato sauce, 1 lb. box of pasta, large yellow onions, 5 lb. bag of flour, individually wrapped roll of paper towels, cloves of garlic, 1 L bottles of soda, brown paper grocery bags. (Any eight items may be used, vary number and weight according to client needs. Avoid glass containers.) One of each item will be in a brown paper grocery bag. The remaining five of each item is stored in a visible location in the room, using varying levels of reaching difficulty. (Activity should be graded to match member skills and abilities.)

Description

Introduction: All of you have discussed with me your difficulties with reaching and handling objects since your illness or injury. The only way to get better at lifting and handling objects is by practicing. Today, we are going to use these grocery items to play a game. This will make exercise and practice more fun.

Warm-Up: Therapist allows each member to choose one item from a grocery bag. Members hold the item with one or both of their hands and briefly discuss the best way to reach for and grasp this item. Taking turns, each member will pass one item to the person on the right and will continue passing the item around the circle. To add a challenge, members may pass more than one item at a time. Continue several times, ask members to keep track of how many times they reached for and grasped each item. Each member will end up holding only one item. Discuss any difficulties members had with this activity.

Activity: For the next part of the game, I'm going to ask each of you to "go shopping" right here in this room. The first part of the game is for each of you to look around the room and locate where I have stored five more of the item you are now holding. Some of them are high up, and you'll have to reach up to get them. Some are eye level, and some are down low. (Members take turns locating and pointing to the stored items. Members may help each other do this.)

Why do you think I put the items where they are? (May process member comments. Pass out grocery bags, encourage/help members to "open" the bags and balance them on their laps.) The goal of this activity is to collect one of each item and place them in your shopping bag. You have 10 minutes to complete this activity. Does everyone understand the directions? Who will volunteer to repeat the directions for the group? (Repeat directions as needed, answer member questions.) I will give you a 1-minute warning. You may begin.

When time is up, return to original circle with grocery bags. Members write names on the grocery bags and count how many items they retrieved and which ones (if any) are missing.

Sharing: Please take turns telling the group how many items you retrieved, what is still missing, and what problems you had in doing this activity. (Encourage members to respond to each other and share some of their problem-solving strategies.)

From Cole, M. B. *Group dynamics in occupational therapy: The theoretical basis and practice application of group intervention* (4th ed.). Thorofare, NJ: SLACK Incorporated. © 2012 SLACK Incorporated.

Grocery Game for Adults With Physical Disabilities (Continued)

Processing:
- How did you feel about playing the grocery game? (Elicit both positive and negative feelings without judgment.)
- What did you like about the activity? What did you dislike? Why?
- What conflicts occurred when more than one of you went for the same item at the same time?
- What help did you receive from or give to other members? How did you feel about that?

Generalizing:
- What physical skills did we need to do this activity?
- What mental skills did we need?
- What was hardest to do? What was easiest?
- What mental and physical strategies did we use to deal with the difficult parts?
- How can we help each other with activities like this?
- What did you learn about yourself from doing this? What did you learn about others?

Application (everyone answers these questions for him- or herself):
- What tasks do you do at home that require these same skills?
- What places in the community require us to do something like this?
- What jobs have you held that require this kind of activity?
- How does where we store different items affect our ability to function at home?
- How could you change where you keep the things you need to do projects at home?
- Who can help you to reach or lift things when you cannot do it yourself?
- Why is it important for you to have the skill and ability to gather items for a project?
- What can you do to practice these skills at home?

Summary (Ask a member to summarize):
- What did we do in group today?
- What skills did we learn or practice?
- Please remember the ways you plan to practice these skills at home.
- I really appreciated how hard everyone worked in group today.
- I especially noticed... (give individual feedback to each member).
- We'll meet again at _____ . See you then.

Chapter 10

A Model of Human Occupation and Other Occupation-Based Models

Occupation-based models, although rooted in the occupational paradigm of OT's founders, represent a relatively recent presence in the profession. Unlike frames of reference, which typically arise from a perspective of remediation and adaptation to disability, occupation-based models incorporate the entire spectrum of health and illness in their proposed inter-relationships of person, environment, and occupation. This chapter focuses on the first of these to be developed, the Model of Human Occupation (MOHO) (Kielhofner, 2008), which mirrors many of Mary Reilly's (1969) principles of occupational behavior. Other prominent models briefly reviewed here are Ecology of Human Performance (EHP), Occupational Adaptation (OA) (Schkade & Schultz, 2003), and the Person-Environment-Occupation (PEO) Model (Law, Cooper, Strong, Stewart, Rigby, & Letts, 1996; Law & Dunbar, 2007). The Canadian Model of Occupational Performance (CMOP) (Townsend & Polatajko, 2007), also an occupation-based model, was discussed in Chapter 3 because of its client-centered focus. Finally, the Kawa Model (Iwama, 2006), a culturally relevant model developed for Japanese OT practice, provides implications for group interventions from a different cultural perspective. Because each of these models is separate and distinct, this chapter makes no attempt to combine them, but describes separate sections for framework focus, basic assumptions, function/dysfunction, change/motivation, and group guidelines. For each model, separate group activity examples from the recent OT literature are described. Only the adaptations for group leadership at the end of the chapter refer to all the occupation-based models together. Generally speaking, all occupation-based models may also draw upon frames of reference when addressing specific disabilities and/or focusing upon specific parts of AOTA Framework-II's domain of concern (AOTA, 2008). For a more in-depth understanding of these models, please refer to Cole and Tufano's *Applied Theories in Occupational Therapy* (2008).

Model of Human Occupation

The MOHO emerged around 1980 as a further definition of the theory of occupational behavior developed by Mary Reilly (1962). The central idea of occupational behavior theory is that engagement in activity or occupation in itself will produce and maintain health. Human achievement and daily occupation are identified as the focal point for the development of the model of human occupation (Kielhofner, 2008). White (1959) is credited with introducing the concept of the human need for competence and achievement. Kielhofner, Burke, and Igi (1980) expanded on these concepts and combined them with general systems theory. They describe the human being as an open system, define the various parts of the system (volitional, habituation, and performance subsystems), and describe how it interacts with other systems (culture, tasks, social norms, human and nonhuman environment). In this fourth edition, MOHO is no longer considered a frame of reference, but represents the first of several recently developed occupation-based models. Other models reviewed here are Ecology of Human Performance (Dunn, 2007); the Person, Environment, Occupation Model (Law & Dunbar, 2007); Occupational

Cole M.B. *Group Dynamics in Occupational Therapy: The Theoretical Basis and Practice Application of Group Intervention (pp 281-314).*
© 2012 SLACK Incorporated.

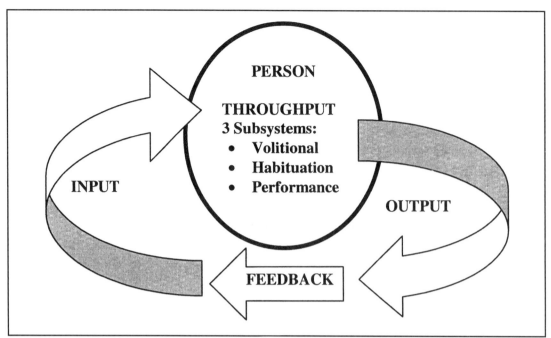

Figure 10-1. The human open system. (Adapted from Kielhofner, G. [Ed.]. [2002]. *A model of human occupation: Theory and application* [3rd ed.]. Baltimore, MD: Williams & Wilkins.)

Adaptation (Schkade & Schultz, 1994), and the Kawa Model (Iwama, 2006). Each of these can be viewed as a superstructure that organizes the concepts of person, environment, and occupation and expresses them in terms that can be readily applied to evaluation and intervention.

Framework Focus

MOHO is sometimes identified as an "overarching" theory because it is so broad. As such, MOHO touches upon just about every domain of the *Occupational Therapy Practice Framework* (American Occupational Therapy Association [AOTA Framework-II], 2008). According to Kielhofner, human occupation is complex and multifaceted. Occupation "encompasses a wide range of doing that occurs in the context of time, space, society, and culture" (2008, p. 5). As a therapeutic approach, it is holistic and universally applicable across ages, cultures, and disabilities. MOHO views the person as an open system, which has the capacity to reorganize itself or be reorganized. Injury or illness can bring about unwelcome change that disrupts both daily occupations and life occupations. The OT evaluates all aspects of the system and facilitates an adaptive reorganization so that order can be restored. The subsystems within the client include volitional, which incorporates occupational choices of performance areas of occupation; habituation, which incorporates occupational performance patterns; and performance, which incorporates both performance skills and client factors. External parts of the system include all of the contexts defined by the AOTA Framework-II

(2008). Perhaps because of its broadness, MOHO "will not address all the problems faced by a client, requiring the therapist to actively use other models along with it" (Kielhofner, 2008, p. 3).

Basic Assumptions

Concepts From Systems Theory

The original assumption in applying systems theory to human functioning was that man is an open system that can change and develop through interaction with the environment (Kielhofner, 1978). The human open system was described as a cyclical process involving output, feedback, input, and throughput (Kielhofner & Burke, 1985). The human being gives output to the environment, receives feedback in the form of input from the environment, and experiences throughput, a process of change and adaptation of the person resulting from the feedback given (Figure 10-1). As systems theory in the sciences and many other disciplines has moved toward greater complexity, so has MOHO. Kielhofner's latest interpretation includes two basic concepts from systems theory: heterarchy and emergence. Heterarchy is the opposite of hierarchy, referring to the seemingly random ways that all parts of the system form a dynamic whole. Emergence is the "principle that complex actions, thoughts, and feelings spontaneously arise out of the interactions of several components" (Kielhofner, 2008, p. 25). Human occupation "encompasses a wide range of doing that occurs in the context of time, space, society, and culture" (p. 5). Although inseparable from the whole, the human system is divided into parts for the purpose of examining (evaluation) and influencing (intervention) its processes.

The Three Internal Subsystems

Following systems theory, throughput occurs within the three internal subsystems: volitional, habituation, and performance capacity, which comprise the internal organization of the human system. These subsystems are consolidated and heterarchical (i.e., they are interdependent with one another, contributing equally to the human system as a whole). The volitional subsystem maintains a belief in oneself and one's values, and exerts influence in choosing one's occupations and initiating occupational behavior. The habituation subsystem organizes and maintains occupational behavior in routines and role patterns (habit maps and role scripts). The performance subsystem has been separated into intrinsic and extrinsic components (Kielhofner, Forsyth, & Barrett, 2003). Performance capacity refers to the status of mental and physical skills and abilities within the individual, while extrinsic performance describes actual engagement in occupational behavior during participation in life. The three subsystems work together in an integrated fashion to maintain the balance of work, play, and self-care activities (see Figure 10-1).

The Volitional Subsystem

The volitional process involves anticipating, experiencing, choosing, and interpreting occupational behavior (Kielhofner, 2008). This system serves to direct and energize the other subsystems toward desired goals. However, this motivating force is highly influenced by the other subsystems (state of fatigue, habitual patterns) as well as external circumstances. Cultural common sense defines one's perceptions of oneself and one's environment and creates the context for occupational choices. Choices for occupation can be immediate (activities for today) or long-term (career choices, committed relationships). The three main components of this subsystem are personal causation, values, and interests. Personal causation refers to a belief in oneself and is related to feelings of competence. A healthy individual is thought to possess needed skills (sense of personal capacity) and to believe himself or herself to be capable of using these skills to have a desired effect on the environment (self-efficacy). A person who believes in himself or herself expects to succeed through the use of his or her own abilities. A person who lacks a sense of personal causation may feel that what happens is controlled by fate or external circumstance. Such a person feels helpless to cope with the functional problems resulting from illness and disability.

Values in the MOHO refer to the meaningfulness of activities. Individuals are thought to spend time doing activities that have meaning and are thought to be good or morally right. For example, if a student thinks that having a college degree is good, he or she may work very hard at reading, writing, and studying, activities that will help him or her achieve that goal. Clients often find themselves unable to perform activities that they consider to be important or meaningful, such as going back to work. A reprioritizing of values might be an intervention goal. Using this model, clients can find alternate ways to perform a work role that are within their capabilities.

Interests in this model are defined as tendencies to find certain occupations attractive and pleasurable. If a person enjoys a particular activity, he or she may be inclined to participate in it frequently or for longer periods of time. Interests are related to work, play, and self-care activities and are not limited to recreational endeavors. Occupational choices are highly influenced by the activities one finds attractive. A healthy individual uses his or her interests to guide present action and to plan the use of time. A person lacking in interests may need help in exploring his or her environment and in finding pleasure in activities.

In summary, the volitional subsystem guides the occupational behavior of the individual in ways that are meaningful and pleasurable and are likely to have a desired effect on the environment.

The Habituation Subsystem

The concept of "habit training" dates back to the practice of Eleanor Clarke Slagle, reflected by the writings of Adolph Meyer. He describes the "systematic engagement of interest and concern about the actual use of time and work (as) an obligation and a necessity" in the treatment of chronic illness (Meyer, 1982, p. 81). The organization of activities throughout the day is the concern of the habituation subsystem, as conceptualized by the MOHO. Roles and habits are its components.

Habits are routine or typical ways in which a person performs tasks. Their familiarity provides a sense of stability and well-being that comes with predictability. For example, a morning routine may involve getting up at 7 a.m., bathing, dressing, and eating breakfast. Habits can decrease the effort required to perform tasks by making them so routine that they are almost automatic. Consider the effort needed to find one's way to a new place of work. After driving the same route for several days, one recognizes familiar landmarks, and the trip requires much less conscious thought. This routine allows the individual to save his or her energy for the more challenging activities of the day.

However, research has shown that habits are not just mindless repetitions of behavior. Rather, they operate as habit maps, or guidelines, which must be improvised to accommodate each new circumstance. Habit maps include thoughts and perceptions as well as action sequences. Young (1988) views habits as internalized intuitive knowledge, which gives us our bearings (orients us) and allows us to anticipate the next step in familiar temporal, physical, and social surroundings. According to Young, habits that are shared by a social group are called "customs" and are the carriers of culture. They are the rules for living that keep us in harmony with our social environment (Young, 1988).

Illness often results in a breakdown of normal routines. Occupational therapy may be needed to relearn and reorganize one's habits after illness. Being in a familiar surrounding may provide a way for people to maintain order in the face of illness or disability. MOHO stresses the importance of a familiar and safe habitat and the necessity of assessing one's habitual ways of doing things. Often, the initial intervention in occupational therapy is to reinforce familiar routines and existing skills.

A role is a position or status within a social group, along with its accompanying obligations and expectations and related cluster of attitudes and actions. Some typical roles are worker, parent, family member, student, and volunteer. Functional individuals generally internalize and enact a variety of life roles and find it necessary to achieve a balance of these if they are to maintain order in their lives. The roles we play have an organizing effect on how we use time. The worker role and the family member role, for example, each require the performance of defined tasks that must be balanced and planned for if the day is to flow smoothly.

According to Kielhofner (2008), every role has a role script. Role scripts guide comprehension of social expectations and construction of performance actions. Similar to habits, roles guide our improvisation of behavior, which changes and adapts continually. The role of a parent in the family, for example, suggests various tasks concerned with providing food and shelter; maintaining the household; and providing instruction, authority, and guidance for the children. The parent role also constrains behavior because parents are expected to set an example for their children and to refrain from activities that would be detrimental (gambling, alcohol abuse) to the family unit. As circumstances change, role expectations may require rethinking and their script adaptation.

Our clients may lack social roles or may find it difficult to meet the obligations and expectations of their roles. The focus of therapeutic intervention may be the development of new roles and/or the planning and modification of activities required within chosen roles. For evaluation and intervention purposes, grouping clients who wish to continue in similar roles, such as returning to work or maintaining a home, allows people with disabilities to share ideas and provide mutual support for adapting their role scripts to accommodate physical, emotional, or cognitive limitations.

In addition to role modification or loss, Hammel (1999) points out the necessity for people with acquired disability to learn a new self-manager role, which involves the management of medical, functional, economic, and social aspects of a disability. The AOTA Framework-II suggests the role of self-advocacy, defined as "understanding your strengths and needs, identifying your personal goals, knowing your legal rights and responsibilities, and communicating these to others" (Dawson, 2007, in AOTA, 2008, p. 675). The degree to which this role is internalized can influence the person's independence in the community and the successful performance of other life roles. An occupational therapist might establish a group for clients with newly acquired disabilities and provide a structure for clients to help one another in learning this new role.

The Performance Capacity Subsystem

Performance capacity is the ability for doing things. This subsystem includes both objective and subjective client factors required to perform purposeful activities. Components, or foundation abilities, include musculoskeletal, neurological, cardiopulmonary, and cognitive processes. Three types of skills are identified as part of subjective experience: perceptual-motor, process, and communication/interaction skills. The intrinsic part of performance has been labeled "performance capacity," and the extrinsic part is called "occupational performance." A person's performance, as linked to the output of the human open system, is called "participation." These updates, adapted from Kielhofner et al. (2003), are diagrammed in Figure 10-2.

The volitional and habituation subsystems can only perform to the extent that existing capacities and skills will allow. Therefore, a lack of skills can prevent the needed organization of roles and habits, the pursuit of interests, and the accomplishment of valued goals. In this area, occupational therapy may treat deficit areas using other frames of reference, such as biomechanical or sensory integration, in a fragmented fashion. Authors of the updated MOHO theory caution against this "reductionistic" practice. The application of physiological, psychological, or biomechanical theory should always be in service to the more basic human need to engage in meaningful occupations.

Interaction With the Environment

The three subsystems discussed above are part of the throughput process of the human open system. Output, feedback, and input define the system's interaction with the environment. Because the health and adaptation of the individual is dependent on this interaction, the environment represents a vital part of the MOHO. The MOHO first defines the influences of the environment on occupational behavior as opportunities, resources, demands, and/or constraints. Second, environments themselves are defined as physical or social and occupation-specific settings.

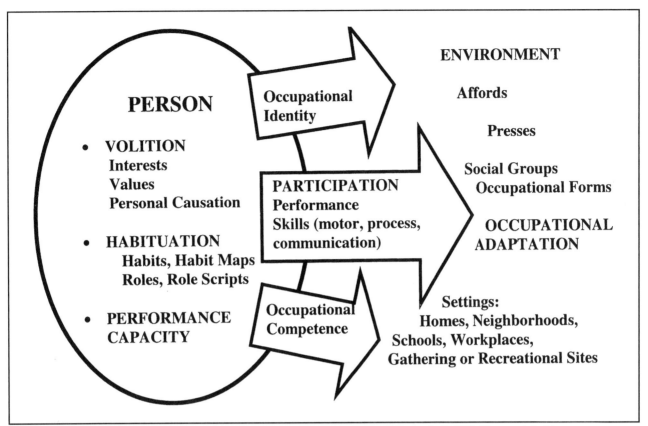

Figure 10-2. Expanded MOHO. (Adapted from Kielhofner, G., Forsyth, K., & Barret, L. [2003]. The model of human occupation. In E. Crepeau, E. Cohn, & B. Boyt Schell [Eds.], *Willard & Spackman's occupational therapy.* Philadelphia, PA: Lippincott, Williams & Wilkins.)

Every environment offers the opportunity for a prescribed range of behaviors. The behavior that is selected depends upon the interaction of the person (intentions, habits, and skills) and the objects and circumstances of the context. Each environment affords opportunities and resources within a range of possibilities. For example, a university environment offers multiple opportunities for academic and technical learning. Classrooms, laboratories, libraries or study areas, and office hours for dialogue with professors all suggest different modes of learning. Environmental press is the expectation of performance or behavior placed on an individual by a given environment (Barris, 1985). For example, a health club environment requires the individual to dress in a defined manner and to demonstrate a certain level of physical skill. Individuals generally seek out environments that fit their interests and their level of skill. Individuals who are disabled may find themselves in environments that do not match their competence level and may need the services of an occupational therapist to help them change either their skill level or their environment.

Environments are described in both physical and social contexts. Physical environments operate according to the laws of science. They may be natural (untouched by humans) or fabricated (buildings, automobiles, roads,

airports). Objects within these environments may also be man-made (clothes, dishes) or may occur naturally (trees, seashells). These environments are organized according to various purposes, and their contents and arrangement greatly influence human occupational behavior.

Social environments consist of social groups and occupational forms. Social groups, which assemble and meet regularly, define and assign occupational roles to individuals within them (a family, a corporation). An occupational form, according to Nelson (1988), is "the preexisting structure that elicits, guides, or structures subsequent human performance" (p. 633). For example, dinner is an occupational form that is accepted across cultures. Each culture has its unique ways of obtaining and preparing food, as well as acceptable ways of consuming it. The obvious purpose of dinner is to sustain life by supplying food to the body, but its purpose is also social, such as a time for a man and woman to get to know one another (dinner date) or for the family to communicate and be together (family dinner). This example demonstrates both the immediate/physical and the symbolic/cultural nature of occupational forms.

Occupational behavior settings combine the physical and social environments in ways recognizable to most people. These include homes, neighborhoods, schools,

Table 10-1

Components of the Model of Human Occupation

Internal	(Components/examples)	External	(Components/examples)
Volitional Subsystem		**Natural Environment**	Mountains, beach
Personal causation	Knowledge of capacity (I can ski) Sense of efficacy (I can learn in college)	**Fabricated Environment**	House, airport, car, factory, supermarket, clothes, dishes, machines, tools
Choices for occupation	Activity choice (I need to buy milk) Occupational choice (I want to be a doctor)	**Social Environment**	
Values	Personal convictions (be kind to others) Sense of obligation (always return what you borrow)	**Social Groups**	Family, corporation
Interests	Attraction (loves reading, conversing) Preference (enjoys the outdoors)	**Occupational Forms**	Driving a car, skiing, shopping, working
Habituation Subsystem		**Settings:**	Homes
Habits	Routines (getting dressed for work) Habit maps (operate a computer, adapt for different uses)		Neighborhoods
			Schools
Roles	Internalized roles (teacher, spouse, parent, friend) Role scripts (teaching = papers, preparing/giving lectures, etc.)		Workplaces
			Gathering or recreational sites
Performance Capacity (mind, body, brain)	Musculoskeletal, neurological, cardiopulmonary, cognitive images	**Occupational Adaptation:** motor, process, communication, interaction skills	Occupational identity, occupational compentence

workplaces, and gathering or recreational sites. These are settings that should be evaluated by occupational therapists when planning and facilitating patient adaptation. Habituation refers to features within these settings that are familiar and that suggest, guide, and sustain purposeful occupational behavior.

A general outline for organizing data about the human occupation system is found in Table 10-1.

For definitions and elaboration of all these terms, the reader is referred to Kielhofner's *A Model of Human Occupation, Fourth Edition* (2008). Additionally, current updates on MOHO may be found at the following Web site www.moho.uic.edu.

Function and Dysfunction

Humans require constant maintenance and reorganization, which is accomplished through the person's ongoing pattern of doing.... Occupation is a dynamic process through which people maintain the organization of their bodies and minds. Engaging in work, play, and activities of daily living serves to organize the self (Kielhofner, 2004, pp. 151-152).

Function in MOHO, therefore, may be defined as the participation, performance, and skill and sustained patterns of engagement in everyday occupations. If a person can describe a typical day at work or home, identify a number of social roles he or she performs, and express satisfaction with these, then he or she is healthy and functional (Kielhofner, 2008). Successful functioning involves the following three outcomes: occupational identity, competence, and adaptation.

According to Kielhofner (2008) occupational adaptation develops from repeated interactions with the environment and consists of two elements: occupational identity and occupational competence. Occupational identity is defined by Kielhofner (2008) as "a composite sense of who one is and wishes to become as occupational being, which is generated from one's history of occupational participation" (p. 153). Sustained patterns of occupational performance lead to a person's occupational competence, which also results from experience. Occupational identity and occupational competence both develop as a result of feedback from the environment.

Dysfunction occurs when occupational adaptation is threatened. Either people's identities do not fit with their possibilities for enacting them or when they become frayed by life circumstances. The causes of occupational dysfunction are multifaceted and can include both intrinsic and extrinsic contributors. Thus, disability may occur because of disorder within the person's volitional, habituation, or performance capacity, or may result from barriers within the physical or social environment. Previously, MOHO, following Reilly's (1974) occupational behavior model, has specified three levels of occupational functioning: 1) exploration, 2) competence, and 3) achievement. These have also been called levels of arousal and accomplishment (Kaplan, 1986; Kielhofner, 1988). Exploration is the lowest level and involves curious investigation of one's self and one's potential for action in conjunction with the properties of the environment. Competence involves striving to meet the demands of a situation through the development of skills and their organization. Achievement includes striving for excellence and the successful performance of roles. Concurrent levels of occupational dysfunction are also described as inefficacy, incompetence, and helplessness. Inefficacy, the least dysfunctional level, implies a reduction of motivation, satisfaction, or control (Bruce & Borg, 2002). While these concepts are no longer mentioned in Kielhofner's latest edition of MOHO (2008), they are nonetheless used as guidelines for group activity selection by Kaplan (1988) and others.

There are many assessment tools originating from this frame of reference, which can help occupational therapists to specify which parts of the system are disordered or malfunctioning. The state of order or disorder is easily observed in the client's occupational behavior.

Change and Motivation

Change in the MOHO involves self-organization in the person's internal and external life structure. In recovering from illness, this often means restructuring a person's daily routines of occupational engagement and re-establishing role performance and participation. For example, Angie's roles were office administrator, wife, and mother of a 5-year-old son. When, at age 35, she was hospitalized for depression following a bitter divorce, all of her roles became inactive. The occupational therapist collaborated with Angie in restructuring her life so that she could resume her roles as worker and mother. Angie was able to volunteer while in recovery to help maintain her administrative skills. She arranged to have dinner with her son each evening and to take him on an outing one day on the weekend. In restoring these roles, Angie was able to organize her already existing skills into a normal daily routine. She showered and dressed each morning, went to her volunteer job each day, and met her son at a relative's house for dinner each evening.

The preceding therapy program addressed the habituation and performance subsystems. Grieving over the loss of her role as spouse was dealt with in counseling and resulted in Angie adding several activities during the week in order to make new social contacts, like joining a tennis club and attending weekly meetings of a church social club.

The therapeutic work involves getting Angie moving toward the regular performance of desired occupational behaviors. Normal, everyday activities are the media used, and the client herself makes the choices of activity, with the help and guidance of the occupational therapist. This work can often be more effective when presenting within the context of OT groups for people with similar circumstances or occupational issues.

Motivation in this frame of reference is attributed to an innate urge to explore and master the environment. Many writers have been credited with the elaboration of this concept, which is said to have a biological basis (Kielhofner, 2008). The best known of these is R. H. White (1960) who contributed the ideas of competence, adaptation, and motivation. Motivation speaks to the meaningfulness of activities. The meaning in occupation is derived not only from the individual, but from the context of his or her social and cultural environment. Part of the OT's job is not only to restore individual task performance but also to identify and restore meaningful roles in society.

A major value of the MOHO lies in its holistic view of the individual and its helpfulness in organizing data about clients' specific dysfunctions. Many examples exist in the literature of the application of the MOHO in identifying patterns of occupational dysfunction.

Group Interventions

A group intervention example given by Kielhofner (2008) is called "Premier Episodes," referring to a program in Quebec City for young adults during their first episode of schizophrenia. The goal for this program was early intervention to prevent the social consequences of prolonged illness that typically involve compromised cognitive, emotional, and social functioning. MOHO was selected as an overall approach because of its focus on occupational performance and its many reliable and valid assessment tools. OTs led a "group workshop therapy" program with two to six members at a time for 90 minutes, focusing on activities chosen by clients. Goals for OT groups were awareness of volitional thoughts and feelings, identifying basic challenges clients wished to undertake, and practicing process and communication skills needed for successful occupational participation. OTs in this program also ran groups combining MOHO with cognitive-behavioral group strategies, such as emotion regulation and psycho-educational groups. Outcomes for 90 clients, as reported by Briand and colleagues (2006) showed improvement in subjective experiences, cognitive and social functioning, and quality of life (Kielhofner, 2008, p. 461). Several aspects of its superstructure are helpful in program planning. For example, a balanced occupational therapy program is ensured when one incorporates group activities addressing the areas of self-care, work, and leisure. Another concept was to organize a program by using the three levels of occupational functioning. Kaplan (1986, 1988) described a group program for short-term psychiatry using group activities at the levels of exploration, competence, and achievement.

Kaplan calls this type of group a "directive group." Exploration level groups incorporate simple activities to help the most severely disorganized clients to develop basic process skills (planning and problem-solving), perceptual motor skills, and communication/interaction skills. The occupational therapist selects the activities and organizes the environment. The group is structured in four stages:

1. Orientation and introductions
2. Warm-up activities
3. Selected activities
4. Wrap-up

An exercise group is an example of an explorative level group. At the competence level, it is assumed that the clients have basic skills but may need to integrate them into habit patterns: "These groups are designed to help patients identify goals, interests, and needs for meaning and action" (Kaplan, 1986, p. 476). Some examples of groups at this level are task groups and activity planning groups. Groups at the achievement level are designed to help clients integrate skills into daily life roles (Kaplan, 1986). Examples of achievement-level groups are assertiveness training and leisure awareness. For more information on the directive group, the reader is also referred to Kaplan's *Directive Group Therapy* (1988).

Group Structure and Limitations

Within the components of the three subsystems of MOHO, the most useful concept for organizing groups is roles. Roles help define the goals for clients and will

dictate the kinds of skills that will need to be restored or strengthened for occupational performance or adaptation within those roles. Therefore, in MOHO, it is best to disregard diagnosis and focus on the social roles people intend to return to or find. Grouping people according to their need to maintain a home, care for children, socialize, participate in recreational activities, or engage in gainful employment allows them to learn from and support each other in adapting their routines, role scripts, and environments to accommodate physical or mental limitations.

It has been stated that the use of the MOHO is not limited by age or diagnosis. Functional levels are organized by levels of arousal and achievement and by the components of the three subsystems that are functioning within the human open system. The focus of occupational therapy in the MOHO is on occupational engagement and not on components or process.

Role of the Therapist

The therapist in MOHO plays the role of an adviser and collaborator. He or she counsels the clients in the various aspects of occupational functioning. Kaplan's "directive group" is so named because of the "active and supportive way in which the group leaders elicit adaptive behaviors and structure the environment to assure maximum participation of all the members" (Kaplan, 1986, p. 477). This role of leader as "director" is necessary for groups that have severely disorganized occupational behavior. However, even at this level, the occupational therapist encourages the active participation of the clients. The occupational therapist continues at higher levels to facilitate, not direct. Thus, the clients' sense of control and personal efficacy is reinforced by the occupational therapist as the client continues to acquire new skills and make personal choices.

Goals

Goals are not discussed as a separate issue in the MOHO. The goal is to restore order in daily functioning, both internal and external. Therefore, the goal of group treatment may be seen as finding and engaging in meaningful occupations and meaningful roles in society. Group intervention goals are concerned with performance of normal daily occupations: work, daily living tasks, and play. They may involve any or all of the three subsystems. In the volitional subsystem, exploration of values and rekindling the urge to explore and master the environment may be goals. Habit formation or the acquisition of new roles may be goals in the habituation subsystem. Learning and practicing the skills necessary to perform the tasks of one's chosen or valued roles can be goals in the performance subsystem.

Examples of MOHO Activities

An updated criterion for placing clients in groups, according to Janice Burke, co-founder of MOHO, is to group them according to their anticipated social roles (1997, personal communication). Common roles, such as homemaker, caregiver, worker, or student, all suggest clusters of skills and tasks that may be selected for group activities. MOHO stresses the use of the client's normal daily activities as the modalities of choice. Groups designed around common roles, as Burke has suggested, can incorporate specific tasks or skills that need to be practiced or adapted. The more common media used in therapeutic groups include cooking, money management, home maintenance skills, parenting skills, leisure planning, and work skills. The client's own interests guide activity selection, and the focus is on the real problems of everyday living. Some kinds of activities necessitate longer sessions. The environment is important in providing feedback to the patient and challenging him or her to further exploration.

Part of the activity planning should address the intended roles and social environments the members will seek out or return to after recovery. Skills and tasks will seem meaningless unless they are connected to meaningful roles that reconnect them with their social groups and help them fulfill a useful purpose. This connection with society and with culture is what sets MOHO groups apart from groups in other frames of reference.

Some occupational therapy group activities used in a program based on the MOHO are described in Activity Examples 10-1 through 10-4.

ECOLOGY OF HUMAN PERFORMANCE MODEL

Originally designed as a model for OT curriculum development and interdisciplinary research and practice at the University of Kansas, EHP's main focus is on contexts (Dunn, 2007; Dunn, Brown, & McGuigan, 1994). Ecology is defined as the transactions between people and their contexts.

Framework Focus

EHP emphasizes the importance of the contexts within which people of all ages perform tasks. The AOTA Framework-II (2008) defines six occupational contexts: personal, physical, social, cultural, temporal, and virtual. The construct of the person in EHP includes most of the client factors described in the Framework-II, physical, sensorimotor, and psychosocial skills (motor and process skills), and the ability to attach meaning to tasks (spiritual) within specific environments. Tasks may fall within any of the occupational performance areas of the Framework-II: self-care, instrumental activities of daily living, work, education, play, leisure, rest and sleep, or social participation. Intervention descriptions within this model also resonate closely with the Framework-II concepts, including establishing or restoring task performance abilities, adapting/modifying the task or context, altering contexts, preventing circumstances that may cause problems, and creating opportunities for task performance that may also take the form of advocating for occupational justice.

Basic Assumptions

There are four basic constructs and four basic assumptions presented within this model. The words task or activity are used to facilitate communication with other disciplines.

Four Basic Constructs

The four main constructs of the EHP model are person, task, context, and performance. Each person brings a unique and complex array of skills, abilities, interests, patterns or doing, and social roles. Tasks are defined as objective sets of behaviors, such as playing a game, writing a check, or driving a car. Tasks are the building blocks of occupations, and the way each person organizes tasks leads to the occupational performance and enactment of social/occupational roles.

Contexts, the interdependent conditions that constitute a person's surroundings, must be carefully evaluated within EHP. Two aspects are specifically defined: temporal and environmental. Temporal contexts refer to the client's age and life stage including life experiences, as well as the timing of task availability and difficulty. For example, children lose the opportunity to go to public school after a certain age, and for adults vocational or career training involves certain time commitments with many steps along the way. The second aspect of context includes physical, social, and cultural environments that define, shape, and expand or limit the range of task availability (Dunn, 2007).

Performance is the person-context-task transaction that "determines what behaviors and level of participation will be possible" (Dunn, 2007, p. 129). The range of occupational performance includes all possible interactions of person and context variables. Because both people and contexts are constantly changing, often the resulting performance is difficult to predict.

Four Basic Assumptions

Some of the initial applications of EHP were applied to OT practice with children (Dunn, Youngstrom, & Brown, 2003). However, these assumptions can also be applied across the lifespan.

1. There is a dynamic relationship between children and their contexts. In order to design relevant OT interventions, practitioners must first understand the child's circumstances, background, abilities, and expectations within his or her specific contexts and demands for performance. In the broader view of the child in context, participation rather than disability becomes the focus of intervention.

2. Contrived and natural contexts are different from each other. Clinical settings, while having the benefit of being specifically designed to elicit optimal task performance, often don't bear enough similarity for the child to perform tasks learned there in natural settings. It is important to analyze the relatively unpredictable attributes of the child's natural settings in order to enable his or her best performance in those settings.

3. Occupational therapy practice promotes self-determination and full inclusion. This assumption takes the client-centered focus into consideration, focusing intervention upon what the child wants or needs to do. Inclusion involves building supports in the child's environment and advocating for the child's rights to full participation. This includes working with families, schools, and other natural settings to overcome contextual barriers.

4. Independence occurs when wants and needs are satisfied. Devices and technology may be necessary tools to promote self-direction and participation in natural settings. Contextual and task adaptations in natural settings should be tried first, so that the child's need for personal adaptation and training can be determined. Dunn (2007) gives the example of changing the seating arrangement in a classroom so that the child can interact with others. From observing the child's performance with this adaptation, his or her need to participate in a social skills training group can best be determined.

Function and Dysfunction

Function may be determined by the range of task being performed. People who are highly functional "have the capacity to perform numerous occupations and roles that match their person variables and natural contexts" (Cole & Tufano, 2008). Dysfunction occurs when mismatches exist between the person and his or her contexts and tasks. The implications for OT intervention, therefore, apply equally to the variables within and outside the person. EHP explains disability as the incongruity between people's abilities or deficiencies and features within the contexts and tasks that prevent or impede performance of important life roles.

Change and Motivation

Personal perceptions of expectations for performance as well as interest in doing specific tasks determine motivation. Through a client-centered collaboration within the therapeutic relationship, the client and OT together will then identify what needs to change. If a child wants to play with other children in a playground setting, the OT then acts as facilitator to enable the child to perform play tasks within that context. The child may

need to learn new skills, the playground equipment may need to be adapted, and the other children and their adult supervisors may need to change their behaviors in order to support the child's inclusion in the playground experience.

Group Intervention

Designing groups always follows a thorough client-centered assessment because the intervention focuses on the client's occupational preferences and priorities. The identified steps in evaluation include the following: 1) Identifying the client's wants and needs, 2) Doing an analysis of identified tasks to understand task demand, 3) Observing and evaluating clients' present capacity to perform selected tasks, 4) Identifying and analyzing desired contexts for task performance, 5) Assessing the person variables, and 6) Assessing the person/task/context match. Group interventions focusing on the overall goal of client engagement in preferred occupations might best be organized around the tasks that are connected with the occupational priorities of members.

Group Structure and Limitations

Several group compositions are implied by EHP:

- Groups of clients with similar interests, needs, situations, and contexts—for example, several children with sensory processing difficulties may practice learning or play tasks together within a natural context they share, such as a classroom or recreational facility.

- The client and his or her peers within a natural context—for example, a group of adolescents participating on a sports team, one of whom may be the client.

- Groups of caregivers or other professional team members in addition to the client—for example, parents, teachers, and other health professionals may meet to discuss possible adaptations of learning tasks and contexts in a school setting.

- People from the community (populations) who wish to maintain health and well-being when faced with occupational challenges—for example, community-living older adults who can no longer drive and need to adapt to the use of public or alternate transportation in order to continue their occupational roles, such as home maintainer, social participant, or volunteer.

The time and place of group sessions vary widely with client needs and circumstances. Natural contexts are preferable so that clients may practice task performance within their own life circumstances. For example, a group of people recovering from substance addiction may meet in a public community setting so that they can appreciate all the ways that they will need to support one another in resisting the temptation to return to their old habits. The OT plans group activities, times, and meeting places in collaboration with group members whenever possible.

Role of the Leader

The OT leadership style can change with group needs. When the OT leader works within another frame of reference, such as developmental or sensorimotor frames, he or she uses a more directive approach in using knowledge and evidence for appropriate task and strategy selection. Facilitative leadership is best used when client input is needed within the group design, in order to ensure that meaningful and relevant tasks and contexts are selected. Advisory or consultant OT roles may be more appropriate when working with families, organizations, or interdisciplinary teams, with goals of education or collaboration when dealing with client occupational performance issues.

Group Goals

For the above groups and others that fit this model, the group interventions may follow one or more of five identified OT goals: 1) establish or restore task performance, 2) alter contexts, 3) adapt or modify tasks or contexts, 4) prevent circumstances that may result in disability, or 5) create task opportunities or enhancements. Goals for groups in the EHP model are highly variable and dependent on the client group along with the assessment results.

Activity Examples

Children's task preferences are often connected with play. Using the EHP model, helping children to expand their ability to play a game of stickball might be more easily done in a group intervention. The OT can help the children and their parents to problem-solve different contextual factors that can make their play safer and easier, such as painting boundary lines on the ground and creating barriers around the play area so that the ball will not so easily go into the street. They might decide to change the rules so as to accommodate different levels of ability, so that a diverse group of children can enjoy the game together in the spirit of fair play.

Young adults who want to lose some weight might form a group to assist one another in changing their diets, resisting temptation, and developing activity plans in contexts where they can socialize with their friends without involving food. Such a group might begin with those recovering from a health condition, such as traumatic brain injury, depression, or diabetes, and the OT's role might be gathering and presenting educational resources, as well as sharing evidence to help members make the best use of the group structure to create an ongoing source of mutual social support. The OT applies therapeutic use of self in facilitating this type of group

so that client members learn supportive interpersonal skills and collaborative decision-making to determine the agenda, the goals, and the activities for each session, using a client-centered group format. The focus on adaptation of tasks and contexts applies the principles of the EHP model.

OCCUPATIONAL ADAPTATION

This occupation-based model was originally developed by faculty at the Texas Women's University as a guide to OT research and curriculum development (Schkade & Schultz, 1992a). With the idea of adaptation as a central focus, first introduced within frames of reference in pediatric practice such as sensory integration (Ayres, 1972) and spatiotemporal adaptation (Gilfoyle, Grady, & Moore, 1981), the occupational adaptation (OA) model expands its application to adults across the lifespan. OA represents one of the most complex of the occupation-based models, incorporating dynamic inter-relationships of multiple factors and subprocesses, with relative mastery and occupational adaptation as the optimal goal.

Framework Focus

The focus of OA encompasses all of the areas of occupation, performance skills and patterns, client factors, activity demands, contexts, and environment. Like other occupation-based models, OA is a holistic, client-focused, and systems-oriented OT approach, reflecting the process of the AOTA Framework-II (2008). Additionally, the importance of therapeutic use of self in the role of facilitator for the client's internal adaptive process is critical to the OA model (Schultz, 2010).

Basic Assumptions

Occupational performance is a part of the normative process of human adaptation. Most models make the assumption that when clients become functional, they can adapt. The OA model assumes the opposite—that when people have the capacity to adapt, they can function (Schultz, 2010).

Three Basic Elements of Adaptation

The process of occupational adaptation involves the interaction of three basic elements, the person, the occupational environment, and the interaction between them. While the model defines each part separately, their inter-relationships in reality are complex and dynamic.

- Each person possesses an internal desire for mastery. The desire for mastery of the environment is viewed as an innate human condition, even at the cellular level. Additionally, each individual brings unique sensorimotor, cognitive, and psychosocial systems that contribute in varying degrees to all occupations.

- Occupational environments are made up of occupational roles (OR) regarding work, play/leisure, and self-care, and occupational contexts (OC) representing physical, social, and cultural influences on occupational performance.
- The person-occupational environment interaction involves several stages or levels: the press for mastery presents an occupational challenge, which then interacts with the occupational role expectations to yield an occupational response. This occupational response is the external observable outcome representing the internal process of occupational adaptation (Schultz, 2010).

Four Subprocesses of Occupational Adaptation

The broader process described within the person-occupational environment interaction is comprised of four subprocesses: adaptive response generation, integration, and evaluation, and evaluation of response outcome. Each subprocess has several components, making the entire process of adaptation exceedingly complex.

1. Adaptive response generation sub process – anticipates the necessary components of an adaptive response. Three mechanisms are involved in this sub process, all of which occur simultaneously to produce an Adaptive Response Gestalt:

   a. Adaptation energy—people use energy at either the primary or secondary level. This concept came originally from Seyle's research on stress responses (1956).
      i. Primary level requires a great deal of cognitive effort and attention.
      ii. Secondary level—cognitive processes continue to work on solving a problem even when the person is engaged in non-related activities.
   b. Adaptive response modes—when presented with an occupational challenge:
      i. Existing responses within the person's repertoire are tried first, and if they fail,
      ii. Modified responses are attempted, and if they fail,
      iii. New responses may then need to be created
   c. Adaptive response behaviors—consist of a classification system adapted from Gilfoyle, Grady, and Moore's (1990) spatiotemporal adaptation frame of reference. Response behaviors, again selected from an internal repertoire, may be either:
      i Hyperstabilized—continuing to attempt the same solution regardless of outcome. These are also called primitive response behaviors.

      ii. Hypermobile—moving rapidly from one response to another with no positive outcome, also called transitional responses.
      iii. Mature—stable, goal-oriented, focused, new behaviors generated with high creative energy and having a higher probability of positive outcome (DeGrace, 2007).
   d. Adaptive Response Gestalt represents the entire process of response generation, which eventually results in a planned response. When the person carries out the plan, the result produces an observable occupational response (Schultz, 2010).

2. Adaptive Response Evaluation Subprocess—occurs when the person evaluates the quality of the occupational response, which OA refers to as the extent of "relative mastery" (Schultz, 2010, p. 467). The judgment of mastery is an internal, highly personal experience, not directly observed or measurable by others. The evaluation of relative mastery reflects the following self-judgments. If the resulting judgment is positive, there is little need for further adaptation.

   a. Efficiency
   b. Effectiveness
   c. Satisfaction to self
   d. Satisfaction to others.

3. Adaptive Response Integration Subprocess—activated when the person's judgment of relative mastery is unsatisfactory. This prompts the individual to try different or new responses to the same occupational challenge and try to produce a better outcome. Integration involves the following reflective processes:

   a. Overall evaluation of the occupational event
   b. Recalling the event and perceived need for change, and
   c. New learning or knowledge about the event that can be applied in future occupational challenges.

4. Evaluation of Response Outcome Subprocess—after the occupational response is generated, the outcome evaluation subprocess is activated. Signs of the outcome of an occupational response may be offered or sought from the physical, cultural, and social environment. Positive and negative features of outcome may enter the reflective process of the person or may indicate aspects of the occupational environment that could also be adapted or changed. This last step allows people to benefit from environmental feedback and thus enables them to raise their level of participation with others through occupational engagement and within desired occupational environments (Cole & Tufano, 2008).

Function and Dysfunction

The continuum of function and dysfunction includes three possible states: occupational adaptation, homeostasis, or occupational dysadaptation. Adaptation is identified through the clients' experience of relative mastery. Further definition of these may be interpreted from the original six basic assumptions of the OA model. Within these statements, functioning is viewed as:

(1) competence in occupation resulting from a lifelong process of adaptation to internal and external performance demands. (2) Demands to perform occur naturally as part of the person's occupational roles and the context (person-occupational context interaction) in which they occur (Schultz, 2010, p. 463).

The OA model views successful occupational performance as the "direct result of the person's ability to adapt with sufficient mastery to satisfy self and others" (Schultz, 2010, p. 463).

(3) Dysfunction occurs because the person's ability to adapt has been challenged to the point at which the demands for performance are not met satisfactorily. (4) The person's adaptive capacity can be overwhelmed by impairment, physical or emotional disabilities, and stressful life events. (5) The greater the level of dysfunction, the greater is the demand for changes in the person's adaptive processes (Schultz, 2010, p. 463).

Change and Motivation

Three sources of motivation are mentioned in the OA model: desire for mastery (person), press for mastery (person-environment interaction), and demand for mastery (environment). These three sources interact to create an occupational challenge, to which the person responds through the process of adaptation. Occupational adaptation has defined several subprocesses (discussed earlier) that result in self-evaluation and the integration of environmental feedback in order to spontaneously make necessary changes to build one's repertoire and refine one's occupational responses. Relative mastery of occupational performance is evaluated in terms of its efficiency, effectiveness, and satisfaction for self and others.

When dysfunction occurs, OT practitioners can influence the person's internal adaptive process through carefully observing client problem-solving while doing tasks that are personally meaningful. The OT and client roles are specifically defined as follows:

1. The OT practitioner is the agent of the occupational environment—selects activities, materials, and other environmental features. Schultz (2010) gives examples of both individual and group contexts for evaluation and intervention.

2. OT practitioner incorporates principles of therapeutic use of self. According to Schultz, "the therapeutic relationship is of critical significance in the theory of occupational adaptation.... It is a partnership in which the client takes the lead (and) the practitioner becomes the facilitator" (Schkade & Schultz, 1993; Schultz, 2010, p. 469).

3. The OT practitioner uses occupation to promote adaptiveness. This requires the OT to carefully analyze tasks and synthesize by matching them with the client's adaptive capacity, considering both strengths and limitations in the sensorimotor, cognitive, and psychosocial person systems.

4. The client becomes the agent of change by activating the internal adaptive subprocesses within the context of doing personally meaningful tasks with guidance and support from the OT and/or others in the occupational environment.

Group Intervention

Both evaluation and intervention may occur in the context of groups. The authors of OA have created a guide to practice, which consists of questions that promote professional reasoning in three areas: OA data gathering, OA programming, and evaluation of the occupational adaptation process. While assessment tools from other models and frames of reference may be used, there are no assessment tools specifically designed for the OA model. However, evaluation of adaptive capacity is best accomplished within the context of occupational performance.

Group Structure and Limitations

OA is clear in setting the focus of intervention on occupational roles. According to this model, without roles, there can be no occupations. "OA theory posits that activities take on meaning only within the context of a role" (Schultz, 2010, p. 468). Therefore clients may be placed in groups according to the meaningful life roles they choose to work on in therapy. Another guideline for structuring groups is that the cognitive and psychosocial abilities of group members be similar, so that the OT may facilitate supportive interactions within the group.

Role of the Leader

The OT group leader designs the group around activities that are connected with the desired roles of group members. In designing groups, the leader carefully plans how the occupational environment will be structured, according to the adaptation capacity of members. Activities or tasks that have a concrete end product work best. The setting, timing, seating arrangement, materials and equipment for the task(s), and other aspects of the occupational environment are set up so as to present a just-right occupational challenge for the group. Tasks may be either individual or group-oriented, and the members of the group become part of the occupational environment. The leader facilitates the group so as to take best advantage of member interactions and especially in eliciting feedback about each member's occupational responses. In Schultz's words, the group leader "arranged the physical space, selected the media, and established the social climate and cultural standards for the therapy group" (2010, p. 471).

Skills in therapeutic use of self, such as questioning, listening, empathizing, guiding, and setting limits, are applied in group leadership and promoting appropriate group interactions. The OT adjusts his or her communication methods to match members' ability to process information. Ideally, in the OA model, the activity itself will provide motivation for occupational engagement and activation of the internal processes of adaptation. Teaching, demonstrating, and directing the task is minimized in OA group leadership, so that members must generate their own adaptive responses and engage in all of the internal subprocesses that will promote positive occupational adaptation.

Occupational Adaptation Group Goals

Goals of any OA intervention are to facilitate improvements in client "adaptiveness." Group goals may not be any more specific, because of the internal nature of the adaptation process and the differences among members' adaptive capacity within a particular group. While the task may produce an end product, the goal of OA groups is more on process and learning, and this will be reflected in the occupational responses of members, their interactions with the leader and each other, and the facilitated discussion that follows. DeGrace discusses two levels of intervention: occupational readiness and engaging in occupational activities. Readiness activities target specific skill deficits, while occupational activities, practiced within the context of the client's occupational roles, focus more on development of better adaptation strategies and producing more acceptable experiences of relative mastery.

Occupational Adaptation Activity Examples

Schultz (2010) describes an open craft group in a school setting, within which members worked mostly in parallel, each doing their own craft project. DeGrace (2007) describes OT evaluation and intervention with family groups based on Werner's (2001) study of five families facing the occupational challenge of caring for a child with autism. DeGrace proposes sample interview questions to stimulate family members to examine and evaluate their collective occupations, such as, "What are some things your family wants (or needs) to do?" "Walk me through a day in your (family's) life. What are some barriers or experiences you know will be challenging?" "At this moment, how happy (satisfied) are you with your family's occupational performance (caregiving, family outing, holiday celebration, other)?" (p. 115). Families with several children in addition to the child with autism indicated that their occupational outcomes were often inefficient, ineffective, and non-satisfying for members. The OA evaluation served as an "empowerment tool" for families to identify which responses are satisfactory and which needed to be modified (p. 120). One outcome of this intervention was the family's realization that they were giving priority to their caregiving for the child with autism at the expense of other family occupations.

A community group example is the Opportunities to Promote Self-responsibility (OPS) program, a sheltered workshop program developed for criminal offenders with mental illness, based on the OA model. The participants were evaluated and, based on their interests and abilities, were assigned to one of three work crews: 1) handmade papermaking crew, 2) leather craft crew, or 3) ceramic craft crew. As members of work teams, workers progressed from trainee to apprentice to master craftsman as their occupational performance improved. The OT facilitated these groups by providing occupational challenges at each worker level. Results showed that the program produced improvements in technical skills, performance behaviors, social skills, and independent functioning within the occupational role of worker (Stelter & Whisner, 2007).

PERSON-ENVIRONMENT-OCCUPATION MODEL

The PEO model is one of several that focus on interactions between person, environment, and occupation. This model is similar to the Canadian Model of Occupational Performance and Enablement (CMOP-E) described in Chapter 3. It differs mainly with respect to the discussion of occupation. "Authors of the PEO model view occupation as part of a hierarchical structure—occupation, task, and activity—whereas CMOP-E discusses the three purposes of occupation: self-care, productivity, and leisure" (Townsend & Polatajko, 2007, p. 29).

A group of faculty at McMaster University in Canada developed the PEO model while researching the effects of environment on occupational performance. The model helps OTs to better understand the dynamic and transactive relationships between persons, environments, and occupations. The Canadian Occupational Performance Measure (COPM; Law, Baptiste, Carswell, et al., 2005) was developed as an analytic tool for assessment and intervention using the PEO model.

Framework Focus

As with other occupation-based models, all of the domains listed in the AOTA Framework-II (2008) fall within this model. The person includes client factors and performance skills, occupation includes occupational performance areas, patterns, and demands, and environment includes contexts. Evaluation focuses on each component of occupational performance, person, occupation, and environment, as well as the transactions among them. Intervention may address one, two, or all three major components. Authors recommend the PEO model as a guideline for OT interventions with individuals or groups, as well as organizations or population programming. The main goal of OT interventions in this model is to maximize the fit between person, environment, and occupation, so as to enable the best possible occupational performance.

Basic Assumptions

Some of the roots of the PEO model come from environmental psychology, architecture, anthropology, and the social sciences. The three main components are person, environment, and occupation.

Person

The person embodies physical, emotional, cognitive, and spiritual characteristics. People use their various skills and capacities to perform occupations connected with a variety of roles throughout life. Both occupations and roles are influenced by one's family and cultural groups. For children, typical roles are child (of parents), learner, player, and friend. In adulthood, worker and citizenship roles are added.

Environment

PEO defines environment very broadly as, "contexts and situations occurring outside individuals that elicit responses from them" (Law & Dunbar, 2007, p. 30). It includes multiple levels of social systems following Bronfenbrenner's (1995) ecological systems model of the contexts within which human social development occurs. The settings within which a person lives change over time and interact to accommodate the needs and desires of the developing person. These contexts include social, political, economic, institutional, physical, and cultural. Contexts shape the person's occupations and roles at the level of household, neighborhood, community, and country in a system of ever-widening spheres of influence.

Occupation

Occupations are groups of self-directed functional tasks and activities in which a person engages over the lifespan. There is an assumption that all humans have an innate need to participate in occupations (Wilcock, 1998). Children and their contexts accommodate each other in an ongoing spiral of growth and development through occupational roles. Patterns of occupation develop over time, and these patterns change with the shifting influence of task demand, environmental press, and the abilities and priorities of the person.

Occupational Performance

In the PEO model, occupational performance is defined as the transaction between the person, occupation, and environment: "a dynamic experience of a person engaged in purposeful activities and tasks within an environment" (Law et al., 1996, p. 16). Furthermore, while occupational performance can be observed, the experience is viewed as subjective (Law & Dunbar, 2007).

Function and Dysfunction

Dysfunction in PEO is a poor fit between person, environment, and occupation. If one views the intersection of three circles representing person, environment, and occupation, occupational dysfunction occurs when the area of overlap is small. Occupational functioning increases when this area of overlap expands, affording the person greater opportunity, better environmental support, and a higher level of competence for occupational engagement.

Change and Motivation

In PEO, people have an intrinsic need for involvement, expression, skill development, and enjoyment. Occupations serve as the means for satisfying this need. When one part of the PEO system changes, all of the others are affected. Czikszentmihalyi (1990) described a dynamic relationship between the challenges of an activity and the person's individual skills. When there is an adequate match between skills and activity demand, the occupational performance will be more satisfying. Conversely, when the person's skill level is inadequate to meet the challenge of an activity, the result will be more anxiety-producing than satisfying. A similar transaction occurs between personal abilities and goals, and demands of the environment. For OT, interventions have the goal of creating a better fit between personal, occupational, and environmental dimensions in order to enable one's optimal occupational performance.

Group Intervention

PEO model supports both individual and group interventions, as well as interventions focused only on environments. Groups have an occupational focus and are directed toward client member goals and priorities.

Group Structure and Limitations

The members may have common roles or occupational issues and, therefore, may select meaningful activities for the focus of group interventions. Preparatory activities using an appropriate frame of reference may also provide guidelines for OT intervention, with the overarching goal of engagement in valued occupations.

Role of the Leader

The style of leadership depends largely upon the ability of group members to process information and make decisions based on information gained through the group experience. Within groups, the leader can organize tasks and contexts to present a just-right challenge that matches the abilities of group members. Groups can meet in natural environments and together problem-solve how to remove barriers to participation and engagement in occupation. The leader orchestrates the components affecting performance to achieve a better fit between the abilities of group members and the task and contextual factors.

Group Goals

Goals are chosen in collaboration with members whenever possible. In some groups, focus will be on building skills of members, while others focus on advocating for environmental changes. For example, a town recreation department worked as a team to develop strategies to make their programs more accessible for people with disabilities.

Person-Environment-Occupation Activity Examples

One recent study used PEO to describe the transactions between clients with Alzheimer's, their caregiving spouses, and the occupations and environments within which they interact. Caregivers experienced "uplifts" or positive outcomes from certain actions and attitudes within their caregiving roles (Donovan & Corcoran, 2010). Activities that provided uplifts were identified as follows:

- Making things organized, such as sorting clothes by color and season, and simplifying table settings during meals.
- Caring for self, such as caregivers eating right, getting exercise, and continuing other roles.
- Maintaining good self-care habits, such as morning routines and bedtime routines.
- Staying engaged with family, friends, co-workers, and paid health workers.
- Engaged in support groups with other caregivers, such as faith-based groups and secular.
- Finding creative ways to communicate with spouse with Alzheimer's, such as non-verbal communication, use of touch or humor.

Some strategies caregivers used to retain positive attitudes were the following:

- Practicing positive approaches to discouraging situations—such as when spouse left the freezer door open all night. Instead of frustration and anger, used as opportunity to "clean out the freezer."
- Using humor instead of outrage—such as making a joke when spouse put together mismatched clothing or added dog food to the casserole.
- Honoring commitment to the marriage—such as continuing family rituals, celebrating holidays and anniversaries, verbally sharing memories, making scrapbooks, showing affection.

Authors of this study suggest that OTs use these guidelines to modify tasks and environments to support uplifting occupations and attitudes to create a better fit between clients and their caregivers. OTs might create a group program for caregivers of clients with Alzheimer's, which focuses on uplifting activities and promotes the positive aspects of caregiving (Donovan & Corcoran, 2010).

THE KAWA MODEL

Kawa means "river" in Japanese. The river serves as a metaphor for the relationships among the variables of occupation in Japanese life and the process of occupational therapy intervention (Iwama, 2006). The model's development in Japan resulted from the realization among Japanese OT educators, practitioners, and students that the occupation-based models, including MOHO, PEOP, and the Canadian Model (CMOP), coming from primarily Western countries did not explain the Japanese practice of OT in a culturally relevant manner. Iwama (2006) writes that Western culture sets occupation in the context of individuals, discrete from nature, separate from social groups, and in an objective and rational manner.

For Western OTs, the real lesson of the Kawa model is the profoundly complex differences that exist between cultures. It is never a matter of simple translation, nor even identifying the ethnic background or religious beliefs of our clients. After many failed attempts to understand and apply Western occupation-based models, Japanese OTs built this theory from the ground up, considering the core beliefs and principles upon which Japanese society is structured. The process of this model's creation attests to the exceedingly complex shifts in thinking that are necessary for the development of true cultural competence.

Framework Focus

For Western OT practice, the Kawa model may apply mainly to working with people from Eastern cultures, as a way to explain the relevance and purpose of OT interventions. The river metaphor communicates the inseparable nature of people from their collective social groups and the inseparable quality of occupations from their natural and spiritual contexts. Clients are defined as inclusive of the individual and other members of the collective. Occupational therapists collaborate with the whole group to assess and design interventions. Occupational challenges occur when internal (client factors) or external (occupational contexts, patterns, or demands) barriers interfere with the working of the group and prevent the river of life from flowing freely. For Japanese clients, occupational performance or engagement may not be the goal. Rather, it is inclusion within the group and the ability to maintain a sense of harmony with others and with nature. This goal might best be achieved through changing social expectations for task performance or changing aspects of the environment. OTs work with individuals facing occupational challenges and their families in order to remove or circumvent barriers and to facilitate participation, so that the life of the collective will continue to flow freely toward its spiritual destiny.

Basic Assumptions

While doing a workshop on occupation-based theory in Japan, Iwama quickly realized that explaining the complex inter-relationships of person, environment, and occupation would have to go beyond merely translating the words. Some of the cultural distinctions he learned from the Japanese OT practitioners were as follows:

- According to Japanese folklore, occupation is "inseparably embedded in nature" and viewed only in cooperation with nature and society (2006, p. 110).

- One person's occupation is not viewed as separate, but collective. Families and social groups have combined identities. An individual's successes and failures, or experiences of health or disability, reflect upon and become the responsibility of the group as a whole.

- Reasoning and reality are situational, making it difficult to apply general theories in all circumstances. The social status of the people involved in any situation has a profound effect upon problem definitions, analytical methods, and decision-making strategies affecting both goal and outcome.

- Ideas and opinions are not accepted on their own merit. The perceptions, thoughts, opinions, or feelings communicated are heard, accepted, or rejected by others according to the status or seniority of the person speaking. Junior members of a group generally defer to more senior members.

Kawa's Grounded Theory Building

A naturalistic research study was designed to build a relevant description of the OT practice, which had been developing for 35 years in Japan. Japanese educators, practitioners, and students formed multiple focus groups, which met monthly, 50 times over 2.5 years in order to discover the shared meaning of occupation, therapy, health, and disability and other relevant concepts within a Japanese cultural framework. Some of the focus group questions were the following:

- How do you as Japanese OTs conceive of the concepts of health, disability, and illness?

- What (if any) role or relationship does OT have with these concepts?

- As an OT, what is your role in Japanese society?

- As an OT, what do you do and why?

- Who are your clients and what are you concerned with?

Even the process of focus groups had its cultural challenges. The groups were kept small in order to minimize barriers of speaking in front of a large group. Groups with members of similar status and OT specialty area, and senior members had to be specifically asked to disregard the typical social hierarchy and to encourage the participation of junior members. Sometimes, ideas had to be written on cards in order to circumvent the socially stratified rules of verbal communication. Sometimes, the groups generated group diagrams in addition to verbal responses. The research investigators also supplemented the focus group format by separately interviewing four senior OT participants.

The various ideas from brainstorming sessions within focus groups were summarized and clustered into categories using methods familiar to Japanese researchers, color coding, sticky notes, using lines and arrows to indicate relational connections, and sorting and arranging index cards to create an "idea map" for the project. Using these methods, five elements were identified:

1. Life flow and health

2. Environmental factors, social and physical barriers, and "ba" (features of social structure)

3. Life circumstances and problems

4. Personal assets and liabilities

5. OT Interventions

Throughout the above analysis, Iwama notes the "complete absence of linearity or directionality" in the relationship of concepts. They simply co-existed, each tied to all others, and no one concept took a central place. All were inseparable from others in a "dynamic rubric" (Iwama, 2006, p. 128). The river metaphor clearly expresses this quality better than linear diagrams.

Meaning of Elements of the River Metaphor

As mentioned earlier, Kawa means river in Japanese. The elements are water, riverbed bottom and sides, rocks, driftwood, and spaces between these.

Water represents life flow and health. I can represent one person's life from birth (the river's source) to death (the mouth where the river meets the sea). Or, the water can represent the life of the whole group or collective.

Rocks represent life circumstance and problems. Rocks vary in size and impede the water's flow. They could be injuries, illnesses, or misfortunes, as well as developmental health conditions.

Driftwood represents personal assets and liabilities, attributes that can help or hinder the water's flow. Driftwood can create log jams in the river, but it can also clear away rocks or other barriers and create new pathways of flow.

River bottom and sides represent external environmental factors, including width and depth (the range and opportunity of flow), and the effect of social factors and relationships.

Spaces between elements provide opportunities for occupational therapy interventions where shifting elements can create new pathways of flow.

The river metaphor is a graphic description of a complex systems perspective of occupation and therapy and accurately depicts the Japanese view of life as a "complex, profound journey that flows through time and space" (p. 143). Although the word "occupation" does not appear in the metaphorical description, it exists everywhere in the Kawa model, because "without water flowing, there can be no river…without occupation, there can be no life" (p. 140).

Function and Dysfunction

In this model, disability is a collective experience. Therefore, the existence of a health condition in one individual does not, in itself, create a disability. Within the metaphor, many situations can disrupt the river's flow: a narrow or shallow riverbed, piles of rocks, piles of driftwood. The person is not represented as a separate element, because the person exists within all the elements. The Japanese "self" is just another manifestation of nature and context. Functioning can be equated with the flow of water in the river; greater speed and volume may represent greater health and well-being. Rather than participation in life through engagement in occupation, functioning in this model is broadly defined as finding ways to "yield to nature and circumstance and find ways to live in harmony with them" (p. 140).

Change and Motivation

According to the Kawa model, people are strongly motivated by the need to be accepted and to belong. This need takes priority over the goals of mastery, independence, or occupational performance. However, occupations can also be the means for the water's flow, that is, a person's occupations define his or her contribution to and status within the social group. Occupations can become a method of change, or a part of a problem's solution. Therefore, clients may desire the ability to engage in occupations that will increase their positive contributions to a collective effort, will restore their sense of belonging within the group, or will increase the overall harmony within the group and with nature.

Additionally, Japanese people have a heightened sensitivity to social status and, within the social structure, feel motivated by a desire for equality with others of their perceived status. This sometimes takes the form of belongings to which they feel entitled, based on status rather than achievement or talent. Occupations that result in a desired end product, which enables them or their families or social groups to gain equality with their neighbors, can be highly motivating.

Group Intervention

Metaphorically speaking, OTs help clients to identify their current status through drawing their "kawa" and identifying those elements that have caused the water to cease flowing. In a group evaluation, the OT may ask clients to "draw the rocks that prevent your life from flowing"—these are the barriers to participation through occupational engagement. The clients' personal and group perspectives are revealed through the drawing. Occupational therapy's role is to find opportunities for intervention within the spaces between elements in the client's "kawa" and to use occupation to impact those elements. The role of OT is "not to control nature and circumstance," but to yield to them and to find ways to increase the flow of life within them (p. 140). Whenever possible, OT uses "the power of the water itself to facilitate nature's course" (p. 193).

Group Structure and Limitations

There are not many published examples of the use of the Kawa model with groups. There are a few ways to structure groups implied in the model, such as working with selected members of a collective, one of whom might be an identified client, or forming a group of individuals within a population, such as people with mental health issues. Given the social nature of relationships within this cultural context, opportunities to form groups based on common roles or occupations might be limited, especially if individual members come from different collectives or hold divergent status within them. Given the cultural limitation described within the focus group used to develop this model, issues of social structure will need to be carefully considered when choosing members of a therapeutic group.

Role of the Leader

The OT leader may find directive leadership styles more appropriate for this model, because the role of the "patient" still implies passive obedience in Japanese health care. The role of educator may be the most acceptable, because clients are motivated to learn occupations and strategies that will increase their river's flow. Group problem-solving has established models in Japan, for example, the KJ method (Kawakita, 1967), which involves brainstorming ideas, writing them in "idea bubbles" on a white board, or writing on cards and pasting them onto a large sheet of paper, forming a graphic view of the ideas of the whole group.

Group Goals

In addition to increasing flow, other analogies can guide the goals of a group. For example, the group might learn and practice social skills, because inadequate social ability might threaten the individual's ability to belong to a group, and social "stigma" might cause people with poor social skills to be denied the opportunity to participate in the mainstream of Japanese society (p. 186). Occupations involving communication and social interaction give group members practice and feedback regarding their ability to become one with the environment or to live in harmony with others. In some examples, Japanese OTs enhanced the Kawa model, using foliage along the river's edge to represent health and human services and resources available to the client. Groups might together explore how and where to access such services. The group might also be organized around transitions, such as clients who are moving from hospital to community settings or from community to institutional settings.

Kawa Model Activity Examples

Moving rocks in the river may not always be possible. Rocks representing personal attributes such as anxiety and physical weakness may be addressed through mobilizing the driftwood, (practicing strength training, learning coping strategies). If the rocks represent social barriers such as stigma, unemployment, or lack of transportation, these rocks may possibly be moved through advocacy for social change or using one's social networks or spheres of influence.

GROUP LEADERSHIP GUIDELINES FOR OCCUPATION-BASED MODELS

In occupation-based models, the activity or occupation itself is considered health-producing, and the need to take great pains to share it or understand its process is de-emphasized. In keeping with the greater emphasis on occupational engagement, Step 2) "sharing" has been eliminated, and Step 3) "processing" is optional. There are longer and more frequent group meetings, and activities tend to be longer or ongoing, so that discussions of general principles and application are not necessary during every session. However, the introduction and summary should be done without fail and should serve the purposes outlined in Chapter 1.

Introduction

Greetings and description of the purpose are done thoroughly at the outset of each activity. A warm-up is optional and can be used to set the mood or energize clients if appropriate. The expectations may be general and somewhat tentative as the members will have input and make choices as the group progresses. The timeframe often varies according to the activity and therefore should be started at the beginning of each session.

Activity

The thrust of all group activities should be moving clients toward meaningful roles in their own social environments. People with similar roles or intended roles are grouped together so that their task choices are likely to be similar also. At the exploratory or occupational-readiness level, the activities selected for groups are generally designed to help clients develop basic life skills. Clients who need to work on these skills are grouped together. For example, those who need to develop routines for self-care might do a series of skill-building sessions, such as maintaining fingernails and toenails; doing laundry; selecting appropriate clothing; applying make-up; shaving; and caring for teeth, hair, and skin.

Clients with similar occupational goals such as returning to work may be encouraged to set their own goals within the group context. For example, the title of the group may be "time management," and within that theme, clients may plan their own individual time schedules with tasks that are meaningful for them in their own social/cultural contexts.

Occupational groups may focus on life roles such as parenting, work re-entry, leisure planning, or home management. Community re-integration might be the desired outcome of members of such groups. Within the context of models, OTs may draw upon other frames of reference to address specific functional problems; they may select activities because of their sensory qualities within the sensory integration frame of reference, for example, as preparatory activity to be followed by a more cognitive task. Clients may practice social skills based on the cognitive-behavioral frame of reference, in preparation for participation in social events in their community.

Processing

While optional, this step may become relevant when emotional issues occur among group members. Discussion of feelings about other group members or group events may be necessary when such emotions create barriers to occupational goal achievement.

Generalizing and Application

The meaning of the activity is discussed with the group as outlined in Chapter 1. This is done after the activity is completed and focuses on how the activity relates to the life roles of the members. Similarities and differences among group members are de-emphasized. For example, in the vocational readiness group described in Activity Example 10-2, the skills learned in doing a leather craft project may be generalized to a client's possible job options. Concentration, efficient use of tools, work neatness, and finishing on time are skills necessary for both. This kind of discussion leads directly into application. A group discussion in the vocational-readiness group will necessarily focus on individual application of skills, as clients' vocational plans are likely to differ widely. Feedback from the occupational therapist on results of the vocational rating scale should also be presented in the group. The group focus is useful to confirm the therapist's observations and give a stronger message to clients. For example, a member may have done very careful work and showed considerable manual skills, but he or she may have taken excessive time to do so. The reality of the workplace is not only to do quality work, but also to meet deadlines. The group discussion may help the client see the necessity to compromise and perhaps curb his or her perfectionist tendencies.

Summary

The summary should review the purpose and goals of the group and should determine what the group accomplished. Focus on individual achievements and strengths should be confirmed. The skills learned may be general or different for each member, and their application should be reinforced in the summary. Future plans, goal achievement, and life roles to which occupational therapy activities apply may be discussed by each member as part of the summary.

REFERENCES

American Occupational Therapy Association. (2008). Occupational therapy practice framework: Domain and process, 2nd ed. *American Journal of Occupational Therapy, 62,* 625-683.

Ayres, A. J. (1972). *Sensory integration and learning disabilities.* Los Angeles, CA: Western Psychological Services.

Barris, R. (1985). Occupation as interaction with the environment. In G. Kielhofner (Ed.), *A model of human occupation: Theory and application.* Baltimore, MD: Williams & Wilkins.

Bronfenbrenner, U. (1995). The bioecology model from a life course perspective: Reflections of a participant observer. In P. Moen, G. H. Elder, & K. Luscher (Eds.), *Examining lives in context: Perspectives on the ecology of human development* (pp. 599-618). Washington, DC: American Psychological Association.

Bruce, M. A., & Borg, B. (2002). Frames of reference in psychosocial occupational therapy. Thorofare, NJ: SLACK Incorporated.

Cole, M., & Tufano, R. (2008) *Applied theories in occupational therapy.* Thorofare, NJ: SLACK Incorporated.

Czikszentmihalyi, M. (1990). *Flow: The psychology of optimal experience.* New York, NY: Harper & Row.

DeGrace, B. W. (2007). The occupational adaptation model: Application to child and family interventions. In S. Dunbar, Ed., *Occupational therapy models for intervention with children and families* (pp. 97-125). Thorofare, NJ: SLACK Incorporated.

Donovan, M., & Corcoran, M. (2010). Description of dementia caregiver uplifts and implications for occupational therapy. *American Journal of Occupational Therapy, 64,* 590-595.

Dunn, W. (2007). Ecology of human performance model. In S. Dunbar, Ed., *Occupational therapy models for intervention with children and families* (pp. 127-155). Thorofare, NJ: SLACK, Incorporated.

Dunn, W., Brown, C., & McGuigan. A. (1994). The ecology of human performance: A framework for considering the effect of context. *American Journal of Occupational Therapy, 48,* 595-607.

Dunn, W., Youngstrom, M., & Brown, C. (2003). Ecological model of occupation. In P. Kramer, J. Hinojosa, & C. B. Royeen, Eds., *Perspectives in human occupation: Participation in life.* Baltimore, MD: Lippincott, Williams & Wilkins.

Gilfoyle, E., Grady, A., & Moore, J. (1990). *Children adapt.* Thorofare, NJ: SLACK Incorporated.

Hammel, J. (1999). The life rope: A transactional approach to exploring worker and life role development. Work: A *Journal of Prevention, Assessment and Rehabilitation, 12,* 47-60.

Iwama, M. K. (2006). *The Kawa Model: Culturally relevant occupational therapy.* Toronto, Canada: Churchill Livingstone.

Kaplan, K. (1986). The directive group: Short-term treatment for psychiatric patients with a minimal level of functioning. *American Journal of Occupational Therapy, 40,* 474-481.

Kaplan, K. (1988). *Directive group therapy.* Thorofare, NJ: SLACK Incorporated.

Katz, N. (1988). Interest checklist: A factor analytical study. *Occupational Therapy in Mental Health, 1,* 45-55.

Kawakita, J. (1967). *Hassou hou; souzu sei kaihatsu no tame ni.* Tokyo: Chou Kouronsha.

Kielhofner, G. (1978). General systems theory: Implications for theory and action in occupational therapy. *American Journal of Occupational Therapy, 32,* 637-645.

Kielhofner, G. (2004). *Conceptual foundations of occupational therapy* (3rd ed.). Philadelphia, PA: F. A. Davis.

Kielhofner, G. (Ed.). (2008). *A model of human occupation: Theory and application* (4th ed.). Baltimore, MD: Williams & Wilkins.

Kielhofner, G., & Burke, J. (1985). Components and determinants of occupation. In G. Kielhofner (Ed.), *A model of human occupation: Theory and application.* Baltimore, MD: Williams & Wilkins.

Kielhofner, G., Burke, J., & Igi, C. (1980). A model of human occupation, part 4. *American Journal of Occupational Therapy, 34,* 572-581.

Kielhofner, G., Forsyth, K., & Barrett, L. (2003). The model of human occupation. In E. Crepeau, E. Cohn, & B. Schell (Eds.), *Willard & Spackman's occupational therapy.* Philadelphia, PA: Lippincott, Williams & Wilkins.

Law, M., & Dunbar, S. (2007). Person-environment-occupation model. In S. Dunbar (Ed.), *Occupational therapy models for intervention with children and families* (pp. 27-50). Thorofare, NJ: SLACK Incorporated.

Law, M., Cooper, B., Strong, S., Stewart, D., Rigby, P., & Letts, L. (1996). *The person-environment-occupation model: A transactive approach to occupational performance.*

Lindquist, J., Mack, W., & Parham, L. D. (1982). A synthesis of occupational behavior and sensory integration concepts in theory and practice, part 2: Clinical applications. *American Journal of Occupational Therapy, 36,* 433-437.

Mack, W., Lindquist, J., & Parham, L. D. (1982). A synthesis of occupational behavior and sensory integration concepts in theory and practice, part 1: Theoretical foundations. *American Journal of Occupational Therapy, 36,* 365-374.

Meyer, A. (1982). The philosophy of occupational therapy. Reprinted from the Archives of Occupational Therapy (Vol. 1, pp. 1-10) in *Occupational Therapy in Mental Health, 2,* 79-89.

Nelson, D. (1988). Occupation: Form and performance. American *Journal of Occupational Therapy, 42,* 633-641.

Reilly, M. (1962). Occupational therapy can be one of the great ideas of 20th century medicine. *American Journal of Occupational Therapy, 16,* 1-9.

Reilly, M. (1974). An explanation of play. In M. Reilly (Ed.), *Play as exploratory learning: Studies of curiosity behavior* (pp. 117-155). Beverly Hills, CA: Sage Publications.

Rogers, J. (1982). Order and disorder in medicine and occupational therapy. *American Journal of Occupational Therapy, 36,* 29-35.

Schkade, J., & Schultz, S. (1992a). Occupational adaptation: Toward a holistic approach to contemporary practice, Part 1. *American Journal of Occupational Therapy, 46,* 829-837.

Schkade, J., & Schultz, S. (1992b). Occupational adaptation: Toward a holistic approach to contemporary practice, Part 2. *American Journal of Occupational Therapy, 46,* 917-926.

Schultz, S. (2010). Theory of occupational adaptation. In E. Crepeau, E. Cohn, & B. Schell (Eds.), *Willard and Spackman's Occupational Therapy* (11th ed., pp. 462-475). Philadelphia, PA: Lippincott, Williams & Wilkins.

Seyle, H. (1956). *The stress of life.* New York, NY: McGraw Hill.

Stelter, L., & Whisner, S. M. (2007). Building responsibility for self through meaningful roles: Occupational adaptation theory applied in forensic psychiatry. *Occupational Therapy in Mental Health, 23,* 69-84.

Townsend, E., & Polatajko, H. (2007). *Enabling occupation II: Advancing an occupational therapy vision for health, well-being, & justice through occupation.* Ottawa: Canadian Association of Occupational Therapy.

White, R. H. (1959). Motivation reconsidered: The concept of competence. *Psychological Review, 66,* 126-134.

White, R. H. (1960). *Competence and the psychosexual stages of development.* Nebraska Symposium on Motivation. Lincoln, NE: University of Nebraska.

Wilcock, A. (1998). Reflections on doing, being, and becoming. *Canadian Journal of Occupational Therapy, 65,* 248-257.

Young, M. (1988). *The metronomic society: Natural rhythms and human timetables.* Cambridge, MA: Harvard University Press.

MOHO Activity Example 10-1
The Special Events Group

This group is designed for exploratory-level clients (chronic mentally ill) whose social relations and daily routines are severely disordered. The purpose is to increase orientation, to expand their level of awareness to the world outside themselves, and to work on time planning and social skills. The focus is on events in people's lives, such as holidays, birthdays, welcomes, and goodbyes and how to celebrate them. The group is organized by the month and begins with a planning session at the beginning of each month. The group meets for 2-hour sessions.

Materials: Poster board with lines drawn up like a monthly calendar. Other materials are colored markers, colored paper, scissors, glue, blank cards and envelopes, cake mixes and frosting ingredients, large sheet cake pan, cake decorating kit, two large punch bowls, ingredients for punch, cake knife, serving ladle, paper supplies for parties, birthday candles, coffee maker, cream and sugar, and access to a kitchen for baking.

Directions: (For a typical month, October.)

October						
Sun	**Mon**	**Tues**	**Wed**	**Thurs**	**Fri**	**Sat**

Figure 10-3. Special events group monthly calendar.

Week 1—Organize monthly calendar (Figure 10-3).

Write name of month and numbers. Therapist begins by writing "1" on the day the month begins. Identify season and decorate calendar with designs appropriate for the season: pumpkins, cornstalks, leaves. Identify holidays for that month, and write on calendar or decorate with appropriate symbols. Survey all patients and staff on ward to find out whose birthday is in October and write on calendar. Identify one day for the whole ward to celebrate October birthdays and Halloween and write on calendar.

Post the calendar in a prominent place on the ward. Other events, such as discharge dates and arrival or departure of staff, may also be added.

Plan what tasks need to be done for the celebration (e.g., make cards, bake cake, shop for supplies, think about masks or costumes for Halloween theme) and decide when to do each.

From Cole, M. B. *Group dynamics in occupational therapy: The theoretical basis and practice application of group intervention* (4th ed.). Thorofare, NJ: SLACK Incorporated. © 2012 SLACK Incorporated.

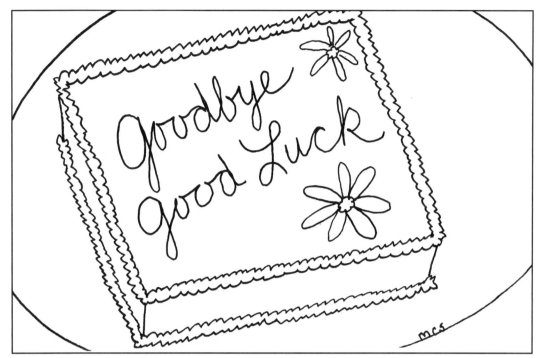

Figure 10-4. Cake decoration.

Week 2—Make cards. Identify birthday people and write names on index cards. Each member makes one card. If there are not enough birthdays, make some for Halloween, too. Each patient designs the card and writes the name and message inside. Stencils and markers, colored paper shapes, scissors, and glue should be available for the less "artistic."

Clients then circulate around the ward gathering signatures for the cards. A shopping list is made for needed refreshment items, eggs and milk for cake, ingredients for punch, etc. (The therapist does the actual shopping.)

Week 3—Bake cake and decorate. Group meets in kitchen. Needed items should be set out on table ahead of time (e.g., bowls, mixing spoons, measuring cups and spoons, eggs, confectioner's sugar, cake decorating supplies, etc.). The large sheet cake pan holds two complete cake mixes, so the recipe should be doubled (assuming a ward size of 20 or more).

The group divides into work teams and roles to accomplish this.

- Cake bakers—Recipe reader, measurer, mixer, timer.

- Frosting makers—Recipe reader, measurer, mixer.

- Designers—Choose motif or theme, border design, colors, and message.

Supply frosting makers with desired food coloring. Trace motif design on paper (jack o' lantern) and cut out. Write out message on paper and check spelling of "Happy Birthday" and "Happy Halloween."

Members learn to use decorating kit to decorate cake, frost in white, do border, trace motif, and write message. All may help with this "fun" part, and all help clean up (Figure 10-4).

When finished, the entire cake is frozen to be used the next week. The ward is informed of the date, and the exact time and place are decided at a ward community meeting. Permission of staff is necessary.

From Cole, M. B. *Group dynamics in occupational therapy: The theoretical basis and practice application of group intervention* (4th ed.). Thorofare, NJ: SLACK Incorporated. © 2012 SLACK Incorporated.

The Special Events Group (Continued)

Week 4—Celebration. Preparation time is 1 hour. Take cake out of freezer 2 hours ahead. Cover a large table with a sheet in the party room. Set up chairs in a large circle. Set out punch bowls, and make punch. Make coffee in coffee maker; set out cream and sugar. Set out plates, forks, cake knife, cake, cups, ladle, spoons, and napkins. Bring the cards. Put the birthday candles on the cake. Bring matches or a lighter. When everything is ready, gather clients and staff.

Party—Estimated time is 30 minutes. Give a toast. Members serve everyone punch, but do not drink it right away, save it for the toast. The whole group is asked to take turns proposing toasts or sharing wishes with honored members. Members lead group in singing "Happy Birthday." Candles are lit. Birthday people must come forward and blow out candles. Group members serve cake to all. Members serve themselves last. Informal socializing occurs while cake is being served. People help themselves to more punch or coffee.

Clean up and discussion—Estimated time is 30 minutes. All members help clean up. When finished, group gathers in a meeting room to discuss and evaluate what roles members played, give feedback, verbalize what skills were learned, and discuss how to apply skills.

MOHO Activity Example 10-2
Vocational Readiness Group

This group uses craft or office activities to explore interests and practice work-related skills. The group runs for 4 weeks and has been used with clients with acute mental health conditions or substance abuse. Appropriate members are those whose goal is to take on a work role after discharge. Group meets in 2-hour sessions. The goals of the group involve all three MOHO subsystems.

1. Volitional—Clients identify and explore their interests by selecting to do craft or office tasks.

2. Habituation—Clients gain and/or maintain good work habits, such as punctuality and following directions, in anticipation of regaining the worker role.

3. Performance—Clients practice basic work skills such as concentration, organization of time and materials, quality of workmanship, and task follow-through. Specific skills like typing and woodworking may also be learned and practiced.

Materials: Two typewriters, access to a copy machine, file cabinet with files and labels, typing tutorial manual, typing paper, workbench with vise, electric drill, band saw, pine boards, plywood, wood patterns, sandpaper, painting supplies, leather work supplies, belt blanks and key fob blanks, buckles, rivets, stamping tools, punch, mallets, bowls of water, sponges, and written directions for making several projects at several different levels of complexity.

Week 1—Evaluation and project choice. Members begin by doing a Work Activity Checklist. The basis for this is Noomi Katz's adaptation of Matsutsuyu's Interest Checklist (Katz, 1988.) For this group, the checklist has been modified to include work-related activities. The scale has been designed to include five work categories as follows.

Vocational Readiness Group (Continued)

1. Office Work
Typing
Using computers
Filing
Answering phones
Using calculator
Accounting and math
Writing letters
Opening mail
Making appointments
Supervising employees

2. Building and Construction
Electrical wiring
Pipe fitting
Assembling parts
Working on cars
Woodworking
Refinishing furniture
Installing carpeting
Landscaping
Gardening
House painting

3. Communications/Teaching
Writing articles
Making posters
Painting signs
Broadcasting news
Introducing people
Reading books
Giving lectures
Giving exams
Taking notes
Teaching children

4. Sales/Service
Showing houses
Selling clothing
Doing make-up
Serving food
Styling hair
Giving sales pitches
Giving fashion shows
Travel planning
Dining with clients
Planning conferences

5. Home Maintenance
Washing dishes
Mopping floors
Cooking
Wallpapering
Arranging furniture
Grocery shopping
Menu planning
Doing laundry
Mixing drinks
Washing windows

Vocational Readiness Group (Continued)

Work Activity Checklist

Activity	INTEREST Some	Casual	None	PAST PERFORMANCE Usual	Some	Never	FUTURE Yes	No
Typing	❑	❑	❑	❑	❑	❑	❑	❑
Electrical wiring	❑	❑	❑	❑	❑	❑	❑	❑
Writing articles	❑	❑	❑	❑	❑	❑	❑	❑
Showing houses	❑	❑	❑	❑	❑	❑	❑	❑
Washing dishes	❑	❑	❑	❑	❑	❑	❑	❑
Using computers	❑	❑	❑	❑	❑	❑	❑	❑
Pipe fitting	❑	❑	❑	❑	❑	❑	❑	❑
Making posters	❑	❑	❑	❑	❑	❑	❑	❑
Selling clothing	❑	❑	❑	❑	❑	❑	❑	❑
Mopping floors	❑	❑	❑	❑	❑	❑	❑	❑
Filing	❑	❑	❑	❑	❑	❑	❑	❑
Assembling parts	❑	❑	❑	❑	❑	❑	❑	❑
Painting signs	❑	❑	❑	❑	❑	❑	❑	❑
Doing make-up	❑	❑	❑	❑	❑	❑	❑	❑
Cooking	❑	❑	❑	❑	❑	❑	❑	❑
Answering phones	❑	❑	❑	❑	❑	❑	❑	❑
Working on cars	❑	❑	❑	❑	❑	❑	❑	❑
Broadcasting news	❑	❑	❑	❑	❑	❑	❑	❑
Serving food	❑	❑	❑	❑	❑	❑	❑	❑
Wallpapering	❑	❑	❑	❑	❑	❑	❑	❑
Using calculator	❑	❑	❑	❑	❑	❑	❑	❑
Woodworking	❑	❑	❑	❑	❑	❑	❑	❑
Introducing people	❑	❑	❑	❑	❑	❑	❑	❑
Styling hair	❑	❑	❑	❑	❑	❑	❑	❑
Arranging furniture	❑	❑	❑	❑	❑	❑	❑	❑
Accounting and math	❑	❑	❑	❑	❑	❑	❑	❑
Refinishing furniture	❑	❑	❑	❑	❑	❑	❑	❑
Reading books	❑	❑	❑	❑	❑	❑	❑	❑
Giving sales pitches	❑	❑	❑	❑	❑	❑	❑	❑
Grocery shopping	❑	❑	❑	❑	❑	❑	❑	❑
Writing letters	❑	❑	❑	❑	❑	❑	❑	❑
Installing carpeting	❑	❑	❑	❑	❑	❑	❑	❑
Giving lectures	❑	❑	❑	❑	❑	❑	❑	❑
Giving fashion shows	❑	❑	❑	❑	❑	❑	❑	❑
Menu planning	❑	❑	❑	❑	❑	❑	❑	❑
Opening mail	❑	❑	❑	❑	❑	❑	❑	❑
Landscaping	❑	❑	❑	❑	❑	❑	❑	❑
Giving exams	❑	❑	❑	❑	❑	❑	❑	❑
Travel planning	❑	❑	❑	❑	❑	❑	❑	❑
Doing laundry	❑	❑	❑	❑	❑	❑	❑	❑
Making appointments	❑	❑	❑	❑	❑	❑	❑	❑
Gardening	❑	❑	❑	❑	❑	❑	❑	❑
Taking notes	❑	❑	❑	❑	❑	❑	❑	❑
Dining with clients	❑	❑	❑	❑	❑	❑	❑	❑
Mixing drinks	❑	❑	❑	❑	❑	❑	❑	❑
Supervising employees	❑	❑	❑	❑	❑	❑	❑	❑
House painting	❑	❑	❑	❑	❑	❑	❑	❑
Teaching children	❑	❑	❑	❑	❑	❑	❑	❑
Planning conferences	❑	❑	❑	❑	❑	❑	❑	❑
Washing windows	❑	❑	❑	❑	❑	❑	❑	❑

Vocational Readiness Group (Continued)

The checklist is discussed with regard to interests, past work history, and satisfaction with current work skills. The expectations for the group are then shared. Members are expected to

- Arrive on time or give prior notification of absence
- Appear well-groomed and dressed in clean work clothes
- Follow directions for project/task
- Respond positively to supervision
- Effectively deal with frustration
- Ask for help when needed
- Work independently
- Learn necessary skills
- Follow through on task (meet deadlines); strive for quality of workmanship.

Several starter projects should be ready with written directions for each client. Members may choose projects based on their interests and skills and get started for the remaining time. Examples of starter craft projects are leather key fobs with stamped initials and border, wood wall plaque made from precut 6" x 8" pine board with picture to decoupage or a wood trivet made from a kit. Examples of starter work projects are typing a short letter or sorting tiles by color. Starter projects are intended to teach basic skills and allow the therapist to evaluate the client's manual and cognitive abilities.

Weeks 2 through 4—Clients complete projects as assigned by the therapist. Each client works independently on a different project. At the end of each session, members are evaluated with the Work Behavior Rating Scale, and results are discussed with the clients.

Vocational Readiness Group (Continued)

Work Behavior Rating Scale					
Name			Dates		
Arrives on time (gives prior notice of valid absence)					
Appropriate appearance (well-groomed, clean work clothing)					
Follows directions					
Responds positively to supervision					
Effectively deals with frustration					
Asks for help when needed					
Works independently					
Learns necessary skills					
Follows through on tasks (meets deadlines)					

Scale: 1 = Independent and correct
2 = Requires some assistance
3 = Requires much assistance
4 = Is dependent or unmotivated

MOHO Activity Example 10-3
The Perfect Parent

This activity is designed for parents who have arthritis or other physical illness involving chronic pain or limitation, who wish to continue being good parents to their young children.

Materials: Worksheets and pencils.

Directions: Have members begin by giving their names and then the names and ages of children living with them. "The purpose of today's activity is to identify some specific concerns involving your ability to care for your children as you deal with the chronic pain and limitations of arthritis." Hand out worksheets and pencils, and give 15 minutes to complete. Areas to consider for parental tasks are meal preparation, dressing, shopping, family events, school-related activities, sports, cultural and social activities, developing special talents or interests, and nurturing/emotional support.

Discussion: The group shares areas of concern from their individual worksheets. Priorities may be discussed, and ideas for coping with conflicts may be shared.

MOHO Activity Example 10-3
The Perfect Parent (Continued)
The Perfect Parent Worksheet

Write name and age of each child:

List and describe five tasks you must perform for your children before 9 a.m. on a typical school day.

1.

2.

3.

4

5.

List five tasks your children would appreciate your doing for them before they return home from school.

1.

2.

3.

4.

5.

List five tasks you must do for your children after 5 p.m. on a typical school day.

1.

2.

3.

4.

5.

Go back over the above lists, and place a * next to those tasks that present potential problems for you in terms of physical exertion or endurance, time constraints, or conflicting obligations.

MOHO Activity Example 10-3
The Perfect Parent (Continued)

The Perfect Parent Schedule Worksheet

Directions: Write the tasks listed on the preceding page in the column "Things I Want to Do for My Children" at the appropriate times. Then, in the next column, schedule in your own needs for rest, exercise, socialization, and other obligations. Put a * next to possible conflicts between these.

Typical School Day	Things I Want to Do for My Children	Things I Want to Do for Myself
6:00 a.m.		
7:00 a.m.		
8:00 a.m.		
9:00 a.m.		
10:00 a.m.		
11:00 a.m.		
12:00 p.m.		
1:00 p.m.		
2:00 p.m.		
3:00 p.m.		
4:00 p.m.		
5:00 p.m.		
6:00 p.m.		
7:00 p.m.		
8:00 p.m.		
9:00 p.m.		
10:00 p.m.		
11:00 p.m. or later		

Conflict areas:

Coping strategies:

From Cole, M. B. *Group dynamics in occupational therapy: The theoretical basis and practice application of group intervention* (4th ed.). Thorofare, NJ: SLACK Incorporated. © 2012 SLACK Incorporated.

MOHO Activity Example 10-4
Forming Good Habits

This activity is designed for people whose daily structure has been disrupted by illness or injury. It starts at the beginning again, with self-care, and assists with building a supportive environment. This activity may require two or three sessions to complete, depending on attention span of members. Contact with family member or caregiver is needed for follow-up.

Materials: 3- x 5-inch cards with pictures of toothbrush, toothpaste, glass, shower or bathtub, bathmat, soap, washcloth, towel, razor, shaving cream, cosmetics, nail file, nail clippers, hand lotion, hairbrush, comb, shampoo, conditioner, and a variety of clothing items appropriate to season and age of members. A second set of cards contains pictures of dishes, utensils, breakfast items, kitchen sink/dishwasher, sponge, broom, dustpan, and trashcan. Duplicate cards should be made for each member. Pictures may be cut out of magazines as needed for this activity. Poster boards, glue or tape, and broad black markers are needed for the second part of this activity.

Directions: Members introduce themselves and discuss familiar morning routines they can remember having in the past. Cards for bathing, dental care, shaving, hair care, and make-up are distributed, and members are asked to select those items used in the morning and place them in sequence in front of them on the table. Items may be sorted into categories and each given separately, depending on the skill level of group members. Dressing and breakfast cards are given in a likewise manner.

Discussion: How can members learn good morning habits? What is the best sequence of tasks for each individual? What is your home environment like? Where can you keep the items pictured on the cards so that you can find them easily each day?

Follow-Up: Poster boards are distributed with labels at the top of each: Grooming and Bathing, Dressing, Eating Breakfast, and Cleaning Up. Each member selects appropriate cards and pastes or tapes them to the poster board in the desired sequence. Members take the poster boards home with them and obtain assistance in gathering the items and finding appropriate storage for the items. The posters serve as reminders until sequences are repeated often enough to form good daily habits of self-care.

From Cole, M. B. *Group dynamics in occupational therapy: The theoretical basis and practice application of group intervention* (4th ed.). Thorofare, NJ: SLACK Incorporated. © 2012 SLACK Incorporated.

PLANNING AN OCCUPATIONAL THERAPY GROUP

This section returns the student to experiential learning. Chapter 11 provides a stepwise structure for the application of theory with client populations, while Chapters 12 and 13 take the form of guided learning experiences.

With the advent of client-centered practice, it is no longer acceptable to simply match theory and technique to a diagnosis. Occupational therapists must take into account client priorities and preferences, activity patterns, and contexts when planning groups for evaluation and intervention. Accordingly, the first step in planning group is to assess client needs. Selecting members for groups was discussed in Chapter 3 as part of the client-centered evaluation. In this section, we will consider designing groups both as intervention and as a part of the process of evaluation.

In Chapter 11, the first learning exercise requires the student to identify a context for occupational therapy intervention. Because occupational therapists work in community as well as institutional settings, a broad range of potential client groups may be considered. For students with limited experience, visits to local community settings are highly recommended. Occupational therapists cannot design effective groups without first gaining a firsthand understanding of the people for whom their groups are designed.

The next step in group planning is selecting a frame of reference that best fits the client needs identified. This sequence reflects both the Occupational Performance Process Model outlined by Fearing, Law, and Clark (1997) and the *Occupational Therapy Practice Framework* (American Occupational Therapy Association [AOTA], 2008). Guidelines are offered for the application of theories discussed in Section Two. This step allows students to review the evidence within the various theoretical perspectives and to consider alternate approaches to client occupational concerns. When an approach is selected, its principles will then guide the process of setting goals, adapting environments, and designing therapeutic group activities.

Concurrently with theory application, the occupational therapist reviews the profession's practice domain to provide a focus for the group design. When client group members have identified specific occupational concerns and priorities, these will guide the selection of group goals, activities, and structure. Groups may be designed to meet multiple goals and to facilitate client involvement in the intervention process. When clients need assistance with sorting out their concerns and priorities, groups may be designed to facilitate self-awareness through learning experiences and group feedback. Observing client occupational performance within the group structure provides valuable insights during the evaluation process as well as intervention.

The group protocol assignment requires the student to design and structure a sequence of six group sessions with a common theme. This gives the student an opportunity to synthesize and integrate the various aspects of clinical thinking that define occupational therapy: client evaluation, theory review and application, consideration of the various domains of occupation, and application of the therapeutic use of the self through the seven steps of group leadership.

Chapter 12, A Group Laboratory Experience, offers a group membership experience as a context for learning about group dynamics. This experience follows the guidelines of the group protocol described in Chapter 11 and thus provides an example of a group intervention designed for students called "Developing Your Professional Self." As a laboratory experience, these sessions can be beneficial for students as they approach the clinical training phase of their education. In the 10 years we have been offering these groups for second-semester juniors, the feedback from students has been excellent. In addition to learning and applying the principles of group dynamics, students have found the feedback for themselves invaluable for their own professional growth.

Respect for diversity is a professional priority, as well as a guiding principle of client-centered practice. To assist students with the application of this principle, Chapter 13, "A Group Experience: Developing Cultural Competence," offers an additional laboratory experience for students. Law and Mills (1998) point out that in client-centered practice:

> ...clients of occupational therapy come from many different backgrounds, have encountered different

life experiences, and have made choices regarding occupation that are unique to them and the situation in which they live. A fundamental concept of client-centered occupational therapy is that therapists show respect for the choices that clients have made, choices they will make, and their personal methods of coping (p. 9).

This chapter applies Black and Wells' (2007) cultural competency model in a series of six group sessions, which can be directly applied in the classroom or as a continuing education series for practicing therapists.

Chapter 14, new to the fourth edition, guides the student in designing group interventions for community groups as possible service learning experiences. Beginning with developing a community profile (Baum, Bass-Haugen, & Christiansen, 2005), followed by a needs assessment (Fazio, 2008), students learn to design and lead focus groups as preparation for their group protocol. Off-site faculty supervisors assist OT students in finding appropriate community contacts and identifying unmet needs. In this way, OT groups serve the community while demonstrating the valuable contributions occupational therapy can offer to organizations and populations outside the umbrella of the medical model.

These experiences facilitate the application of theory in practice. The process of this text has gone from concrete (the seven-step format), to abstract (the frames), and then back to concrete (the protocol). This is not unlike the clinical reasoning process itself, which swings back and forth between the empirical and the hypothetical as the therapy process progresses. A good group plan involves the empirical collection of data about clients' occupational functioning in disability and health, the formation of a hypothesis about what kind of group

activity might be helpful, and a method for evaluation of treatment outcome after implementation (empirical again). The laboratory experiences for students demonstrate this process.

Finally, as part of the practical application of theory to group planning, the student is encouraged to think about how Cole's seven-step group leadership is changed and adapted with each frame of reference. As a learning guide, a chart comparing group leadership in the six frames of reference is presented in Appendix E.

REFERENCES

American Occupational Therapy Association. (2008). Occupational therapy practice framework: Domain and process. *American Journal of Occupational Therapy, 63,* 623-685.

Baum, C., Bass-Haugen, J., & Christiansen, C. (2005). Person-environment-occupation-performance: A model for planning interventions for individuals and organizations. In C. Baum, J. Bass-Haugen, & C. Christiansen (Eds.), *Occupational therapy: performance, participation, and well-being* (3rd ed., pp. 375-388). Thorofare, NJ: SLACK Incorporated.

Black, R., & Wells, S. (2007). *Culture & occupation: A model of empowerment in occupational therapy.* Bethesda, MD: American Occupational Therapy Association.

Fearing, V., Law, M., & Clark, J. (1997). An occupational performance process model: Fostering client and therapist alliances. *Canadian Journal of Occupational Therapy, 64,* 7-15.

Fazio, L. (2008). *Developing occupation centered programs for the community* (2nd ed.). Upper Saddle River, NJ: Pearson Prentice Hall.

Law, M., & Mills, J. (1998). Client-centered occupational therapy. In M. Law (Ed.), *Client-centered occupational therapy* (pp. 1-18). Thorofare, NJ: SLACK Incorporated.

Chapter 11

WRITING A GROUP PROTOCOL

The group protocol is an extensive and detailed outline of a group to be planned by the occupational therapist for a specific client population. Recent group theory suggests that careful planning greatly influences group outcome (see Gersick (2003) study in Chapter 2). This exercise is intended to prepare students and therapists to plan effective programs to meet the needs of clients with a wide variety of characteristics, using multiple frames of reference.

This method of group intervention planning fits well with the *Occupational Therapy Practice Framework's* concept of designing group interventions for populations (American Occupational Therapy Association [AOTA], 2008). The members selected for groups should have common population characteristics (e.g., young mothers with arthritis or unemployed workers with depression) so that their occupational needs and priorities can be evaluated as a group, and interventions can be designed that will have meaning for all members. Given the importance that the framework process places on collaboration, client profiles should be formed as a part of the group member selection process. Care should be taken to orient each member to the format and purpose of the group prior to its inception, leaving no doubt as to why he or she has been assigned to a particular group. The introduction to the group session can then serve as a reminder of the group's intended purpose, and the summary serves as an outcomes review as described in Chapter 1.

PROFESSIONAL REASONING AND THE ART OF GROUP DESIGN

Aside from the scientific reasoning needed when addressing health conditions of participants, designing groups draws primarily upon creativity, which is the art of occupational therapy. Pierce (2003) has studied this creative aspect of practice in her book, Occupation by Design. She reminds us that all people design activities and occupations throughout their daily lives, and so do clients. Yet, in the art of occupational therapy, practitioners can benefit from a more organized approach. Some of the steps Pierce describes are "divergent," or expanding one's thinking through "brainstorming" or an unrestrained flow of group ideas, without the limitations of practicality. Alternately, there are convergent steps in the design process, in which priorities are set and decisions made that will narrow the choices listed in previous steps. Pierce outlines seven phases within the design process:

1. *Motivation*—Recognizing a problem and the need for change, and making a commitment to change. For designers of groups with specific health conditions or other common characteristics, collaborating with group members in a focus group format might be a good place to gather ideas about what potential clients feel most compelled to change in their lives. Motivation is a convergent phase, because it narrows the scope of the problems to those that are client priorities and/or those that are known issues for the chosen population.

Cole M.B. *Group Dynamics in Occupational Therapy: The Theoretical Basis and Practice Application of Group Intervention (pp 317-332).*
© 2012 SLACK Incorporated.

2. *Investigation*—A divergent phase, involving looking for ideas in books, on the internet, and through personal discussions with others, as possible ways to address the identified problem area. A skilled designer looks for as many ways to address the problem as possible in order to have the broadest choice.

3. *Definition*—Brings the design out of the exploratory stage by clustering ideas and comparing them with the previous convergent phase, motivation. In the definition phase, summarize the issue to be addressed in a few words, and establish the criteria the activities must meet to reach the goal. Pierce gives the example of "annual house party" as an activity, and the criteria are it should be fun for guests, seasonal, memorable, include music and dancing, and not too expensive.

4. *Ideation*—Another divergent phase, ideas are gathered using the defined criteria, in a brainstorming fashion, but armed with the resources discovered in the investigation phase. For example, party ideas for each holiday of the year might be matched with other criteria. One can revisit good books, stores, or websites found previously as further sources of ideas.

5. *Idea selection*—As the name implies, this phase requires a decision. Pierce suggests listing pros and cons or creating a rating system using the criteria in the definition to see which idea best addresses the problem.

6. *Implementation*—Setting the date, performing all of tasks in preparation, and actually giving the party. This step parallels the group session outlines required for the group protocol. While the groups will not actually occur, all of the details for a planned hourly session will be written down.

7. *Evaluation*—A most neglected phase of the creative process, this requires reflection on not only the outcome but all of the previous phases leading up to it. Feedback from group members (or party participants) can serve as a good source of feedback, along with suggestions about what could be changed for a better outcome when next designing a similar group.

These steps in creative design of occupations apply directly to the creation of a group protocol. A recent example of the application of Pierce's design approach is described by Egan and Joseph (2010), working with residents of a transitional living facility for people who struggle with HIV/AIDS, homelessness, and substance abuse issues. They designed an OT group to address the emotional problem expressed by clients of feeling "boxed-in," a metaphor for the confinement of the 12-step program they were required to attend as well as other house

rules and requirements within the recovery model. In the 1) motivation phase, they surrounded their office with boxes in various forms, bird cages, fish bowls, etc. 2) Investigation took the form of creating a large poster board with the word "box" in the center; they began "ballooning" out from there, writing many ideas to address the problem through occupational engagement. From this effort, they identified themes such as boxes that provide protection (a playpen), organization (a filing cabinet), enjoyment (a swimming pool), nourishment (cereal box), as well as confinement. 3) Definition, a convergent phase, yielded the following criteria for the group design: have fun, address 12-step requirement, appropriate for adults, cost-effective, just right challenge for 1-hour session, and a feasible, "metaphorically dense" occupation that could continue in the future. In the 4) ideation phase, they considered many activities, narrowed down in the idea selection phase to step-aerobics, swimming, and square dancing, After careful analysis, the 5) idea selected was square dancing. 6) Implementation was accomplished with careful planning and the help of one of the home's board members, who was a square dance caller. Upon 7) evaluation, members continued the metaphor in giving feedback, with comments such as:

- Not paying attention to the contents of her box—A metaphor for self-discovery.

- Not realizing how much fun the box could be—A tendency to always dwell upon the negative, or

- Neither the 12 steps nor recovery are easy—Learning the square dance steps wasn't easy either, but they get easier with practice (adapted from Egan & Joseph, 2010).

This example of the creative process of group design emanated from a client-centered evaluation within which potential group members expressed their issues and concerns with the occupations of group living in the recovery model.

While for students it will not be possible to interview potential clients, the process of indentifying problem areas for a chosen population, investigating potential resources, further narrowing the choices through problem definition, and creating suitable group experiences to address it fall within the scope of this chapter assignment.

Several steps have been outlined to prepare students for writing a group protocol:

- Identifying your client population

- Selecting a model and/or frame of reference

- Selecting a focus for intervention (general problem area)

- Writing a group intervention outline

- Planning individual sessions

IDENTIFYING YOUR CLIENT POPULATION, SETTING, AND LEVEL OF CARE

For the purposes of learning, the student should choose one of the interventions settings (listed in Worksheet 11-1) in which occupational therapists typically work with clients. This will be the client population around which you will plan your group. Star the services and/or level of care from the list of settings and populations that are of interest to you. Investigate the different types of services by using your various textbooks, faculty experts, related OT articles, program descriptions found on the internet, prior personal and professional knowledge and experience, and public marketing resources. For those students who are unfamiliar with some of the diagnoses mentioned or implied in the list of populations, a short research assignment may be appropriate prior to attempting Worksheet 11-1. Once the clients in a given setting are defined with respect to diagnosis, one or two of the most common illnesses can be researched in medical textbooks. In a real-life setting, a needs assessment is the preferred format for defining the population because it includes collaboration with potential clients.

Settings should be chosen on the basis of interest, prior experience, or curiosity. The planning will incorporate a process of familiarization with the chosen population. Because most students do not have much experience, it is advisable to contact a local intervention center and arrange a visit. Prior fieldwork and volunteer experience is also helpful. It is impossible to plan an effective group intervention without some knowledge of the population for which it is intended.

Another way to become more familiar with the population you choose is to do some reference reading. Many excellent books are available describing specific diagnostic categories, such as Alzheimer's disease, multiple sclerosis, drug abuse, eating disorders, and mental retardation. Reading case studies of people with these disorders is particularly helpful.

Probably the most motivating way to choose a client population is personal experience. Many students have friends or relatives who may have a disorder that fits one of the listed categories. Writing a group protocol for a specific individual and others with the same disorder gives the student the advantage of greater personal understanding. It may be easier to imagine the impact of certain group activities and the barriers that may need to be addressed.

HOW TO DO A NEEDS ASSESSMENT

Some students may have the opportunity to work with organizations in the community or to work with nontraditional populations. For these settings, the student should perform a needs assessment in lieu of a population worksheet. Brownson (2001) outlines some helpful steps in performing a needs assessment at schools, worksites, community agencies, and assisted living or other health-care environments for the proposed population for whom your group will be directed. The purpose of community interventions with well populations is to educate and strive to achieve preplanned objectives, such as changes in lifestyle; changes in knowledge, attitudes, skills, or behaviors; and maintenance of improvement in function or health.

A needs assessment is a systematic set of procedures to identify and describe specific areas of need for a given population, which leads to a clear set of goals and objectives for the program (group). The steps are as follows:

1. *Gather background data:* Do an internet search or literature search on the organization for which you are designing a group. Research various aspects of the population you already know, such as adolescents and discipline problems if you are working with a local high school. Choose at least three topics to summarize.

2. *Identify participants for a survey:* Involve the potential participants by collaborating with them concerning their perceptions of the needs, problems, or circumstances that you might potentially address. There are several methods for eliciting potential participant input. Students should choose one of the following:

3. *Written survey:* Design a one-page survey containing both closed- (yes/no) and open-ended questions about the topics of concern. Give it to 20 people, and make arrangements for returning it by having someone collect it or by mail. Because participation is voluntary, you can expect less than half the surveys to be returned.

4. *Face-to-face interviews:* Arrange to meet with a limited number (five or six) of potential participants one at a time. Come prepared with specific questions that will serve as both a guideline and a reminder to gather all the information you intended.

5. *Telephone interviews:* Although this is not the preferred method, it may be more time-efficient. Be sure you have specific questions and a quick way to record the answers before calling. Interview 10 people, and keep track of answers to consider for later analysis.

Worksheet 11-1
Population, Setting, and Level of Care

1. **Setting**—Select one choice for this assignment and circle it below:

- Community mental health programs
- Hospice
- Sheltered workshops/vocational training centers
- Partial hospitalization
- Supported employment
- Child/adolescent day program
- Long-term care (physical and mental health)
- Child/adolescent inpatient program
- Adult day services (social, medical, dementia)
- Child/adolescent residential
- Skilled nursing units—Transitional care
- Community wellness programs
- Assisted living facilities
- Senior centers
- Inpatient rehabilitation
- Home health
- Outpatient rehabilitation

- Psychiatric hospital
- Community transition and re-integration
- Aquatic therapy
- Inpatient psychiatry (adult)
- School systems
- Inpatient rehabilitation
- VA Hospital
- Outpatient rehabilitation
- Hippo therapy
- Developmental disability group homes
- Assistive technology
- Adolescent/adult substance use—Inpatient
- Work hardening/work-related
- Adolescent/adult substance use—Outpatient
- Sober house program
- Support groups (physical, mental, social)

2. **Population Definition**—What population is most likely to benefit from this level of care or service? Gather as much background data as you can find at this time.

   a. Who is most likely to benefit from this type of care (epidemiological factors)? Could they benefit from a group model of care?

   b. What are common health conditions or diagnostic categories associated with this type of care? List client factors and typical client characteristics (etiological factors).

   c. What are common risk factors associated with this population—precautions for care?

   d. What is the rehabilitation potential of this population? What is the typical length of stay? What is the verbal and non-verbal communication capacity like for this population? What is the cognitive capacity of this population?

3. **Context**—What will be the context for your group intervention?

   a. Describe the typical health-care setting in your chosen category by considering the following components:
      o Referral source and requirements for admission
      o Length of stay
      o Typical services offered
      o Any legislative and funding resources or restrictions
      o Discharge disposition of clients

   b. Describe the type of OT services found at this level of care or service.

   c. What is OT's specific role in this setting?

From Cole, M. B. *Group dynamics in occupational therapy: The theoretical basis and practice application of group intervention* (4th ed.). Thorofare, NJ: SLACK Incorporated. © 2012 SLACK Incorporated.

(Adapted by Roseanna Tufano, 2010)

6. *Key informants:* Ask your contact person to identify people who would be most helpful in identifying needs of your potential population, and limit your surveys or interviews to just a few people (three or four).

7. *Focus group:* Invite a small group (eight or less) of potential participants to meet for a brief discussion of their perceptions, problems, and needs relative to your group intervention idea. This is the preferred way to assess the needs of a group of participants because you can also observe their social skills and modes of interaction in a group.

8. Use secondary data, such as archives, prior surveys, and reports by related organizations or agencies. If other "volunteers" or "fieldwork students" have worked with this population before, consult their notes, reports, or summaries. Find out what has already been tried so that you do not repeat past errors. If you cannot find data, interview your contact person (fieldwork supervisor) regarding what group strategies have been effective in the past.

9. *Analyze the data:* Look at answers to survey/interview questions, and find a way to summarize this information for the purposes of group planning. It is not necessary to do a statistical analysis, but charts or graphs are an easy way to get a visual picture of the results. For example, if you would like to do a weight control group for overweight adolescents at a local school, your survey questions might address issues of self-image; facts of height, weight, and diet; and amount of and attitude toward physical activity. Part of your summary will confirm the extent of obesity in this specific group and compare that with information you have previously gathered from the internet regarding adolescent obesity in the general population. Another issue to summarize is the strength of interest your responses indicate in attending a group that focuses on weight control. Self-esteem might be a factor that motivates adolescents to attend such a group, and that can be a part of your "marketing" strategy.

10. Write a profile of the "typical" participant. Include gender, age, educational and cultural factors, diversity factors, family background, and client factors such as verbal and problem-solving skills, functional capacities, and barriers to participation. In a real community setting, you will need to define the inclusionary and exclusionary criteria for membership in your proposed group and share this information with potential sources of member referral.

The needs assessment is included here as a possible alternative to the Population Worksheet. If opportunities exist for planning community groups, students have much to gain from designing a group protocol for a "real" population rather than an imagined one.

Students who choose this option should now move on to the next step, choosing a frame of reference.

SELECTING A MODEL AND/OR FRAME OF REFERENCE

After you describe your client population, the next decision to make is what frame of reference to use (Worksheet 11-2). There are several factors to consider in this decision. The preceding six chapters can be consulted for a better understanding of the choices. While there are many frames of references in occupational therapy, for this assignment, try to stick with one of those included in this text. While personal beliefs usually have some influence over model or frame of reference selection, students should become competent in using all of them.

The major factor in the selection should be what is likely to work best for the clients. Sometimes, the intervention setting has an identified frame of reference, and, if so, the occupational therapist should find an occupational therapy approach that is compatible with it. Some helpful factors to consider include the following:

- View of function and dysfunction
- Client physical and cognitive level of function
- Change strategies
- View of motivation
- Intervention time frame
- Intervention options

View of Function and Dysfunction

Each frame of reference has its unique point of view of disability. Looking at your client population, compare their abilities and disabilities with the explanations of function and dysfunction given in each frame of reference. Which frame best explains the function and dysfunction you see in your clients? Why?

Client Physical and Cognitive Level of Functioning

Some frames of reference have a greater usefulness for higher-functioning clients, while some relate better to lower levels of functioning. Which frame offers intervention guidelines that have been effective for your clients' level of functioning? Summarize guidelines given to your clients.

Worksheet 11-2
Theoretical Framework

Directions: Based on data from Worksheet 11-1, select an occupational therapy model (MOHO, Ecology of Human Performance, Occupational Adaptation, PEO) OR a frame of reference that will be the best fit for your population needs, setting and level of care, domain of concern, and therapeutic activities and occupations. Use the information from other textbooks or class notes as well as Section II of this book to answer the following questions.

The following theory is the best choice for this protocol assignment: _____.

I. Briefly state why you have selected this theory for your protocol assignment.

II. Briefly describe the function/dysfunction continuum of this theory.

III. Briefly describe how this theory defines motivational factors and the "change" process.

IV. What are typical OT assessments that match this theory?

V. What are typical intervention guidelines that relate to this theory?

From Cole, M. B. *Group dynamics in occupational therapy: The theoretical basis and practice application of group intervention* (4th ed.). Thorofare, NJ: SLACK Incorporated. © 2012 SLACK Incorporated.

(Adapted by Roseanna Tufano, 2010)

Change Strategies

Another way the frames of reference differ is in their view of the change process. Some depend on the therapeutic relationship or on group interaction to facilitate change, while others rely more heavily on the components of tasks and activities or on the environment. Think about what changes your clients need to make. Then, look at the explanations given by the frames of reference on how change takes place. Which do you think might work the best for your clients? Why?

View of Motivation

How motivated are your clients? What forces do you think might motivate them to make positive changes? Each frame of reference explains motivation differently. The existential/humanistic view is freedom from anxiety and self-actualization. The ego adaptive, developmental, and neurophysiological frames of reference and Model of Human Occupation describe a drive toward mastery, but each defines something different to be mastered. The cognitive-behavioral approach looks at various forms of reinforcement as the motivator. The goal of most of our occupational therapy groups is to help clients achieve a higher level of function or adaptation. However, it is not enough for the therapist to be motivated. We need to think about our clients' motivation as well. Which frame of reference best explains how our clients could be motivated? Why?

Intervention Timeframe

Some frames of reference work best for long-term intervention that encourages the development of relationships and insight, while others lend themselves to more immediate goals. For the purposes of this assignment, the intervention runs for six 1-hour sessions. But these could be spread out once a week for 6 weeks or condensed into two sessions a day for 3 days. If there is no center mentioned, what would be the most likely setting for the client population you have chosen? Acute settings can be assumed to average 10 days to 2 weeks. Substance abuse programs are generally 1 to 4 weeks of intensive intervention. Day treatment can go on for a year or more, and chronic conditions can be treated for a lifetime. How long are your clients likely to be in treatment? Which frame of reference best fits the timeframe at your identified intervention center?

Intervention Options

Each frame of reference has different guidelines for activity selection. Some have specific suggestions, while others are more flexible and able to be adapted. Which frame of reference offers intervention options that would interest you? What are they? Which frame of reference offers intervention options that would interest your clients and/or best meet their needs? What are some options you might choose?

Combining a Model and a Frame of Reference

Because the occupation-based models have a broad perspective, they provide the overall guidelines for adjusting the best fit of person, occupation, and environment. Models are often used when working with communities or on wellness and prevention with populations. Within that perspective, there may be occupational issues with individuals for which a frame of reference that addresses specific disabilities would be appropriate. An example might be working on fitness or fall prevention with older adults in the community. One could begin by framing the program using the person-environment-occupation model, looking at the environments within which older adults navigate on a daily basis and their overall mobility within those parameters. The groups might also focus on building strength and endurance, using a biomechanical frame of reference. For the purposes of the group protocol, it is acceptable to use no more than one Model and one Frame of Reference. In practice, sometimes more than one frame of reference is used within groups, but never more than one model simultaneously.

SELECTING A FOCUS FOR INTERVENTION

The *Occupational Therapy Practice Framework* (AOTA, 2008) outlines the domains of concern for occupational therapy and the process of evaluation, intervention, and outcomes that enables "engagement in occupation" and "supports participation in life."

The framework domain lists and defines six categories related to human occupation. The order in which the terms are presented has no bearing on their relative importance (see Appendix D).

1. Performance in areas of occupation includes activities of daily living, instrumental activities of daily living, rest and sleep, education, work, play, leisure, and social participation.

2. Performance skills include sensory perceptual skills, motor and praxis skills, emotional regulation skills, cognitive skills, and communication/interaction skills.

3. Performance patterns include habits, routines, roles, and rituals.

4. Seven contexts are specified: cultural, physical, social, personal, spiritual, temporal, and virtual.

5. Activity demands are listed as follows: objects used and their properties, space demands, social demands, sequencing and timing, required actions, required body functions, and required body structures.

6. Finally, client factors are specified as body functions, body structures, values, beliefs, and spirituality.

The document goes on to define each of the terms. For definitions, please refer to the original 2nd edition publication (AOTA, 2008). All of the above-mentioned areas can potentially shape group interventions.

The best strategy is to go over the document in Appendix D and decide what parts of the domain your clients most need to work on or improve. In practice, occupational therapists would collaborate with clients in choosing the most meaningful options. Group evaluations using the focus-group format described in Chapter 1 could be used when time and setting permits. When adapted for OT, focus groups use a client-centered approach, allowing potential group members to verbalize their needs, preferences, and perspectives about occupational issues. The format of focus groups can also help build rapport by conveying an attitude of respect for member individuality. Most clients have more than one occupational priority, and activities in occupational therapy can be designed to address several of the areas identified.

For this assignment, however, you will not have the benefit of client input and will have to rely upon your best judgment. After looking over the framework document, use Worksheet 11-3 to list 10 areas that your client population may need to work on.

The *Occupational Therapy Practice Framework* process lists five intervention approaches:

1. Create, promote (health promotion)

2. Establish, restore (remediation, restoration)

3. Maintain

4. Modify (compensation, adaptation)

5. Prevent (disability prevention)

Using these intervention approaches, write a statement about each domain area you have listed, incorporating one of these five approaches on the worksheet. For example, a group of home maintainers with arthritis might work on instrumental activities of daily living to establish energy-conservation strategies. Statements may be either general or specific. These statements will help the therapist define the scope of the group. For example, sessions might include several instrumental activities of daily living, such as child rearing, home establishment and management, shopping, meal preparation and cleanup, and care of pets, or its focus may be modifying the activity demands for only one of these areas, such as

meal preparation and cleanup for all six sessions. In the next section, these identified aspects of intervention can help us to formulate goals for our group.

Writing a Group Intervention Outline

Once the client population is chosen and the frame of reference and aspects of intervention have been identified, the next step is to write a general outline. The outline should include all the factors inherent in designing a group. The general outline includes the following headings:

- Group title
- Author
- Frame of reference
- Purpose
- Group membership and size
- Group goals and rationale
- Outcome criteria
- Method
- Time and place of meeting
- Supplies and cost
- References

This outline is intended to include not only the ingredients of an effective group intervention protocol but also factors that will be of interest to administrators. Often, occupational therapists are asked to present a group protocol to administrators prior to implementation. Administrators will need to consider factors such as group size, space, scheduling, and cost. The plan you present must not only be therapeutically sound, but also cost-effective.

Group Title

The name of a group is often the client's first impression of the role occupational therapy will play in treatment. Choose it with care. Not only should a title accurately reflect the goals and content of the group, but it should also attract the client's interest. Some examples of good titles are "Developing Self-Identity" (a group for substance abusing adolescents), "Art for Social Skills" (a group for people with chronic mental illness), and "Re-Entering Your Kitchen" (a group for postoperative cardiac clients).

Author

This includes your name and professional title (e.g., Jane Doe, OTS).

Worksheet 11-3
OT Domains and Therapeutic Activities/Occupations

Directions: Based on Worksheets 11-1 and 11-2, identify 10 occupational therapy domains of concern that reflect your population needs, setting, and level of service. Refer to the Framework document as a guide for OT-related concerns. From this list, you will identify general activities and occupations that could match your populations' needs and could be delivered in a group context. Consider activities and occupations that promote health, prevent injury or disability, maintain health, foster safety, restore functioning, and/or remediate for loss of functioning.

1. List 10 performance areas, skills, patterns, etc, that your clients may want or need to work on based on their health condition. Identify three to five therapeutic activities and/or occupations that would relate to these concerns.

OT Domain of Concern	Therapeutic Activities/Occupations
1. _____	_____
2. _____	_____
3. _____	_____
4. _____	_____
5. _____	_____
6. _____	_____
7. _____	_____
8. _____	_____
9. _____	_____
10. _____	_____

2. Review the list above. Now, select one domain of concern for the purpose of this protocol. You may cluster similar concerns into one theme for this assignment. Here is an example. Interpersonal communication can be a theme for people in a mental health partial hospitalization program that includes diagnoses such as mood disorders, substance use, personality disorders, etc. OT intervention strategies for this theme can include verbal and non-verbal written and oral expression, assertiveness training skills, conflict resolution, seeking trustworthy relationships, safe sex practices, etc.

My final selection for this protocol is the _____ domain of concern.

My current ideas for OT interventions include _____

_____

_____

_____ .

From Cole, M. B. *Group dynamics in occupational therapy: The theoretical basis and practice application of group intervention* (4th ed.). Thorofare, NJ: SLACK Incorporated. © 2012 SLACK Incorporated.

(Adapted by Roseanna Tufano, 2010)

Frame of Reference or Model

State the frame of reference you have decided to use to guide your approach to clients, organization of intervention groups, and selection of activities. A single sentence on why this frame of reference is appropriate will suffice. For example: "The cognitive-behavioral approach has been widely used with substance abuse clients, and it seems to help them change their own behavior by learning new ways of thinking about their lives."

Purpose

The purpose of the group is the group's general intent. Overall goals of the group should be stated, as well as the general nature of the activities to be used. This section should be short, preferably no longer than three sentences, and should summarize the overall scope of the group plan. For example, "The purpose of a leisure planning group might be to assist clients whose disability requires a loss of the worker role in identifying and planning leisure activities to meet their social and emotional needs. Clients will complete written exercises, participate in group discussions, and plan and carry out individual leisure activities as part of group requirements."

Group Membership and Size

The client population for which your group is intended should be described in as much detail as possible. Not only general diagnostic factors but factors like age, functional level, gender, and role identity might be included. For purposes of referral, both inclusionary and exclusionary criteria should be described here. Inclusionary criteria describe characteristics that are appropriate for your group. Exclusionary describes characteristics that are not appropriate. Some activities are appropriate for specific groups only, while others encompass a wide variety of characteristics. A target population should always be identified to give the group a focus. Broader applicability of the protocol should be described in a separate paragraph.

For the purposes of this assignment, the size of groups will be limited to three to eight members. It is generally not cost-effective to treat groups of less than three and not effective intervention for more than eight. The size of a group will depend on many factors, such as the degree of impairment, the need for individual attention, and the complexity of the tasks, to name a few. Group membership may be open or closed. A closed group includes all the same clients at every session for the duration of the group. An open group allows members to be added or dropped from session to session. It is generally easier to plan for closed groups, because the membership is predictable and a sense of belonging is developed. Open groups are more practical for most intervention settings and are a necessity in acute settings in which clients come and go rapidly. This assignment requires you to plan a closed group. This allows the student to plan specific sessions without having to adapt to unexpected changes in membership.

Group Goals and Rationale

The goals of a group are the specific intervention aims that are intended to be met by individuals participating in the group. No less than three and no more than eight goals should be stated. Less than three usually means that goals are too vague and therefore not useful in planning specific activities. More than eight gives the group too broad of a focus. Ideally, there should be at least one specific goal for each individual session planned. However, because there is usually more than one goal met with any given activity, the exact number will vary.

Goals should be stated in measurable terms. They should state what the client will do (i.e., define, discuss, report, demonstrate). Vague terms like "learn," "understand," and "develop" should be avoided; "attend" and "participate" are generally not enough of a description to be meaningful. Well-written goals are the backbone of any well-designed group. They will make the rest of the group easier to plan and the outcome easier to measure. For example, the goals of a money management group might be the following:

- Recognize the need for a budget.
- List monthly income and expenses.
- Demonstrate ability to follow a budget for 1 week.
- Demonstrate specific banking skills.
- List anticipated needs and expenses.
- Practice comparative shopping techniques and skills to reduce impulse buying.

Once these goals are identified, the activities used to reach the goals will logically follow. Perhaps each group session can focus on a different goal, or several sessions can include more than one goal. For example, the fourth goal can be addressed by giving each client samples of a check register, check, deposit slip, and withdrawal slip. Simple addition and subtraction can be practiced and included when appropriate. Use of a banking machine or telephone banking can be taught and practiced. The outcome of this activity can be measured by examining the completed forms and watching the demonstrated procedures. Specific activities and measured outcomes should follow logically from each stated goal. Rationale for goal selection should relate goals to the chosen client population and its inherent problems. This section should explain why the goals you selected are appropriate. Limitations of the group should be mentioned—for which clients are these goals inappropriate? For example, clients who will be institutionalized may not need the skills. Precautions that may need to be taken should also be mentioned in the rationale. Adaptations that can be made to make the group useful to a wider variety of clients, perhaps in settings other than the target setting, should be mentioned here as well. For example, in the case of the money management group, the same goals can be applied to any group of clients with the goal of living independently.

Outcome Criteria

The desired results of the group should be stated in behavioral terms. By the end of the group, each client should be able to show how he or she has progressed. The therapist needs to develop a measurable way to demonstrate the effectiveness of the group to the client, the administrator, and to those responsible for payment of services. Specific procedures should be outlined, such as a pre-/post-questionnaire or a pre-/post-rating scale for each client. An appropriate assessment tool can be identified, if one exists, or evaluation can be specific for the group.

Outcome criteria have a direct relationship to the client goals. However, the outcomes also need to relate in some way to engagement in occupations and participation in life. This necessitates greater emphasis on the application part of group discussion during each session, where clients discuss how they will apply this particular group experience to their own lives. It would be appropriate for the therapist to take this opportunity to remind group members how their comments relate to outcome. The topic could be introduced as a discussion question, and feedback from the therapist and other members could occur spontaneously. However, if verbal feedback is used, the therapist should specify where and how this information is to be recorded. The easiest way to keep track of session-by-session progress is to create an observation check sheet or brief comment form ahead of time.

Therefore, for learning purposes, both pre-/post-test, assessment, or questionnaire (such as the Group Member Progress Rating outlined in the next chapter) and a weekly outcomes documentation worksheet must accompany your group outline as separate worksheets.

Methods

An outline of the media to be used and the kind of leadership offered are key elements here. Media can be as simple as structured discussions and as complex as learning to build a small engine. Most activities are fair game. However, complex media that require special training, such as biofeedback, systematic desensitization, bioenergetics, and psychodrama, should not be used. Therapeutic interventions that are the traditional roles of other disciplines, such as family therapy, unstructured verbal psychotherapy, or dietary planning, should also be avoided.

The kind of leadership offered depends upon the therapist's frame of reference. If a psycho-educational format is used, the therapist may include short lectures on skills to be learned (see Chapter 13 for example). The therapist's frame of reference will determine the type of introduction and explanation given to clients during each session. The group protocol should reflect a consistent frame of reference. If a psychoanalytic, developmental, or cognitive behavioral approach is used, more emphasis may be placed on group interaction. Cognitive perceptual, cognitive disabilities, or sensorimotor groups for lower-level clients require more structured environments with carefully planned therapist assistance.

Time and Place of Meeting

Several design elements should be described in this section. For the purposes of this assignment, the time will be limited to six 1-hour sessions. The scheduling of sessions will vary according to the intervention setting. Chronic settings will accommodate weekly sessions. Acute settings may require daily meetings. The length of sessions will vary with client attention span and type of activity chosen.

The place of meeting should be chosen with specific requirements in mind. In an actual intervention setting, a room can be identified. For the purposes of this assignment, only the characteristics of the setting should be described. The following environmental factors could be included:

- Size of room
- Contents (tables, chairs, cabinets, sink, etc.)
- Lighting, windows
- Visual factors (bare walls or more home-like)
- Door opened or closed
- Noise factors (not next to gym or bathroom)
- Accessibility of medical assistance (special telephone equipment needed, if any; kitchen for cooking activities)
- Availability of assistance from therapist
- Safety factors

This assignment will not limit any of these factors. A good room description will take into consideration the characteristics of the client population chosen, as well as the activities to be included.

Supplies and Cost

The sum total of all materials and supplies and their total cost is listed here. It is recognized that copies of forms and paper and pencils or pens are generally available in most settings at no cost. Items other than these should be listed. If specific items such as videotapes or assessment materials are to be used, the name and address of the source of these should also be listed. This section will probably have to be done after specific sessions are outlined.

References

List all references that were used to create the material for the group sessions, including short lectures, forms to be used as worksheets, and other copyrighted materials. References should be in the format of the American Psychological Association (2001):

- *Books:* Author, date, title, publisher, place of publication.
- *Articles:* Author, date, title of article, journal name, volume, and pages.
- *Materials:* Name of item (such as videotape, if used), name and address of source, company, center or hospital, telephone number, and approximate cost.

PLANNING INDIVIDUAL SESSIONS

A group session outline should be written for each of the six sessions of your group.

Headings are as follows:
- Session
- Group title
- Session title
- Format (time sequence)
- Supplies
- Description: Each of the seven steps numbered in order: 1) introduction, including warm-up, educational concepts, or purpose; 2) activity including instructions; 3) sharing including procedures used; and 4 through 7) discussion questions in processing, generalizing, application, and summary.

Sessions 1-6

The session number (session _____ of 6) out of total number of sessions planned indicates sequence. Your group sessions should be planned in logical order, from simple to complex, superficial to deep, general to specific, etc. In a closed group, the sessions should build on one another so that general group principles can be applied. It would make sense for the first session to be somewhat introductory, so that members begin to know not only the subject of the group, but each other as well. Subjects of a more personal nature should be saved for later in the sequence when members know one another better. The last session needs to deal with summary and termination of the group. The way you sequence the sessions will depend somewhat on your chosen population.

Group Title

This is the title of the group as a whole (e.g., "Money Management").

Session Title

Like the group title, each session should be labeled with a word or phrase describing either the content or the goal for that session.

Format

This is a short outline stating what will happen when. For example, a session in "Balancing Your Checkbook" might have the following format:
- 15 minutes—Review last week
- 15 minutes—Introductory short lecture
- 15 minutes—Complete sample checkbook worksheet
- 10 minutes—Check answers with calculator
- 20 minutes—Discuss specific problems and summarize importance of balancing checkbook
- 75 minutes—Total

You need not include this last total figure, but make sure your timing fits the total time allotted for the group.

Supplies

This category includes a complete list of what is needed to complete the group. Do not assume clients will be carrying pens and pencils with them or will be wearing a watch. The supply list should include the correct number of each item needed. For a "Balancing Your Checkbook" session, supplies for a group of five clients would include the following:
- 5 worksheets (attach copy)
- 5 pencils
- 5 pocket calculators
- 1 large pad and 1 marker (for therapist to illustrate process)

Description

This is a step-by-step description of what will be included:
1. The introduction should be fully described, including warm-up (if appropriate), explanation of purpose, expectations, and timeframe. If there are educational concepts that illuminate the purpose, these must be outlined.
2. Activity: If worksheets are to be written, a copy must be attached. Activities must be fully described including directions, choices, timing. If the activity was selected from a text or prior experience, reference should be given.

3. Sharing: Procedures for how individual work is to be shared/discussed with the group is given.

4 through 6. For the discussion part, a list of questions to be asked is included for each of the categories: processing, generalizing, and application. Refer to Chapter 1 for a description of these phases of the group. Your discussions will vary depending on the frame of reference you are using. It is wise to be prepared with more questions than you will need. Also, keep in mind the goals of the group when choosing discussion questions. An activity is generally more effective when the clients feel it has meaning for them. Relating each session's activity back to the original goals will help keep both clients and therapist on track.

7. A verbal summary at the end of each session is important. Include for each session some points to remember for the summary.

INSTRUCTIONS FOR PREPARING THE GROUP PROTOCOL

When you have written the entire protocol, you should type it using a computer. Each session should start a new page. When typing the protocol on the computer, use the exact headings in the order described. Capitalize the headings; use single spacing and 1-inch margins. It is not necessary to indent. Skip a line between each section or heading.

When rating sheets or worksheets are used, a copy should be attached to the outline or session to which it relates. Use the following forms to write your first draft of your Group Intervention Plan Protocol (see Worksheet 11-3).

The next two chapters provide examples of group protocols. The first has a developmental focus, while the second has a cognitive-behavioral focus. For each of these, the role of the leader is facilitator. However, each has a different frame of reference.

REFERENCES

American Occupational Therapy Association. (2008). Occupational therapy practice framework: Domain and process. *American Journal of Occupational Therapy, 62,* 625-683.

American Psychological Association. (2001). *Publication manual of the American Psychological Association.* Washington, DC: Author.

Brownson, C. (2001). Program development for community health: Planning, implementation and evaluation strategies. In M. Scaffa (Ed.), *Occupational therapy in community based practice settings.* Philadelphia, PA: F. A. Davis.

Egan, B. E., & Joseph, M. (2010). *Using Pierce's seven phases of the design process to understand the meaning of feeling "Boxed in": A community-based group.*

Pierce, D. (2003). *Occupation by design: Building therapeutic power.* Philadelphia, PA: F. A. Davis.

Acknowledgments: The author acknowledges Professor Roseanna Tufano of Quinnipiac University, Hamden, Connecticut, for classroom testing and adapting Worksheets 11-1 through 11-3 in this chapter.

Note: James P. Klyczek was co-author of Chapter 11 in the first and second editions. Dr. Klyczek originated the concept of the group intervention plan assignment with the six-session outlines in 1985 and very kindly shared his group dynamics course materials with me. Dr. Klyczek is Assistant Professor and Clinical Coordinator in the Occupational Therapy Program, Division of Health and Human Services, D'Youville College, Buffalo, NY.

Worksheet 11-4
Group Intervention Plan Outline

Group title:

Author:

Frame of reference:

Purpose:

Group membership and size:

Group goals:

1.

2.

3.

4.

5.

6.

7.

8.

Group Intervention Plan Outline (Continued)

Rationale, limitations, adaptations:

Outcome criteria (attach separate sheet as needed):

Method:

Time and place of meeting:

Supplies and cost:

References:

Worksheet 11-5
Session Outlines

Group Session Outline

Session _____ of 6*

Group title:

Session title:

Format:

Supplies:

Description (includes discussion questions as applicable):

*A separate copy of this outline must be used for each of the six sessions of the group.

From Cole, M. B. *Group dynamics in occupational therapy: The theoretical basis and practice application of group intervention* (4th ed.). Thorofare, NJ: SLACK Incorporated. © 2012 SLACK Incorporated.

Chapter 12

A GROUP LABORATORY EXPERIENCE

The following is an example of a group protocol. It is a group designed as a laboratory experience for professional students. Ideally, it is done in groups of eight students, with the instructor as the leader. It addresses some of the most common professional issues for students and serves as a context for the discussion of the principles of group dynamics described in Chapter 2. The series of six sessions is planned in a sequence that moves toward greater intimacy as the group develops. The leadership is also intended to change from directive in the beginning toward a democratic, facilitative style at the end. The group leader models therapeutic interventions with various problem behaviors and fosters the exploration of here-and-now relationships. Members have the opportunity to take on various roles and to practice group interaction skills. Process illumination should be discussed as a part of each session, with a goal of learning and personal growth.

Although this is a six-session sequence, it has been suggested by my students that three open sessions be interspersed. An open session has no planned activity, and its purpose is to discuss the process of prior sessions. After Session 3 in my group, for example, there seemed to be little time to discuss the many issues and feelings resulting from giving and receiving feedback. An open group following this session would give the members a chance to discuss their concerns and to better understand their relationship to each other. Session 4 seemed to be too structured, and several of the groups felt the need to voice their urge to rebel against the structure and/or the directive leadership style. An open session following this one would allow for the discussion of group development and the significance of their rebellion in the context of group development theories. Another interesting addition to the sequence is a leaderless group. This forces the group members to take on leadership roles and further illuminates the group process. This semester, many of the groups decided to end their group with a "termination" activity. One group brought in brunch, another had a pizza party, and another decided on a goodbye collage. With these additions, the group lab experience is expanded to 10 weekly sessions.

Cole M.B. *Group Dynamics in Occupational Therapy:
The Theoretical Basis and Practice Application
of Group Intervention (pp 333-352).*
© 2012 SLACK Incorporated.

GROUP INTERVENTION PROTOCOL

Group title: "Developing Your Professional Self"

Author: Marilyn B. Cole, MS, OTR/L

Frame of reference: The frame of reference for this group is developmental. Students experiment with new ideas and behaviors in anticipation of the next phase of their lives, which involves taking on a professional identity. The assumption is that members are intrinsically motivated to know themselves better and to become competent professionals.

Purpose: This group is designed to help junior occupational therapy students to make the transition from a student role to a professional role. The six group activities are selected to deal with the most common areas of difficulty for students, such as being assertive, accepting feedback, and setting priorities in their lives.

Group membership and size: "Developing Your Professional Self" is designed for second-semester junior occupational therapy students. Most of these students are between 20 and 22 years of age, although several are adults coming back to school. The majority are women who have lived independent of their families for at least 2 years, although there are several men and several students who commute from home. Having entered the junior year in an occupational therapy academic program, these students have all achieved and maintained a high academic average and have survived at least one semester of difficult and challenging professional coursework. All have had at least one semester of clinical Fieldwork I experiences, allowing them a taste of what it is like to work with clients (a few hours per week). In choosing to become occupational therapists, these students have set a goal and are working to achieve it. This will be a closed group of no more than eight members. The same members will be expected to attend all six sessions with no absences (Worksheet 12-1).

Group goals and rationale: The student will do the following:
1. Discuss awareness of professional self in relation to clients and peers.
2. Demonstrate ability to problem solve, behave assertively, and set goals and priorities.
3. Identify strengths and weaknesses of self and others.
4. Express feelings directly and offer respectful feedback to others.
5. Accept feedback from others and use it constructively.
6. Clearly state professional values.
7. Demonstrate ability to interact effectively with peers.
8. Identify group behaviors and group process.

Students in the junior year are learning many of the skills necessary to treat clients. However, in order to use those skills effectively, the student needs to feel comfortable in the professional role. The "Developing Your Professional Self" group is designed to promote a needed self-awareness associated with professionalism. As a professional team member, future occupational therapists will need to interact effectively, behave assertively when necessary, share in group problem-solving, and learn constructively from other team members. Factors other than academic ones will influence professional effectiveness, such as warmth and empathy, flexibility and openness, ability to express feelings, and appropriate self-disclosure. The group format gives students an opportunity to explore and practice needed skills and attributes in preparation for their Fieldwork II experiences. This group design, although planned for occupational therapy students, may also be useful for students in other disciplines. Adaptations would be minimal, simply substituting for "occupational therapy," nursing, physical therapy, social work, etc. The group and interpersonal skills needed by many health professionals are quite similar.

Worksheet 12-1
Contract for Group Membership

This contract should be reviewed and signed by each member of the group before beginning the first session.

I understand I am involved in a developmental process, and, therefore, it is necessary to attend all sessions to benefit fully from the process. I realize that in order for me to be an effective member, it is important that I complete all assignments and arrive on time. I agree to participate as openly, honestly, and responsibly as I am able to, realizing that I am not under any group pressure to reveal personal data that I would regret sharing with the group. I agree to speak personally and make "I" statements as objectively and specifically as I can, trying not to generalize or talk in abstractions. I realize that no personal information about any group member should ever be discussed outside of the group.

Signed: _____

Date: _____

From Cole, M. B. *Group dynamics in occupational therapy: The theoretical basis and practice application of group intervention* (4th ed.). Thorofare, NJ: SLACK Incorporated. © 2012 SLACK Incorporated.

Outcome criteria:

1. The student will demonstrate interpersonal skills by verbal participation at least three times in each weekly session.

2. Students within the context of each session will discuss and demonstrate the skills required for self-disclosure, problem-solving, giving and receiving feedback, empathizing with or confronting others, behaving assertively, and setting goals and priorities.

3. The progress of each student may be rated twice on a five-point scale, one being poor ability and five being excellent ability. The first rating should be before the first session, the second rating after the sixth session. This pre-/post-group rating will then show progress made by each student in each skill required. The Group Member Progress Rating chart (Worksheet 12-2) may be used to measure progress in each of these factors: self-disclosure, problem-solving, giving feedback, receiving feedback, empathizing with others, confronting others, behaving assertively, setting personal goals, and understanding dynamics.

Method: Structured group activities and discussions will occur each week. The activities will be graded from a superficial and safe level to a deeper level interpersonally. The activities will also be graded so as to encourage more group interaction and less dependence on the leader as each week progresses. Group development and interpersonal learning will be encouraged, and an understanding of the process of the group will be facilitated.

Time and place of meeting: The group will meet for 1 hour each week for 6 weeks. The rooms are selected to be free of noise distraction and to preserve the confidentiality of the group. A large table and nine chairs are preferable, so that members can work on group projects. On days when only discussion takes place, chairs may be arranged in a circle without the table. For the 1-hour meeting, it is important that no one leaves or comes late and that there are no interruptions. The door should be closed, and a sign saying, "Do Not Disturb, Group in Session" should be displayed outside.

Worksheet 12-2
Group Member Progress Rating

Rating 1 (low) to 5 (high)	Session 1	Session 6 (or last)
Self-disclosure		
Problem-solving		
Giving feedback		
Receiving feedback		
Empathizing with others		
Confronting others		
Behaving assertively		
Setting personal goals		
Understanding dynamics		

Supplies and Cost

	Unit Price	Total
9 sheets of white drawing paper 12 x 18 inches	Donated	$0.00
16 assorted magazines	Donated	$0.00
5 jars of glue	$1.50	$7.50
9 pairs of scissors	$2.50	$22.50
10 marking pens (set)	$2.50	$2.50
10 pencils (pack)	$1.50	$1.50
1 package 3- x 5-inch index cards	$1.25	$1.25
10 Xerox copies	$0.10	$2.00
9 sheets of typing paper	Donated	$0.00
Total cost		**$37.25**

Adapted from Rider, B., & Gramblin, C. (2000). *Activities card file.* Kalamazoo, MI: Author.

Session 1 of 6

Group title: "Developing Your Professional Self"

Session title: "Professional Self-Awareness Collage" (adapted from Rider & Gramblin, 1987)

Format:
Warm-up—3 minutes
Introduce group lab—2 minutes
Instructions for activity—2 minutes
Collage activity—20 minutes
Sharing—10 minutes
Discussion—20 minutes
Summary—3 minutes

Supplies:
9 sheets white drawing paper 12 x 18 inches
5 jars of glue or 9 glue sticks
9 pairs of scissors
16 uncut magazines
10 marking pens, assorted colors

Description:
1. Introduction
- Warm-up—Ask each person in turn to give his or her name and something he or she likes and does not like about occupational therapy.

- Introduce group lab—Group outline will be shared with the group.

- Purpose—The purpose of this activity is to help us think about ourselves as professionals.

2. Activity
Give out bags and markers. "We will begin by signing our name at the top like this 'Jane Doe, OTS.'" Magazines, glue, and scissors are placed in the center of the table. "Look through the magazines and cut out pictures that represent qualities you have as a professional. We all have some characteristics that we will want to share and have others know about. These may be characteristics that will help us as professionals. Fold the drawing paper in half and paste the pictures representing these on the outside of the folder you have made. You may use both front and back covers.

"We also have some characteristics we would rather not share. These may be a hindrance to our professional identity. Cut out pictures representing these, and paste them on the inside of the folder you have made. When you are finished pasting the pictures, use markers to label each with the characteristic you intend it to represent. You have about 20 minutes to complete this task. We will discuss the collages when we are finished. This will be a good way to get to know each other better."

Give warning when 5 minutes are left. After 5 minutes, collect all materials and place out of reach.

3. Sharing:
Ask for a volunteer to start sharing the collages. Once started, go around the group in order, forcing no one to share more than he or she wants.

4. Processing:
Questions for discussion:
1. How did you feel about doing this activity?
2. How many of us felt comfortable sharing the inside vs. the outside of the folder?

Session 1 of 6 (Continued)

5. Generalizing:

1. How well do you know your professional self?

2. What did you learn about yourself from doing this activity?

3. What did you learn about others?

4. How difficult was it to decide which parts of yourself are "professional"?

6. Application:

1. How will an activity like this help people build a professional identity?

7. Summary:

Points to remember are to be taken from comments of members. Some might be

- The "face" we show to the public is not what is really inside.

- The outside represents what we wish to be, the inside what we fear we may be.

- Students do not find it easy to think of themselves as professionals.

- Some common characteristics are the wish to play a helping role and fondness and empathy for other people.

SESSION 2 OF 6

Group title: "Developing Your Professional Self"

Session title: "Difficult Decisions"

Format:
   Warm-up—5 minutes
   Introduce activity—5 minutes
   Instructions for activity—5 minutes
   Difficult decision writing—10 minutes
   Discussion—30 minutes
   Summary—5 minutes

Supplies:
   8 index cards 3 x 5 inches
   8 pencils
   Basket or box ("hat")

Description:
1. Introduction:
   - Warm-up—Ask members to give names and recall one characteristic about their professional self from last session.

2. Activity:
   "Today, we will discuss difficult professional decisions or problems. Each of you take an index card and a pencil and write on the card a professional problem or decision you have experienced in the past year. You may draw on Fieldwork I experiences, volunteer experiences, or situations in the classroom, as long as they concern some aspect of your chosen profession.

   "You can write about a problem you had difficulty with or had trouble making a decision about. Give necessary background and detail, but you need not identify yourself. We will be putting the cards in a hat and drawing out someone else's problem to solve. You have 10 minutes to write your problem." Give 1 minute warning.

3. Sharing:
   Collect all cards after 10 minutes, and shuffle them. Put them back in "hat," and ask each member to draw one out. If someone draws his or her own, he or she has the option of putting it back and drawing another. "Now think about the problem on the card you drew, and get ready to share with the group how you would solve it. Take turns sharing solutions and discuss."

   For this activity, discussion will be during the sharing rather than afterward. Members have the option of identifying their problem and asking the group for additional help.

4. Processing:
   Questions for discussion:
   1. What feelings are involved in making difficult decisions?
   2. How did you feel hearing someone else address your problem?
   3. What parts of this activity did you find difficult? Easy?
   4. How does it feel to need/ask for help? Receive help?

Session 2 of 6 (Continued)

5. Generalizing:
1. What did you learn from today's activity?
2. Who owns the problems discussed? Who should take responsibility?
3. What did you/others contribute?
4. What is the worst/best thing you could do?
5. If decision, what are pros and cons?
6. Whose decision is it? Should it be?
7. What additional information is needed to decide/solve?

6. Application:
1. What can we learn from each other as professionals?
2. How can we help each other as professionals?

7. Summary:
This activity usually produces much discussion, and often members own up to their own problem. They have become a group of peers working together and trusting one another. A parallel should be drawn to the ideal in practice where no one should feel afraid to ask for the help of his or her colleagues in facing a difficult problem.

SESSION 3 OF 6

Group title: "Developing Your Professional Self"

Session title: "Giving and Receiving Feedback"

Format:
  Warm-up—5 minutes
  Introduce activity—5 minutes
  Instructions for activity—5 minutes
  Writing activity—15 minutes
  Discussion—25 minutes
  Summary—5 minutes

Supplies:
  9 sheets of paper 8½ x 11 inches
  9 pens or pencils

Description:
1. Introduction:
- Warm-up—Begin by asking members to say a few words about how they are feeling today.
- Educational concepts—"Today, we will be working on communication, self-awareness, and accepting feedback from others. Often, the success of our professional interactions will depend on how well we understand our own feelings and express them to others. Even negative feelings can be expressed in positive terms. For example, if you are studying for a test, and your roommate is talking loudly on the phone, you might say to her: 'I know you're enjoying talking to your friend, but I'm having a hard time concentrating on my work. Would you mind calling your friend back later?'"

  "Most people have an easier time giving positive feedback than negative. However, avoiding negative comments can cause all kinds of problems, especially when two people have to work together. This exercise is designed to practice giving positive and negative feedback to each other."

2. Activity:
  Pass out paper and pencils. "Fold paper in half. Put name on the outside folded half at the top. On the inside, write some ways you feel you need to grow professionally (skills needed, issues to deal with, etc.). Fold paper over so what you have written is not visible. Pass folded paper around circle. Each person writes on the outside how he or she feels the person whose name is on the paper could grow professionally. To make this chore less difficult, you may also write one thing you admire about the person. Both positive and 'change needed' comments should be expressed constructively. Even if you do not know everyone that well, do the best you can."
  Give 15 minutes for this part. After that, stop, even if not finished. Each reads own paper for a few minutes.

3. Sharing:
  Members share the results with the group. If possible, each should read a few positive and growth comments to the group.

4. Processing:
  Questions for discussion:
  1. How do you feel about the feedback you received?
  2. How did you feel about giving feedback to others?
  3. What problems did you encounter in doing this exercise?

5. Generalizing:
  1. How do the comments about yourself compare with comments of others?
  2. What feedback from others do you agree/disagree with?
  3. What did you learn from doing this exercise?

Session 3 of 6 (Continued)

6. Application:

1. Whom would you like feedback from in your professional role?

2. How can you use feedback in everyday life?

3. How can you become more comfortable in giving constructive feedback to others? To clients?

7. Summary:

Ask members to summarize.

SESSION 4 OF 6

Group title: "Developing Your Professional Self"

Session title: "Professional Values"

Format:
   Warm-up—5 minutes
   Introduce activity—5 minutes
   Instructions for activity—5 minutes
   Activity—15 minutes
   Discussion—25 minutes
   Summary—5 minutes

Supplies:
   9 pencils
   9 Values worksheets (Worksheet 12-3)

Description:
1. Introduction:
- Warm-up—Begin by summarizing last week's activity. How are people left feeling about the group? Is there any unfinished business? (Any comments, either negative or positive, should be accepted by the leader without judgment and acknowledged.)
- Educational concepts—"Knowing our professional values can help us set priorities and use our time at work and away from work more constructively. For example, if I want to balance my career with a meaningful relationship with my family, then I will be careful not to work overtime or make work-related commitments on weekends. Professional values should also guide our behavior at work. If you believe a good rapport with clients is important, you may take extra time with them to show your concern."

   Pass out Worksheet 12-3 and pencils. Follow instructions on top of sheet. Allow 15 minutes to complete. When finished, each member shares his or her responses with the group.

2. Activity:
   The discussion guidelines written on the sheet are to come up with a group consensus on values held in common. One group member can be a recorder and allow group to collaborate on what professional values they can agree on. A separate Values worksheet may be used for note taking of group values.

3. Sharing:
   Done during the activity.

4. Processing:
   1. How did the group perform without leader intervention?
   2. How did you feel about doing the activity on your own?
   3. How did the structure affect your interaction?

5. Generalizing:
   Done during the activity.

6. Application:
   1. How do values affect your interpersonal relationships?
   2. What role do values play in your professional life?
   3. How do values determine how you spend your time?

7. Summary:
   In summary, the recorder can read his or her notes back to the group and accept final revisions and/or comments.

Worksheet 12-3
Values

Directions: Complete the following sentences in your own words. Then, compare your responses to those of the other members of your group in order to generate a set of commonly held values in interpersonal relations. In the discussion, you have four tasks:

1. To make yourself heard
2. To hear others accurately
3. To listen for themes
4. To collaborate on the group consensus

A professional should

A professional should not

A supervisor:

A student:

A colleague:

A spouse or boyfriend/girlfriend:

I want to be remembered as a person who

Our group:

SESSION 5 OF 6

Group title: "Developing Your Professional Self"

Session title: "Assertiveness Role Play"

Format:
  Warm-up—5 minutes
  Introduce activity—2 minutes
  Instructions for activity—3 minutes
  Activity writing—10 minutes
  Sharing (role playing)—25 minutes
  Discussion—10 minutes
  Summary—5 minutes

Supplies:
  8 index cards 3 x 5 inches
  8 pencils

Description:
1. Introduction:
- Warm-up—Define assertive, passive, and aggressive and discuss the differences between these.
- Educational concepts—"One of the most common problems students have in making the transition to professionals is not acting assertively. Lack of assertiveness can lead to difficulty even on fieldwork experiences, as many of you have already discovered. For example, one student on a Fieldwork I experience overheard a discussion by staff members who were setting up a family conference in the client lounge at 2:00 p.m. This student was already scheduled to run an occupational therapy group in that room at 2:00 p.m. However, she did not say anything about it to the staff group. The student was left without a place to run group and became very frustrated. Afterward, when staff became aware of the problem, they wondered why the student did not speak up! They could have met in several other places. This situation could have been avoided if the student had behaved more assertively."

2. Activity:
Pass out index cards and pencils. "You will now write down on the card a professional situation in which you would like to have responded more assertively but did not. You may either have been too passive or overly aggressive instead. On the front of the card, describe the situation: who, what, where, when, and whatever background information is necessary. On the back, state what your actual response was (if possible, give a quote) and state how you felt afterward."

3. Sharing:
Each member shares the situation written on the front of the card. Then, members decide as a group which situations they would like to role-play. Group chooses first, second, and third choices, using group decision-making techniques to do this.
Role-play one to three situations as time allows:
- Allow protagonist to direct role play.
- Protagonist chooses members of group to play significant characters.
- Protagonist sets up room, props.
- Role-play situation as it really happened first, then discuss.
- Reverse roles, and play situation using assertive behavior as discussed by the group.
- Allow a few alter egos to present feelings and/or alternate responses.

Session 5 of 6 (Continued)

4. Processing:
1. How did you feel about doing the role-play?

2. Which characters did you identify with?

3. How do you feel about being assertive? Passive? Aggressive?

4. What are you feeling about the protagonist's situation?

5. Generalizing:
1. What passive, assertive, and aggressive behaviors can you identify in the role play?

2. What are the advantages of assertive behavior?

6. Application:
1. What did you learn about being assertive professionally?

2. What steps do you personally need to take to be able to behave assertively in the professional setting? As a student? As an occupational therapist?

7. Summary:
Summarize by reinforcing assertive behaviors, reviewing the role of feelings and habits, and thanking role-players for their participation.

SESSION 6 OF 6

Group title: "Developing Your Professional Self"

Session title: "Group Evaluation"

Format:
    Warm-up—5 minutes
    Introduce activity—5 minutes
    Instructions for activity—5 minutes
    Activity—15 minutes
    Discussion/Summary of all six sessions—20 minutes
    Summary—10 minutes

Supplies:
    9 Group Evaluation worksheets (Worksheet 12-4)
    9 pencils

Description:

1. Introduction:

- Warm-up—Begin by stating that this will be the final group of the series, and ask members to say how they feel about ending the group.

- Educational concepts—"An important part of the termination of groups is to review all the sessions and summarize what has been valuable. As professionals, we will all need to evaluate our client groups, so this will be good practice. Worksheet 12-4 has been designed to help you think specifically about this group and to apply some of what you have learned about group dynamics."

2. Activity:

Give out worksheets.

"First, you are asked to identify the roles your fellow members played in the groups, and for this you will have to name names. In our discussion, these questions will serve as the basis of giving one another feedback about our participation. Next, we will look at the events of the group. These are emotionally charged situations that often emerge unexpectedly. In the context of activities, often, it is the conflicts and problems groups encounter that become the turning points from which we learn the most. You are asked to identify three such events over the last five sessions.

"Norms are the 'ground rules' of behavior in groups. You are asked to identify the implicit or implied norms over the course of the group. The stage of development is sometimes difficult to identify in the short time this group has been meeting. We will use Schutz's stages of inclusion, control, and affection as a guide (see Chapter 2). Sometimes, the characteristics of stages overlap, and this can be confusing, so you are asked to justify your choice with behaviors you see or have seen in this group. Your feeling about the group may be an important clue about what stage the group has achieved.

"Finally, you are asked to look at the group leadership. What style was used, and how has it changed over the course of the group? You have 15 minutes to complete the worksheet."

3. Sharing:

Members share their answers to some or all of the questions on the sheet, as time allows. After each question, ask the group to discuss their answers and come to a consensus. Be sure to leave the last 15 minutes to summarize and to reflect on the past six sessions.

4. Processing:

1. How do you feel about the group as a whole? Specific members? The leader?
2. What parts of the group experience are most memorable?
3. Which experiences did you like best/least?
4. How do you feel about your role in the group?

Worksheet 12-4
Group Evaluation

Directions: Answer the following questions about your group as it has developed from Session 1. Be sure to identify members by name.

Participation and Roles:
1. Who are the most outspoken participants?

2. Who are the least frequent participants?

3. Who talks to whom? What patterns have you observed? (Identify any subgroups that exist.)

4. Who keeps the ball rolling?

5. Who/what has blocked the group?

6. What rivalries have you observed during the group? Who has challenged the leadership?

Events: Name three interactions or situations that were high points or turning points for the group. Describe each situation briefly.
   1.

   2.

   3.

Norms:
1. What behaviors are acceptable to the group today?

2. What behaviors are not acceptable today?

3. How have norms changed from the beginning of the group?

From Cole, M. B. *Group dynamics in occupational therapy: The theoretical basis and practice application of group intervention* (4th ed.). Thorofare, NJ: SLACK Incorporated. © 2012 SLACK Incorporated.

Worksheet 12-4
Group Evaluation (Continued)

Stage of Development:
1. What stage of development has this group achieved? Justify your answer.
   a. Inclusion
   b. Control
   c. Affection

2. How do you feel about the group right now?
   a. It means a lot to me. I'm sorry it's ending.
   b. I feel good about the other members.
   c. I feel indifferent.
   d. It feels uncomfortable. I'm glad it's ending.
   e. I strongly dislike the group.

Leadership:
1. What was the leader's style of leadership? Why?
   a. Directive
   b. Facilitator
   c. Leader as adviser

2. How has the role of the leader changed over the course of the group?

Other Process Observations:

From Cole, M. B. *Group dynamics in occupational therapy: The theoretical basis and practice application of group intervention* (4th ed.). Thorofare, NJ: SLACK Incorporated. © 2012 SLACK Incorporated.

Session 6 of 6 (Continued)

5. Generalizing:

    1. What did you learn about yourself from being a part of this group?

6. Application:

    1. What parts of this group experience can you take with you and apply to future roles both personally and professionally?

7. Summary:

End by summarizing results and asking each person to say in his or her own words what parts of this group experience he or she values and feels good about.

Chapter 13

A GROUP EXPERIENCE
DEVELOPING CULTURAL COMPETENCE

Cultural competence is essential if occupational therapists are to practice effectively in a growing multicultural society (Evans, 1992). With diverse populations on the rise across the United States, the importance of cultural competency for occupational therapy professionals has only gained prominence during the past two decades. Many professional students do not fully appreciate the meaning of culture. In its broadest sense, culture may be understood as the "sum total of a way of living, including values, beliefs, standards, linguistic expression, patterns of thinking, behavioral norms, and styles of communication that influence behaviors of a group of people and are transmitted from generation to generation" (Wells & Black, 2007, p. 5). Culture includes notions of health and illness and ways of doing everyday tasks.

There is a growing body of evidence supporting the need for increased cultural competence for health-care providers. Much of this research has occurred outside the profession. Caffrey, Neander, Markle, and Stewart (2005) found that a 5-week international immersion experience proved much more effective in instilling cultural competence for nursing students than cultural content within a curriculum. Studies of nursing faculty found that most scored very low on the cultural knowledge variable, and the majority had little experience working with diverse backgrounds (Sealey, Burnett, & Johnson, 2006). In an OT study, Gray and McPherson (2005) found generational differences in cultural attitudes, with older-generation therapists having greater attitude change than younger OT practitioners. These researchers noted that people who had traveled and/or had personal experiences with discrimination were more culturally responsive. In a systematic literature review, Beach et al. (2005) found "excellent evidence" that culturally competent training improved knowledge, attitudes, and skills of health professionals. From a client perspective, Napoles-Springer, Santoyo, Houston, Perez-Stable, and Stewart (2005) identified positive and negative factors influencing medical encounters. Negative factors included a lack of sensitivity to complementary or alternative medicine, ethnic discordance between provider and client, and discrimination related to health insurance, social class, and age. Positively influencing health encounter were

- Positive values, beliefs, and attitudes
- Effective communication skills
- Patient- and family-centered decision-making
- Respect for privacy and modesty
- Openness to immigration
- Nutritional awareness
- Language and ethnic concordance
- Lack of discrimination
- Promotion of empowerment
- Complementary and alternative medicine recognition
- Respect for spirituality

In a study of health professionals working with Latino and African-American families, Karner and Hall (2002) identified the following behaviors as "vital aspects of culturally competent care" (p. 129): building trust,

Cole M.B. *Group Dynamics in Occupational Therapy:
The Theoretical Basis and Practice Application
of Group Intervention (pp 353-380).*
© 2012 SLACK Incorporated.

addressing language and cultural issues, providing clear expectations and consistent service, and individualizing services to better meet unique needs and concerns.

Black and Wells (2007) define cultural competence as a "broad term that includes cultural awareness and cultural knowledge (cognitive domain), cultural skills (behavioral domain), cultural sensitivity (affective domain), and cultural encounter (environment domain) (Callister, 2005)" (p. 33). With both education and motivation, these abilities become integrated into one's professional repertoire only with time and experience. The process may begin in an educational setting, but will continue throughout one's life and career. Some of the components of cultural competence include the following:

- Self-awareness and reflection
- Culture-generic knowledge and skills applicable across cultural groups
- Culture-specific knowledge and skills relating to specific groups
- Cross-cultural communication
- Appropriate and effective interactions with diverse others (Black & Wells, 2007)

Cultural understanding results from learning and experiencing cultural differences (Black & Wells, 2007). It is hoped that the mix of students in each group laboratory will provide enough diversity of experience for students to learn and practice strategies and skills for effectively communicating with potential clients from a variety of cultural backgrounds.

This group laboratory uses Black and Wells' Cultural Competency Model (2007), which incorporates many of the ideas from the field of multicultural education. Some of the principles of multicultural education are equality, mutual respect, acceptance, understanding, and a moral commitment to social justice. This concurs with AOTA's position paper (Hansen & Hinojosa, 2004), which states that "by embracing the concepts of non-discrimination and inclusion, we will all benefit from the opportunities afforded in a diverse society" (p. 668). The purpose of the model is to provide a structured approach for developing cultural competency and involves three components (Black & Wells, 2007, p. 60):

1. *Self-exploration*—Awareness of one's own cultural perspective and how it influences self and others

2. *Knowledge*—Recognition of differences and similarities among groups and an openness to learning and growth through multicultural experiences

3. *Skills*—Communication/interaction skills and strategies including expression of empathy and ability to form trusting connections with diverse others.

These components provide the theoretical basis for the group intervention strategies used in this group protocol. As a beginning point, self-awareness of one's own culture, beliefs, and biases are emphasized. The students' cultural perspectives consist of attitudes, perceptions, and behaviors, which are defined by their own culture and have been passed on to them by their families or others in their culture. Cultural awareness refers to knowledge of one's own culture: what beliefs and values we hold and how we define what is ordinary for us. Sometimes, it is necessary to take ourselves away from our own everyday routines and get out of our home territory in order to recognize the cultural idiosyncrasies that make us truly unique. Therefore, the first step in developing cultural competence is to become aware of our own cultural uniqueness.

In the groups, cultural knowledge will be imparted via short educational introductions at the beginning of each session, while self-exploration will be encouraged through the worksheets and exercises. Students will also learn and use group interaction skills such as empathy, active listening, and open questions in learning about the cultures of other members. Cultural sensitivity assumes a certain level of cultural awareness. McGruder (2003) defines cultural sensitivity as a "readiness to explore other cultures non judgmentally. Contact with empowered people whose cultural, racial, ethnic, class, gender, or sexual orientation is different from one's own is the most highly valued sort of activity for increasing cultural sensitivity. The learner must be willing to leave his or her own comfort zone and enter environments in which he or she will have the experience of being the numerical minority" (p. 93). Collectively, members will develop skill in using verbal and non-verbal communication to create an atmosphere of non-judgmental acceptance in exploring the cultures of others.

The following group protocol was designed to introduce professional students to the concept of cultural competence. Each session begins with a didactic component that reviews current thinking on the subject from a variety of sources. The group activities for each session flow from the introductory topic to promote self-awareness and allow members to learn from each other's experiences. This group protocol uses the seven-step, client-centered format for group facilitation, interaction, and learning.

GROUP INTERVENTION PLAN OUTLINE

Group title: "Developing Cultural Competence"

Author: Marilyn B. Cole, MS, OTR/L, FAOTA

Frame of reference: A cognitive-behavioral frame of reference is chosen because it encourages students to examine their own thinking process regarding cultures of self and others. This frame of reference teaches students to use reasoning to question and dispute some of their beliefs regarding cultures different from their own.

Purpose: This group laboratory is intended to broaden the cultural perspective of students and to prepare them to practice and to live in a changing world of diverse cultures and people. The laboratory exercises will teach members to recognize their own biases and to explore cultural differences without judgment or prejudice. It will prepare students to create an atmosphere of acceptance and open-mindedness wherever they go, both professionally and socially.

Group membership and size: This group intervention was designed for professional students. Groups of eight members are ideal. An effort should be made to include a mix of people from different cultures in each group whenever possible.

Goals and rationale: Eight specific goals are outlined for this laboratory experience. Students will
1. Fully appreciate the meaning of culture (beyond ethnicity) in the broadest sense.
2. Develop an awareness of one's own culture.
3. Recognize and verbalize one's own attitudes and biases toward others.
4. Explore and verbalize similarities and differences among group members.
5. Demonstrate nonjudgmental acceptance.
6. Define "otherness" as it pertains to one's own culture.
7. Develop and communicate empathy with others different from oneself.
8. Demonstrate cultural awareness and sensitivity through group interactions and journal writing.

Much can be learned about culture using the members' own cultural backgrounds and experiences. Attitude change is often best accomplished through interaction with peers rather than lectures or individual assignments. During group discussions, members will be encouraged to share their beliefs through open and honest self-disclosure.

Outcome criteria: The achievement of goals can be measured through self-ratings, written answers to essay questions, and personal journals. Please refer to Worksheet 13-1 to be given as a pre-/post-test. In addition, members will write a journal entry (minimum two handwritten pages) immediately following each session, using guidelines as follows:
- What I learned about myself from today's session.
- What I learned about other members (give names).
- One positive aspect of the group session.
- One negative aspect of the group session.
- What are my personal barriers to nonjudgmental acceptance of others?
- What goal can I set for myself during the next session and why?
- Other issues as assigned.

Methods: The instructor begins each session by imparting educational concepts about one aspect of culture, followed by experiential learning. Sessions use structured group activities to explore various aspects of culture. The instructor then facilitates discussion of the group activity, using the seven-step format outlined in Chapter 1. During discussions, instructors will model nonjudgmental acceptance and open self-disclosure.

Worksheet 13-1
Outcome Criteria Pre-/Post-Test:
Developing Cultural Compentence

Directions: Please answer these questions as best you can. Do not skip any questions.

1. Define culture.

2. Give an example of cultural awareness.

3. Describe your own cultural background.

4. Name five ways that members of this group are different from each other.

5. Rate your own attitude toward diversity on a scale of 1 to 10 (1 = negatively biased, 10 = positively biased) for each of the following:
___African American
___Homosexual male
___Adult with cerebral palsy
___Asian American
___Homeless person
___Hispanic (Mexican)
___White American
___Person with moderate mental retardation
___Person imprisoned for sexual assault
___Catholic priest
___Muslim anti-American demonstrator
___Female with extreme obesity

6. Give an example of how you could show empathy and sensitivity toward a client whose culture evokes negative feelings in you.

7. Write three questions you could ask to learn more about someone's culture.

From Cole, M. B. *Group dynamics in occupational therapy: The theoretical basis and practice application of group intervention* (4th ed.). Thorofare, NJ: SLACK Incorporated. © 2012 SLACK Incorporated.

GROUP INTERVENTION PLAN OUTLINE (CONTINUED)

Time and place of meeting: Group meets once a week for 90 minutes. This allows ample time for both educational learning and group experiences. Either day or evening time is suitable. The room should allow for privacy and freedom from distractions. Members may sit in comfortable chairs arranged in a circle. During written exercises, members seated around one large table may be preferable.

Supplies and cost: This group is relatively inexpensive to run, using mainly copies of worksheets and pencils. Index cards (3 x 5 inches) and a roll of adhesive tape are also needed. In addition, the following are required for each member:

- Sets of eight colored markers
- Glue sticks
- 12- x 18-inch drawing paper
- Scissors
- 2 magazines
- Bound notebooks for journal writing may also be provided

The cost is estimated at $10 per member.

GROUP SESSION OUTLINE (1 OF 6)

Group title: "Developing Cultural Competence"

Session 1: "Your Cultural Heritage"

Format (90 minutes total):
  Introduce members—5 minutes
  Educational concepts, introduction to cultural competence—15 minutes
  Instructions for activity—5 minutes
  Worksheets—20 minutes
  Sharing—10 minutes
  Discussion—30 minutes
  Summary—5 minutes

Supplies:
- Worksheets
- Pencils with erasers for each member

Description:

1. **Introduction:**
   - Warm-up—Ask each person to state his or her name and give national/ethnic origin.
   - Educational concepts—As a beginning step in developing cultural competence, we will first explore our own cultural heritage and share some information about our families with the group. We will define the key terms for this exploration: culture, ethnicity, race, and socioeconomic status. Then, we will look at a model for developing cultural competence (Black & Wells, 2007).
   - Culture—In its broadest sense, culture may be understood as the "sum total of a way of living, including values, beliefs, standards, linguistic expression, patterns of thinking, behavioral norms, and styles of communication that influence behaviors of a group of people and are transmitted from generation to generation" (Black & Wells, 2007, p. 5). Culture also includes notions of health and illness and ways of doing everyday tasks. Another definition comes from Krefting and Krefting (1991, p. 102) in McGruder (2009): culture is "a learned, shared experience that provides 'the individual and the group with effective mechanisms for interacting both with others and with the surrounding environment'" (p. 56).
   - Ethnicity—Culture is not the same as ethnicity or race, although some people use it that way. According to Weber's classic definition (1968) in McGruder (2009), ethnic groups are those that "entertain a subjective belief in their common descent because of similarities of physical type, or of customs, or both, or because of memories of colonization and migration" (p. 58).
   - Race—According to McGruder (2009), both race and ethnicity are socially constructed categories, concepts agreed on in public and private discourse that can only be understood in the context of the history of their use at a specific time and place. Neither ethnicity nor race has a biological basis. Groups categorized by skin color (blacks), linguistics (Hispanics), or religion (Jews) have been shown to be more biologically diverse and heterogeneous than homogeneous. In other words, there are no common racial characteristics that can be validated statistically. Yet, as McGruder points out, the categories are psychologically and socially real. In every corner of the globe, humans are denied or given rights and privileges based on race. Therefore, psychologically, a history of privilege or oppression within an ethnic or racial group can, to a great extent, shape one's culture.
   - Socioeconomic status—Socioeconomic status is historically based on three factors: occupational, educational, and income achievements. These three factors determine our social position within a society. To a great extent, our social position influences our values, beliefs, and view of the world. Our "class" (i.e., lower, middle, or upper income level) often determines the material resources and opportunities available to us and to our clients (Lysack, 2009). People might be upwardly mobile, in relation to their parents, or downwardly mobile, as might be the result of illness or other life events. Social status has a profound effect on a person's attitudes and beliefs and shapes culture in ways of which he or she might not be aware or cannot easily explain.

GROUP SESSION OUTLINE (1 OF 6) (CONTINUED)

While speaking about issues of culture is socially acceptable, issues of ethnicity, race, and social status are often not acceptable topics of discussion in polite society. Therefore, one of the goals of this group is to recognize the sensitive nature of these issues and to explore our own backgrounds and attitudes, so that we will not offend our clients unintentionally by making assumptions about them based on our own cultural baggage.

We will begin this process by first developing cultural awareness (i.e., the exploration and recognition of our own cultural uniqueness).

Before we begin, are there any questions or comments members would like to share?

2. Activity:

The worksheet you will fill out is called My Cultural Heritage. (Hand out Worksheet 13-2 and pencils). You will trace your ancestry for three generations, using a method called a genogram (McGoldrick & Gerson, 1985). On the worksheet diagram, triangles represent males, circles represent females. You will first identify yourself as either a circle (if you are female) or a triangle (if you are male) at the bottom of the diagram. Write your name in the circle or triangle. You may draw additional triangles or circles for your brothers and sisters, and write their names also. Spaces for your parents and grandparents are labeled. Follow the instructions written on the worksheet for additional information about each ancestor. Then, on the reverse side of the worksheet, write the answers to the questions outlined on the bottom of the sheet. Feel free to add information that you think is meaningful or important to share. For example, if someone's parents or grandparents are divorced, you might want to add a stepmother or stepfather or an additional set of grandparents. If any of your grandparents have died, you can add a date of death and perhaps a cause of death. You have 20 minutes to complete the worksheet. Any questions? May I have a volunteer paraphrase these instructions?

3. Sharing:

When time is up, collect pencils. Ask for a volunteer to begin sharing. In the interest of time, members should restrict their sharing to facts that have special meaning for them. Other ways to limit sharing might be to choose the relative who had the most influence on a member's cultural identity. Questions on the back should be discussed one at a time.

4. Processing:

1. How did it feel to create the three-generation genogram?

2. What was hard for you? What was easy?

3. How did it feel to share information about your family with the group?

4. What questions do members have about each other's families or culture?

5. Generalizing:

1. What are some things members have in common?

2. What are some cultural differences?

3. What did you learn about culture from doing this activity?

4. What did you learn about each other?

6. Application:

1. After hearing about each other's families, what do you think is unique about your own culture that makes you different from other members?

2. What did you learn about yourself from doing this genogram?

3. How do you think your own cultural heritage affects your ability to communicate with people from cultures different from your own?

4. What are the most important values you learned from your parents/grandparents?

Worksheet 13-2
My Cultural Heritage

Directions: Create a three-generation genogram using the diagram below (McGoldrick & Gerson, 1985). Write each person's name, date of birth, and primary occupation on the diagram.

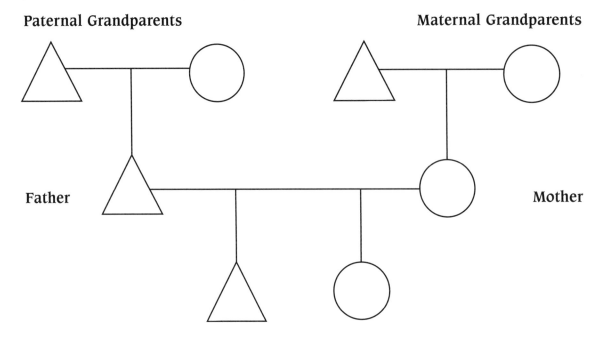

Paternal Grandparents

Maternal Grandparents

Father

Mother

You and your brothers and sisters (add circles/female or triangles/male, as needed)

List the following characteristics for parents and grandparents below: Name, place of birth, religion, special talents or abilities, and most important life achievement.

On the back of this worksheet, please answer the following questions:
- What ethnic identities do you hold?
- How are you like/unlike your parents?
- What do you believe the role of a grandparent should be?
- What values did you learn from your family about working, learning, spending money, marriage, aging, or any other significant issue?

GROUP SESSION OUTLINE (1 OF 6) (CONTINUED)

7. Summary:

1. "May I have a volunteer to summarize our first group session?"

2. Leader gives feedback to group on how well they accomplished the task.

3. May give preview to next week's group topic.

4. Journal entry: What cultural beliefs and values have been passed on to you from your ancestors? What is your family's socioeconomic status, and how does it affect your own beliefs and expectations of yourself?

GROUP SESSION OUTLINE (2 OF 6)

Group title: "Developing Cultural Competence"

Session title: "Gender Roles"

Format (90 minutes total):
  Warm-up—5 minutes
  Educational concepts—15 minutes
  Worksheet—25 minutes
  Discussion—40 minutes
  Summary—5 minutes

Supplies:
  Worksheets and pencils for each member, colored markers to share.
  List of values for warm-up: Write on a sheet large enough for all members to read from a distance:
  - A good love relationship
  - Financial security
  - Satisfying religious faith
  - Freedom to do what I want
  - Meaningful family life
  - Success at my chosen career
  - Excitement and adventure
  - Power and fame

Description:
1. Introduction:
  - Warm-up—Each member states name and chooses one of the values on the list that has special meaning for him or her. Members tell group why the value they chose is important for them.

  - Educational concepts—Cultural awareness refers to our knowledge of our own culture. What values and beliefs do we hold, and how do we define what is ordinary for us? One way to organize our thinking about what we value is to define the life roles we play. Mary Reilly used roles such as worker, housewife, student, player, and retiree to provide conceptual structure for occupational therapy's theory and practice (Jackson, 1998). Each role we play has tasks or occupations associated with it and, thus, serves to define our occupational patterns or lifestyles. Furthermore, roles imply both an intrinsic and an extrinsic perspective. Roles are the parts that people play in a larger social system. One's role in a family, for example, might be a son or daughter, a spouse, a caregiver, or a breadwinner. The role carries with it not only occupational choices for the individual, but social expectations as well. The tasks of a caregiver might be to feed, clothe, or comfort a young child or an aging parent. These occupations have meaning for both the caregiver and the recipient of care. Thus, role theory takes into account the social and cultural contexts within which occupations are performed.

    "Role expectations are the rules and the enabling and constraining forces defined by cultures in specific social situations. For example, what are the role expectations of a group leader?" Comments from members can be processed. "Some expectations might be to set the boundaries of time and place, to provide structure, or to allow members to have choices about the topics discussed or group activities. In fact, each of you may have different expectations of a leader. Your expectations of me will have a great deal to do with your own cultural beliefs about how a good group leader should behave. Because I understand this fact, that each of you comes to the group with a different cultural perspective, I will be careful not to judge you and not be too offended if you criticize my leadership. If this were a client group, I would need to take their cultural perspectives into account also. To do otherwise would be culturally insensitive."

    Role identification occurs when a role is internalized. We see ourselves as students, workers, or family members because we see ourselves occupying these social positions and performing the occupations associated with these roles (Kielhofner, 2008).

GROUP SESSION OUTLINE (2 OF 6) (CONTINUED)

Role theory helps to explain a few problems with occupational performance. Role conflict occurs when a person takes on overlapping roles and finds him- or herself having to choose between meeting one role expectation or another. The mother who is called home from work to care for a sick child is an example of a role conflict. She must either ignore the sick child or leave her work undone. Role overload can occur when a person takes on more roles than he or she can handle. Some of you might know people who work night and day, yet never seem to be able to meet all of the obligations demanded by their multiple social roles.

Roles can provide scripts that define our social interactions and behaviors. For example, our occupations, mode of dress, and style of interaction will be different when we are at work than when we are home with our families. Role confusion can occur when you and your spouse start a business together or when your boss invites you out for dinner.

How are roles related to values or to culture? The answer to that question is different for each individual. Each of us chooses roles that are meaningful for us or that we perceive as helping us achieve valued goals. For example, why are all of you currently in the role of a student? (May process answers from members.) Because you perceive that role as a stepping stone to achieving the status of a professional. Roles help us organize and sequence the occupations we need to perform in order to achieve a higher social status.

To illustrate, during our warm-up, some of you chose a meaningful family life as an important value for you. What roles do you play relative to that value? (May process comments from members.) You might show your appreciation to your parents for paying for your college education by studying hard and getting good grades in your courses. That is what a good son or daughter should do, right? Discuss.

Our cultural background shapes our perceptions of the roles we choose and our own expectations of how those roles should be enacted.

2. Activity:

"Today, we will explore one type of role, gender roles. Beliefs about the roles of males and females have been instilled in most of us from when we were very young. The toys we are given to play with, for example, might be seen as early lessons preparing us for our roles as adults. That is the topic of today's worksheet." Pass out Worksheet 13-3 and pencils. "Please follow the instructions written on the top. You may use colored markers for your drawings. No one needs to be an artist, but please don't draw a stick figure. We will have an opportunity to explain our drawings during our discussion. You have 25 minutes to complete the worksheets."

3. Sharing:

Ask for a volunteer to start. Pictures and information in the boxes may be discussed during the first go around. Answers to essay questions should be shared one at a time, with discussion and interaction on each separate topic. Facilitator should take care to allow each member to answer each question. This could take up to half the time allotted for discussion.

4. Processing:

1. How did it feel to share your drawings?

2. Which was easier, drawing or writing?

3. What did you feel about each other's drawings and comments?

4. How do you feel you measure up to your ideal (woman or man)?

Worksheet 13-3
My Cultural Heritage

Directions: Use pencil and/or markers to draw an ideal man and ideal woman in the space provided. Then, answer the essay questions below and on the back of the worksheet.

Draw an ideal man	Draw an ideal woman
Describe some of the characteristics of your ideal man:	Describe some of the characteristics of your ideal woman
What are the roles of men in your family?	What are the roles of females in your family?
Describe a typical day for your father:	Describe a typical day for your mother:

1. How are you similar to your parent of the same gender? How are you different?
2. How have gender roles in your family affected your own roles and expectations of yourself? Who else has provided major role/gender identification for you?
3. What did your parents tell you a good girl always does? Never does?
4. What did your parents tell you a good boy always does? Never does?
5. How well have you followed your parents' advice? What happens when you do not?
6. As a child, were you treated differently because you were female/male? Give some examples.
7. What are some cultural stereotypes regarding gender role?
8. What are some actual male/female differences vs. myths?
9. Compare the status of men and women in your own culture with that of other cultures.
10. How does gender affect career choices and opportunities for power or leadership?

From Cole, M. B. *Group dynamics in occupational therapy: The theoretical basis and practice application of group intervention* (4th ed.). Thorofare, NJ: SLACK Incorporated. © 2012 SLACK Incorporated.

GROUP SESSION OUTLINE (2 OF 6) (CONTINUED)

5. Generalizing:

1. What are some of the lessons learned from today's activity?
2. What are some ways that different cultures define the roles of men vs. women?
3. What occupations are required by the roles each of us holds?
4. How are role expectations different according to gender in the following examples: parent, military personnel, authority figure, athlete, corporate executive?
5. In addition to gender, what other roles are defined by culture? Give some examples.
6. What is the relationship between culture, roles, and occupations?

6. Application

1. Why might understanding gender roles be important when working with clients?
2. Which gender is more likely to provide caregiving?
3. How do gender roles influence the occupations we enable our clients in doing?
4. How does gender affect our role as an occupational therapist?
5. What can we do to learn about our client's values and beliefs about gender?
6. What are some gender differences in the way we express emotions? Handle stress?

7. Summary

- Ask for volunteer to summarize.
- What are some new things members learned today?
- Facilitator provides feedback to members about their participation.

GROUP SESSION OUTLINE (3 OF 6)

Group title: "Developing Cultural Competence"

Session title: "Customs, Traditions, and Rituals"

Format (90 minutes total):
   Warm-up—5 minutes
   Educational concepts—20 minutes
   Worksheet—20 minutes
   Discussion—40 minutes
   Summary—5 minutes

Supplies:
   Worksheets and pencils, index cards for warm-up, on which the following are written:
- Introduce yourself to a potential employer.
- Introduce yourself to a new client.
- Greet your best friend from home who has come to visit for the weekend.
- Say hello to someone of the opposite sex at a singles bar.
- Greet your grandmother at her home when you arrive for Thanksgiving dinner.
- Greet your doctor at his office.
- Introduce yourself to a stranger seated next to you on an airplane or train.
- Greet your sister or brother the day after the two of you have had a heated argument.

Description:
1. Introduction:
- Warm-up—Each member draws an index card. Ask members to stand and greet the person to their right, according to the role-play situation on the card they have drawn.

- Educational concepts—"Today we're going to explore some of the more subtle aspects of culture. As you observed in the warm-up, even the simple act of greeting one another is bound by social rules applying to different situations. These expectations are based on our culture."

Ethnocentrism refers to the lack of understanding or appreciation of another culture. It is rooted in the belief that one's own way of life is superior. For example, someone might visit a foreign country and be offended that they do not speak English or they do not accept the American dollar (Hasselkus, 2002). Who has traveled to a foreign country? What were some of your thoughts and experiences regarding cultural differences? (Members' comments may be processed.) Even within the United States, there are differences between north and south, east and west. For example, how is a "southerner" different from a "Connecticut Yankee"? Or a "Kansas farmer" different from a "New Yorker"? Who is from another part of the United States? Discuss. Cultural sensitivity assumes a certain level of cultural awareness. The first step is to become aware that our own ways of doing things are not the only way and may not even be the best way. Perhaps there are things that other cultures do better than ours. We need to move away from the position of egocentrism and adjust our attitude about another person's culture. McGruder (2009) defines cultural sensitivity as a "readiness to explore other cultures non-judgmentally."

One aspect of culture that is easily recognized and communicated is tradition. Webster's Dictionary (1992) defines a tradition as "a long-established or inherited way of thinking or acting." Traditions may be passed on to you by your families or by others of your culture. Organized religions are often said to embody traditions regarding the celebration of holidays (holy days). These religious rituals have been expanded and interpreted by many subcultures. For example, how a Christian family celebrates Christmas might have many variations depending upon which nationality or branch of Christianity one belongs to. Life events like weddings, baptisms, and funerals also differ according to the religious beliefs of one's culture."

GROUP SESSION OUTLINE (3 OF 6)

Webster's Dictionary defines a custom as "a habitual practice; the usual way of acting in given circumstances...applied to an individual or a community...reinforced by traditions and social attitudes." Hasselkus (2002) tells us that "social rules for behavior in our everyday lives are part of the shared beliefs and shared webs of significance that make up our culture" (p. 47). She uses a kindergarten classroom as an example of defined social norms as to behaviors that are acceptable and not acceptable. Kindergarten children quickly learn to conform to the expectations of the teacher. What are some customs that affect your behavior in this classroom? How do we address each other? What would happen if...(add an unacceptable behavior)?

Customs often define our choices and preferences and how we react to different contexts. For example, the foods we eat and how we eat them are defined by our culture. What do some of you consider appropriate foods for breakfast? While traveling in Europe, I noticed that the buffet breakfasts served at our hotel included many cheeses, cold cuts, and varieties of fish. In the southern United States, grits may be a common addition to a traditional breakfast. Customs can become so automatic that they can influence us in ways that we are not aware. For example, what do you say when someone sneezes? What do you say when someone accidentally bumps into you?

Customary behaviors may be organized into routines, habits, and rituals. Hasselkus (2002) uses these three words to describe the repetitive, predictable patterns of behavior in daily life (p. 49). Habits and rituals offer stability to an otherwise chaotic existence. Clark (2000) makes a distinction between habits and routines. Habits are "relatively automatic things a person thinks or does repeatedly," while routines are "higher-order habit(s) that involve sequencing and combining processes" and are related to specific outcomes. Rituals, although characterized by repetition like habits and routines, have the added feature of "drama, symbolism, and meaning-centeredness" (Crepeau, 1995, in Hasselkus, 2002). In other words, what makes a ritual different from a habit or routine is its meaning.

"In order to begin to explore cultures different from our own, I'm going to ask you to share some of the cultural differences represented right here in this room. All of us come from somewhat different cultures. Let's explore some ways that our cultures might differ from each other by sharing some of our customs, traditions, and rituals."

2. Activity:
Hand out Worksheet 13-4 and pencils. "You have 20 minutes to answer the questions on this worksheet. Some have choices, and some do not, so please read the questions carefully. We will be sharing our answers with the group."

3. Sharing:
Ask for a volunteer to start. Go in order around the group sharing one category at a time. Allow members to ask each other questions at the end of sharing in each category.

4. Processing:
1. How did you feel about answering these questions about your culture?
2. What feelings did you have about sharing your answers?
3. Does anyone want to ask the leader some questions? (Answer them.)
4. How do you feel about other member responses to what you shared?
5. What was hardest/easiest about doing the worksheet?

5. Generalizing:
1. What did you learn about culture from today's activity?
2. How would you define your own culture as compared with others in the group?
3. What do members have in common? What are some differences you observed?
4. What different cultures are represented in this group? (List them.)

Worksheet 13-4
Customs, Traditions, and Rituals

Directions: Please take the next 20 minutes to answer some of the questions in each category as specified. Do not skip any categories. You may continue on the back of the sheet or use additional sheets as needed.

Customs (choose 1)

- How does your family typically celebrate a favorite holiday? Choose a specific holiday and give details.
- How are birthdays celebrated in your family? Describe your most memorable birthday celebration.

Rituals (choose 1)

- Describe one daily ritual that has meaning for you. How did you get started doing this, and what are some symbolic meanings connected with this ritual?
- What task do you routinely do for/with someone else? What does this act symbolize?

Traditions (choose 1)

- What is your religion? How do you practice this religion?
- Describe the customs and rituals connected with one of the following in your culture: a wedding, a death in the family, or the birth of a child.

Subtleties

- How do you express anger, joy, grief? Give an example of each.
- How did you learn to do or say these things? Which are cultural vs. individual?

From Cole, M. B. *Group dynamics in occupational therapy: The theoretical basis and practice application of group intervention* (4th ed.). Thorofare, NJ: SLACK Incorporated. © 2012 SLACK Incorporated.

GROUP SESSION OUTLINE (3 OF 6)

6. Application:

1. How do traditions, customs, and rituals define a person's behavior?

2. How do traditions, customs, and/or rituals help people in times of crisis?

3. What customs or traditions are liberating for you. Which are burdensome?

4. Which of your personal attitudes about these aspects of culture have changed? How?

7. Summary:

- Ask members to summarize.
- Thank members for their honesty and self-disclosures.
- Encourage members to write further thoughts in their journal entries.
- Next week: outsiders versus insiders.

Journal entry: What customs, traditions, and/or rituals have you experienced in your own family (holidays, special foods, etc.)? In practicing your religion (marriage, baptism, funerals, etc.)? What do you like about these traditions? What is their meaning for you? What social purpose do they serve for those of your culture?

From today's exercise, what can you say about the cultural differences of members?

SESSION OUTLINE (4 OF 6)

Group title: "Developing Cultural Competence"

Session title: "Diversity Collage"

Format (90 minutes total):
  Warm-up—5 minutes
  Educational concepts—15 minutes
  Collage—30 minutes
  Discussion—35 minutes
  Summary—5 minutes

Supplies:
  - Stack of assorted magazines (two per person) to share
  - The following for each member:
    o Scissors
    o Glue stick
    o 12- x 18-inch white paper
    o Pencil
    o Set of eight colored markers

Description:

1. Introduction:

  - Warm-up—Members seated around a large table extend one hand, palm down, toward the center of the table so that hands and arms resemble the spokes of a wheel. Middle fingers may touch in the center. Each member states name and answers the following question: "What features make your own hand/arm distinctive and unique?" Members may consider skin, size, shape, and decorative features such as nail polish, jewelry, and clothing. A short discussion may follow in which members comment on each other's responses.

  - Educational concepts—Today's topic is diversity. The warm-up exercise highlighted only a few ways that people can be different from each other. What are some other ways that people are diverse? (List on board.) Black and Wells (2007) refer to diversity as the varied national or ethnic backgrounds of U. S. citizens and also categories of class, gender, age, ability, and sexual orientation. Health status may be added to this list of ways people differ.

    People sometimes feel uncomfortable when they talk about issues of diversity. That may be because we have learned that we should be politically correct (PC). This term became popular around 1990 and is defined as "a set of ideas, concerns, principles, and directives that stress social non-oppressiveness, inclusiveness, and sensitivity to diverse groups of people" (Herbst, 1997, p. 183). The focus of correctness is to limit sexist, racist, or otherwise offensive language when discussing diversity issues. Language is one way that people convey elitist attitudes about non-dominant groups in society.

    But there is a problem with always being politically correct. It teaches us to be color-blind. Has anyone heard this term? (May process comments from members.) We are not talking about an inability to see red and green traffic lights. Rather, it comes from the directive that we must treat everyone the same and to minimize our awareness of diversity. But is everyone the same? Of course not. That's why we've taken so much time doing exercises to make you more aware of your own culture. If we are to become culturally competent, culture cannot be invisible to us. So today, in this group, let's leave political correctness on the other side of the door. Race and skin color are not topics to avoid; they are two of many aspects of culture that we can learn to explore and appreciate. Let us acknowledge how people are different, without stereotypes or prejudice.

    The context in which we hear about things like race or skin color usually involves some incidence of discrimination. Discrimination is the action resulting from stereotyping and prejudice. Prejudice is defined as "an erroneous judgment, usually negative, which is based on incomplete or faulty information. Any preconceived opinion or feeling, either favorable or unfavorable. Unreasonable feelings, opinions, or attitudes, especially

SESSION OUTLINE (4 OF 6) (CONTINUED)

of a hostile nature, directed against any group of persons" (Black & Wells, 2007, p. 86). Does prejudice apply only to race? What might be some prejudices regarding fat people, old people, crazy people, or homeless people? May process comments from members.

Stereotyping involves putting people into categories based on some external or perceived characteristic (e.g., "Old people can't drive" or "White men can't jump"). Categorization is the brain's natural tendency to sort out information to facilitate storage and retrieval. It is useful to categorize much of what we learn, so that we can cluster information about different topics and remember it when we take a test or have an intelligent conversation. But when it comes to people, we should try to refrain from categorizing them too quickly. If we are to become culturally competent, we must remind ourselves that each person, whether friend, potential client, or associate, is an individual.

While prejudice and stereotyping are attitudes, discrimination is a social action. Discriminatory actions may be individual (choice of friends), community level (racial profiling by local police), or national level (better health care for those with private insurance). Most people in American society would say that discrimination is not a good thing. Yet, in many ways, we tolerate discrimination by looking the other way. One of our objectives for this group is to heighten our sensitivity to discriminatory acts at every level of society. The first step in reaching that sensitivity is to become aware of our own unacknowledged prejudices and stereotypes and those we have observed in our communities and in society.

2. Activity:

"Today's activity may be difficult for you if you have been taught to be politically correct. But acknowledging the prejudices and stereotypes held by many mainstream Americans is a necessary step in developing cultural sensitivity. I'm going to ask you to be honest in constructing a diversity collage from pictures you find in these magazines. You'll need to examine the social attitudes you have observed, both in others and within yourself, and to think about the stereotypes and labels that might be given to diverse groups of people." Hand out scissors, glue sticks, paper, pencils, and sets of markers; place stack of magazines in the center of the table.

"There are four steps to this task:

1. Find six pictures in these magazines of people who are different from yourself in some way. Think about the list we made earlier about the ways in which people differ. Cut out the pictures and glue them onto the paper, leaving space to write under each one.

2. Make up a name for each picture, and write it with a marker.

3. List under each name, four or five adjectives, labels, or stereotypes that might be given to that person by society. Here is where I'm asking you to put aside political correctness and acknowledge the possibility of stereotypes and prejudice. What you write down does not necessarily represent your own attitudes, and we will need to agree as group that members are not to judge each other by what we write down. You may use pencil to write your list, so that you can change your mind without worry.

4. Last, write three questions you might like to ask this person about his or her culture. Remember, not everyone is as aware of his or her culture as you are. Be subtle in the wording of your questions, and make them reflect an open, nonjudgmental curiosity. Try to use open questions that cannot be answered by 'yes' or 'no.'

You have 30 minutes to complete your collage, labels, and questions."

3. Sharing:

Ask for a volunteer to start. Members explain their collages to the group, including names and list of characteristics. In a separate go-around, each member may choose one picture for which to read his or her questions and discuss the reasons for asking them.

4. Processing:

1. How did it feel to do this collage?

2. What parts were hard? Easy?

3. What internal barriers did you discover when naming and labeling the pictures?

SESSION OUTLINE (4 OF 6) (CONTINUED)

5. How did you feel about writing questions?

6. How did you perceive other members responded to your collage?

7. What was it like to share your collage with the group?

8. What feelings do you have about my asking you to do something like this?

5. Generalizing:

1. What types of diversity did the collages represent? (List.)

2. What common themes did you see?

3. What common feelings did members express about doing the collage?

4. What are some differences among the collages?

5. What parts of this exercise affected you the most?

6. What might be some reasons for doing a diversity collage?

7. What did you learn about yourself?

8. What did you learn about other members?

6. Application:

1. What does your collage reveal about you personally?

2. How has this exercise raised your awareness of your own attitudes toward diverse groups? How has it raised your awareness of the attitudes of others?

3. Which diverse groups interest you the most? Least?

4. What people in your own life are similar to those represented in your collage?

5. What experiences have you had interacting with someone who is different from yourself?

7. Summary:

Ask for volunteers to summarize. Thank members for their honesty. Remind members of confidentiality and not to disclose the content of the group to others outside the group. Members write their names on collages; collect collages and keep for further discussion.

Journal entry: Discuss your feelings about today's activity. What might be some reasons for these feelings? What labels have been applied to you or someone you love? Tell about one experience you have had with someone of another culture.

GROUP SESSION OUTLINE (5 OF 6)

Group title: "Developing Cultural Competence"

Session title: "Insider versus Outsider"

Format (90 minutes total):
Warm-up—5 minutes
Educational concepts—15 minutes
Activity—20 minutes
Sharing—5 minutes
Discussion—40 minutes
Summary—5 minutes

Supplies:
- Adhesive tape
- Scissors
- Index card (3 x 5 inches) with the following labels written in large letters: Blame Me, Protect Me, Laugh at Me, Put Me Down, Worship Me, Ignore Me, Fear Me, Listen to Me, Call Me Stupid, Agree with Me. These labels should be kept out of sight until they are anonymously taped by the leader on members' heads.
- Clipboard with pad and pencil

Description:
1. Introduction:
- Warm-up—Members stand in tight circle, arm to arm. Members take turns being "odd man out" and from outside the circle, physically try to break in. The game ends when each member has successfully broken into the group. Briefly discuss strategies used by members to "break in" vs. "keep out."
- Educational concepts—Everyone wants or needs to be accepted. We first seek acceptance by the people around us, our family, our friends, our neighbors, our classmates. Acceptance generally means matching our own behavior to the behavior of the other members of the group to which we wish to belong. As the song says, everyone wants to be "in with the in-crowd." Sometimes being an insider is a good thing, and sometimes it isn't. What might be some reasons being an "insider" is good? What might be some reasons not to belong? (May process member comments.)

  You may be familiar with Abraham Maslow's (1968) hierarchy of needs, which are the following:
  a. Physiological
  b. Safety
  c. Belonging and love
  d. Self-esteem
  e. Self-actualization

  Belonging is the third greatest human need after safety and is equal in importance to love needs. According to Schutz (1958), a child's need for inclusion is initially met by his or her family. This early acceptance (or rejection) forms the basis for later behaviors with regard to inclusion or exclusion from social groups.

  On a societal level, Black and Wells (2007) define inclusion as the "belief that all individuals should be able to participate fully in activities of life with the same benefits and opportunities" (p. 164). This value is consistent with the philosophy and ethical principles of occupational therapy. The National Association for Multicultural Education (NAME) (2003) views the multicultural approach as "a philosophical concept built on ideals of freedom, justice, equity, and human dignity...(which are) attitudes and values necessary for a democratic society." The stated purpose of NAME is to challenge all forms of discrimination in schools and society through the promotion of democratic principles of social justice.

GROUP SESSION OUTLINE (5 OF 6) (CONTINUED)

Why do you think we need a national association to wipe out discrimination? Who is being discriminated against in this country? (May process member comments.) Minority groups in this country might be of as African American, Native American, Hispanic, and others. What is the difference between a minority group and a non dominant group? (May process member comments.) What is the dominant group in the United States? Domination has to do with the unequal distribution of power. McIntosh (1988) states that "white privilege is like an invisible weightless knapsack of special provisions: assurances, tools, guides, codebooks, passports, visas, clothes, a compass, emergency gear, and blank checks" (pp. 1-2). Black and Wells (2007) call this an "unearned privilege" that results from simply being born into a dominant group. What do you think about this statement? Is it true? (May process member comments.) How do you think white people feel about this? Wells and Black suggest that white people in positions of authority (e.g., teachers) have an obligation to promote the following goals:

- Respect human rights for all diverse peoples
- Promote the strengths and values of cultural diversity
- Accept alternate lifestyle choices for people
- Promote social justice and opportunity for all
- Attempt to equalize power among all ethnic groups

What do you think might be some special obligations for occupational therapists with regard to these goals?

2. Activity:

Imagine that you are creating the rules, regulations, policies, and procedures for an exclusive club to which only people exactly like you can belong. As a group, your goal is to make a list of 10 qualifications members must meet in order to be eligible. Does everyone understand the task? (May process questions and clarify, but don't give any specific advice.)

To add a bit more challenge, I'm going to give each of you a label, which I will tape to your forehead so the rest of the group can easily see it. You will see everyone else's label, but not your own. After the group completes its task, we will each try to guess what our label is. (Instructor randomly selects labels and tape to member's foreheads, taking care to make sure the words are visible but not seen by the member him- or herself.)

Do your best to role play what the labels say while you complete the group task. Please don't anyone take offense at what anyone says because we know that this is only pretend. So we can say whatever we like to each other during the next 20 minutes, without worrying about being polite. Agreed? Can everyone see each person's label? (May ask members to pin back hair or other obstructions or rearrange seating.) You have about 20 minutes to come up with your list of inclusionary qualifications. Here is a pad to record your list. (Place pad and pencil in center of the table, but don't say anything else. Stop the group after 20 minutes, whether or not they have completed the list.)

3. Sharing:

Before members remove their labels, ask for a volunteer to start guessing what their labels say. Allow discussion of feelings if this happens spontaneously. Each member can remove the card after he or she has guessed, even if the guess is incorrect.

4. Processing:

1. How did it feel to have a label?
2. How did you feel about treating each other according to the labels?
3. How did you like being asked to do this task?
4. What made it hard? Easy?
5. What feelings did you have toward each other as a result of role playing?
6. Who was left feeling badly? Why?
7. What do you need to say to each other to resolve these feelings?

GROUP SESSION OUTLINE (5 OF 6) (CONTINUED)

5. Generalizing:
  1. How did the labels affect the way you completed the task?
  2. What do you think about the list you created?
  3. Who did most of the work in creating the list?
  4. How did you choose who would record the list?
  5. What lessons did you learn from this experience?
  6. How does this experience relate to being an outsider or an insider?
  7. How does this experience relate to the concept of white privilege?

6. Application:
  1. What are some social parallels with aspects of this experience?
  2. What experiences in your own life are you reminded of?
  3. What insights did you gain about yourself from this experience?
  4. How can you apply this experience to your own life?

7. Summary:
  - Ask for a volunteer to summarize.
  - Thank members for their honesty and self-disclosures.
  - Congratulate members on being able to put aside political correctness.
  - Remind members to keep member disclosures confidential.
  - Include members in reviewing important lessons learned.
  - Next session will be the last.

Journal Entry: Describe two experiences you have had in the recent past: one which made you feel like an "insider" and one that made you feel like an "outsider." Describe your thoughts about termination of the group. What unfinished issues would you like to discuss?

GROUP SESSION OUTLINE (6 OF 6)

Group title: "Developing Cultural Competence"

Session title: "Exploring Another Culture"

Format (90 minutes total):
  Warm-up—5 minutes
  Educational concepts—15 minutes
  Worksheets—10 minutes
  Sharing—20 minutes
  Discussion—25 minutes
  Pre-/post-test—10 minutes
  Summary—5 minutes

Supplies:
- Worksheets
- Pencils
- Pre-/post-test copies for each member

Description:
1. Introduction:
- Warm-up—Introduce yourself as if you were answering your telephone at your place of work. Explain where you work and who might be calling you there. In a second go-around, answer the phone as you would at home. How is this different from work, and why?

- Educational concepts—People hold multiple cultural identities in the United States. This happens because each setting in which we perform occupations of daily life has its own set of norms, roles, and expectations, which are based on shared attitudes and beliefs. Some cultural environments may even have a unique language or a unique set of tools and equipment. Consider the differences in culture between a restaurant and hospital emergency room. How are the missions of these two workplaces different? What other differences come to mind? (May process member comments.) How does one's behavior change when entering these settings as a client? What other work cultures can members describe? (Discuss a few examples.)

  What are some other cultures with which you are familiar? What is the culture of your college campus or educational setting? What are the roles people hold, and how are they defined? What religious groups do members belong to? (Discuss some examples, including physical setting, what occupations are involved, who organizes and structures meetings and how, what are the traditions and/or rituals, and what is their meaning?)
  How do people begin to learn about an unfamiliar culture? The process involves taking the risk of leaving one's own cultural comfort zone and a willingness to become the numerical minority. Traveling to another country might be one way of doing this. What other countries have members visited? (May discuss member comments.) What cultural conflicts did you encounter while traveling? What happens if you enter an environment where you don't speak the same language? How do you feel when others can't understand you? This experience may give you some empathy for clients who do not understand your questions on an evaluation or who ask you questions that you don't understand.

  Empathy may be defined as "a way of seeing with the eyes of others, to appreciate their views of the world" (Egan, 2001). Rogers (1975) writes of empathy, "It means entering the private world of the other and becoming thoroughly at home in it.... It means temporarily living in his or her life, moving about in it delicately without making judgments." Earlier, we defined cultural sensitivity as a readiness to explore the cultures of others non-judgmentally. Empathy is one way of developing an understanding of a person from another culture. As professionals, we may communicate empathy by identifying the feelings clients express both verbally and nonverbally. But Peloquin (2003) states that true empathy transcends procedures, calling it "not a fusion with the pain of another, but a connection with the person of another" (p. 159).

GROUP SESSION OUTLINE (6 OF 6) (CONTINUED)

Developing empathy means taking certain risks. Rogers (1975) writes that, "In some sense it means that you lay aside yourself, and this can only be done by a person who is secure enough in himself that he knows he will not get lost in what may turn out to be the strange and bizarre world of the other" (p. 3). As professionals, we never know what the world may look like through the eyes of our clients. That is why we need to be aware of our own multiple cultures, whatever they may be, before attempting to explore cultures unfamiliar to us. This is another way of saying we need to be comfortable with ourselves, with who we are. Cultural awareness strengthens our own identity and sense of self and, therefore, gets us ready to be open to others.

Cultural sensitivity includes the quality of empathy for individuals who are different from ourselves. A related concept from Carl Rogers (1961) is nonjudgmental acceptance; the client is accepted for the human being that he or she is, regardless of his or her feelings or behaviors. Our responses to clients need to be both respectful and genuine. These are not techniques we learn as therapists; they are attitudes we may need to work hard to develop. Because if we have not done the work of examining ourselves and recognizing our own biases, our verbal and nonverbal behaviors may communicate our prejudices to clients without our realizing it. All of the client-centered concepts discussed in Chapter 3 apply in forming therapeutic relationships with our clients, regardless of their cultural differences. Bonder, Martin, and Miracle (2004) recommend paying close attention to one's own interactions with diverse clients together with reflection on the meaning and outcomes, in order to improve one's skills. Similarly, Black and Wells (2007) suggest "Looking for culture through careful observation of and interaction with others coupled with introspection of self enables the establishment of accurate empathy between practitioner and client" (p. 94).

Egan (2001) describes a way of communicating empathy by first identifying the feeling being expressed and then summarizing the situation that is perceived to have caused it. The primary accurate empathy statement essentially entails filling in the blanks in the following sentence: "You feel _____ because _____ ." (see Chapter 3). For example, if I'm rushing in to this meeting late and out of breath, and I tell you I've just come from a very intense meeting, how might you communicate empathy for me using this format? (May process answers from members). Perhaps you'd say, "You feel distressed (tense/upset) because of something that happened in the meeting you just left." That kind of statement would tell me several things. It would tell me you didn't judge me negatively because I was late, which would be a relief. It would also tell me that you would be open to hearing about what I might be distressed or upset about. This is how an expression of empathy builds trust between you and your client. You are not only reflecting back your understanding but also your caring and concern for him or her. This opens the door for deeper, more meaningful communication.

The activity for today was designed to help us practice exploring each others' cultures in ways that show respect, genuineness, empathy, and nonjudgmental acceptance. We will role play, asking questions and responding to each other, and we will examine the messages we convey about our own hidden biases or our openness and empathy with one of our peers.

2. Activity:
Today's activity has two parts: a worksheet and a role-play exercise. First, we will describe one of several cultures with which we identify. (Pass out Worksheet 13-5 and pencils.) These will be briefly shared, and the group may decide which culture to explore as a group. One of you will then become the "client," while the other group members ask questions and/or express empathy while exploring the culture you have briefly described. You have 10 minutes to complete the worksheets.

3. Sharing:
Ask for a volunteer to start, and each member describes one cultural identity. We will choose one cultural identity to explore as a group. Which one interests you most? (Can take several suggestions, and then take a vote).

Members take turns asking questions to learn more about the culture of the member chosen. Allow this process to continue for about 10 minutes.

Worksheet 13-5
Cultural Identities

Name at least three cultural identities you currently hold (educational, work, religious, recreational, community, family, alternate family, social activist, ethnic, etc.):

1.

2.

3.

Choose one specific identity to describe in-depth:

- Name of setting:

- Purpose or mission:

- Physical setting:

- Social/occupational roles:

- Norms or rules of social conduct:

- Power structure (who is in charge, what is the hierarchy):

- Tools and equipment, dress codes, and special vocabulary:

- Rituals and traditions and their meaning:

- Any other culturally meaningful factors:

From Cole, M. B. *Group dynamics in occupational therapy: The theoretical basis and practice application of group intervention* (4th ed.). Thorofare, NJ: SLACK Incorporated. © 2012 SLACK Incorporated.

4. Processing:

First, ask person chosen to role play:

    1. How did it feel to be asked all these questions?

    2. Which questions made you feel most accepted?

    3. Which questions were hardest to answer?

Then, ask group members:

    1. Which questions might have implied judgment or bias? Why?

    2. How did members feel about each other's questioning style?

    3. What made this activity hard? Easy?

    4. How do members feel about not being chosen to role play?

5. Generalizing:

    1. What questions demonstrate genuine curiosity?

    2. How does the language we use convey our attitude?

    3. How did members convey empathy?

    4. What nonverbal messages did you observe during the role play?

    5. What level of understanding did you achieve about the chosen culture?

    6. How is this culture different from your own?

    7. What can you learn from doing an exercise like this?

6. Application:

    1. What did you learn about your own style of asking questions?

    2. What did you avoid asking? Why?

    3. Which questions taught you the most about cultural sensitivity?

    4. How culturally sensitive do you think you are?

    5. What feedback can you give each other about respectfulness, genuineness, and nonjudgmental acceptance during the role play?

    6. Why do you need to practice your skills in exploring other cultures?

    7. Where in your own life can you apply this exercise?

Pre-/post-test:

Because this is the last session, we will take a short post-test. If you don't finish it in the next 10 minutes, you may have extra time after the session ends. The reason for doing it now is to become aware of what we have learned from all six sessions. This knowledge may contribute to our summarizing all six sessions. (10-minute limit.)

7. Summary:

- What are some lessons you have learned since this group began?

- What activities were most meaningful to you? Least meaningful?

- What feelings do members wish to share about our time together?

- What are some ways you might apply the lessons you learned?

Thank members for their participation.

Congratulate members on their trust, self-disclosure, and openness with each other.

Final journal entry (collect journals after completed): Describe any feelings you have about ending the group. What were the most meaningful parts of this group for you? What parts didn't work so well for you? What changes would you suggest, and why?

End note: This group could be enhanced by incorporating field trips, travel, or volunteer experiences that bring members into contact with different cultures. The focus of the preceding group activities is on self-awareness and cultural awareness. Developing sensitivity is expected to be an ongoing process.

REFERENCES

Beach, M. C., Price, E. G., Gary, T. L., Robinson, K. A., Gozu, A., Palacio, A., Smarth, C., et al. (2005). Cultural competence: A systematic review of health care provider educational interventions. *Medical Care, 43,* 356-373.

Black, R., & Wells, S. (2007). *Culture and occupation: A model of empowerment in occupational therapy.* Bethesda, MD: American Occupational Therapy Association.

Caffrey, R. A., Neander, W., Markle, D., & Stewart, B. (2005). Improving the cultural competence of nursing students: Results of integrated cultural content in the curriculum and an international immersion experience. *Journal of Nursing Education, 44,* 234-240.

Callister, L. C. (2005). What has the literature taught us about culturally competent care of women and children? *American Journal of Maternal & Child Nursing, 30,* 380-388.

Clark, F. A. (2000). The concepts of habit and routine: A preliminary theoretical synthesis. *Occupational Therapy Journal of Research, 20(Suppl.),* 1235-1375.

Crepeau, E., Cohn, E., & Boyt Schell, B. (2003). *Willard & Spackman's occupational therapy* (10th ed.). Philadelphia, PA: Lippincott, Williams & Wilkins.

Egan, G. (2001). *The skilled helper: A problem management and opportunity development approach to helping.* Monterrey, CA: Wadsworth Publishing.

Evans, J. (1992). What OT's can do to eliminate racial barriers to health care access. *American Journal of Occupational Therapy, 46*(8), 679-683.

Hansen, R. H., & Hinojosa, J. (2004). AOTA Position Paper: Occupational Therapy's commitment to nondiscrimination and inclusion. *American Journal of Occupational Therapy, 60,* 679.

Hasselkus, B. (2002). *The meaning of everyday occupation.* Thorofare, NJ: SLACK Incorporated.

Herbst, P. H. (1997). *The color of words: An encyclopedic dictionary of ethnic bias in the United States.* Yarmouth, ME: Intercultural Press.

Jackson, J. (1998). Contemporary criticisms of role theory. *Journal of Occupational Science, 5,* 49-55.

Karner, T. X., & Hall, L. C. (2002). Successful strategies for serving diverse populations. In R. J. V. Montgomery (Ed.), *A new look at community based respite programs* (pp. 107-131). New York, NY: Haworth Press.

Kielhofner, G. (2008). *A model of human occupation: Theory and application* (4th ed.). Baltimore, MD: Lippincott, Williams & Wilkins.

Krefting, L. (1992). Strategies for the development of occupational therapy in the third world. *American Journal of Occupational Therapy, 46*(8), 758-761.

Krefting, L., & Krefting, D. (1991). Cultural influences on performance. In C. Christiansen & C. Baum (Eds.), *Occupational therapy: Overcoming human performance deficits* (pp. 101-124). Thorofare, NJ: SLACK Incorporated.

Lysack, C. (2009). Socioeconomic factors and their influence on occupational performance. In E. Crepeau, E. Cohn, & B. Boyt Schell (Eds.), *Willard & Spackman's occupational therapy* (11th ed., pp. 68-79). Philadelphia, PA: Lippincott, Williams & Wilkins.

Maslow, A. H. (1968). *Toward a psychology of being* (Rev. ed.). New York, NY: Van Nostrand Reinhold.

McGoldrick, M., & Gerson, R. (1985). *Genograms in family assessment.* New York, NY: W. W. Norton & Company, Inc.

McGruder, J. (2009). Culture, race, ethnicity, and other forms of human diversity. In E. Crepeau, E. Cohn, & B. Boyt Schell (Eds.), *Willard & Spackman's occupational therapy* (11th ed., pp. 55-67). Philadelphia, PA: Lippincott, Williams & Wilkins.

McIntosh, P. (1988). *White privilege and male privilege: A personal account of coming to see correspondences through work in women's studies.* Working paper No. 189. Wellesley, MA: Wellesley College Center for Research on Women.

Napoles-Springer, A. M., Santoyo, S., Houston, K., Perez-Stable, E. J., & Stewart, A. L. (2005). Patients' perceptions of cultural factors affecting the quality of their medical encounters. *Health Expectations, 8*(1), 4-17.

National Association for Multicultural Education. (2003). www.nameorg.org. Accessed November 19, 2004. Washington, DC: Author.

Peloquin, S. (2003). The therapeutic relationship: Manifestations and challenges in occupational therapy. In E. Crepeau, E. Cohn, & B. Boyt Schell (Eds.), *Willard & Spackman's occupational therapy* (10th ed.). Philadelphia, PA: Lippincott, Williams & Wilkins.

Rogers, C. (1961). *On becoming a person.* Boston, MA: Houghton Mifflin.

Rogers, C. (1975). Empathic: An unappreciated way of being. *The Counseling Psychologist, 5*(2), 2-9.

Schutz, W. (1958). The interpersonal underworld. *Harvard Business Review, 36,* 123-135.

Sealey, L. J., Burnett, J., & Johnson, G. (2006). Cultural competence of baccalaureate nursing faculty: Are we up to the task? *Journal of Cultural Diversity, 13*(3), 131-140.

Weber, M. (1968). *Economy and society: An interpretive sociology.* (Originally published in 1922.) New York, NY: Bedminster.

Webster's college dictionary. (1992). New York, NY: Random House.

Wells, S., & Black, R. (2000). *Cultural competency for health professionals.* Bethesda, MD: American Occupational Therapy Association.

Chapter 14

COMMUNITY INTERVENTION
A SERVICE LEARNING EXPERIENCE
FOR STUDENTS

Community service learning for OT students often occurs in role-emergent settings, where no organized OT role or program has previously existed (Bossers, Cook, Polatajko, & Laine, 1997). These community sites serve as service learning opportunities for OT students to design and implement an OT program using a university faculty member as an offsite advisor.

One example of such a service learning project is the "Facing Up" project in Cape Town, South Africa. The goal of the Facing Up program was to establish OT health promotion programs for young, at-risk adolescents at mainstream schools. By way of background, it is significant to note that despite 10 years of South African liberation, outlying communities still reflected racially segregated living areas typical of the previous apartheid government. The service learning OT students from the University of Cape Town were primarily white and were working with primarily black adolescents for 8 weeks. The students designed and ran groups aimed at enabling the black teens to build occupational skills and divert their attention away from harmful occupations. A typical group included nine boys ages 10 to 12 years who were in grade 6. One leader describes playing a game of charades, with a goal of working on listening and communication skills. The boys formed teams and acted out scenarios from their experience. One team acted out finding a man who had be shot and helping him to receive medical attention. The other team enacted robbing a drug merchant. These choices troubled the student leaders, who were not familiar with such dangerous situations. In subsequent sessions, the power structure of the school playground and dress code are discussed, and the boys became aware of idealizing gangsters in their dress and play (Joubert, Galvaan, Lorenzo, & Ramugondo, 2006). What social issues put these boys at risk in their everyday lives? What can be done to change the direction of their aspirations? What might be their choices for occupations as they approach adulthood? The challenge for program planners was to design group activities that are respectful of their culture, but to also promote social change.

DEFINING COMMUNITY HEALTH

Scaffa (2002) defines community health as "the physical, emotional, social, and spiritual well being of a group of people who are linked together in some way, possibly though geographical proximity or shared interest." Practice in communities requires a paradigm shift away from the medical model and redefines the role of OT professionals as facilitators and educators rather than decision-makers. The focus of intervention is on social and environmental determinants of health. Some of the features of a healthy community include the following:

- Access to affordable, high-quality health care
- Social and environmental supports for healthy lifestyles
- Clean air and water
- Access to affordable, high-quality schools
- Recreational facilities and opportunities for people of all abilities to participate

Cole M.B. *Group Dynamics in Occupational Therapy: The Theoretical Basis and Practice Application of Group Intervention (pp 381-388).*
© 2012 SLACK Incorporated.

- Opportunities to experience and express creative arts
- Safe and accessible work and community environments
- Religious freedom in an atmosphere of mutual respect for diversity (adapted from Scaffa, 2005)

Scaffa (2005) summarizes the following guidelines for community programming from theories of health promotion:

- Comprehensive approaches relating to how economic, social, and political factors affect health are more effective than traditional educational approaches
- Changing community norms (culture change) is an effective way to raise health standards
- Community-level approaches contribute more to reducing health risks than individual approaches
- Programs are more effective if at-risk community members and community organizations are actively involved in prioritizing, developing, and implementing intervention programs
- Intervention strategies based on needs of and input from the community work best
- Multiple strategies will increase effectiveness (flyers, lectures, sponsored activities)
- Clearly defined and mutually agreed upon goals are essential to success
- Effective interventions also require ongoing evaluation and adjustment of strategies

Although social factors that put people at risk may be obvious, enacting social change is exceedingly difficult. Culture change is a slow, and sometimes frustrating, process, and often leaders must be content with small gains. The focus of OT group interventions in the community is mostly on prevention.

Fazio (2008) defines communities as local webs of relationships around locally relevant functions through formal and informal networks. Communities can be defined by locale (a town, a neighborhood) or interest groups (virtual communities, religious communities). In the transient world of today, communities provide a sense of stability, unity, and belonging. Other professionals, such as nurses, have addressed several threats to community wellness and have designed strategies to intervene, for example offering immunizations to children and recognition and prevention of societal violence, abuse, and neglect (Fazio, 2008). Increasing a sense of community by facilitating connections between members and getting them involved in shared activities that foster group morale and pride is known as "community building." Some features of community building are identifying common interests, building membership in groups based on interests, creating rituals for group inclusion, such as pledges or songs, refreshments at meetings,

patterns of interaction, common "jargon," and shared memories. Possible community-building interventions for OT are creating sports teams to compete with other communities, sponsoring running marathons, group walks, or other group recreational activities, advocating for public arenas for socialization and regular interactions, advocating for safe and accessible recreational facilities for youth, organizing volunteer transportation for older adults who no longer drive to engage in community activities, or providing tutoring or mentoring for children who are academically challenged. For example, one town recruited overweight volunteers from a local fast-food restaurant to compete in a "biggest loser" contest, emulating the popular TV show. Members formed teams, participated in diet and fitness activities over 8 weeks, then weighed in. As in the TV show, the team who lost the most pounds overall won. The losing team had to provide a service to the winners (washing their cars, cleaning their homes, preparing meals for a week, throwing a party). Both winners and losers benefited by increasing fitness, losing weight, and building relationships and team spirit. This is the essence of a community-building activity.

Reducing disparities is another common goal of interventions. The creation of inclusive communities involves reducing ageism, social stigmas for minority groups (disabled people, people with mental health issues), and access to public areas, activities, and health services. Often, clients choose to participate in communities, but "inclusion may not be their choice to make" (Fazio, 2008, p. 13). Often, changing attitudes, knowledge, and behaviors of the larger community is required to overcome barriers to participation, and this requires building collaborations and partnerships with existing community groups.

A Framework for Quality Service Learning

To make the most of service learning opportunities, a quality framework for learning and supervision needs to be developed. As in all groups, the interactions among students, educators, community entity onsite supervisor, and recipients of service are dynamic and complex. To ensure that outcomes become more predictable, general standards need to be agreed upon and policies set in place (Duncan & Lorenzo, 2006). At the center of a model of the dimensions of practice education in context lies the power and potential of both learners and service recipients. Neither students nor service recipients may be aware of their potential at the outset of a service learning assignment. Service settings must create enabling environments in order for learning to occur, while off-site educators have the responsibility for maintaining academic and professional standards.

"Potential and power operate in creative tension during the learning process" (2006, p. 53). Power represents the amount of control student learners and the people with whom they work are able to control the learning process. Empowerment increases the potential to learn and effect positive change. Cultural and social history can impose internalized oppression in certain segments of society who may be the recipients of service, and this effect may be difficult to undo.

Around the power and potential center of the model are the four key players: the student learner, the educator who ensures that OT students meet specified competencies and standards, the onsite supervisor, whose ultimate responsibility is the welfare of recipients of service, and the individuals or group members receiving interventions in identified domains of health or social need. Questions of power among these players include who is setting the agenda for service learning and need and how learning and the needs of recipients can be balanced in a way that is beneficial for all? Among the duties of the educator are negotiating entry for students to organizations as learning sites, assisting students in formulating specific learning goals, and assisting students in translating theory into practice through OT program interventions. The onsite supervisor communicates the standards of the organization and ensures that clients are satisfied with the services and attitudes of student learners. Educators and on-site supervisors form a collaborative partnership for student service learning. Learning requires more than professional competence in the OT student. It also requires interpersonal skills, problem-solving, clinical reasoning, technical skills, and "a special type of professionalism embracing culturally responsive attitudes and values" (Duncan & Lorenzo, 2006). Throughout and following the service learning project, students' performance is evaluated, including both student actions and the effects of the learning environment. Feedback from the onsite supervisor and educator promote competence development in specific roles. Some of the responsibilities of onsite supervisors and educators is to role-model best practice standards, ensuring that the OT services provided by students are both evidence-based and client-centered.

One of the many benefits of community service learning is to promote OT practice within communities so that interventions can occur within the natural contexts in which clients live, work, play, and learn.

DESIGNING PROGRAMS FOR COMMUNITIES

The first step in designing community programs is to identify a population with an unmet need. The needs of populations within a community are numerous, and there are many choices for students. Consider the many ways that different ages, genders, diversity dimensions,

social roles, work status, health status, and educational levels effect disparities in access to occupational engagement and inclusive participation in community life. Some suggestions for populations are:

- People who are homeless and/or unemployed (employment agencies, homeless shelters, soup kitchens)
- Independent living older adults with chronic health conditions (senior centers, adult day care centers, some senior public housing centers)
- People in recovery from mental illness or addiction (group homes, clubhouse peer support centers, mental health outpatient clinics)
- People with post-traumatic stress experiences (veterans organizations, organizations that shelter or treat stress-related disorders, local support groups)
- Teenage parents and their families (child wellness centers, public schools)
- Parents of children with disabilities (school systems; local rehabilitation centers)
- Caregivers of people with Alzheimer's or other dementias (adult day care centers)
- Children with learning disabilities or other physical challenges in school settings (public schools, special education services)
- Adolescents with dysfunctional families/homes (high school guidance counselors)
- Foster children transitioning to work or independent living (welfare or department of children and families local agencies)
- People transitioning to retirement (local corporations, churches, senior centers)
- Older adults living alone or in senior public housing (churches, town housing centers)

Entrance into a community organization is best pre-arranged by an OT professional or educator. However, the student first needs to do some background research. Places where students might look for the populations listed are suggested above. The student or practitioner will need to develop a community profile for the potential community group that will be the recipients of OT services. Baum, Bass-Haugen, and Christiansen have developed a structural analysis for organizations, populations, and communities based on the Person-Environment-Occupation-Performance Model (PEOP) (Baum, Bass-Haugen, & Christiansen, 2005).

DEVELOPING A COMMUNITY PROFILE

Organization and population information gathering included both general information and identifying issues of concern relative to occupational therapy. The process includes the following steps (adapted from Baum, Bass-Haugen, & Christiansen, 2005):

1. A general description of the community includes size, characteristics, census issues related to population, education, employment, ages, diversity, socio-economic status, income level, cultural issues, beliefs attitudes, ethnicity, and religion.

2. Areas of concern include critical issues such as unemployment, homelessness, crime, accessibility, sometimes available through local broadcasts, websites, and press releases. For each issue, determine prevalence, institutional environment, stakeholders (interested parties), influencing factors, and behaviors observed.

3. Identify issues related to OT—Look for general concerns and how they affect a population's ability to participate or engage in occupations, as well as effects on health and well-being. Determine what community activities occur, who participates, and the level of community engagement by its citizens.

4. Population or community general goals, both immediate and long-term.

5. Population or community occupational goals.

6. Match between population or community goals and OT professional domain. Is there a match? If OT is not deemed relevant, the issues are better referred to a more appropriate entity.

After creating a profile and identifying one or more unmet occupational needs, the analysis begins by identifying the constraints and barriers that prevent this need from being met. The OT develops a client-centered plan to address occupational and related general goals for the population or community. At this point, it is important to find out what other services are already being provided for the target population, so that OT is not duplicating what others have already done. What public or charitable services are available to this population? What are their resources, and how are they being used? Building partnerships with organizations that have access to the population is an important prerequisite to the success of any OT intervention.

CONDUCTING FOCUS GROUPS

The need for the proposed intervention must now be checked out by engaging potential clients in a collaborative process to identify their occupational needs and goals and to obtain feedback from them regarding the proposed interventions. This can be done via interviews or focus groups (see Chapter 1 for more information on focus group leadership).

Contacting and recruiting people to participate in focus groups begins the process of communicating and developing relationships with people from the targeted population. Their input during the focus group provides valuable information about their life perspective as well as their own preferences and priorities, necessary information to the development of a relevant intervention plan. The questions proposed in the focus group should be minimal and open-ended, allowing the group to self-direct, respond to one another, and freely express their opinions and feelings about the issues you are proposing. For an example of open-ended questions, refer to Chapter 10, the Kawa Model, which was developed from a series of focus groups.

The group idea you propose should fall within the domains of occupational therapy, according to AOTA's Framework-II (2008) (see Appendix E). Issues addressed should have an intellectual component and an activity component in order to provide an adequate guide for your group design.

POLITICAL ACTIVITIES OF DAILY LIVING MODEL

There is much we can learn about enacting social change from countries like South Africa. Theirs is perhaps a more clear-cut dilemma, with 80% of the population historically marginalized, those with power and education feel a responsibility to improve the conditions of the freed but impoverished majority. What are the lessons of the "Facing Up" project described at the beginning of this chapter? Are there similar at-risk populations locally that could benefit from OT group intervention? Or look at the "culture change" example in Chapter 4. What situations can you identify in local institutions that might benefit from culture change interventions to promote fuller participation and occupational engagement?

Authors from the United Kingdom and the Netherlands have suggested that OTs add "political competency" to their repertoire of skills to better prepare them to advocate for occupational justice and social change to remove barriers to participation for populations (Pollard, Sakellariou, & Kronenberg, 2009). Political competence is defined as the dynamic set of critical knowledge, skills, and attitudes that enables one to engage effectively in situations of conflict and cooperation in responding to people's (clients') needs and demonstrating the relevance of the profession. Examples of components of political competence are "political reasoning (pADL), strategic planning and decision making, networking, lobbying, and debating" (p. 23). The acronym pADL begins with a small "p" denoting the nonaffiliation with any specific political party, government, administration, state, or ideology. The term refers to OTs' preparation for political engagement and strategic involvement in conflict and cooperation when responding to local conditions, the intricacies of accountability, inter-professional relationships, and user and carer needs and motivations—issues that are often managerial concerns (Pollard, Kronenberg, & Sakellariou, 2009). These authors further describe pADL in terms of three Ps—personal, professional, and political values that define what one "stands for as a person and as a professional" (2009, p. 4).

Tiffany Boggis, an OT educator from Pacific University, used the pADL model to design student service learning experiences regarding health-care disparities in Oregon. She points to the evidence that medical care contributes relatively little to health when compared to social and environmental factors, health behaviors, and genetics (Boggis, 2009). She challenged OT students to investigate health disparities and to promote equalization of opportunity, social integration, and inclusion for people with disabilities. In order to address physical, social, and cultural environmental barriers to participation and inclusion for clients, OTs will need advocacy skills and a broader understanding of how people can influence or change public policies that create disparities. This service learning experience was designed to teach OT students these political skills. The project began with a seminar addressing occupational injustice, cultural competency, the workings of the democratic process, and the professional and ethical responsibilities of OTs as health-care professionals. Boggis found that while students could readily describe examples of occupational "apartheid" in far-off lands, they had a difficult time identifying "relevant examples within their own lives and communities" (p. 148). Small groups of students then interviewed leaders of four community agencies that worked with underserved populations in Oregon. Leaders within these agencies identified individual constituents who were willing to share their stories with the OT students. "By honing their interview skills and employing culturally sensitive behaviors within these social networks, students gained an understanding of the unmet needs of Oregonians who experience limited opportunities to engage in occupations that promote health and wellness" (p. 148). The students derived from their interviews some general themes that constituted barriers, such as lack of access to resources, education, and employment opportunities. Student groups engaged in political reasoning and reflected upon the three Ps (personal, professional, and political values), in preparation for a visit to the state capitol.

At the Oregon state capital, students kept two goals of pADL in mind: 1) to enable people-centered empowerment and 2) to encourage occupational justice. They accompanied 20 low-income Latina women to meet with state officials to learn how these elected officials are dealing with health-care disparities and to deepen their understanding of the legislative process. Students and participants demonstrated leadership by sharing the

women's stories of how health-care disparities affected their lives. The OT students and community members challenged the social norms and dominant cultural forces that create disparities in occupational opportunity and engaged in a provocative dialog with legislators. Some legislators considered this a "significant political action," a good example of combined professional and community group advocacy.

Students concluded that engagement in this political process provided them with "the social, cultural, and analytical skills necessary to participate effectively in the American democratic system to address health policy issues" (Boggis, 2006, p. 150). This project demonstrates how the pADL model guides OT interventions at the local and global systems levels.

How could a project such as this be replicated in your locale? What agencies could you identify in your community as sources of information about health disparities and occupational injustice? What questions could you ask them to better understand their roles and position within the larger health or social service systems? What populations could you gain access to through these agencies?

PRACTICE GROUP PROTOCOL

Using the guidelines in Chapter 11, create a group protocol for one community population, using educational, wellness, or prevention intervention strategies. Begin with the Worksheet 14-1: Focus Group Plan. From client responses or information gained from relevant case studies, develop a theme for intervention, including a model, frame of reference, outcome measure, and estimated cost for equipment and supplies.

Use Worksheets 11-3, 11-4, and 11-5 to write your group design and six group activity sessions. If you have the opportunity to conduct a focus group, use the feedback from it to create the session outlines.

COMMUNITY GROUP ACTIVITY EXAMPLE

The goal of this community intervention is to address the unmet need of retired older adults who are unable to find meaningful volunteer occupations in their community. The project design includes the following steps:

- Meet with local senior center directors to discuss the feasibility of recruiting groups of retired men and women who are interested in a time-limited volunteer project to benefit their community. Focus group questions might include, "What volunteer roles are currently available in this community? How does your staff currently recruit volunteers?

Worksheet 14-1
Focus Group Plan

Directions: Decide on an underserved population or a community group with an unmet occupational need. Identify the following:

- *Inclusionary Criteria*—What characteristics qualify people to be potential recipients of service? For example, what should be their age range, gender, health status, employment status, etc.
- *Exclusionary Criteria*—What characteristics would prevent people from benefiting from your proposed service? For example, what problems with cognition, communication, or social skills would make it difficult to participate? Which health conditions would make the group inappropriate (deafness, blindness, paralysis, psychosis)?
- *Identify Source of Participants*—Where will you look for representative members of your chosen population to participate in a focus group? (Schools, homeless shelters, senior centers).
- How will you recruit them? (Personal contact, volunteer sign up, referral source).
- *Locate Convenient Place and Time for the Meeting*—Where can you find a local meeting room for no cost? What time would be convenient for potential participants?
- *Incentives for Participation*—What will you offer in return for their participation? Refreshments? A free meal? Money? Transportation? Without a connection to other members, people have little incentive to participate and usually need some enticement.
- *Proposed Theme of OT Intervention*—What domains of the OT Practice Framework will you address in this intervention? What will be the theme of your group? The title?

Write four open questions to ask the group below, related to their issues, needs, and opinions about your proposed idea:

1.

2.

3.

4.

How will you communicate the time and place of your focus group meeting?

Follow the guidelines for focus group leadership discussed in Chapter 1.

What do you think of the idea of using a team approach? What service projects can you think of that teams of retirees might organize and accomplish within 6 to 8 weeks? How can this organization help with such a project?"

- Recruit retired men and women through the local senior or recreational centers to form a team of six to eight members for a pilot project. Ask for a meeting room and access to newsletters, bulletin boards, and other ways to market your pilot group project.

- Hold a planning meeting to identify unmet needs in the communities to which members belong. Assign members to explore the feasibility of their ideas during the week. Examples: river cleanup, beach gardening/planting, providing services for homeless, joining another organization to provide short-term services, tutoring or supervising youth activities, providing services to independent living elderly.

- Next meeting, group chooses one idea to pursue. Project will be planned and completed over a 6-week time period.

While the team will be given ample freedom with which to self-organize, the OT will facilitate weekly discussion/wrap-up sessions to help participants to discover the meaning of their occupational participation and appreciate how it benefits their community and society, as well as themselves. These sessions could include group problem-solving or conflict-resolution as needed as well as offering resources and guidance to members who ask for this. Meaningful productive occupations in retirement have been shown to help older adults to maintain health and well-being as they age (Knight, Ball, Corr, Turner, Lowis, & Ekberg, 2007). Within these sessions, the OT will educate participants about how their occupations help them stay healthy and maintain their sense of well-being. These sessions also serve as social support for participants, and one of the goals is to teach members to accommodate their differences and to provide support for one another in their roles as volunteers.

An outcomes measure will be designed to assess the effectiveness of this pilot project in meeting the needs of the community and the volunteer team members. For example, use a five-point rating scale for members to rate their satisfaction with various aspects of the project.

This group example uses a client-centered approach, allowing the group members to choose their own activity within preset limits and encouraging the team to self-organize and direct its own processes. A developmental frame of reference best justifies the goal of wellness and prevention for retired older adult members. Following

Laslett's (1989) Third Age theory, older adults in this stage of development are retired, but are still healthy, active, and resourceful. They are seeking self-fulfillment in ways that also serve society. Having left paid employment, they are looking for new ways to use their interests and skills and to maintain their social identity. Service projects such as this one provide the means to apply their skills while also meeting their own social needs and making a contribution to the well-being of themselves and society.

REFERENCES

Baum, C., Bass-Haugen, J., & Christiansen, C. (2005). Person-environment-occupation-performance: A model for planning interventions for individuals and organizations. In C. Baum, J. Bass-Haugen, & C. Christiansen (Eds.), *Occupational therapy: performance, participation, and well-being* (3rd ed., pp. 375-388). Thorofare, NJ: SLACK Incorporated.

Boggis, T. (2009). Enacting political activities of daily living in occupational therapy education: Health care disparities in Oregon. In N. Pollard, D. Sakellariou, & F. Kronenberg (Eds.), *A political practice of occupational therapy*. New York, NY: Churchill Livingstone Elsevier.

Bossers, A., Cook. J., Polatajko, H., & Laine, C. (1997). Understanding the role of emerging placement. Canadian *Journal of Occupational Therapy, 64,* 71-81.

Duncan, M., & Lorenzo, T. (2006). A quality framework for practice education and learning. In T. Lorenzo, M. Duncan, H. Buchanan, & A. Alsop (2006). *Practice and service learning in occupational therapy: Enhancing potential in context* (pp. 50-67). Chichester, UK: John Wiley & Sons, Ltd.

Fazio, L. (2008). *Developing occupation centered programs for the community* (2nd ed.). Upper Saddle River, NJ: Pearson Prentice Hall.

Joubert, R., Galvaan, R., Lorenzo, T., & Ramugondo, E. (2006). Reflecting on contexts of service learning. In T. Lorenzo, M. Duncan, H. Buchanan, & A. Alsop (2006). *Practice and service learning in occupational therapy: Enhancing potential in context* (pp. 50-67). Chichester, UK: John Wiley & Sons, Ltd.

Knight, J., Ball, V., Corr, S., Turner, A., Lowis, M., & Ekberg, M. (2007). An empirical study to identify older adults' engagement in productivity occupations. *Journal of Occupational Science, 14,* 145-153.

Laslett, P. (1989). *A fresh map of life.* Cambridge, MA: Harvard University Press.

Pollard, N., Kronenberg, F., & Sakellariou, D. (2009). A political practice of occupational therapy. In N. Pollard, D. Sakellariou, & F. Kronenberg (Eds.), *A political practice of occupational therapy.* New York, NY: Churchill Livingstone Elsevier.

Pollard, N., Sakellariou, D., & Kronenberg, F. (2009). A political competence in occupational therapy. In N. Pollard, D. Sakellariou, & F. Kronenberg (Eds.), *A political practice of occupational therapy.* New York, NY: Churchill Livingstone Elsevier.

THE TASK-ORIENTED GROUP
AS A CONTEXT FOR TREATMENT

Gail S. Fidler, OTR

Increasing recognition of the influence of man's social and cultural environment on behavior has extended the parameters of patient treatment. Such developments are manifested in the gradual melding of sociologic, psycho-analytic, and learning theories and the emerging focus on ego functions and adaptive skills. This appendix explores concepts of the task-oriented group within this context, offering a definition and delineation of purpose for its use in occupational therapy as a remedial-learning experience for the schizophrenic patient.

Returning the hospitalized psychiatric patient to an acceptable productive role in the community and appreciably reducing the rate of recidivism is a complex problem. Such concern has led to intensive studies of both psychotherapeutic procedures and organizational structures of the mental hospital. The impact of socio-logic inquiry into the mental hospital has been to add another dimension to our theoretical constructs regarding both individual feeling and behavior and conditions under which such behavior may be altered to the benefit of the patient.

Understanding the significance of the social matrix in which the patient functions has brought more sharply into focus factors influencing ego function in addition to the intrapsychic and intrapersonal. As early as 1931, Harry Stack Sullivan spoke of the importance of the social setting to the behavior of schizophrenic patients (Sullivan, 1931). Literature from the past 15 years is replete with the investigations and analyses of the import of environment on patient functioning (Caudill, 1958; Jones, 1953;

Stanton & Schwartz, 1954). This focus has inevitably led to theoretical and practical attempts to relate concepts of ego psychology to social theories of the environment (Cummings & Cummings, 1963; Edelson, 1964). Such linkage, as well as the social scientist's interest in group phenomena, has given impetus to increased exploration of the many facets of group process and group therapy.

GROUP PROCESS AND
GROUP PSYCHOTHERAPY

Group psychotherapy is firmly established as a meth-od of treatment for mental illness. It has its foundation in psychodynamic personality theories and emerged in America essentially from a psychoanalytic frame of refer-ence stressing personality change through exploration of intrapsychic and interpersonal pathology believed to be at the root of conflicts and problems (Bach, 1954; Mullan & Rosenbaum, 1962; Slavison, 1964; Wolf, 1949). The group has been seen as a setting in which the individual, with the help of the therapist and through sharing with other members, could explore and work through those unconscious conflicts and problems that inhibited per-sonality change and growth. Such a frame of reference places primary importance on unconscious phenomena and explores "here-and-now" feelings and behavior as a means to arriving at an awareness and understanding of intrapsychic conflict. The role of the therapist is to

Cole M.B. *Group Dynamics in Occupational Therapy:
The Theoretical Basis and Practice Application
of Group Intervention (pp 389-394).*

facilitate such awareness and elicit the involvement and help of members in exposing and working through personal conflicts and problems.

The social scientist's interest in groups emanated from a sociologic orientation rather than from personality theories. This frame of reference stresses the impact of society and the group on individual behavior and seeks to explain behavior based on the nature of the society in which a man lives. This ideology is exemplified by Lewin (1945) who theorized that behavior was determined by the situation in which it occurred as well as by personality factors. The sociologist's beginning involvement with groups was via his interest in organizational structure, and this was reflected in an early focus on the use of the group to accomplish a task or to effect a change in management (Schien & Bennis, 1965). Such experimentation inevitably led to the development of theories regarding the use of such groups in teaching and learning (Bradford, Gibb, & Benne, 1964).

Theories and practice in the field of group dynamics have focused on the group as a dynamic force in facilitating learning and behavioral change. Emphasis on "the group" as the primary change-producing agent thus accentuates the importance of exploring the dynamic forces within the here-and-now group to both understand and facilitate such change. Group structure and membership roles become significant, and individual feeling and behavior is viewed only as it contributes to or deters from cohesive structure and contributory roles.

As the group therapist, the psychiatrist, and the social scientist work collaboratively in an attempt to resolve some of the complex problems of the mentally ill, these two seemingly disparate theories have moved closer together. There are increasing efforts to integrate not only practice of group psychotherapy and group dynamics but also the more apparently divergent concepts of each. One has but to survey current literature to be impressed with the ubiquity of these efforts.

EXPERIMENTAL STUDIES

In *Social Psychology in Treating Mental Illness*, Fairweather (1964) describes an experimental approach combining the psychodynamic doctrine of patient treatment with theories of social psychiatry, sociology, and the small group. This program was focused around patient-led, small task-oriented groups for the chronic regressed schizophrenic. Such an approach, Dr. Fairweather points out, "called for an altered perception of the patient's role from that of a subordinate to that of a peer group member with responsibilities to himself and his group members, and away from that of a passive recipient within the limits of his abilities, despite existing psychopathology" (Fairweather, 1964). Tasks around which these autonomous patient-led groups were organized concerned the

current and future living of each member. Thus, task levels ranged according to the capacity of the patient from personal care and ward responsibility to responsibility for vocational planning and placement. These groups provided the opportunity for patients to explore and develop their capacities for independent function, creating patient roles within the hospital that were more consistent with those of the outside community.

This study made an important contribution to patient programming and treatment. Although it concerned itself entirely with problems of the chronic regressed schizophrenic, there is much that would seem to be directly applicable to other patient categories and most certainly to patient groups in rehabilitation settings.

Marshall Edelson's experimental study at the University of Oklahoma was concerned with "making possible the meaningful integration of both group experience and individual psychotherapy in an intensive treatment program designed to accomplish fundamental alteration in characterological disorder rather than solely rapid relief of acute secondary symptomatology and restoration of an ability to function marginally in the community" (Edelson, 1964). This work combines ego psychology and group dynamics in a therapeutic community as the basis for intensive psychotherapy. The focus of this study is aptly stated by Dr. Edelson in these words: "The therapeutic community (and small group) is organized to provide opportunities for the appearance of the patient's characterological difficulties or way of life as these are expressed in activities and other aspects of group living and for the confrontation of the patient and the group with these difficulties and their consequences to the life of the (hospital) community."

A third innovative experiment was Robert Morton's use of the laboratory method with psychiatric patients (Morton). This study describes the design and use of the group process laboratory training program for hospitalized mental patients. The laboratory is a structured, small group experience designed to bring about change by establishing conditions whereby participants are forced to test their assumptions regarding interpersonal and group relations. Not only is the application of the laboratory experience to hospitalized psychiatric patients a creative innovation, but it is even more provocative to learn that they were autonomous, staff-leaderless, patient groups. Morton agrees with Fairweather that cohesive decision-making groups with psychotics cannot be explored if a professional leader is present. It is their contention that even the most permissive therapist-leader reinforces dependency for the psychotic to a detrimental extent. This experiment provides some useful and creative postulates regarding small group experiences for psychiatric patients and should stimulate further research and study in the adaptation of this technique in treatment and rehabilitation programs.

It is interesting to note that, in follow-up studies on the Morton experiment, only two findings seemed to be suggestive (Johnson, Hanson, Rothaus, Morton, Lyle, & Moyer). Training laboratory patients were employed a mean of 5.92 months during the 9-month follow-up period whereas the group therapy patients were employed 4.70 months. In the Fairweather study, patients participating in the small-group program were significantly better than the control group in community adjustment with regard to areas of employment, verbal communication with others, and friendships.

These three experimental studies are examples of the way in which the small group is being used and adapted to meet treatment needs and essentially bridge the apparent gap between theories of individual psychodynamics and sociology.

The Task Group in Occupational Therapy

Development of task-oriented treatment groups approximately 4 years ago within the occupational therapy program at New York State Psychiatric Institute emanated from several not unrelated observations. First, the increasing conviction that as patients engaged in activities or created objects they expressed characterological difficulties and that attention to these problems as they emerged and were operant in the here-and-now seemed to be of benefit to the patient. The second observation was a seemingly evident relationship between problems evidenced by the patient in his activity experiences and difficulties he encountered in the workday world. Third, the nature of the occupational therapy setting, which expects active involvement in doing, provides a microcosm of life-work situations that can be seen and explored as they occur rather than in retrospect. Fourth, there was recognition of the relationships between verbal skills and learning and our experience, which indicated that learning and concomitant growth were enhanced when problems in doing were identified and explored. Finally, it is our belief that the shared, small group experience is conducive to the exploration and amelioration of some problems in ego function.

Groups were organized with approximately eight members selected on the basis of their particular difficulties in doing and being productive as well as their readiness and need for a small group experience. All patients admitted to these early groups were male schizophrenics, and placement in a given group was determined by the level of ego function. Meetings were held three to four times a week for periods of 1.5 hours. Each group was responsible for choosing its own common task and arriving at a consensus regarding procedures for accomplishing that task.

Definition and Purpose

Task as it relates to such groups is defined as any activity or process directed toward creating or producing an end product or demonstrable service for the group as a whole and/or for people outside of the group. Some examples of tasks chosen by these groups were publishing a newspaper, cooking, building a playhouse for the children's service, gardening, organizing a patient council, play reading, and ward decoration and improvement.

The intent of the task-oriented group is to provide a shared working experience wherein the relationship between feeling, thinking, and behavior; their impact on others and on task accomplishment; and their productivity can be viewed and explored. Alternate patterns of functioning can be considered and tested within the context of the here-and-now, to the end that such learning may induce ego growth and improve function. Task accomplishment is not the purpose of the group but hopefully the means by which purpose is realized. It is seen as the catalytic agent that elicits behavior and interaction, brings into focus both functional capacities and limitations, facilitates collaboration in working through problems, and provides a concrete reality factor against which to measure learning and achievement. Furthermore, the task provides a frame of reference, which helps to keep in focus what is relevant to explore and work through and what conflicts and issues belong more appropriately in other treatment settings. In such a group, issues and problems that directly affect the cohesiveness and/or task accomplishment are the appropriate agenda items.

Such groups are not unique in eliciting or diagnosing conflicts of the schizophrenic but it would seem that use of a common task within a small group setting does facilitate delineation of certain problems and their amelioration. Responsibility for selecting and accomplishing a task provides an opportunity for the group to explore problem-solving and decision-making skills, to have concrete evidence of their ability to function as well as to identify those expectations that give rise to conflict. The expectation that an activity needs to be chosen and implemented makes it necessary for the group to look at concepts regarding self and others who have impaired problem-solving skills and gives impetus to working toward their resolution.

The ability to perceive cause-and-effect relationships is a well-recognized problem of the schizophrenic, and learning in this area requires consistent, repeated opportunities to see and have evidence of cause and effect. The task-oriented group with its focus on the relationship between feelings, thinking, behavior, and task achievement thus creates excellent learning opportunities. Following through on a task procedure, the nature of doing or not doing, gives ample confirmation of cause and effect regarding behavior and function. When task responsibility must be shared, and when the nature of one's doing is viewed in terms of its contribution to the group, such learning is further amplified.

Reality testing through consensual validation is an essential process in every group and is of particular value to the schizophrenic. In addition to the shared reality indigenous to group structure and interaction, a clearly delineated task with standard procedures and techniques provides a shared reality from which perceptions can be tested and shared. Shared participation in an activity, the necessary interdependence, makes possible an objective, demonstrable assessment of one's capacities and limitations. One of the values of the task-oriented group is the consensual validation of the patients' capacity to grow and change as evidenced in the accomplishment of a task.

The need to work together, as well as talk together about one's doing, contributes to learning to conceptualize and verbalize more accurately and directly. Identification of problems in functioning and discussion of these as well as exploration of alternatives combines feeling, behavior, and cognition and provides the necessary components of learning and change. The shared decision-making, working experiences available in these groups, and the opportunity to explore and work through problems that interfere with satisfactory function make integrated learning possible. If we are to teach new and better ways of functioning, then we need to combine the patient's doing with his thinking and bring such relationships into awareness in order that he may integrate such learning.

Collaboration on a concrete, clearly defined task encourages more direct and clear communication and, coupled with group support, provides a safe area in which to practice such skills. In addition, experiences in working and sharing help the schizophrenic to begin to perceive and conceptualize his needs within the context of gratification potential with increasing awareness of his own potential for obtaining gratification rather that the expectation of rejection or frustration outside himself.

The task-oriented group, with its focus on function related to here-and-now tasks and doing their corresponding responsibilities, bears a closer resemblance to living in the outside community and provides learning that correlates more directly with those skills and expectations required in community adjustment.

It would seem useful at this time to make some distinction between these groups and verbal psychotherapy and delineate some values to the patient when both experiences are correlated. Within the task-oriented group setting, issues concerning feelings, perceptions, and behavior are discussed and explored only insofar as they are shared by others and impede or contribute to the problem-solving and/or activity accomplishment of the group. Personal, intrapsychic, and historical determinants are not emphasized but are reserved for investigation in psychotherapy. Many personal and interpersonal perceptions and responses are elicited but not dealt with

in the group. Psychotherapy provides an opportunity to explore these in depth, inter-relating the unconscious, the historical, the personal, and the interpersonal to the here-and-now. Likewise, the task-oriented group provides a life-like action and doing setting in which insights gained in psychotherapy can be tested and consolidated through performance. The extent to which the task-oriented group and psychotherapy is correlated and the degree that the purpose of each and their relationship is understood by both staff and patients may well determine the extent to which treatment potential will be realized.

LEADERSHIP

The role of staff leader or therapist is an important determinant in the group. The function of the leader is to facilitate a process and milieu that will be conducive to the kind of learning and growth to which these groups are directed. The role of the leader is to make learning possible and not to assume responsibility for the group. Fulfillment of objectives will depend in good measure on the leader's concepts of the mental patient and himself, as well as his skill in group and interpersonal processes.

Confidence in the inherent capacity of the group to be constructively self-determining, in its ability to ultimately recognize problems and reach realistic solutions to these, is a basic requirement. The foundation for such an attitude is belief in the right of the patient to be self-determining and a trust sufficient to allow exercise of freedom in exploring and testing his capacities. The group needs to be perceived as a therapeutic agent in its own right and leadership not as giving treatment but rather as the agent that helps to maximize the therapeutic and learning potential of the group.

It would seem that we tend to see patients as more fragile and thus needing more guidance and direction than seems warranted, at least on the basis of our experience. Perhaps this view of the patient is sustained by our need to be needed and important to the patient and to be recognized as having expertise. Autocratic leadership confirms for the patient his dependent position and tends to reaffirm his concept of self as inept and inadequate, while hesitant, aloof permissiveness increases his sense of vagueness, unpredictability, and limitlessness. Jay W. Fidler (1965) defines the nature and extent of leader activity as it pertains to working with groups of psychotics, emphasizing the importance of active interventions based on sensitivity and understanding of the schizophrenic's particular problems with reality testing and other ego functions.

Such understanding and attitude sets, however, are not the only basis of leadership skills for these groups. An intimate knowledge of and skill in problem-solving procedures is essential if the group is to be helped toward learning and developing such capacities. The extent to which problem-solving skills are an inherent part of the leader's way of thinking and functioning and his ability to make these appropriately apparent in identifying and dealing with issues will, by and large, determine the extent to which the group will be able to learn these processes and incorporate them into their functioning.

The extent and quality of the leader's receptivity to looking at himself and his relations to others, his freedom to participate in the learning and growth process, his ability to share perceptions, and his openness to exploring all aspects of his functioning in the group, will either make learning and growth possible and a less threatening expectation for members, or will confirm the many doubts and distortions they bring to the experience. The leader cannot expect from his group what he is not willing or able to do himself.

Problems of the Schizophrenic

Several aspects of the task-oriented group seem to bring into focus particular problems of the schizophrenic patient. First, decision-making is particularly difficult, especially the decision regarding task choice. There seems to be little question that groups expect the staff leader to make the choice for them. Some groups have insisted that this be done while others have behaved as though this was what they both wanted and expected. Groups have discussed their anxieties and conflicts about decision-making, and these discussions suggest that problems in this area are related to dependency needs, fear of responsibility, and the ultimate unacceptability of any decision they might make. It would seem that, because they conceptualize themselves as worthless and "bad," any decision they make as well as its implementation will be worthless and "bad" and will reflect basic ineptness and inadequacy. It would also seem they expect authority (the parental figure) to find any decision they make unacceptable and inadequate. However, groups resent and may forcefully reject any task choice suggestion made by the leader. Ambivalence with regard to dependency, coupled with problems related to self-concept, compose one of the major conflictual areas that need to be worked through before meaningful growth can occur. Some of these findings would seem to support Fairweather's hypothesis that the dependency needs of the psychotic contraindicate staff leadership in task-oriented groups.

More recently, we have been experimenting with a standard task for each beginning group in an effort to assess the extent to which decision-making problems may be altered or reduced when task choice is not an initial requirement. It is further hoped that such a procedure may lead to the development of a group diagnostic implement. However, the issue is not so much whether we deny or gratify the patient's dependency needs but rather how we can teach decision-making. It seems reasonable to conjecture that teaching such skills is a problem because of our limited understanding of the full nature of blocks to learning and thus our inability to identify and use techniques and procedures that facilitate learning.

Second, expectations of a shared group are frightening. It is as though fluid ego boundaries and difficulties in perceiving self as separate from others makes the closeness inherent in the small group an additional threat to identity. For some patients, there is also the expectation that narcissistic needs will be frustrated and that sharing in a group will deny dependency needs. In addition, anticipation of shared doing seems to represent a threat to the schizophrenic's defenses and orientation. However, the structured, predictable aspects of the task and engagement with non-human objects increase opportunities for supportive consensual validation of observable abilities and facilitate identification of those perceptions that they share in common.

Third, great difficulty is experienced in problem-solving. Although some of the dilemmas operant in problem-solving are obviously related to dependency needs and authority relationships, difficulties that emerge in these groups suggest also that many patients have never learned even the basic procedures for identifying problems and exploring possible solutions, or have lost the ability to appropriately perceive and organize perceptions into logical concepts.

The combined thinking and doing, the cognitive perceptual skills at both the motor and verbal level inherent in the product of these groups, seem to bring clearly into focus disturbances and abilities in thinking and learning.

Fears associated with learning and related conflicts, disturbances in cognition, and resultant dysfunction become readily evident. By the same token, the structure and focus of these groups make possible a sense of competence and learning less conflictual, the task providing evidence of movement toward achievement. Furthermore, task activity furthermore creates opportunities to engage and relate in a more concrete way, making it possible to be involved at a conceptual level commensurate with current capacities rather than consistently requiring a higher symbolic thinking order. The task also facilitates gradation of learning. As we become more knowledgeable about blocks to learning and their impact on function, we should be able to articulate more meaningfully related learning experiences and use more fully the potential of the task-oriented group.

Finally, two generalized responses have been evident in these groups. There are those who find expectations of doing, the intrinsic action, learning, and responsibilities, very threatening. These patients place a high premium on talking about their problems, and intellectualization is used as a way of avoiding the more hazardous and fearful doing of a task. These groups have great difficulty arriving at a choice of task, and such a decision may be prolonged for an inordinate period of time. Other patients seem driven to an excessive emphasis on the task, to a flight into activity as a means of avoiding bringing problems into awareness and working them through. Furthermore, there would seem to be a correlation between the leader's characteristic way of functioning, what he perceives as the more important "therapeutic set," and a group's sustained focus or movement toward a more equitable balance between these two responses.

One further observation would seem to be useful, and this relates to the kind of task choices made by groups. There seems to be an identifiable relationship between the task selected by a group, the level and nature of their primary emotional needs, and the conflicts surrounding those needs. Furthermore, task choice seems to reflect the group's progress or regression. Further study of this phenomenon should increase our understanding of need-gratifying processes and enhance our ability to make growth potential opportunities available to the patients.

Returning the schizophrenic patient to the community as a potentially productive, contributing member with an increased capacity to sustain such a role, is a multi-faceted, complex problem. The task-oriented group represents one of many attempts to reduce the problem. It seems that at least it provides a structure wherein dysfunction can be observed and explored. Hopefully, these and other explorations will make it possible to ultimately articulate more clearly the essential factors of remedial processes. As we become increasingly able to inter-relate psychodynamic and sociologic concepts, as we enhance our knowledge of the cognitive process and its relationships to intrapsychic phenomena and overt behavior, our efforts may come closer to realizing the ultimate goal of satisfactory community living for our patients.

ACKNOWLEDGMENT

The author is indebted to Dr. Lothar Gidro-Frank and Dr. Eugene Friedberg for their interested support and to Patricia Mayer, OTR, whose creative thinking and skillful leadership contributed so much to our learning.

REFERENCES

Bach, G. (1954). *Intensive group psychotherapy*. New York, NY: The Ronald Press.

Bradford, L., Gibb, J., & Benne, K. T. (1964). *Group theory & laboratory method*. New York, NY: John Wiley & Sons.

Caudill, W. (1958). *The psychiatric hospital as a small society*. Cambridge, MA: Harvard University Press.

Cummings, J., & Cummings, E. (1963). *Ego and milieu*. New York, NY: Atherton Press; 1963.

Edelson, M. (1964). *Ego psychology, group dynamics and the therapeutic community*. New York, NY: Grune & Stratton.

Fairweather, G. W. (1964). *Social psychology in treating mental illness*. New York, NY: John Wiley & Sons.

Fidler, J. W. (1965). Group psychotherapy of psychotics. *Am J Orthopsychiat, 35,* 4.

Johnson, D. L., Hanson, P. G., Rothaus, R., Morton, R. B., Lyle, E., & Moyer, R. Follow up evaluation of human relation training for psychiatric patients. In: *Personal and Organizational Change Through Group Methods*.

Jones, M. (1953). *The therapeutic community: A new treatment method in psychiatry*. New York, NY: Basic Books.

Lewin, K. (1945). *Dynamic theory of personality*. New York, NY: McGraw Hill.

Morton, R. B. The uses of the laboratory method in a psychiatric hospital. In: *Personal and Organizational Change Through Group Methods*.

Mullan, H., & Rosenbaum, M. (1962). *Group psychotherapy, theory and practice*. Glencoe Free Press.

Schien, E., & Bennis, W. (1965). *Personal and organizational change through group methods*. New York, NY: John Wiley & Sons.

Slavison, S. (1964). *Group psychoanalytic psychotherapy*. New York, NY: International University Press.

Stanton, A. H., & Schwartz, M. S. (1954). *The mental hospital*. New York, NY: Basic Books.

Sullivan, H. S. (1931). Socio-psychiatric research: its implications for the schizophrenic problem and mental hygiene. *Am J Psychiat, 10.*

Wolf, A. (1949). The psychoanalysis of groups. *Am J Psychother, 3.*

THE CONCEPT AND USE OF DEVELOPMENTAL GROUPS

Anne Cronin Mosey, PhD, OTR

Developmental groups are task-oriented groups structured in such a manner as to stimulate the various types of nonfamilial groups usually encountered in the normal development process. Five types have been identified:

1. Parallel
2. Project
3. Egocentric-cooperative
4. Cooperative
5. Mature

The concept of developmental groups was formulated in an attempt to apply recapitulation of ontogeny in the treatment of patients who are deficient in their ability to interact effectively in small groups. In dealing with this area of dysfunction, consecutive participation in the various types of developmental groups provides a framework for planned change. Group experiences are graded so as to provide opportunities for acquisition of basic group interaction skills. It is suggested that learning occurs through reinforcement of behaviors or approximation of behaviors that are necessary for successful participation in a given type of developmental group and non-reinforcement of behaviors that are inconsistent with successful participation.

A subtle change in orientation seems to be taking place among practitioners and scientists. There is movement away from the medical model, with its focus on concepts of pathology, toward an organization of thinking and effort around the concepts of growth. Scientists have shown renewed interest in exploring the development of various mature human capacities (here referred to as skills) and identifying factors that promote or cause development of these skills. Practitioners are beginning to think in terms of lags, deficits, or deviations in the normal developmental process. Classical diagnostic categories are being discarded for a more functional delineation of areas of adequate development and areas in which there is need for continued or redirected development.

Treatment that emphasizes the nurturing of growth rests upon three major postulates:

1. Deviations in development can be altered.
2. Subskills fundamental to mature adaptive skills must be acquired in a sequential manner.
3. Mature adaptive skills can be acquired through participation in situations that simulate those interactions between individual and environment believed to be responsible for the sequential development of a given adaptive skill.

It is out of this orientation, of treatment as recapitulation of ontogeny, that the concept of "developmental groups" has been formulated. It is presented principally as a heuristic device for discussing one facet of patient care.

Cole M.B. *Group Dynamics in Occupational Therapy:*
The Theoretical Basis and Practice Application
of Group Intervention (pp 395-398).
© 2012 SLACK Incorporated.

DESCRIPTION OF DEVELOPMENTAL GROUPS

Developmental groups are clinical simulations of the various types of nonfamilial groups usually encountered in the normal developmental process. These groups and their community-based counterparts are described as task-oriented and primary. Task-oriented refers to members' active engagement in the accomplishment of a definable project or task. "A primary group is a face-to-face organization of individuals who cooperate for certain common ends, who share some common ideas and patterns of behavior, who have confidence in and some degree of affection for each other, and who are aware of their similarities of bonds of association." The family (in its ideal form) is one example of a primary group. However, there are many nonfamilial groups that have the above-listed characteristics. It is this type of group that is of concern here.

Five types of developmental groups have been identified: parallel, project, egocentric-cooperative, cooperative, and mature. In a clinical setting, they would be described as follows:

A parallel group is made up of an aggregate of patients who are involved in individual tasks with minimal necessity for interaction. Group members may act as sources of stimulation for one another or tentatively test the effect of their behavior on others. However, task accomplishment does not require interaction. The therapist provides assistance with tasks and takes responsibility for meeting the social-emotional needs of each member.

In a project group, members are involved in common, short-term tasks that require some interaction, cooperation, and competition. The task is paramount. Mutual interaction outside the task is not expected. The therapist provides or assists the group in selecting tasks that require interaction of two or more people for completion. He or she responds to the social-emotional needs of group members.

Egocentric-cooperative groups are characterized by group members selecting, implementing, and executing relatively long-term tasks through joint interaction. The task remains central, but satisfaction of some social-emotional needs of fellow group members is encouraged. There is emphasis on the reciprocal satisfaction that can be gained by responding to others' needs. The therapist gives support and guidance relative to the task and continues to satisfy a considerable portion of each member's emotional needs.

In a cooperative group, members are encouraged to identify and gratify each other's social-emotional needs in conjunction with task accomplishment. This type of group often includes only members of the same gender. The therapist acts primarily in the role of an advisor and may not be present at all group meetings.

A mature group is heterogeneous in composition and is characterized by members taking those task and social-emotional roles that are required for adequate group functioning. Maintenance of a proper balance between productivity and personal need satisfaction is stressed. The therapist interacts as a coequal group member.

Division of developmental groups into five types is arbitrary—an attempt to provide demarcation points. It is more accurate to perceive these groups as being on a continuum. Thus, in the clinical setting, a given group may be best described as standing somewhere between two adjacent types of developmental groups.

When used in the treatment process, developmental groups are seen as agents of planned change. It is postulated that change occurs through the individual experiencing the consequence of his behavior in the group setting. Developmental groups are so structured that adaptive behavior leads to a positive reinforcing stimulus while maladaptive behavior does not. A positive reinforcing stimulus is an event that causes need reduction. The need may be outer-directed as in the need for companionship or inner-directed as in the need to be competent.

TREATMENT OF GROUP INTERACTION SKILL DEFICIENCY

The concept of developmental groups was formulated originally to delineate and describe a method of treating deficiency in group interaction skill. It grew out of the attempt to apply recapitulation of ontogeny in the treatment of patients who were deficient in their ability to interact effectively in small groups. Although developmental groups may be used in other areas (which will be briefly discussed later), they are seen as particularly useful in treatment of inadequate development of group interaction skill.

Group interaction skill is here considered to be an adaptive skill. It is defined, in its mature form, as the ability to participate in a variety of groups in a manner that is satisfying for oneself and for one's fellow group members. It is postulated that this skill develops sequentially, each stage in its development being marked by acquisition of behavior that is required for adequate participation in the community-based counterpart of the five types of developmental groups. It is further postulated that group interaction skill is acquired through participation in these various types of groups in conjunction with the opportunity to experience the consequences of appropriate and inappropriate behavior.

It is beyond the scope of this appendix to give a detailed description of evaluative methods for group interaction skill. Ideally, the therapist and patient collaborate in identifying what stages of this skill the patient has successfully integrated. Pertinent information may be acquired by observation of the patient in a group situation and discussion with the patient about his participation in groups outside the clinical setting. Evaluation also involves identifying what behavior the patient needs to acquire for successful interaction in small groups and current behavior that is interfering with successful participation.

The therapist must determine when deficiency in group interaction skill will be dealt with in the treatment process. The criterion suggested for making this judgment in treatment is initiated when the patient shows evidence of having acquired those abilities or skills that are normally learned prior to involvement in nonfamilial groups. The first step in treatment is engagement of the patient in that type of developmental group that is compatible or nearly compatible with his current capacity for meaningful group interaction.

Briefly, the treatment process consists of providing positive reinforcers for behaviors or approximation of behaviors that are necessary for successful participation in a given type of developmental group and withholding positive reinforcers for behaviors that are inconsistent with successful participation. These predetermined consequences are believed to be the central factor in bringing about change. The developmental group provides the structure; it sets and defines classes of behavior that are to be learned. Participation in a developmental group in and of itself is not conducive to planned behavioral change. Participation must be concurrent with deliberate and controlled reinforcement.

There are several methods that the therapist may use to increase the probability of the patient emitting desirable behaviors so that they can be reinforced. The method or methods selected will be determined primarily by the other adaptive skills available to the patient and his fellow group members. The most primitive method is simply to wait until the patient exhibits an approximation of the behavior he needs to acquire. This behavior is differentially reinforced as it moves in the direction of becoming an affective behavior pattern. Other initiating methods include the following:

1. Encouraging imitation of the therapist or other group members.

2. Suggesting specific patterns of behavior to the patient.

3. Identifying the patient's ineffectual responses, and encouraging him to experiment with other forms of behavior.

4. Group discussion regarding the behavior of self and others with mutual encouragement for engaging in appropriate and effective group behavior.

5. Experimentation with various behaviors through role-playing exercises.

Pragmatically, the therapist uses those initiating methods that appear to be successful.

An effort is made in all developmental groups to engage the patients in helping each other to acquire group interaction skill. Patients are encouraged to give and withhold reinforcers on the basis of the behavior exhibited by fellow group members. In order for patients to function as ancillary therapists, they must be able to comprehend what behavior is appropriate for a given type of developmental group and have sufficient self-control to give and withhold reinforcing stimuli. If it is deemed appropriate, the initial phase of treatment may be devoted to helping group members take on this ancillary therapist role.

Treatment continues to take place within the context of a specific type of developmental group until the patient has acquired the ability to function effectively in that group. He is then ready to begin learning the behavior that is necessary for competent functioning in the next, sequentially more advanced, developmental group. Depending upon the particular clinical situation and the extent to which the patient's fellow group members have progressed in an analogous manner, the patient is either placed in a new group or his original group as a whole is altered in the direction of the next type of developmental group. Treatment continues as previously outlined.

The treatment of deficiency in group interaction skill is terminated when any of the following criteria are met:

1. The patient has attained the ability to function in the type of group that is typical for his age.

2. He is able to participate in the kinds of groups that he is likely to encounter in his community environment (given its culture and the patient's preferred lifestyle).

3. The patient appears to be able to continue the development of group interaction skill outside the treatment situation.

ADDITIONAL COMMENTS

The concept of developmental groups was formulated in the attempt to apply recapitulation of ontogeny in the treatment of patients who were deficient in their ability to interact effectively in small groups. This concept may prove useful in three other areas:

1. Treatment of deficiency in other adaptive skills.

2. Meeting mental health needs.

3. Describing the evolution of small groups.

Many of the subskills that are fundamental to the development of mature, adaptive skills are acquired through interaction in the familial group. These are usually the most basic or primitive subskills. However, more advanced subskills are often learned in the context of nonfamilial groups. The familial group may, indeed, continue to play a strongly supportive role, but interaction in nonfamilial groups is essential for adequate learning. (Treatment of those subskills that are usually developed within the family group is outside the scope of this paper.) In regard to those subskills that are partially or completely acquired through interaction in nonfamilial groups, it is suggested that they can be learned most easily through participation in a group that is structurally similar to the type of group in which the subskills are normally acquired. The concept of developmental groups could be used as a guide for selecting and forming appropriate groups. The difference between using developmental groups in the treatment of group interaction skill deficiency and deficiency in other adaptive skills is one of focus. The therapist would be primarily concerned with regulating reinforcement of behavior specific to the skill being learned as opposed to concentrating on helping the patient to learn how to function in the group. These two foci are not mutually exclusive, but it may be useful to deal with them as such to clarify treatment goals and methods.

That area of patient care here identified as meeting mental health needs refers to patient-therapist-nonhuman object interactions that are directed toward satisfying the normal human needs of the patient and maintaining his ability and desire to function. The majority of mental health needs are most successfully met in a small group situation. However, needs cannot be satisfied unless there is synchronization of the individual's capacity to function in a particular group and the demands inherent in the structure of that group. In attempting to meet mental health needs, it is suggested that the therapist structure groups along a developmental continuum and that patients be encouraged to become involved in the type of group that is compatible with their group interaction skill. When a developmental group is oriented to satisfying mental health needs, the therapist is not concerned with bringing about a predetermined change in the patient's behavior. Therefore, the process of providing and withholding reinforcement is minimally important. The purpose of the group is to give pleasure, to have fun, to enjoy.

Preliminary, and somewhat superficial, observation indicates that the concept of developmental groups could be a useful tool in describing the evolution of task-oriented groups. This observation is not restricted to patient groups. As a task-oriented group moves toward becoming an effective working unit, there appear to be sequential patterns of interaction that are similar in many respects to the five types of developmental groups. Further study of this phenomenon may provide useful information for those people who are concerned with facilitating the maturation and productivity of task-oriented groups.

The concept of developmental groups has been presented as a heuristic device. It is meant to stimulate interest and to encourage discovery. Its usefulness will be confirmed or refuted as we learn more about the human growth process, this entity that we call illness or dysfunction, and the effectiveness of treatment founded on the principles of recapitulation of ontogeny.

REFERENCES

Ayres, A. J. (1964). *Perceptual motor dysfunction in children.* Presented at the Ohio Occupational Therapy Association Conference.

English, H., & English, A. (1958). *A comprehensive dictionary of psychological and psychoanalytic terms.* New York, NY: David McKay Co.

Erikson, E. (1950). *Childhood and society.* New York, NY: W.W. Norton and Co.

Ferster, C., & Perrott, M. (1961). *Behavior principles.* New York, NY: Appleton-Century-Crofts.

Fidler, G. (1969). The task-oriented group as a context for treatment. *American Journal of Occupational Therapy, 23.*

Fidler, G., & Fidler, J. (1963). *Occupational therapy: A communication process in psychiatry.* New York: The Macmillan Company.

Flavell, J. (1963). *The developmental psychology of Jean Piaget.* New York, NY: D. Van Nostrand Company.

Freud, A. (1965). *Normality and pathology in childhood.* New York, NY: International University Press.

Kimble, T. (1961). *Hilgard and Margis' conditioning and learning.* New York, NY: Appleton-Century-Crofts.

Mead, G. (1934). *Mind, self and society.* Chicago, IL: University of Chicago Press.

Mills, T. (1963). *The sociology of small groups.* Englewood Cliffs, NJ: Prentice-Hall.

Mosey, A. (1968). *Occupational therapy: Theory and practice* (printed through support of R.S.A. Training Grant No. 543-T-65). Medford, MA: Pothier Brothers.

Overly, K. (1968). *Developmental theory and occupational therapy-considerations for research.* Presented at the American Occupational Therapy Association Convention, Portland, Oregon.

Parsons, T., & Bales, R. (1955). *Family, socialization and the interaction process.* Glencoe, IL: The Free Press.

Parsons & Bales. (1934). *Family, socialization, and the interaction process.*

Pearce, J., & Newton, S. (1963). *The conditions of human growth.* New York, NY: Citadel Press.

Pines, M. (1969). Why some 3-year olds get A's-and some get C's. *The New York Times Magazine, July 6.*

Sechehaye, M. (1965). *A new psychotherapy in schizophrenia.* New York, NY: Grune and Stratton.

Skinner, B. F. (1953). *Science and human behavior.* New York, NY: The Macmillan Co.

Smith, A., & Tempone, V. (1968). Psychiatric occupational therapy within a learning theory context. *American Journal of Occupational Therapy, September-October.*

Spence, K. (1956). *Behavior theory and conditioning.* New Haven, CT: Yale University Press.

SUMMARY OF MOSEY'S ADAPTIVE SKILLS

Sensory Integration Skill: The ability to receive, select, combine, and coordinate vestibular, proprioceptive, and tactile information for functional use.

1. The ability to integrate the tactile subsystems (birth to 3 months).
2. The ability to integrate primitive postural reflexes (3 to 9 months).
3. Maturation of mature righting and equilibrium reactions (9 to 12 months).
4. The ability to integrate the two sides of the body, to be aware of body parts and their relationship, and to plan gross motor movements (1 to 2 years).
5. The ability to plan fine motor movements (2 to 3 years).

Cognitive Skill: The ability to perceive, represent, and organize sensory information for the purpose of thinking and problem solving.

1. The ability to use inherent behavioral patterns for environmental interaction (birth to 1 month).
2. The ability to inter-relate visual, manual, auditory, and oral responses (1 to 4 months).
3. The ability to attend to the environmental consequence of actions with interest, to represent objects in an exoceptual manner, to experience objects, to act on the bases of egocentric causality, and to seriate events in which the self is involved (4 to 9 months).
4. The ability to establish a goal and intentionally carry out means, to recognize the independent existence of objects, to interpret signs, to imitate new behavior to apprehend the influence of space, and to perceive other objects as partially causal (9 to 12 months).

5. The ability to use trial-and-error problem-solving, to use tools, to perceive variability in spatial positions, to seriate events in which the self is not involved, and to perceive the causality of other objects (12 to 18 months).
6. The ability to represent objects in an image manner, to make believe, to infer a cause given its effect, to act on the bases of combined spatial relations, to attribute omnipotence to others, and to perceive objects as permanent in time and place (18 months to 2 years).
7. The ability to represent objects in an endoceptual manner, to differentiate between thought and action, and to recognize the need for causal sources (2 to 5 years).
8. The ability to represent objects in a denotative manner, to perceive the viewpoint of others, and to decenter (6 to 7 years).
9. The ability to represent objects in a connotative manner, to use formal logic, and to work in the realm of the hypothetical (11 to 13 years).

Dyadic Interaction Skill: The ability to participate in a variety of dyadic relationships.

1. The ability to enter into trusting familial relationships (8 to 10 months).

Cole M.B. *Group Dynamics in Occupational Therapy: The Theoretical Basis and Practice Application of Group Intervention (pp 399-400).*
© 2012 SLACK Incorporated.

2. The ability to enter into association relationships (3 to 5 years).

3. The ability to interact in an authority relationship (5 to 7 years).

4. The ability to interact in a chum relationship (10 to 14 years).

5. The ability to enter into a peer, authority relationship (15 to 17 years).

6. The ability to enter into an intimate relationship (18 to 25 years).

7. The ability to engage in a nurturing relationship (20 to 30 years).

Group Interaction Skill: The ability to engage in a variety of primary groups.

1. The ability to participate in a parallel group (18 months to 2 years).

2. The ability to participate in a project group (2 to 4 years).

3. The ability to participate in an egocentric group (9 to 12 years).

4. The ability to participate in a cooperative group (9 to 12 years).

5. The ability to participate in a mature group (15 to 18 years).

Self-Identity Skill: The ability to perceive the self as a relatively autonomous, holistic, and acceptable person who has permanence and continuity over time.

1. The ability to perceive the self as a worthy person (9 to 12 months).

2. The ability to perceive the assets and limitations of the self (11 to 15 years).

3. The ability to perceive the self as self-directed (20 to 25 years).

4. The ability to perceive the self as a productive, contributing member of a social system (30 to 35 years).

5. The ability to perceive the self as having an autonomous identity (35 to 50 years).

6. The ability to perceive the aging process of oneself and ultimate death as part of the life cycle (45 to 60 years).

Sexual Identity Skill: The ability to perceive one's sexual nature as good and to participate in a relatively long-term sexual relationship that is oriented to the mutual satisfaction of sexual needs.

1. The ability to accept and act on the basis of one's pregenital sexual nature (4 to 5 years).

2. The ability to accept sexual maturation as a positive growth experience (12 to 16 years).

3. The ability to give and receive sexual gratification (18 to 25 years).

4. The ability to enter into a sustained sexual relationship characterized by the mutual satisfaction of sexual needs (20 to 30 years).

5. The ability to accept the sex-related physiological changes that occur as a natural part of the aging process (40 to 60 years).

Reprinted with permission from Mosey, A. (1986). *Psychosocial components of occupational therapy* (pp. 416-418). New York, NY: Raven Press.

EXCERPTS FROM THE
AOTA PRACTICE FRAMEWORK-II

Table D-1

Part I: Occupational Therapy Domains of Concern

Areas of Occupation	Client Factors	Performance Skills	Performance Patterns	Context and Environment	Activity Demands
Activities of daily living (ADL)	Values, beliefs, spirituality	Sensory perceptual skills	Habits	Cultural	Objects used and their properties
Instrumental Activities of daily living (IADL)	Body functions	Motor and praxis skills	Routines	Personal	Space demands
Rest and sleep	Body stuctures	Emotional regulation	Roles	Physical	Social demands
Education		Cognitive skills	Rituals	Social	Sequencing and timing
Work (volunteering)		Communication and social skills		Temporal	Required actions
Play				Virtual	Required body functions
Leisure					Required body structures
Social participation					

Adapted from American Occupational Therapy Association. (2008). Occupational therapy practice framework: Domain and process. *American Journal of Occupational Therapy, 63,* 623-685.

Table D-2

Part II: Process of Occupational Therapy

Evaluation	Intervention	Outcomes
Occupational profile	Intervention plan Types of intervention: • Therapeutic use of self • Therapeutic use of occupations and activities • Consultation process • Education process	Supporting health • Health and wellness • Adaptation • Prevention • Participation
Analysis of occupational performance	Intervention implementation Intervention approaches: • Create/promote • Establish/restore • Maintain • Modify (compensation, adaptation) • Prevent	Supporting participation in life • Occupational performance • Quality of life • Self-advocacy • Occupational justice • Role competence
	Intervention review	Engagement in occupation

Adapted from American Occupational Therapy Association. (2008). Occupational therapy practice framework: Domain and process. *American Journal of Occupational Therapy, 63*, 623-685.

THEORY-BASED GROUP LEADERSHIP GUIDELINES

Table E-1

Group Guidelines From Five Frames of Reference

	Structure	Goals	Leadership	Activities
Psychodynamic	Loosely structured, task-oriented	Develop ego skills, gain insight, emotional and spiritual dimensions	Facilitative	Creative, expressive, free choice of tasks or activities
Behavioral and Cognitive Frames	Highly structured	Specific, observable, measurable goals; learning skills; changing thoughts and behaviors	Directive	Educational sessions, worksheets, learning and practice, reinforcements, social learning sessions
Allen's Cognitive Disabilities	Highly structured, groups of similar cognitive level	Ongoing evaluation, problem solving in activities of daily living, building safe environments and habits	Directive	Crafts and tasks of daily life in specific, structured environments
Developmental Frames	Group by similar life stage; structure around stage-specific tasks, skills, and challenges	Skill mastery, altering life structure, making successful transitions, establishing growth facilitating environments	Directive or facilitative	Graded tasks and age-appropriate activities, life review, transitional adaptations
Sensorimotor Frames	Highly structured sequence of sensory motor activities	Stimulate development of central nervous system, normalize movement patterns, sensory modulation and integration, increasing adaptive responses	Directive	Movement activities, sensory stimulation, activities and games with minimal or graded cognitive demands, creating "just right" challenges

Cole M.B. *Group Dynamics in Occupational Therapy: The Theoretical Basis and Practice Application of Group Intervention (pp 403-404).*
© 2012 SLACK Incorporated.

Table E-2

Group Guidelines From Five Occupation-Based Models

	Structure	Goals	Leadership	Activities
Model of Human Occupation (MOHO)	Members grouped by common roles, members choose structure	Restore order in daily occupations, re-establish roles, develop healthy routines	Facilitator, advisor, or consultant	Everyday tasks, work, play, and self-care; establishing or restoring meaningful roles in families, social groups, and the community
Ecology of Human Performance (EHP)	Groups based on common task interest and skill level	Alter contexts to facilitate task choices and skill building within optimized natural contexts	Director or facilitator, depending on age of clients and group goals	Activities chosen through collaboration with client groups, related to their preferred interests and roles
Occupational Adaptation (OA)	Clients placed in groups according to meaningful life roles	Increasing adaptiveness by learning through the process of engagement in occupations	Facilitator	Readiness activities or therapeutic occupations of the client's choosing; the OT leader carefully sets up an adaptation-facilitating environment
Person-Environment-Occupation Model (PEO)	Members select preferred activities and may form groups based on common interests or occupational issues	Find and facilitate best fit between person, task, and environment	Director, facilitator, or advisor	Activities that match the skill level of clients are more satisfying; interventions that impact context at various levels may require advocacy as well as negotiation with others
Kawa Model	In this Eastern cultural model, clients and their immediate families engage in therapy together to overcome the client's disability	Restore harmony with families, social groups, and with nature; occupational engagement may not be a goal, but the means to restore a social role or status within the group	Director or facilitator	Family group problem solves together to adjust the task, environment, or social expectation for a client with disabilities so they can make a meaningful contribution to the group

OVERVIEW OF
THE *INTERNATIONAL CLASSIFICATION OF*
FUNCTION, DISABILITY, AND HEALTH,
SECOND EDITION

The purpose of the *International Classification of Function, Disability, and Health* (ICF) is to provide a common language and framework for the description of health and health-related states. The two key terms, "functioning" and "disability," are defined as follows. Functioning refers to body functions, activities, and participation. Disability refers to impairments, activity limitations, and participation restrictions. The definitions of all components of health domains and contexts enable health-care workers of many disciplines (including occupational therapy) to provide a complete picture of clients with health conditions and to share useful information with others throughout the world. The classification system provides a basis for the global collection of health statistics and research and a tool for clinicians, social policymakers, and educators.

In 2001, the World Health Organization (WHO) updated its classification system to include both positive and negative aspects of health. Formerly, this global classification document focused on impairments, disabilities, and handicaps as a way to identify people needing health-care services. The updated version particularly relates to occupational therapy in its consideration of well-being and prevention in addition to the consequence of disease. Much of the language of ICF was incorporated into the *Occupational Therapy Practice Framework* (American Occupational Therapy Association [AOTA], 2002), including a broad range of activities, a hierarchy of task demands, a focus on participation, and an acknowledgment of contextual factors.

The ICF is divided into two parts, each with two components. Part 1, Functioning and Disability, includes (1) body functions and structures and (2) activities and participation. Part 2, Contextual Factors, includes (1) environmental and (2) personal factors. The global paradigm shift in health care is apparent in the ICF's inclusion of both positive and negative factors of each health or contextual factor identified. This new, holistic perspective moves beyond the medical model to the public health arena where environmental factors within the system may act as facilitators or barriers to an individual's full participation in life. The classification system lists, codes, and defines each component and, in some cases, provides a rating scale for the status of a component with percentages or ranges of severity, such as the extent of vision loss or the degree of difficulty with climbing stairs. The eight components of the ICF are as follows:

1. Body functions—Mental (learning) and physical (walking) functions of the body systems that are categorized under "client factors" in the *Occupational Therapy Practice Framework*.

2. Body structures—Include the body's anatomy (organs, limbs), also a part of "client factors."

3. Impairments—Problems with body functions or structures that are the result of some health condition and may or may not cause a disability for the client.

4. Activity—The execution of a task. The *Occupational Therapy Practice Framework* refers to this concept as "occupation."

Cole M.B. *Group Dynamics in Occupational Therapy:
The Theoretical Basis and Practice Application
of Group Intervention (pp 405-406).*
© 2012 SLACK Incorporated.

5. Participation—"Involvement in a life situation" (p. 123), a definition that is adopted by the *Occupational Therapy Practice Framework*.

6. Activity limitations—Refers to the negative aspect of activity, formerly called occupational performance deficits in the occupational therapy literature.

7. Participation restriction—The negative aspect that is known in occupational therapy as a "barrier."

8. Environmental factors, including physical, social, and attitudinal environments, are recategorized in the *Occupational Therapy Practice Framework* as the seven occupational performance contexts.

Occupational therapists need to be familiar with the language and categories of ICF, in order to:

- Perform needs assessments.
- Match treatments with specific conditions.
- Document accurately for reimbursement sources.
- Substantiate the need for intervention.
- Plan for community or job market re-entry.
- Evaluate intervention outcomes.

- Advocate effectively for client needs.
- Communicate effectively with other disciplines, clients, and public policymakers.

In reviewing the ICF, it becomes apparent that there are many parallels between this document and the occupational therapy profession. Global recognition of these familiar concepts (activity demand, participation, contextual facilitators, and barriers) provides an inspiration to occupational therapists everywhere to expand the role of occupational therapy and to make others aware of the broad range of skills and services we offer as a profession.

REFERENCES

American Occupational Therapy Association. (2002). Occupational therapy practice framework: Domain and process. *American Journal of Occupational Therapy, 56,* 609-639.

World Health Organization. (2001). *International classification of functioning, disability, and health* (2nd ed.). Geneva, Switzerland: Author.

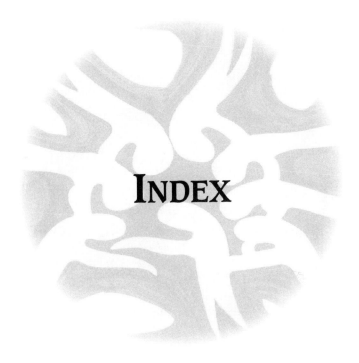

INDEX

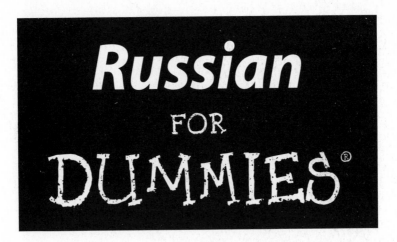

Russian
FOR
DUMMIES®

**by Andrew Kaufman, PhD, and
Serafima Gettys, PhD, with Nina Wieda**

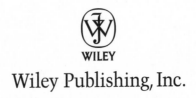

WILEY

Wiley Publishing, Inc.

Russian For Dummies®

Published by
Wiley Publishing, Inc.
111 River St.
Hoboken, NJ 07030-5774
www.wiley.com

For general information on our other products and services, please contact our Customer Care Department within the U.S. at 800-762-2974, outside the U.S. at 317-572-3993, or fax 317-572-4002.

For technical support, please visit www.wiley.com/techsupport.

Wiley also publishes its books in a variety of electronic formats. Some content that appears in print may not be available in electronic books.

Library of Congress Control Number: 2006920617

ISBN-13: 978-0-471-78001-4

ISBN-10: 0-471-78001-4

Manufactured in the United States of America

10 9 8 7 6 5

1B/RS/QU/QW/IN

WILEY

About the Authors

Andrew Kaufman, PhD, is currently a Visiting Lecturer in the Department of Slavic Languages and Literatures at the University of Virginia. He holds a PhD in Slavic Languages and Literatures from Stanford University, and he has recognized success as both a published scholar and an innovative, award-winning teacher of Russian language, literature, and culture at some of the country's top universities. Dr. Kaufman has worked as a Russian language and literature expert for "Oprah's Book Club," he has discussed Russian literature and culture on the national television show *Democracy Now!*, and he has been heard as a featured guest on Talk America Radio and on Silver Rain Radio in Russia. A fluent speaker of Russian, Dr. Kaufman has lived extensively in Russia, where he studied at Moscow State University and also worked as an interpreter, translator, and management consultant. To learn more about Dr. Kaufman, please visit his website at www.professorandy.com.

Serafima Gettys, PhD, earned her doctorate degree in Foreign Language Education from Gertzen State Pedagogical University, Leningrad, USSR. She is currently a Coordinator of the Foreign Language Program at Lewis University, where she also teaches Russian. Prior to coming to Lewis University, she taught Russian at Stanford University. Gettys is also a member of a number of professional language associations.

Nina Wieda is a doctoral student in Slavic Languages and Literatures at Northwestern University in Chicago. She is committed to bringing Russian language and culture into the lives of her readers and students, because, as the Latin proverb goes, "With each new language, you live a new life." A trained linguist with an MA in Social Sciences, Nina also has a book of poetry published in Russian, and a number of scholarly articles on Chekhov and contemporary drama published in English.

Authors' Acknowledgments

Andrew Kaufman: First and foremost, I would like to thank my colleague, former Stanford professor, and co-author, Serafima Gettys, one of the most original and inspired Russian language teachers I know. Her grace, infectious love of Russian, and professionalism were instrumental in making this book happen — and a joy to write. A sincere thanks, too, to Nina Wieda, who stepped up to the plate when we needed her and who performed marvelously.

A hearty thanks to Georgette Beatty at Wiley for her expert guidance and her constant encouragement throughout the writing process, and to Tracy Boggier at Wiley for her supervision and coordination, and for making this book possible. I'd also like to thank Sarah Faulkner, the copy editor, and Thomas Garza, the technical reviewer, for helping to make sure that every sentence in the book is both accurate and readable.

An immediate and heartfelt thanks to my agent, Margot Maley-Hutchison of Waterside Productions, for trusting me with this book, and for her expert representation and skillful problem resolution throughout.

Thanks to all my colleagues and students in the Department of Slavic Languages and Literatures at the University of Virginia for helping to create a supportive and stimulating environment in which to share our common passion for Russian language and culture.

I also owe a tremendous debt to my former professors at Stanford University (especially Professors Lazar Fleishman, Gregory Freidin, Joseph Frank, Monika Greenleaf, and Stephen Moeller-Sally) and at Amherst College (especially Professors Stanley Rabinowitz and Stephanie Sandler) for their mentorship and their faith in me, and for igniting my early passion for all things Russian.

And a very special and warm thank you to Professor Aida Borisovna Lominadze, whom I first met as a student at Moscow State University, and whose compassion, humanism, and extraordinary creativity have remained an inspiration to me throughout the years.

And finally, a loving thanks to my wonderful parents and to my family for their unwavering love and support, for their wisdom, and for their always impressive, behind-the-scenes marketing efforts on my behalf.

Serafima Gettys: Many thanks to Andy Kaufman for bringing this project to my attention and for taking on the responsibility of organizing and managing the project.

Many thanks go to Stanford University for bringing Andy and me together at an earlier point in our lives, first as a teacher and student, later as colleagues, and now finally as co-authors. Warm thanks also to my past and current students of Russian at various schools, both in Russia and the United States, who constantly challenge and inspire me and without whom this book would not have been written.

A loving thanks also to my family, husband Steve and daughter Anna. Their love has been an inspiration throughout.

Nina Wieda: Great thanks to Andy Kaufman and Serafima Gettys for making this project happen, and for being wonderful co-authors.

Many thanks to the Northwestern University Slavic Department for creating an excellent educational environment.

Special thanks to Andrew Wachtel for inspiring me to enter the field of Slavic Languages and Literatures, and to Elizabeth Elliott for awakening my pedagogical talents.

Great thanks to my mother, Alla, and my husband, John, for being a great team, and to my two-month-old daughter, Nadia, for being my muse.

Publisher's Acknowledgments

We're proud of this book; please send us your comments through our Dummies online registration form located at www.dummies.com/register/.

Some of the people who helped bring this book to market include the following:

Acquisitions, Editorial, and Media Development

Project Editor: Georgette Beatty

Acquisitions Editor: Tracy Boggier

Copy Editor: Sarah Faulkner

Editorial Program Coordinator: Hanna K. Scott

Technical Editor: Thomas J. Garza

Editorial Manager: Michelle Hacker

Editorial Assistants: Erin Calligan, Nadine Bell

Cartoons: Rich Tennant (www.the5thwave.com)

Composition Services

Project Coordinator: Kristie Rees

Layout and Graphics: Joyce Haughey, Stephanie D. Jumper, Julie Trippetti

Proofreader: Mildred Rosenzweig

Indexer: Joan Griffitts

Special Help Jennifer Bingham, Josh Dials, Her Voice Unlimited, LLC

Publishing and Editorial for Consumer Dummies

> **Diane Graves Steele,** Vice President and Publisher, Consumer Dummies
>
> **Joyce Pepple,** Acquisitions Director, Consumer Dummies
>
> **Kristin A. Cocks,** Product Development Director, Consumer Dummies
>
> **Michael Spring,** Vice President and Publisher, Travel
>
> **Kelly Regan,** Editorial Director, Travel

Publishing for Technology Dummies

> **Andy Cummings,** Vice President and Publisher, Dummies Technology/General User

Composition Services

> **Gerry Fahey,** Vice President of Production Services
>
> **Debbie Stailey,** Director of Composition Services

Contents at a Glance

Table of Contents

Introduction

Speaking more than one language is like living more than one life, one of the ancient philosophers said. And it's true — traveling in a foreign country such as Russia suddenly becomes a lot more exciting when you can engage in elegant small talk with a hotel receptionist, compliment your tour guide's dress, or actually read the menu and order the food that you really want. Being able to ask for things instead of pointing at them and getting directions from the locals instead of staring at a map are some of the little things that make you feel at home.

You don't even need to cross the ocean to immerse yourself in Russian culture; you can find little Russian neighborhoods (or even pretty big ones!) in many American cities. Whether your colleagues, your neighbors, or your friends speak Russian, the best way to win their hearts is to speak their language to them.

Now, *Russian For Dummies* won't make you a fluent reader of Dostoevsky in the original (most Russians themselves need somewhat of a preparation for that). It will, however, equip you with phrases necessary to function in many life situations, from shopping to visiting the theater. And little gems of cultural wisdom offered throughout the book help you not only translate the language, but also understand Russians so much better. So, buckle up, and good luck on your journey! Or, as the Russians like to say, **Zhelayem vam udachi!** (zhih-*lah*-eem vahm oo-*dah*-chee; We wish you good luck!)

About This Book

The best thing about *Russian For Dummies* is that you don't have to read all the way through it to get the information you need. You can open the table of contents, find the section that interests you at the moment, and start talking! You don't have to read the previous chapters to understand any of the sections of this book. And if you decide that you want more information about something, a convenient system of cross-references takes you to just the right place.

Another thing you don't need to do is memorize long vocabulary lists or grammar rules. We give you ready-made phrases; you just need to read them and start using them right away to impress your Russian friends!

Conventions Used in This Book

Here are some conventions that allow you to navigate through this book with maximum ease:

- ✔ We present Russian phrases in *transliteration* (Russian sounds represented with English characters). You can see the Cyrillic alphabet in Chapter 1. Russian terms are easily found in the text because they are set in **boldface.**

- ✔ Each Russian word is followed by its pronunciation and English translation in parentheses. In each pronunciation, the stressed syllable is in *italics.*

A little example to give you an idea of what we mean: The phrase for "I love you" in Russian is **Ya tebya lyublyu.** (ya tee-*bya* lyu-*blyu*; I love you.)

The meaning of a phrase doesn't always equal the sum of the individual words the phrase consists of. In this case, we talk about a *literal meaning* (the meaning of the individual words) and an *idiomatic meaning* (the actual meaning of the phrase in conversation). If the literal translation of a phrase differs from its idiomatic meaning, we give you both the literal and the idiomatic meanings in parentheses. For instance: **Kak dyela?** (kahk dee-*lah*; How are you? *Literally:* How is business?)

In each chapter, look for the following elements:

- ✔ **Talkin' the Talk** — These real-life dialogues illustrate how native speakers use words and phrases in a particular section of the book. These informal dialogues are the actual conversations you may hear in similar situations. And the CD has the audio version of these dialogues to help you grasp them even faster!

- ✔ **Words to Know** — This section follows every **Talkin' the Talk** and provides pronunciation and transcription of new words and expressions encountered in the dialogue.

- ✔ **Fun & Games** — Find this section at the end of each chapter. These fun activities allow you to use the new words and phrases encountered in each chapter to answer questions and solve puzzles.

Foolish Assumptions

When we started writing this book, we tried to imagine what our future reader was going to be like. In the end, we came up with a list of foolish assumptions about who we think wants to read this book. Do you recognize yourself in these descriptions?

- ✔ You know no Russian — or if you took Russian in high school, you don't remember a word of it.

- ✔ You're not looking for a book that will make you fluent in Russian; you just want to know some words, phrases, and sentence constructions so that you can communicate basic information in Russian.

- ✔ You don't want to have to memorize long lists of vocabulary words or a bunch of boring grammar rules.

- ✔ You want to have fun and learn a little bit of Russian at the same time.

How This Book Is Organized

Russian For Dummies consists of five parts and an audio CD. Each part of the book offers something different.

Part 1: Getting Started

In this part, find the basic essentials of the Russian language. Chapter 1 shows you that you already know some Russian, although it may be a surprise to you. We introduce the Russian alphabet and also give you an idea of how to use your knowledge of English to decipher some Russian words. Chapter 2 gives you a crash course on Russian grammar; it's also the right place to turn to if you want to know Russian numbers. And finally, find your first Russian words — greetings and introductions — in Chapter 3.

Part 11: Russian in Action

Part II prepares you for most social situations that you need to handle in Russian. Chapter 4 shows you how to make small talk; Chapters 5 and 6 prepare you to talk about food and shopping. When you have the essentials covered, find out how to talk about fun things, such as going out (Chapter 7), and

sports, reading, and other hobbies (Chapter 8). Chapter 9 equips you with the necessary phrases to make phone calls and send mail. For navigation through serious situations like getting a job or finding an apartment, refer to Chapter 10.

Part III: Russian on the Go

This part covers all the aspects of traveling, from planning your trip (Chapter 11) and discussing transportation (Chapter 12), to arranging for a place to stay (Chapter 13) and settling your financial matters (Chapter 14). Chapter 15 also shows you how to ask for directions, and Chapter 16 prepares you for handling emergencies.

Part IV: The Part of Tens

The Part of Tens is an unusual part of this book; it gives you lists of fun things to know, such as ten ways to pick up Russian quickly, ten holidays that Russians celebrate, and ten things never to do or say in Russia or to Russians. This part is also the place to find ten favorite Russian expressions and to pick up ten phrases that make you sound authentically Russian.

Part V: Appendixes

Russian For Dummies also includes four appendixes, which bring together some useful information. In Appendix A, find Russian verb tables. Appendix B is a convenient mini-dictionary for your quick reference. Appendix C offers the answer key to the Fun & Games sections of each chapter. And Appendix D helps you navigate through the attached audio CD; it contains the description of all the dialogues on the CD and tells you in which chapter you can find the text of the dialogue.

Icons Used in This Book

For your convenience, we marked some information in this book with special icons. Check out this guide to the icons, and the next time you see one of them, you'll know what to expect!

This icon indicates which Talkin' the Talk dialogues are included on the audio CD that comes with this book. This CD allows you not only to read but also to hear real conversational Russian.

From famous Russian writers to a polite way to decline an invitation, this icon marks a wide variety of curious and useful facts about Russian culture.

If you're curious about how the Russian language works, and if you want to expand your command of Russian to the extent of making up your own phrases, these bits of grammatical information may be of interest to you.

This icon points out some important information about Russian that's worth remembering.

This icon signals a useful bit of information that can make life easier for you, whether it's a handy way to remember a useful word or an insider's advice on how to better handle a certain situation.

This icon attracts your attention to something you need to know to avoid a common mistake.

Where to Go from Here

Now that you're familiar with the anatomy of *Russian For Dummies,* you can embark on your journey. You can start anywhere, and you don't have to go in a specific order. Just choose a topic that seems appealing, find the corresponding chapter in the table of contents, and start speaking Russian!

If you're at a loss about where to start, Chapter 2 may be a good place to get a grasp of the essentials of Russian grammar. Another good starting point is Chapter 1, which quickly boosts your confidence by pointing out all the Russian words you already know. Or, you can go straight to the sections that deal with something you need urgently: Ordering ice cream is covered in Chapter 5, for example.

Wherever you decide to start, you can find plenty of useful phrases to get you speaking Russian and exploring the benefits that your language skill brings. And now we wish you **Schastlivogo puti!** (shees-*lee*-vuh-vuh poo-*tee*; bon voyage!)

Part I
Getting Started

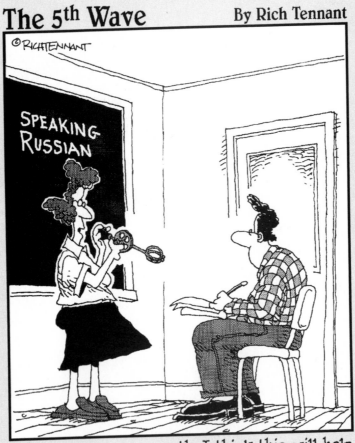

The 5th Wave   By Rich Tennant

SPEAKING RUSSIAN

"If you open your mouth, I think this will help you get the feel for rolling your r's."

In this part . . .

Part I is the beginning of your exciting journey. Here you get the essential information you need to take you through the rest of the book. Chapter 1 puts you at ease as you breeze through the Russian alphabet and discover that you actually already know quite a few Russian words. Chapter 2 gives you the basics of Russian grammar, which you may want to refer to throughout the rest of the book. And in Chapter 3, you start putting your new-found knowledge to work right away with popular greetings and introductions in Russian. So, get ready to start speaking **po-russki** (pah *roos*-kee; Russian)!

Chapter 1

You Already Know a Little Russian

In This Chapter

▶ Getting a grip on Russian words you know

▶ Understanding the Russian alphabet

▶ Pronouncing words properly

▶ Discovering popular expressions

▶ Reading Russian with confidence

*W*elcome to Russian! Whether you want to read a Russian menu, enjoy Russian music, or just chat it up with your Russian friends, this is the beginning of your journey. In this chapter, trust your eyes, ears, and intuition, and you quickly discover that Russian isn't that hard after all. When you're done with this chapter, you'll be able to recognize all the letters of the Russian alphabet, discover the basic rules of Russian pronunciation, and be able to say some popular Russian expressions and idioms.

Scoping Out Similarities between English and Russian

You may be surprised to find out that English and Russian are very distant relatives. They both come from the same ancestor — Sanskrit — and both belong to the same family of Indo-European languages. The similarities don't stop there. If you know English, you already know many Russian words.

In this section, you discover Russian words that are already part of English, and you find out about Russian words that have the same meaning and pronunciation as their English counterparts. We also warn you about a few words that sound similar in both languages but have very different meanings.

Identifying Russian words in English

As the world becomes more and more international, languages and cultures are constantly borrowing from and lending to one another, and Russian is no exception. Many Russian words that now appear in English either describe food and drinks or came into use during important historical periods.

Eating and drinking up

If you drink **vodka,** then you can already speak some Russian, because the word, like the drink, came from Russia. Maybe you can even rattle off the differences between **Smirnoff** (smeer-*nohf*) and **Stoly.** If so, you're already on your way to sounding like a real Russian, because **Smirnoff** is a Russian person's last name, and **Stoly** is an abbreviation for the word **Stolichnaya** (stah-*leech*-nuh-ye), which means "metropolis" in Russian.

When you go out to eat, do you like to order a great big bowl of **borsh'** (bohrsh'; beet soup) with sour cream? Well, then you're eating one of the most famous Russian dishes, and when you order it, you're using a completely Russian word.

Hearing historical terms

If you're interested in world history, then you probably know that the head of the Russian state in previous centuries was not the president or the king, but the **tsar,** which is just what they called him in Russia, too: **tsar'** (tsahr').

Some of the best-known Russian words actually came into English during the Cold War period, when the Soviet Union was competing with the United States in the areas of science, technology, military, and education. Who would've thought that a short and simple Russian word, **sputnik** (*spoot*-neek; traveling companion), which refers to the first Soviet artificial Earth satellite, would become a household word in English and even lead to a revolution in American space education? And if you've ever used the word **sputnik,** then you were speaking Russian. **Sputnik** means "companion" in Russian.

Maybe you followed world news in the 1980s. If so, you may remember a guy by the name of Mikhail Gorbachev, who reformed Russian Soviet society. He also added two new words to the English language: **glasnost** and **perestroika,** or in Russian: **glasnost'** (*glahs*-nuhst'; openness) and **pyeryestroika** (pee-ree-*strohy*-kuh; restructuring). These words have become part of American speech. Even Ronald Reagan, who was president during Gorbachev's era, liked to repeat the famous Russian phrase, **Dovyeryai, no provyeryai!** (duh-vee-*ryahy,* noh pruh-vee-*ryahy;* Trust but verify!), when talking about the new nuclear weapons treaties he was negotiating with the Soviet Union.

Recognizing English words in Russian

Russian today is filled with words that came from English. Words that have a common ancestry are called *cognates.* Cognates are like foreign political refugees or immigrants. They settle down in their new country and start to adapt to their new life, and even begin to look and behave like native words of their new country.

Your ability to recognize English cognates when you read or hear Russian will be very helpful to you. Cognates are your allies, and they greatly increase your Russian vocabulary. Here are some examples of common cognates you should recognize:

- **aeroport** (ah-eh-rah-*pohrt*; airport)
- **akadyemiya** (uh-kuh-*dye*-mee-ye; academy)
- **algyebra** (*ahl*-geeb-ruh; algebra)
- **amyerikanyets** (ah-mee-ree-*kah*-neets; American man)
- **astronomiya** (uhs-trah-*noh*-mee-ye; astronomy)
- **bank** (bahnk; bank)
- **biologiya** (bee-ah-*loh*-gee-ye; biology)
- **biznyes** (*beez*-nehs; business)
- **biznyesmyen** (beez-nehs-*mehn*; businessman)
- **boks** (bohks; boxing)
- **dyemokrat** (dee-mah-*kraht*; democrat)
- **diryektor** (dee-*ryek*-tuhr; director)
- **doktor** (*dohk*-tuhr; doctor)
- **dokumyent** (duh-koo-*myent*; document)
- **effyektivnyi** (eh-feek-*teev*-nihy; effective)
- **fyermyer** (*fyer*-meer; farmer)
- **filarmoniya** (fee-luhr-*moh*-nee-ye; philharmonic)
- **futbol** (foot-*bohl*; football)
- **gamburgyer** (*gahm*-boor-geer; hamburger)
- **gyenyetika** (gee-*neh*-tee-kuh; genetics)
- **gyeografiya** (gee-uhg-*rah*-fee-ye; geography)

- ✔ **gimnastika** (geem-*nahs*-tee-kuh; gymnastics)
- ✔ **gol'f** (gohl'f; golf)
- ✔ **intyeryesnyj** (een-tee-*ryes*-nihy; interesting)
- ✔ **istoriya** (ees-*toh*-ree-ye; history)
- ✔ **kommunizm** (kuh-moo-*neezm*; communism)
- ✔ **kosmonavt** (kuhs-mah-*nahft*; astronaut)
- ✔ **kosmos** (*kohs*-muhs; cosmos)
- ✔ **kryedit** (*kree*-deet; credit)
- ✔ **lityeratura** (lee-tee-ruh-*too*-ruh; literature)
- ✔ **muzyka** (*moo*-zih-kuh; music)
- ✔ **nos** (nohs; nose)
- ✔ **profyessor** (prah-*fye*-suhr; professor)
- ✔ **sotsiologiya** (suh-tsih-ah-*loh*-gee-ye; sociology)
- ✔ **sport** (spohrt; sports)
- ✔ **sportsmyen** (spahrts-*myen*; sportsman or athlete)
- ✔ **stadion** (stuh-dee-*ohn*; stadium)
- ✔ **studyent** (stoo-*dyent*; student)
- ✔ **styuardyessa** (styu-uhr-*deh*-suh; stewardess)
- ✔ **tyeatr** (tee-*ahtr*; theater)
- ✔ **tyelyevizor** (tee-lee-*vee*-zuhr; TV)
- ✔ **tyennis** (*teh*-nees; tennis)
- ✔ **tyeoriya** (tee-*oh*-ree-ye; theory)
- ✔ **univyersityet** (oo-nee-veer-see-*tyet*; university)
- ✔ **viski** (*vees*-kee; whiskey)
- ✔ **viza** (*vee*-zuh; visa)
- ✔ **vollyejbol** (vuh-leey-*bohl*; volleyball)
- ✔ **zhiraf** (zhee-*rahf*; giraffe)
- ✔ **zhurnal** (zhoor-*nahl*; journal)
- ✔ **zoologiya** (zuh-ah-*loh*-gee-ye; zoology)

Watching out for words that may seem similar but aren't

Beware of *false cognates!* These are words that look and sound like allies (cognates) but aren't. You won't find too many of them, but they can be tricky. And when used incorrectly, they can lead to some funny and even embarrassing situations. Here's a list of the false friends that trip English speakers up the most:

- ✔ **simpatichniy** (seem-puh-*teech*-nihy; good-looking) — This word doesn't mean "sympathetic," so be careful who you say it to!

- ✔ **normal'no** (nahr-*mahl'*-nuh; okay, fine) — This word doesn't mean "normally"!

- ✔ **klass** (klahs; classroom) — This word is the room where a class takes place but doesn't refer to the academic course itself. It also indicates a group of kids in the same grade.

- ✔ **banda** (*bahn*-duh; band of gangsters) — This word has nothing to do with a musical band, so be careful when you use it!

- ✔ **magazin** (muh-guh-*zeen*; store) — This word doesn't mean "magazine," but you can buy one there!

- ✔ **familiya** (fuh-*mee*-lee-ye; last name) — This word isn't your family, but your family name.

Talkin' the Talk

Vladimir and Irina are talking about their new university. How many English cognates can you recognize?

Vladimir:	Irina, ya schitayu, chto biologiya, astronomiya, i gyeografiya ochyen' intyeryesnyye pryedmyety.
	ee-*ree*-nuh, ya sh'ee-*tah*-yu shtoh bee-ah-*loh*-gee-ye, uhs-truh-*noh*-mee-ye, ee gee-uhg-*rah*-fee-ye *oh*-cheen' een-tee-*ryes*-nih-ee preed-*mye*-tih.
	Irina, I think that biology, astronomy, and geography are very interesting subjects.

Irina: **Nye soglasna. Samyye intyeryesnyye pryedmyety v etom universityetye sotsiologiya, istoriya, algyebra, muzyka i tyeatr.**

nee-sahg-*lahs*-nuh. *sah*-mih-ee een-tee-*ryes*-nih-ee preed-*mye*-tih v *eh*-tuhm oo-nee-veer-see-*tye*-tee suh-tsih-ah-*loh*-gee-ye, ees-*toh*-ree-ye, *ahl*-geeb-ruh, *moo*-zih-kuh ee tee-*ahtr*.

I disagree. The most interesting subjects at this university are sociology, history, algebra, music, and theater.

Vladmir: **A tvoj profyessor po lityeraturye intyeryesnyj?**

ah tvohy prah-*fye*-suhr puh lee-tee-ruh-*too*-ree een-tee-*ryes*-nihy?

Is your literature professor interesting?

Irina: **Da, intyeryesnyj, no u nyego bol'shoj nos i on vysokij kak zhiraf.**

dah, een-tee-*ryes*-nihy, noh oo nee-*voh* bahl'-*shohy* nohs i ohn vih-*soh*-keey kahk zhih-*rahf*.

Yes, he's interesting, but he has a big nose, and he's as tall as a giraffe.

Words to Know

ya schitayu	ya sh'ee-<u>tah</u>-yu shtoh	I believe that
ochyen'	<u>oh</u>-cheen'	very
pryedmyety	preed-<u>mye</u>-tih	academic subjects
nye soglasna	nee sahg-<u>lahs</u>-nuh	I disagree
u nyego	oo nee-<u>voh</u>	he has

Looking at the Russian Alphabet (It's Easier than You Think)

If you're like most English speakers, you probably think that the Russian alphabet is the most challenging aspect of picking up the language. The idea of having to memorize all those letters, some of them weird-looking, can be a little bit daunting to the newcomer. But not to worry. The Russian alphabet isn't as hard as you think. In fact, compared to some other features of Russian, such as case ending and verbs (see Chapter 2 for details on those), the alphabet is a piece of cake. When you're done with this section, you'll be able to recognize and pronounce all the letters of the Russian alphabet.

From A to Ya: Making sense of Cyrillic

The Russian alphabet is based on the Cyrillic alphabet, which was named after the ninth-century Byzantine monk, Cyril (see the sidebar "Who was this Cyril guy, anyway?" later in this chapter). Throughout the centuries, Cyril's original alphabet went through many attempts to shorten it from its original 43 letters. Today the alphabet is still pretty lengthy — 33 letters in all, compared with the 26 letters in the English alphabet. But don't panic. You don't have to master every letter. Throughout this book, we convert all the letters into familiar Latin symbols, which are the same symbols we use in the English alphabet. This process of converting from Cyrillic to Latin letters is known as *transliteration*. We list the Cyrillic alphabet below for those of you who are adventurous and brave enough to prefer reading real Russian instead of being fed with the ready-to-digest Latin version of it. And even if you don't want to read the real Russian, check out Table 1-1 to find out what the whole fuss is about regarding the notorious "Russian alphabet."

Notice that in most cases a transliterated letter corresponds to the way it's actually pronounced. As a rule, you may assume that the transliteration fairly well represents the actual pronunciation. The biggest exceptions to this are the letter **Йй**, which is transcribed as **j** but pronounced like an English *y,* and the soft sign **ьь,** which is transcribed as ' but only softens the preceding consonant.

As we walk you through the Russian alphabet, pay attention to the way the alphabet is transliterated, because that's how we spell out all the Russian words throughout the rest of the book. Table 1-1 has the details on Cyrillic letters, their transliteration, and their pronunciation. You can also find a guide to pronunciation on the audio CD that comes with this book.

Scholars do not agree on the letter **j**. Some believe that it's a consonant; others think that it's a vowel. We don't want to take sides in this matter and are listing it both as a consonant and a vowel.

Table 1-1	**The Russian Alphabet in Cyrillic**		
The Letter in Cyrillic	*Transliteration (The Corresponding Letter or Sound in the English Alphabet)*	*Pronunciation*	*Vowel or Consonant*
Аа	**A**	*ah* if stressed as in f**a**ther; *uh* if appearing in any unstressed syllable, as in hum**a**n	Vowel
Бб	**B**	*b* as in **b**ook; *p* if at the end of the word	Consonant
Вв	**V**	*v* as in **V**ictor; *f* if at the end of the word	Consonant
Гг	**G**	*g* as in **g**reat; *k* if at the end of the word	Consonant
Дд	**D**	*d* as in **d**uck; *t* if at the end of the word	Consonant
Ее	**Ye**	*ye* as in **ye**s; *ee* as in s**ee**k if appearing in any unstressed syllable	Vowel
Ёё	**Yo**	*yo* as in **yo**ke	Vowel
Жж	**Zh**	*zh* as mea**s**ure; *sh* if at the end of the word	Consonant
Зз	**Z**	*z* as in **z**ebra; *s* if at the end of the word	Consonant
Ии	**I**	*ee* as in p**ee**k	Vowel
Йй	**J**	very short *y* as bo**y** or Ma**y**	Vowel or Consonant
Кк	**K**	*k* as in **K**ate	Consonant
Лл	**L**	*l* as in **l**amp	Consonant

The Letter in Cyrillic	Transliteration (The Corresponding Letter or Sound in the English Alphabet)	Pronunciation	Vowel or Consonant
Мм	**M**	*m* as in **m**om**m**y	Consonant
Нн	**N**	*n* as in **n**ote	Consonant
Оо	**O**	*oh* as in as in talk; *ah* as in park, if appearing one syllable before the stressed syllable; *uh* as in Morm**o**n, if appearing in any other unstressed syllable	Vowel
Пп	**P**	*p* as in **p**ort	Consonant
Рр	**R**	flap *r*, similar to trilled r in Spanish, as in "madre," for example	Consonant
Сс	**S**	*s* as in **s**ort	Consonant
Тт	**T**	*t* as in **t**ie	Consonant
Уу	**U**	*oo* as sh**oot**	Vowel
Фф	**F**	*f* as in **f**act	Consonant
Хх	**Kh**	*kh* like you're clearing your throat, or like the German "ch"	Consonant
Цц	**Ts**	*ts* as in ca**ts**	Consonant
Чч	**Ch**	*ch* as in **ch**air	Consonant
Шш	**Sh**	*sh* as in **sh**ock	Consonant
Щщ	**Sh'**	soft *sh*, as in **sh**eep	Consonant
ъ	**"**	hard sign (makes the preceding letter hard)	Neither
Ыы	**Y**	*ih*	Vowel
ь	**'**	soft sign (makes the preceding letter soft)	Neither
Ээ	**E**	*e* as in **e**nd	Vowel
Юю	**Yu**	*yu* as in **u**se	Vowel
Яя	**Ya**	*ya* if stressed as in **ya**rd; *ee* if unstressed and not in the final syllable of the word; *ye* if unstressed and in the final syllable of the word	Vowel

Who was this Cyril guy, anyway?

Picture this: The year is sometime around AD 863. Two Byzantine monks and brothers, Cyril and Methodius, were commissioned by their emperor to Christianize the East European pagan tribes. To carry out the emperor's order, the two brothers had to transcribe the Bible into Slavic. This task was very daunting because the Slavs didn't have any written language at the time and the Slavic dialect they were working with contained a lot of bizarre sounds not found in any other language.

One of the brothers, Cyril, came up with an ingenious idea: create a Slavic alphabet from a mishmash of Greek, Hebrew, and old Latin words and sounds. That was a clever solution because by drawing on different languages, Cyril's alphabet contained practically every sound necessary for the correct pronunciation of Russian.

In honor of Cyril's clever idea, the alphabet became known as the Cyrillic alphabet. The Cyrillic script is now used by more than 70 languages, ranging from Eastern Europe's Slavic languages (Russian, Ukrainian, Belorussian, Bulgarian, Serbian, and Macedonian) to Central Asia's Altaic languages (Turkmen, Uzbek, Kazakh, and Kirghiz).

I know you! Familiar-looking, same-sounding letters

You may notice that some of the Russian letters in the previous section look a lot like English letters. The letters that look like English and are pronounced like English letters are:

- Aa
- Kк
- Mм
- Oo
- Tт

Whenever you read Russian text, you should be able to recognize and pronounce these letters right away.

Playing tricks: Familiar-looking, different-sounding letters

Some Russian letters look like English letters but are pronounced differently. You want to watch out for these:

✔ **Вв:** It looks like English Bb, at least the capital letter does, but it's pronounced like the sound *v* as in *victor* or *vase*.

✔ **Ее:** This one's a constant annoyance for English speakers, who want to pronounce it like *ee,* as in the English word *geese.* In Russian, it's pronounced that way only if it appears in an unstressed syllable. Otherwise, if it appears in a stressed syllable, it is pronounced like *ye* as in *yes.*

✔ **Ёё:** Don't confuse this with the letter **Ее.** When two dots appear over the Ее, it's considered a different letter, and it is pronounced like *yo* as in *yoke.*

✔ **Нн:** It's not the English Hh. It just looks like it. Actually, it's pronounced like *n* as in *Nick.*

✔ **Рр:** In Russian it's pronounced like a trilled *r* and not like the English letter *p* as in *Peter.*

✔ **Сс:** This letter is always pronounced like *s* as in *sun* and never like *k* as in *victor.*

✔ **Уу:** This letter is pronounced like *oo* as in *shoot* and never like *y* as in *yes.*

✔ **Хх:** Never pronounce this letter like *z* or *ks* as in the word *Xerox.* In Russian the sound it represents is a coarse-sounding, guttural *kh,* similar to the German *ch.* (See "Surveying sticky sounds," later in this chapter, for info on pronouncing this sound.)

How bizarre: Weird-looking letters

As you've probably noticed, quite a few Russian letters don't look like English letters at all:

✔ Бб

✔ Гг

✔ Дд

✔ Жж

✔ Зз

✔ Ии

✔ Йй

✔ Лл

✔ Пп

✔ Фф

✔ Цц

✔ Чч

✔ Шш

✔ Щщ

✔ ъ

✔ Ыы

✔ Ь

✔ Ээ

✔ Юю

✔ Яя

Don't panic over these letters. Just because they look weird doesn't mean they're any harder to say than the others. It's just a matter of memorizing their proper pronunciations. (Refer to Table 1-1 for details on how to say each letter.)

You may recognize several of these weird letters, such as **Ф, Г, З, Л, П,** from learning the Greek alphabet during your fraternity or sorority days.

Sounding Like a Real Russian with Proper Pronunciation

Compared to English pronunciation, which often has more exceptions than rules, Russian rules of pronunciation are fairly clear and consistent. In this section, you discover some of the basic rules and patterns of Russian pronunciation and find out about important irregularities with vowels and consonants. In addition, we show you how to say some of the more difficult letters and sounds.

Understanding the one-letter-one-sound principle

Russian is a *phonetic language,* which means that for the most part one Russian letter corresponds to one sound. For example, the letter **K** is always pronounced like *k,* and the letter **M** is always pronounced like *m.* This pattern is different from English, where a letter can be pronounced in different ways depending on where it shows up in a word. For instance, consider the two different pronunciations for the letter *c* in the words *cat* and *race.* This difference almost never happens in Russian.

Giving voice to vowels

Vowels are the musical building blocks of every Russian word. If you flub a consonant or two, you'll probably still be understood. (To avoid such flubs, though, check out "Enunciating consonants correctly," later in this chapter.) But if you don't pronounce your vowels correctly, there's a good chance you won't be understood at all. So it's a good idea to get down the basic principles of saying Russian vowels, which we cover in the following sections.

That's stretching it: Lengthening out vowels

If you want to sound more Russian, don't shorten your vowels like English speakers often do. When you say **a, o,** or **u,** open your mouth wider and purposefully stretch out the sounds to make them a little bit longer. Imagine, for example, that you're in your room on the second floor, and your mom is downstairs in the kitchen. You call her by saying "Mo-o-o-m!" That's the way Russians say their vowels (except for the shouting part!).

Some stress is good: Accenting the right vowels

Stress is an important concept in Russian. Putting a stress in the wrong place isn't just a formal mistake. It can hinder communication, because the meaning of a word can change based on where the stress is. For example, the word **zamok** (*zah*-muhk) means "castle." However, if you shift the stress from the first syllable to the last, the word **zamok** (zuh-*mohk*) now means "lock."

Unfortunately, no (hard and fast) rules about stress exist. Stress in Russian is unpredictable and erratic, though you begin to recognize some patterns as you learn more. The harsh truth, however, is that each word has its own stress pattern. What happens if you stress the vowel in the wrong place? Certainly, nothing terrible: the earth will continue to rotate around its axis. What may happen, however, is that your interlocutor will have a hard time understanding you and take longer to grasp what you really mean. Before learning a new Russian word, find out which vowel to stress. Look in any Russian-English dictionary, which usually marks stress by putting the sign ´ over the stressed syllable. In a dictionary, **zamok** (*zah*-muhk; castle) is written за́мок, and **zamok** (zuh-*mohk*; lock) is written замо́к.

Vowels misbehavin': Reduction

Some Russian letters change their behavior depending on whether they're in a stressed or an unstressed syllable. The vowels **a, o, ye,** and **ya** do this a lot. When stressed, they behave normally and are pronounced in the usual way, but when they're in an unstressed position, they go through a process called *reduction*. This deviation in the vowels' behavior is a very important linguistic phenomenon that deserves your special attention. Not knowing it is like a double-edged sword: not only does it take other people longer to understand you (they simply won't recognize the words you're saying), but you also may find it hard to recognize the words you think you already know (but unfortunately store in your own memory with the wrong stress).

- ✔ **O,** which is normally pronounced like *oh,* sounds like *ah* (like the letter **a** in the word *father*) if it occurs exactly one syllable before the stressed syllable, and like a neutral *uh* (like the letter **a** in the word *about*) if it appears in any other unstressed syllable.

  A, which is pronounced like *ah* when it's stressed, is pronounced like a neutral *uh* (like the letter **a** in the word *about*) if it appears in any unstressed syllable.

The honest-to-goodness truth is that when the letter **a** appears in the syllable preceding the stressed syllable, its pronunciation is somewhere between *uh* and *ah*. We don't, however, want to burden you with excessive linguistic information, so we indicate the letter **a** as *uh* in all unstressed positions, even though we realize that some persnickety Russian language phonologists (pronunciation specialists) may take issue. Moreover, in conversational speech, catching the distinction is nearly impossible. If you say an unstressed **a** as *uh,* people will fully understand you.

✔ **Ye,** which is pronounced like *ye* (as in *yet*) in a stressed syllable, sounds like *ee* (as in *seek*) in any unstressed syllable.

When it appears at the end of a word, as in **viditye** (*vee*-dee-tee; (you) see; formal singular and plural), or after another vowel, as in **chayepi-tiye** (chah-ee-*pee*-tee-ee; tea drinking), an unstressed **ye** is actually pronounced somewhere between *ee* and *ye*. Russian phonologists (pronunciation experts) still debate which sound it's closer to. So for the sake of simplicity, we always render an unstressed **ye** as *ee*. If you say it that way, any Russian will understand you.

✔ An unstressed **ya** sounds either like *ee* (as in *peek*) if it's unstressed (but not in the word's final syllable) or like *ye* (as in *yet*) if it's unstressed and also in the final syllable of the word.

Here are some examples of how vowel reduction affects word pronunciation:

✔ You write **Kolorado** (Colorado) but say kuh-lah-*rah*-duh. Notice how the first **o** is reduced to a neutral *uh* and the next **o** is reduced to an *ah* sound (because it's exactly one syllable before the stressed syllable), and it's reduced again to a neutral *uh* sound in the final unstressed syllable.

✔ You write **khorosho** (good, well) but say khuh-rah-*shoh*. Notice how the first **o** is reduced to a neutral *uh,* the next **o** is reduced to *ah* (it precedes the stressed syllable), and **o** in the last syllable is pronounced as *oh* because it's stressed.

✔ You write **napravo** (to the right) but say nuh-*prah*-vuh. Notice that the first **a** is reduced to a neutral *uh* (because it's not in the stressed syllable), the second **a** is pronounced normally (like *ah*) and the final **o** is pronounced like a neutral *uh,* because it follows the stressed syllable.

✔ You write **Pyetyerburg** (Petersburg) but say pee-teer-*boork.* Notice how **ye** is reduced to the sound *ee* in each case, because it's not stressed.

✔ You write **Yaponiya** (Japan) but say ee-*poh*-nee-ye. Notice how the unstressed letter **ya** sounds like *ee* at the beginning of the word and like *ye* at the end of the word (because it's unstressed and in the final syllable).

Saying sibilants with vowels

The letters **zh, ts, ch, sh,** and **sh'** are called *sibilants,* because they emit a hissing sound. When certain vowels appear after these letters, those vowels are pronounced slightly differently than normal. After a sibilant, **ye** is pronounced like *eh* (as in *end*) and **yo** is pronounced like *oh* (as in *talk*). Examples are the words **tsyentr** (tsehntr; center) and **shyol** (shohl; went by foot; masculine). The sound *ee* always becomes *ih* after one of these sibilants, regardless of whether the *ee* sound comes from the letter **i** or from an unstressed **ye.** Take, for example, the words **mashina** (muh-*shih*-nuh; car) and **bol'shye** (*bohl'*-shih; bigger).

Enunciating consonants correctly

Like Russian vowels (see the previous section), Russian consonants follow certain patterns and rules of pronunciation. If you want to sound like a real Russian, you need to keep the basics in the following sections in mind.

Say it, don't spray it! Relaxing with consonants

When pronouncing the letters **p, t,** or **k,** English speakers are used to straining their tongue and lips. This strain results in what linguists call *aspiration* — a burst of air that comes out of your mouth as you say these sounds. To see what we're talking about, put your hand in front of your mouth and say the word "top." You should feel air against your hand as you pronounce the word.

In Russian, however, aspiration shouldn't happen because consonants are pronounced without aspiration. In other words, say it, don't spray it! In fact, you should totally relax your tongue and lips before saying Russian **p, t,** or **k.** For example, imagine somebody who's just had a stroke. She won't be able to put too much effort into her consonants. Believe it or not, that's almost the way you should say your Russian consonants. Relax your speech organs as much as possible, and you'll say it correctly. To practice saying consonants without unnecessary aspiration, again put your hand in front of your mouth and say Russian cognates **park** (pahrk), **lampa** (*lahm*-puh), and **tank** (tahnk). Practice until you don't produce a puff of air with these words!

Cat got your tongue? Consonants losing their voice

Some consonants (**b, v, g, d, zh,** and **z**) are called *voiced consonants* because they're pronounced with the voice. Practice saying them out loud and you'll see it's true.

But when voiced consonants appear at the end of a word, a strange thing happens to them: They actually lose their voice. This process is called *devoicing.* They're still spelled the same, but in their pronunciation, they transform into their devoiced counterparts:

- **B** is pronounced like *p*.
- **V** is pronounced like *f*.
- **G** is pronounced like *k*.
- **D** is pronounced like *t*.
- **Zh** is pronounced like *sh*.
- **Z** is pronounced like *s*.

Here are some examples:

- You write **Smirnov** but pronounce it as smeer-*nohf* because **v** at the end of the word is pronounced like *f*.
- You write **garazh** (garage) but say guh-*rah***sh**, because at the end of the word, **zh** loses its voice and is pronounced like *sh*.

Nutty clusters: Pronouncing consonant combinations

Russian speech often sounds like an endless flow of consonant clusters. Combinations of two, three, and even four consonants are quite common. Take, for example, the common word for *hello* in Russian — **zdravstvujtye** (*zdrah*-stvooy-tee), which has two difficult consonant combinations (**zdr** and **vstv**). Or take the word for *opinion* in Russian — **vzglyad** (vzglyat). The word contains four consonants following one another: **vzgl**.

How in the world do Russians say these words without choking? They practice, and so should you. Here are some words that contain consonant clusters you may want to repeat at leisure:

- **obstoyatyel'stvo** (uhp-stah-*ya*-teel'-stvuh; circumstance)
- **pozdravlyat'** (puh-zdruhv-*lyat'*; to congratulate)
- **prestuplyeniye** (pree-stoo-*plyen*-ee-ye; crime)
- **Rozhdyestvo** (ruzh-deest-*voh*; Christmas)
- **vzdor** (vzdohr; nonsense)
- **vzglyanut'** (vzglee-*noot'*; to look/glance)

Surveying sticky sounds

Some Russian letters and sounds are hard for speakers of English. Take a look at some of them and find out how to pronounce them.

The bug sound zh

This sound corresponds to the letter **Жж.** It looks kind of like a bug, doesn't it? It sounds like a bug, too! In pronouncing it, try to imitate the noise produced by a bug flying over your ear — zh-zh-zh . . . The sound is similar to the sound in the words "pleasure" or "measure."

The very short i sound

This sound corresponds to the letter **Йй.** This letter's name is *i kratkoye,* which literally means "a very short i," but it actually sounds like the very short English *y.* This sound is what you hear when you say the word bo**y.** You should notice your tongue touching the roof of your mouth when you say this sound.

The rolled sound r

This sound corresponds to the letter **Рр** in the Russian alphabet. To say it correctly, begin by saying an English *r* and notice that your tongue is rolled back. Now begin moving your tongue back, closer to your upper teeth and try to say this sound with your tongue in this new position. You'll hear how the quality of the sound changes. This is the way the Russians say it.

The guttural sound kh

The corresponding Russian letter is **Хх.** To say it, imagine that you're eating and a piece of food just got stuck in your throat. What's the first reflex you body responds with? Correct! You will try to cough it up. Remember the sound your throat produces? This is the Russian sound *kh.* It's similar to the German *ch.*

The revolting sound y

To say this sound correctly, imagine that you're watching something really revolting, like an episode from *Fear Factor,* where the participants are gorging on a plate of swarming bugs. Now recall the sound you make in response to this. This sound is pronounced something like *ih,* and that's how you pronounce the Russian **ы** (the transliteration is *y*). Because this letter appears in some of the most commonly used words, including **ty** (tih; you; informal), **vy** (vih; you; formal singular and plural), and **my** (mih; we), it's important to say it as best you can.

The hard sign

This is the letter **ъ.** While the soft sign makes the preceding sound soft (see the next section), the hard sign makes it — yes, you guessed it — hard. The good news is that this letter (which transliterates to ") is rarely ever used in contemporary Russian. And even when it is, it doesn't change the pronunciation of the word. So, why does Russian have this sign? For two purposes:

- ✔ To harden the previous consonant
- ✔ To retain the hardness of the consonant before the vowels **ye, yo, yu,** and **ya**

Without the hard sign, these consonants would normally palatalize (or soften). When a hard sign ъ separates a consonant and one of these vowels, the consonant is pronounced without palatalization, as in the word **pod"yezd** (pahd-*yezd*; porch), for example. However, don't worry too much about this one if your native language is English. Native speakers of English rarely tend to palatalize their Russian consonants the way Russians do it. In other words, if you're a native English speaker and you come across the situation described here, you probably make your consonant hard and therefore pronounce it correctly by default!

The soft sign

This is the letter ь (transliterated to '), and it doesn't have a sound. Its only mission in life is to make the preceding consonant soft. This sound is very important in Russian because it can change the meaning of a word. For example, without the soft sign, the word **mat'** (maht'; mother) becomes **mat,** which means "obscene language." And when you add a soft sign at the end of the word **von** (vohn; over there), it becomes **von'** (vohn') and means "stench." See how important the soft sign is?

So, here's how you can make consonants soft:

1. Say the consonant — for example, **l, t,** or **d.** Note where your tongue is. What you should feel is that the tip of your tongue is touching the ridge of your upper teeth and the rest of the tongue is hanging in the mouth like a hammock in the garden on a nice summer day.

2. While you're still pronouncing the consonant, raise the body of your tongue and press it against the hard palate. Can you hear how the quality of the consonant has changed? It sounds much "softer" now, doesn't it? That's how you make your consonants soft.

Using Popular Expressions

Using popular expressions is one way to make a great first impression when speaking Russian. We recommend that you memorize the phrases in the following sections because they can come in handy in almost any situation.

Speaking courteously

The way to say "please" and "you're welcome" in Russian is **pozhalujsta** (pah-*zhahl*-stuh). You often use the word **pozhalujsta** just after the verb when making a polite request, as in the following sentences:

- ✔ **Povtoritye, pozhalujsta.** (puhf-tah-*ree*-tee pah-*zhahl*-stuh; Please repeat what you said.)

- ✔ **Govoritye, pozhalujsta, pomyedlyennyeye.** (guh-vah-*ree*-tee pah-*zhahl*-stuh pah-*myed*-lye-nee-ee; Please speak a little more slowly.)

- ✔ **Skazhitye, pozhalujsta, kak proiti do myetro?** (skah-*zhih*-tee pah-*zhahl*-stuh kahk prahy-*tee* duh meet-*roh;* Please tell me how to get to the subway station.)

After somebody answers your polite request or does you a favor, you say **spasibo** (spuh-*see*-buh; thank you) or **spasibo bol'shoye** (spuh-*see*-buh bahl'-*shoy*-ee; thank you very much).

When you want to say "you're welcome," you simply use the word **pozhalujsta** by itself.

Excusing yourself

The most common way to say "excuse me" in Russian is **izvinitye** (eez-vee-*nee*-tee). To be even more polite, you can add the word **pozhalujsta** (pah-*zhahl*-stuh; please), as in the following sentences:

- ✔ **Izvinitye, pozhalujsta, mnye pora.** (eez-vee-*nee*-tee pah-*zhahl*-stuh mnye pah-*rah;* Excuse me, it's time for me to go.)

- ✔ **Izvinitye, pozhalujsta, ya vas nye ponimayu.** (eez-vee-*nee*-tee pah-*zhahl*-stuh yah vahs nee puh-nee-*mah*-yu; Excuse me, I didn't understand what you said.)

Arming yourself with other handy phrases

You can also put the following phrases to good use in Russian:

- ✔ **Dobro pozhalovat'!** (dahb-*roh* pah-*zhah*-luh-vuht'; Welcome!)

- ✔ **Pozdravlyayu vas!** (puhz-druhv-*la*-yu vahs; Congratulations!)

✔ **Zhyelayu udachi!** (zhih-*lah*-yu oo-*dah*-chee; Good luck!)

✔ **Nichyego.** (nee-chee-*voh*; It's all right/no problem.)

✔ **Vsyego khoroshyego!** (vsee-*voh* khah-*roh*-shih-vuh; All the best!)

✔ **Priyatnogo appyetita!** (pree-*yat*-nuh-vuh uh-pee-*tee*-tuh; Bon appetit!)

✔ **Zhal'!** (zhahl'; Too bad!)

✔ **Khorosho.** (khuh-rah-*shoh*; It's all right.)

Reading Russian with Ease

Reading in Russian is an important skill to have. If you want to read a Russian magazine, menu, or train schedule, or if you want find your way around Russian-speaking places, you have to know how to read some Russian.

Suppose that you're walking in the Russian district of an American city and are suddenly in the mood for food. Being able to read Russian is a big help when you see a building with the sign **РЕСТОРАН** (ree-stah-*rahn*) on it. You'll understand that the building is exactly what you're looking for — a restaurant! (We give you the lowdown on talking about food in Chapter 5.)

Or imagine that you booked a trip to Moscow with your favorite travel agent and you've just gotten off the plane. The big sign on the airport building reads **Санкт-Петербрг.** If you know how to read some Russian, you're able to understand that the sign says **Sankt-Peterburg** (sahnk pee-teer-*boork*; St. Petersburg) and not **Москва/Moskva** (mahs-*kvah*; Moscow), which means you've come to the wrong place, and it's time to find a new travel agent! (You can find out all about planning a trip to Russia and navigating the airport in Chapters 11 and 12.)

The first step to reading Russian is recognizing Cyrillic letters (see "From A to Ya: Making sense of Cyrillic," earlier in this chapter, for info on these letters). Try sounding out each word, and you may be surprised that you recognize quite a few of them because they're similar to words you know in English or other languages. Then you can look up the ones you're unsure of in the Russian-English dictionary. You don't need to know every word in a sentence to get the sense of what you're reading. At least try to locate and understand the nouns and the verbs, and you'll be off to a good start (see Chapter 2 for info on nouns and verbs).

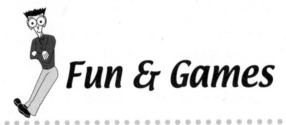

Fun & Games

Match the Russian letters in the first column with the sounds they correspond to in the second column. You can find the answers in Appendix C.

1. **Н**   a. r

2. **Р**   b. n

3. **Г**   c. ee

4. **Я**   d. ya

5. **И**   e. g

Below are Russian cognates used in English. Sound out each word and see whether you can recognize its meaning. The answers are in Appendix C.

1. **Водка**

2. **Борщ**

3. **Перестройка**

4. **Гласность**

5. **Спутник**

6. **Царь**

Chapter 2

The Nitty Gritty: Basic Russian Grammar and Numbers

Grammar is the glue that ties together all the words in a sentence in any language. Not knowing grammar can be very frustrating and sometimes even embarrassing, so getting the basics of Russian grammar down is worth your time. Russian has more grammar than English does, but fortunately it's all very structured, and you can easily learn it if you put in a little effort.

You may be surprised to find out that English and Russian are very distant relatives. Both come from the same ancestor — Sanskrit — and both belong to the same family of Indo-European languages. Although they're distantly related, they have one big difference: Unlike English, Russian is a *flectional language,* which is a fancy way of saying that it has lots of different word endings.

English words don't have too many different flections, or endings. As far as verbs go, you have the -ed ending for past tense verbs (worked) and the -ing ending for some present tense verbs (working). And you also know the singular present verb form -(e)s (goes, walks), and the -er and -est endings for comparative and superlative adjectives (bigger, biggest). And singular nouns don't have any flections at all. A table is a table is a table, no matter how you use it in a sentence.

But in Russian, the same noun can take several different endings! The ending depends on the case of the noun, which is determined by how the noun is

used in the sentence. And a Russian verb in the present tense can take up to six different endings, depending on who the subject of the sentence is.

In this chapter, you find out about cases and the different noun and verb endings. You discover how to spice up your speech with pronouns, adjectives, and adverbs. You also find out how to ask questions and how to form other complete sentences that make you sound like a real Russian. As a bonus, you also discover how to count in Russian and use numbers with nouns.

Making the Russian Cases

In a Russian sentence, every noun, pronoun, and adjective takes a different ending depending on the case it's in. What's a case? In simple terms, *cases* are sets of endings that words take to indicate their function and relationship to other words in the sentence. If you've studied languages such as Latin or German, you know that different languages have different numbers of cases. Russian has six cases, which isn't that bad compared to Finnish, which has fifteen! English speakers, on the other hand, never have to bother with cases.

In the following sections, you discover the six different cases in Russian and how to use them. (Later in this chapter, we explain the specific endings that nouns, pronouns, and adjectives take in each case.)

Nominative case

A noun (or a pronoun or an adjective) always appears in the nominative case in an English-Russian dictionary. Its main function is to indicate the subject of the sentence.

As a rule, the subject behaves the same way in Russian as it does in English. It answers the question "Who or what is performing the action?"

For example, in the sentence **Bryenda izuchayet russkij yazyk** (*brehn*-duh ee-zoo-*chah*-eet *roos*-keey ee-*zihk*; Brenda studies Russian), the word **Bryenda,** indicating a woman who (like yourself) studies Russian, is the subject of the sentence and consequently is used in the nominative case.

Genitive case

You usually use the genitive case to indicate possession. It answers the question "Whose?" In the phrase **kniga Anny** (*knee*-guh *ah*-nih; Anna's book), **Anna** is in the genitive case (**Anny**) because she's the book's owner.

Genitive case also is used to indicate an absence of somebody or something when you combine it with the word **nyet** (nyet; no/not), as in **Zdyes' nyet knigi** (zdyes' nyet *knee*-gee; There's no book here). **Knigi** (*knee*-gee; book) is in the genitive case because the book's absence is at issue.

Russian uses genitive case after many common prepositions, such as **okolo** (*oh*-kuh-luh; near), **u** (oo; by, by the side of), **mimo** (*mee*-muh; past), **iz** (ees; out of), **vmyesto** (*vmyes*-tuh; instead of), and **byez** (byes; without). For more info on prepositions, see Chapter 15.

Accusative case

The accusative case mainly indicates a direct object, which is the object of the action of the verb in a sentence. For example, in the sentence **Ya lyublyu russkij yazyk** (yah lyu-*blyu roo*-skeey ee-*zihk*; I love Russian), the phrase **russkij yazyk** is in the accusative case because it's the direct object.

Some frequently used verbs like **chitat'** (chee-*taht'*; to read) **vidyet'** (*vee*-deet'; to see), **slushat'** (*sloo*-shuht'; to hear), and **izuchat'** (ee-zoo-*chaht'*; to study) take the accusative case. Like in English, these verbs always take direct objects.

The accusative case is also required in sentences containing verbs of motion, which indicate destination of movement. For instance, if you want to announce to your family that you're going to **Rossiya** (rah-*see*-ye; Russia), **Rossiya** takes the form of the accusative case, which is **Rossiyu** (rah-*see*-yu; Russia). Chapter 12 is full of info on verbs of motion.

You also use the accusative case after certain prepositions, such as **pro** (proh; about) and **chyeryez** (*chye*-rees; through).

Dative case

Use the dative case to indicate an indirect object, which is the person or thing toward whom the action in a sentence is directed. For example, in the sentence **Ya dal uchityelyu sochinyeniye** (yah dahl oo-*chee*-tee-lyu suh-chee-*nye*-nee-ee; I gave the teacher my essay), **uchityelyu** (oo-*chee*-tee-lyu; teacher) is in the dative case because it's the indirect object. ("My essay" acts as the direct object, which we cover in the previous section.)

You also use the dative case after certain prepositions such as **k** (k; toward) and **po** (poh; along).

Some frequently used verbs, such as **pomogat'** (puh-mah-*gaht'*; to help) and **pozvonit'** (puh-zvah-*neet'*; to call), force the nouns that come after them into the dative case. The implication with these verbs in Russian is that you're giving help or making a call *to somebody*, which suggests an indirect receiver of the action of the verb.

Instrumental case

As the name suggests, the instrumental case is often used to indicate the instrument that assists in the carrying out of an action. So, when you say that you're writing a letter with a **ruchka** (*rooch*-kuh; pen), you have to put **ruchka** into the instrumental case, which is **ruchkoj** (*rooch*-kuhy).

Use the instrumental case after certain prepositions such as **s** (s; with), **myezhdu** (*myezh*-doo; between), **nad** (naht; over), **pod** (poht; below), and **pyeryed** (*pye*-reet; in front of). For more information on prepositions, see Chapter 15.

Prepositional case

Prepositional case got its name because it's used only after certain prepositions. Older Russian textbooks often refer to it as the locative case, because it often indicates the location where the action takes place. No wonder it's used with the prepositions **v** (v; in) and **na** (nah; on).

The prepositional case is also used after the prepositions **o** (oh; about) and **ob** (ohb; about). So when you say to that special someone, "I am constantly thinking about you," make sure to put **ty** (tih; you; informal singular) in the prepositional case, which is **tyebye** (tee-*bye*): **Ya postoyanno dumayu o tyebye** (yah puhs-tah-*ya*-nuh *doo*-muh-yu uh tee-*bye*).

By the way, you may wonder why the English preposition "about" is translated by two different Russian equivalents: **o** and **ob**. For your information, **o** is used if the following word begins with a consonant. Use **ob** if the following word begins with a vowel.

Building Your Grammar Base with Nouns and Pronouns

Nouns and pronouns are the building blocks of any sentence. In the following sections, you find out about the three different genders for nouns. You also

discover how to change the ending of nouns and pronouns depending on their function in a sentence and how to form plurals of nouns.

Getting the lowdown on the gender of nouns

A noun can be a person, an animal, a place, a thing, an event (Easter, funeral), an idea (truth, virtue), or even a feeling (envy, love). Unlike English nouns, every Russian noun has what's called a *grammatical gender:* either masculine, feminine, or neuter. All nouns have gender, and not just humans or living beings.

Knowing the grammatical gender of a noun is important, because gender determines how the noun changes for each of the six cases.

In the following sections, we explain how to determine the gender of nouns in Russian and warn you about some tricky-looking nouns.

Which one is it? How to tell the gender of a Russian noun

Determining the gender of a Russian noun is simple and a lot of fun. To truly enjoy determining the gender of a noun, you need to know that it's the ending of a noun that in most cases indicates the noun's gender. In their dictionary form (the nominative case), Russian nouns may end with only one of the following: a consonant; **-j** (an unusual letter — see Chapter 1); the vowels **-a**, **-ya**, **-o**, **-ye**, and **-yo**; or the soft sign (').

To define the gender of a noun, just follow the rules in Table 2-1.

Table 2-1	Determining the Gender of a Russian Noun
If a Noun in Nominative Case Ends In	**The Noun's Gender Is**
A consonant	Masculine
-j	Masculine
-a or -ya	Feminine
-o, -ye, or -yo	Neuter
Soft sign (')	Either feminine or masculine; look up this word in the dictionary to be sure

Grammatical gender for words denoting living beings, in the majority of cases, coincides with biological gender. The word **mal'chik** (*mahl'*-cheek; boy) is a masculine noun and the word **dyevushka** (*dyeh*-voosh-kuh; girl) is a feminine noun, just as you'd expect.

When it comes to inanimate objects, grammatical gender seems to have no relationship to the meaning of the word. The word **dvyer'** (dvyer'; door) is feminine, while **pol** (pohl; floor) is masculine noun. **Okno** (ahk-*noh*; window) is neuter, while **zanavyeska** (zuh-nuh–*vyes*-kuh; curtain) is feminine.

Gender deviants: Masculine nouns that look feminine

A number of common Russian nouns denoting male beings can be confusing, because their grammatical gender is actually feminine. These nouns are considered feminine, because they have the feminine ending **-a**:

- **muzhchina** (moo-*sh'ee*-nuh; man)
- **papa** (*pah*-puh; dad)
- **dyedushka** (*dye*-doosh-kuh; grandfather)
- **dyadya** (*dya*-dye; uncle)

These gender deviants behave just like feminine nouns when their endings change for each of the cases. Memorizing them is a good idea, because they're words you use a lot.

Checking out cases for nouns

Noun declension is when you change the case endings for nouns. Table 2-2 shows you the declension for masculine, feminine, and neuter singular nouns for all the cases. This table shows declension for singular nouns only. For plural noun declension, see the next section.

Table 2-2	Declension of Singular Nouns				
If a Noun In Its Dictionary Form (Nominative Case) Ends In	To Form Genitive	To Form Accusative	To Form Dative	To Form Instrumental	To Form Prepositional
A consonant	Add -a	Add -a if the noun is a living being; otherwise, don't do anything	Add -u	Add -om	Add -ye

If a Noun In Its Dictionary Form (Nominative Case) Ends In	To Form Genitive	To Form Accusative	To Form Dative	To Form Instrumental	To Form Prepositional
-a	Replace -a with -y	Replace -a with -u	Replace -a with -ye	Replace -a with -oj	Replace -a with -ye
-iye	Replace -iye with -iya	Don't do anything	Replace -iye with -iyu	Replace -iye with -iyem	Replace -iye with -ii
-iya	Replace -iya with -ii	Replace -iya with -iyu	Replace -iya with -ii	Replace -iya with -iyej	Replace -iya with -ii
-j	Replace -j with -ya	Replace -j with -ya if the noun is a living being; otherwise, don't do anything	Replace -j with -yu	Replace -j with -yem	Replace -j with -ye
-o	Replace -o with -a	Don't do anything	Replace -o with -u	Replace -o with -om	Replace -o with -ye
-ye	Replace -e with -ya	Don't do anything	Replace -ye with -yu	Replace -ye with -yem	Don't do anything
-ya	Replace -ya with -i	Replace -ya with -yu	Replace -ya with -ye	Replace -ya with -yej	Replace -ya with -ye
Soft sign (')	If the noun is feminine, replace the soft sign with -i If the noun is masculine, replace the soft sign with -ya	If the noun is feminine, don't do anything If the noun is masculine and a living being, replace the soft sign with -ya; otherwise, don't do anything	If the noun is feminine, replace the soft sign with -i If the noun is masculine, replace the soft sign with -yu	If the noun is feminine, replace the soft sign with -yu If the noun is masculine, replace the soft sign with -yem	If the noun is feminine, replace the soft sign with -i If the noun is masculine, replace the soft sign with -ye

Russian nouns in the nominative case never end in the letters **-i, -u, -y, -e,** or **-yu.** A small number of nouns end in **-yo,** but they're special cases and we deal with them as they come up.

This table may look kind of scary at first, but it's actually easy to use. Imagine you want to brag to your Russian friends about your new car by saying "I bought my friend a car." The first part of the sentence is **ya kupil** (ya koo-*peel*; I bought). But what should you do with the nouns "car" and "friend"? In this sentence, **mashina** (muh-*shih*-nuh; car) is a direct object of the action expressed by the verb **kupil** (koo-*peel*; bought). That means you have to put **mashina** into the accusative case. (For more info on cases, see "Making the Russian Cases" earlier in this chapter.)

The next step is to find the appropriate ending in Table 2-2. You find this ending in the second row, third column. The table says to replace **-a** with **-u.**

Now what about **drug** (drook; friend)? Because "friend" is the indirect object of the sentence (the person to whom or for whom the action of the verb is directed), it takes the dative case in Russian. Table 2-2 indicates that if a noun ends in a consonant (as does **drug**), you form the dative case by adding the letter **-u** to the final consonant. The correct form for **drug** in this sentence is **drugu** (*droog*-oo). So here's your complete sentence: **Ya kupil drugu mashinu** (yah koo-*peel droog*-oo muh-*shih*-noo; I bought my friend a car).

Congratulations! You just created your first Russian sentence!

Putting plurals into their cases

As you probably guessed, Russian plural nouns take different endings depending on the case they're in. In the following sections, you find out about all the different rules for forming the plural. We start with the nominative plural and then look at plural declension for all the other cases.

Forming plurals in the nominative case

Table 2-3 shows you the rules for plural formation in the nominative case.

Table 2-3	Forming the Plural of Nouns in the Nominative Case
If a Noun In Its Dictionary Form (Nominative Case) Ends In	*To Form the Nominative Plural*
A consonant	Add -y
-a	Replace -a with -y
-iye	Replace -iye with -iya

If a Noun In Its Dictionary Form (Nominative Case) Ends In	To Form the Nominative Plural
-iya	Replace -iya with -ii
-j	Replace -j with -i
-o	Replace -o with -a
-ye	Replace -ye with -ya
-ya	Replace -ya with -i
Soft sign (')	Replace soft sign with -i

Practice using this table. Take the word **komp'yutyer** (kahm-*p'yu*-tehr; computer). If you want to say "computers" in Russian, first ask yourself what the word **komp'yutyer** ends in: the consonant **r.** When you look at the first row and first column of Table 2-3, you see that if a noun ends in a consonant, to form the plural you need to add the letter **y** at the end. So "computers" in Russian is **komp'yutyery** (kahm-*p'yu*-teh-rih).

The rules in Table 2-3 have a few important exceptions. Some consonants, namely **zh, sh, sh', g, k,** and **kh,** are very touchy. They just don't tolerate the letter **y** after them and prefer an **i** instead. Take, for example, the word **kniga** (*knee*-guh; book). According to Table 2-3, **kniga** should replace the final **-a** with **-y** to form its plural. But the touchy **g** doesn't tolerate the **-y** ending. It takes an **-i** ending instead. So the plural of **kniga** is **knigi** (*knee*-gee; books).

Changing plurals into the genitive case

Forming the plurals of nouns in the genitive case is a little trickier than in the other cases, so we deal with it first in Table 2-4.

Table 2-4   Forming the Plural of Nouns in the Genitive Case

If a Noun In Its Dictionary Form (Nominative Case) Ends In	To Form Genitive Plural
A consonant other than -zh, -sh, -sh', -ch, or -ts	Add -ov: **studyent** (stoo-*dyent*; male student) becomes **studyentov** (stoo-*dyen*-tuhf; male students)
-zh, -sh, -sh', -ch, or soft sign	Add -yej: **klyuch** (klyuch; key) becomes **klyuchyej** (klu-*chyey*; keys)
-ts	Add -yev: **myesyats** (*mye*-seets; month) becomes **myesyatsyev** (*mye*-see-tsehf; months)

(continued)

Table 2-4 *(continued)*

If a Noun In Its Dictionary Form (Nominative Case) Ends In	To Form Genitive Plural
-a	Drop the final –a
	If the resulting genitive plural form has two consonants at the end, the fill vowel -o or -e is often added between the consonants: **sosyedka** (sah-*syed*-kuh; female neighbor) becomes **sosyedok** (sah-*sye*-duhk; female neighbors)
-iye or -iya	Replace -iye or -iya with -ij: **stantsiya** (*stahn*-tsih-ye; station) becomes **stantsij** (*stahn*-tsihy; stations)
-j	Replace the final -j with -yov if the ending is stressed, or with -yev if the ending is not stressed: **popugaj** (puh-poo-*gahy*, parrot) becomes **popu-gayev** (puh-poo-*gah*-eef; parrots)
-o	Drop the -o: **myesto** (*myes*-tuh; place) becomes **myest** (myest; places)
-ye	Add -j: **morye** (*moh*-ree; sea) becomes **moryej** (mah-*ryey*, seas)
Consonant + -ya	Replace -ya with the soft sign: **nyedyelya** (nee-*dye*-lye; week) becomes **nyedyel'** (nee-*dyel'*, weeks)

Now, try to apply Table 2-4 to a real-life situation. Imagine that your friend asks you whether you have a pencil: **U tyebya yest' karandash?** (oo tee-*bya* yest' kuh-ruhn-*dahsh*; Do you have a pencil?)

You, being by nature a very generous person, say that you have a lot of pencils, meaning that your friend is free to use all of them. It may come as a surprise to you, but when you make this statement, the word **mnogo** (*mnoh*-guh; many/a lot of) requires that the noun used with it take the genitive plural form. In your sentence, the word **karandashi** (kuh-ruhn-duh-*shih;* pencils) should take the form of genitive plural. What does Table 2-4 say about the ending **-sh**? That's right; you need to add the ending **-yej.** You say **U myenya mnogo karandashyej** (oo mee-*nya mnoh*-guh kuh-ruhn-duh-*shyey*; I have many pencils).

Setting plurals into other cases

Table 2-5 shows how to form the plurals of nouns for all the other cases.

Table 2-5   Forming the Plural of Nouns in the Accusative, Dative, Instrumental, and Prepositional Cases

If a Noun In Its Dictionary Form (Nominative Case) Ends In	To Form Accusative Plural	To Form Dative Plural	To Form Instrumental Plural	To Form Prepositional Plural
A consonant	If the noun is a living being, it looks just like the genitive plural (see Table 2-4); otherwise, it looks just like the nominative plural (see Table 2-3)	Add -am	Add -ami	Add -akh
-a or -ya	If the noun is a living being, it looks just like the genitive plural (see Table 2-4); otherwise, it looks just like the nominative plural (see Table 2-3)	Add -m	Add -mi	Add -kh
-iye	Replace -iye with -iya, like the nominative plural (see Table 2-3)	Replace -ye with -yam	Replace -iye with -yami	Replace -ye with -yakh
-iya	Replace -iya with -ii, like the nominative plural (see Table 2-3)	Add -m	Add -mi	Add -kh
-j	If the noun is a living being, it looks just like the genitive plural (see Table 2-4); otherwise, it looks just like the nominative plural (see Table 2-3)	Replace -j with -yam	Replace -j with -yem	Replace -j with -yakh
-o	If the noun is a living being, it looks just like the genitive plural (see Table 2-4); otherwise, it looks just like the nominative plural (see Table 2-3)	Replace -o with -am	Replace -o with -ami	Replace -o with –akh
-ye	Replace -ye with -ya, like the nominative plural (see Table 2-3)	Replace -ye with -yam	Add -m	Replace -ye with -yakh
A soft sign (')	If the noun is a living being, it looks just like the genitive plural (see Table 2-4); otherwise, it looks just like the nominative plural (see Table 2-3)	Replace the soft sign with -yam	Replace the soft sign with -yami	Replace the soft sign with -yakh

Imagine that you ask your friend, a Russian professor, whether he has a book that you want to borrow. It appears he does, but unfortunately, he can't give it to you because he has already given it to his students. He says **Ya dal knigu studyentam** (ya dahl *knee*-goo stoo-*dyen*-tuhm; I gave the book to the students).

Why did your friend use the form **studyentam?** It's the plural dative form of the word **studyenty** (stoo-*dyen*-tih; students), the indirect object of the sentence. The singular nominative form of this word is **studyent** (stoo-*dyent*), and he just added **-am** as shown in Table 2-5.

Picking out pronouns

Pronouns are words like *he*, *she*, and *it*. They're used in place of nouns to refer to someone or something that's already been mentioned. In the following sections, we show you the basic pronouns in Russian and how to place them into the correct cases. We also give you the scoop on possessive and interrogative pronouns.

Recognizing basic pronouns

Major Russian pronouns include the following:

- **ya** (ya; I)
- **ty** (tih; you; informal singular)
- **on** (ohn; he)
- **ona** (ah-*nah*; she)
- **my** (mih; we)
- **vy** (vih; you; formal singular and plural)

So what about "it"? In English, inanimate objects are usually referred to with the pronoun *it,* but in Russian, an inanimate object is always referred to with the pronoun corresponding to its grammatical gender. (For more about noun gender, see "Getting the lowdown on the gender of nouns" earlier in this chapter.) You translate the English pronoun *it* into Russian with one of these pronouns:

- **on** (ohn) if the noun it refers to is masculine
- **ona** (ah-*nah*) if the noun it refers to is feminine
- **ono** (ah-*noh*) if the noun it refers to is neuter
- **oni** (ah-*nee*) if the noun it refers to is plural

For example, in the phrase **Eto moya mashina. Ona staraya** (*eh*-tuh mah-*ya* muh-*shih*-nuh ah-*nah stah*-ruh-ye; That's my car. It's old), the pronoun *it* is translated as **ona,** because it refers to the Russian feminine noun **mashina.**

Placing basic pronouns into cases

Like nouns, Russian pronouns have different forms for all the cases. Table 2-6 shows the declension for pronouns.

Table 2-6	Declension of Russian Pronouns				
Pronoun in the Nominative Case	*Genitive*	*Accusative*	*Dative*	*Instrumental*	*Prepositional*
ya (ya; I)	myenya (mee-*nya*; me)	myenya (mee-*nya*; me)	mnye (mnye; me)	mnoj (mnohy; me)	mnye (mnye; me)
ty (tih; you informal singular)	tyebya (tee-*bya*; you)	tyebya (tee-*bya*; you)	tyebye (tee-*bye*; you)	toboj (tah-*bohy*, you)	tyebye (tee-*bye*; you)
on (ohn; he or it)	(n)yego ((n)ee-*voh*; him/it)	(n)yego ((n) ee-*voh*; him/it)	(n)yemu ((n) ee-*moo*; him/it)	(n)im ((n)eem; him/it)	nyom (nyom; him/it)
ona (ah-*nah*; she or it)	(n)yeyo ((n) ee-*yoh*; her/it)	(n)yeyo ((n)ee-yoh; her/it)	(n)yej ((n)yey; her/it)	(n)yej ((n)yey; her/it)	nej (nyey; her/it)
ono (ah-*noh*; it)	ono (ah-*noh*; it)	ono (ah-*noh*; it)	(n)emu ((n) ee-*moo*; it)	(n)im ((n)eem; it)	(n)im ((n)eem; it)
my (mih; we)	nas (nahs; us)	nas (nahs; us)	nam (nahm; us)	nami (*nah*-mee; us)	nas (nahs; us)
vy (vih; you formal singular and plural)	vas (vahs; you)	vas (vahs; you)	vam (vahm; you)	vami (*vah*-mee; you)	vas (vahs; you)
oni (ah-*nee*; they)	(n)ikh ((n)eekh; them)	(n)ikh ((n)eekh; them)	(n)im ((n)eem; them)	(n)imi ((*n*)ee-mee; them)	nikh ((n)eekh; them)

Imagine that somebody asks you if you saw Nina today: **Ty vidyel Ninu?** (tih *vee*-deel *nee*-noo; Did you see Nina?) You didn't. In preparing to answer this question, you may decide not to use the word "Nina" again but to replace it with the pronoun "her." Because "Nina" is a direct object, you have to use the accusative case in translating the word "her." Using Table 2-6, you discover that accusative case of **ona** (ah-*nah*; she) is **yeyo** (ee-*yo*; her). You respond **Ya yeyo nye vidyel.** (ya ee-*yo* nee *vee*-deel; I didn't see her.)

You add the letter **n** to the beginning of pronouns whose first letter is a vowel when the pronoun is used right after a preposition. Refer to Table 2-6 for the pronouns that do this.

Surveying possessive pronouns

Possessive pronouns indicate ownership or possession. Words like *my, mine, your, yours, his, her, hers, our, ours, their*, and *theirs* are English possessive pronouns. In Russian, a possessive pronoun must always agree in number, gender, and case with the noun it's referring to. Table 2-7 shows you how to form the possessive pronouns in the nominative case, which is by far the case you'll use most.

Table 2-7	Forming Possessive Pronouns in the Nominative Case			
English Possessive Pronoun	*When It Modifies a Masculine Noun*	*When It Modifies a Feminine Noun*	*When It Modifies a Neuter Noun*	*When It Modifies a Plural Noun (All Genders)*
My/mine	moj (mohy)	moya (mah-*ya*)	moyo (mah-*yo*)	moi (mah-*ee*)
Your/yours (informal singular)	tvoj (tvohy)	tvoya (tvah-*ya*)	tvoyo (tvah-*yo*)	tvoi (tvah-*ee*)
His	yego (ee-*voh*)	yego (ee-*voh*)	yego (ee-*voh*)	yego (ee-*voh*)
Her/hers	yeyo (ee-*yo*)	yeyo (ee-*yo*)	yeyo (ee-*yo*)	yeyo (ee-*yo*)
Our/ours	nash (nahsh)	nasha (*nah*-shuh)	nashye (*nah*-sheh)	nashi (*nah*-shih)
Your/yours (formal singular and plural)	vash (vahsh)	vasha (*vah*-shuh)	vashye (*vah*-sheh)	vashi (*vah*-shih)
Their/theirs	ikh (eekh)	ikh (eekh)	ikh (eekh)	ikh (eekh)

Say you're getting ready to go out on the town and you notice you lost your favorite shirt. You want to say, "Where's my shirt?" Because **rubashka** (*roo-bahsh*-kuh; shirt) ends in **-a,** it's a feminine noun. (For information on determining a noun's gender, see "Which one is it? How to tell the gender of a Russian noun" earlier in this chapter.) Because *my* modifies the feminine noun **rubashka,** it's written **moya** (mah-*ya*; my) according to Table 2-7. The phrase you want is **Gdye moya rubashka?** (gdye mah-*ya* roo-*bahsh*-kuh; Where's my shirt?)

Now say you can't find your tie either. You want to ask, **Gdye moj galstuk?** (gdye mohy *gahl*-stook; Where's my tie?) Notice how *my* is now written **moj** (moy), because in this sentence, it modifies the masculine noun **galstuk.**

A possessive pronoun changes its endings in all the cases. Its declension is totally dependent on the way the noun it is attached to declines. So the phrase **moya kniga** (mah-*ya knee*-guh; my book) declines differently from the phrase **moj tyelyefon** (moy tee-lee-*fohn*; my telephone) for one simple reason: **Kniga** is a feminine noun and **tyelyefon** is a masculine noun.

Investigating interrogative pronouns

Interrogative pronouns are question words like *who, whose,* and *which.* "Who" in Russian is **kto** (ktoh), and you're likely to hear or use this word in phrases like

- ✔ **Kto eto?** (ktoh *eh*-tuh; Who is that?)
- ✔ **Kto on?** (ktoh ohn; Who is he?)
- ✔ **Kto vy?** (ktoh vih; Who are you?)

Kto changes its form depending on the case it's in. It becomes **kogo** (kah-*voh*; whom) in the genitive case, **kogo** (kah-*voh*; whom) in the accusative case, **kom** (kohm; whom) in the dative case, **kyem** (kyem; whom) in the instrumental case, and **kom** (kohm; whom) in the prepositional case. But you hear and use the basic nominative case form **kto** in most situations. And just as in English, you use **kto** no matter what the gender of the noun is.

"Whose" in Russian is **chyej** (chyey), and "which" is **kakoj** (kuh-*kohy*). **Chyej** and **kakoj** change their endings depending on the gender, number, and case of the noun they modify. For now, you just need to know the nominative case endings in Table 2-8.

Table 2-8	Nominative Case Endings for Chyej (Whose) and Kakoj (Which)			
Interrogative Pronoun	When It Modifies a Masculine Noun	When It Modifies a Feminine Noun	When It Modifies a Neuter Noun	When It Modifies a Plural Noun
chyej (chyey; whose)	chyej (chyey)	ch'ya (ch'ya)	ch'yo (ch'yo)	ch'i (ch'yee)
kakoj (kuh-kohy; which)	kakoj (kuh-kohy)	kakaya (kuh-kah-ye)	kakoye (kuh-koh-ee)	kakiye (kuh-kee-ee)

Here are examples of some phrases you may hear or say using the interrogative pronouns **chyej** and **kakoj**:

- **Chyej eto dom?** (chyey *eh*-tuh dohm; Whose house is that?) **Dom** (house) is masculine, so you use **chyej**.

- **Ch'ya eta kniga?** (ch'ya *eh*-tuh *knee*-guh; Whose book is that?) **Kniga** (book) is feminine, so you use **ch'ya**.

- **Kakoj magazin ty pryedpochitayesh'?** (kuh-*kohy* muh-guh-*zeen* tih preed-puh-chee-*tah*-eesh'; Which store do you prefer?) **Magazin** (store) is masculine, so you use **kakoj**.

- **Kakoye blyudo ty pryedpochitayesh'?** (kuh-*koh*-ee *blyu*-duh tih preed-puh-chee-*tah*-eesh'; Which dish do you prefer?) **Blyudo** (dish) is neuter, so you use **kakoye**.

The question words **kogda** (kahg-*dah*; when), **gdye** (gdye; where), and **chto** (shtoh; what) are also sometimes used as interrogative pronouns. The good news is that **kogda** and **gdye** never change their form. **Chto** changes its form for all cases.

Decorating Your Speech with Adjectives

Adjectives spice up your speech. An adjective is a word that describes, or modifies, a noun or a pronoun, like *good, nice, difficult,* or *hard.* In the following sections, you discover how to use adjectives, how to change their endings for different cases, and what to do about the articles "the" and "a."

Always consenting: Adjective-noun agreement

A Russian adjective is like a jealous lover. It can't live without the noun or the pronoun it describes. In English, an adjective never changes its form no matter what word it modifies or where it's used in a sentence, but a Russian adjective always agrees with the noun or pronoun it modifies in gender, number, and case. Table 2-9 shows how to change adjective endings in the nominative case, which is the case you're likely to see and use the most.

Table 2-9	Adjective Formation in the Nominative Case	
If an Adjective Modifies	**The Adjective Takes the Ending**	**Examples**
A masculine noun/pronoun	-oj//ij/yj	**bol'shoj myach** (bahl'-*shohy* myach; big ball) **sinij pidzhak** (*see*-neey peed-*zhahk*; blue jacket) **krasivyj mal'chik** (kruh-*see*-vihy *mahl'*-cheek; beautiful boy)
A feminine noun/pronoun	-aya/yaya	**bol'shaya kniga** (bahl'-*shah*-ye *knee*-guh; big book) **sinyaya shuba** (*see*-nee-ye *shoo*-buh; blue fur coat) **krasivaya rubashka** (krah-*see*-vuh-ye roo-*bahsh*-kuh; beautiful shirt)
A neuter noun	-oye/yeye	**bol'shoye zhivotnoye** (bahl'-*shoh*-ee zhih-*voht*-nuh-ee; big animal) **sinyeye okno** (*see*-nee-ee ahk-*noh*; blue window) **krasivoye myesto** (krah-*see*-vuh-ee *myes*-tuh; beautiful place)
A plural noun	-yye/iye	**bol'shyye zhivotnyye** (bahl'-*shih*-ee zhee-*voht*-nih-ee; big animals) **siniye okna** (*see*-nee-ee *ohk*-nuh; blue windows) **krasivyye myesta** (krah-*see*-vih-ee mees-*tah*; beautiful places)

Dictionaries list adjectives in their singular and masculine form (the first row in Table 2-9). The trick is correctly selecting the ending for the adjectives' feminine, neuter, and plural forms; dictionaries don't provide these forms because dictionary compilers assume that you know how to do it. You're not on your own; we're going to provide you with some general rules:

> ✔ If an adjective in its masculine form ends in **-oj/-yj:**
>
>> • Replace the original ending with **-aya** to make it feminine
>>
>> • Replace the original ending with **-oye** to make it neuter
>>
>> • Replace the original ending with **-yye** to make it plural
>
> ✔ If an adjective in its masculine form ends in **-ij:**
>
>> • Replace the original ending with **-yaya** to make it feminine
>>
>> • Replace its original ending with **-yeye** to make it neuter
>>
>> • Replace the original ending with **-iye** to make it plural

Now put the rule to work. Take the word **poslyednij** (pahs-*lyed*-neey; last). As you see, in its dictionary (singular and masculine) form, the adjective has the ending **-ij.** How are we going to change the ending of this adjective to say "the last word" in Russian?

Figure out the gender of the word "word" (sorry!). Its Russian equivalent is **slovo** (*sloh*-vuh; word). The ending in this word is **-o.** The ending **-o** in a noun indicates neuter gender (refer to Table 2-1). What ending does **poslyednij** take when it's used with a neuter noun? Yes, the ending is **-yeye.** So "the last word" in Russian is **poslyednyeye slovo** (pahs-*lyed*-nee-ee *sloh*-vuh).

A lot in common: Putting adjectives into other cases

Table 2-10 shows how to change adjective endings for all the cases other than nominative. (Work with Table 2-9 to figure out which particular ending to use in each case.) Notice how masculine and neuter nouns take the same endings in the genitive, dative, instrumental, and prepositional cases. The feminine endings are the same for all cases except accusative. And the plural genitive and plural prepositional endings are the same.

Table 2-10   Adjective Declension in the Genitive, Accusative, Instrumental, and Prepositional Cases

If the Adjective Modifies	To Form Genitive	To Form Accusative	To Form Dative	To Form Instrumental	To Form Prepositional
A masculine noun	Replace -oj/ij/yj with -ogo/ yego/ogo	If the noun is a living being, it looks just like the genitive; otherwise, it looks just like the nominative (see Table 2-9)	Replace -oj/ij/yj with -omu/ yemu/ omu	Replace -oj/ ij/yj with -ym/im/ym	Replace -oj/ij/yj with -om/im/om
A feminine noun	Replace -aya/yaya with -oj/ yej/oj	Replace -aya/yaya with -uyu/ yuyu/uyu	Replace -aya/yaya with -oj/ yej/oj	Replace -aya/yaya with -oj/ yej/oj	Replace -aya/yaya with -oj/yej/oj
A neuter noun	Replace -oye/yeye with -ogo/ yego	It looks just like the nominative (see Table 2-9)	Replace -oj/ij/yj with -omu/ yemu/omu	Replace -oj/ij/yj with -ym/im/ym	Replace -oj/ij/yj with -om/im/om
A plural noun	Replace -yye/iye with -ykh/ikh	If the noun is a living being it looks just like the genitive; otherwise it looks just like the nominative (see Table 2-9)	Replace -yye/iye with -ym/im	Replace -yye/iye with -ymi/imi	Replace -yye/iye with -ykh/ikh/

Nowhere to be found: The lack of articles in Russian

The English words *the, a,* and *an* are called articles. You use articles all the time in English, but these words don't exist in Russian, so you don't need to worry about how to say them. When you want to say *the, a,* or *an,* all you have to do is say the noun you mean. "The store" and "a store" in Russian are simply **magazin** (muh-guh-*zeen*; *Literally:* store). "The girl" and "a girl" are simply **dyevushka** (*dyeh*-voosh-kuh; *Literally:* girl).

Adding Action with Verbs

If nouns and pronouns are the building blocks and adjectives the flavoring in a Russian sentence, then the verb is the engine. Without the verb, you can't express a complete thought. A Russian verb carries loads of important information. It can reveal whether an action was completed or resulted in something and whether the action occurs on a regular basis or is a one-time event. Russian verbs also reveal the number (and, in the past tense, the gender) of the person or thing performing the action.

In the following sections, we show you how to spot the infinitive of a verb, and how to form verbs in the past, present, and future tenses. We also tell you about a basic but unusual verb often used in Russian.

Spotting infinitives

Spotting Russian infinitives is easy, because they usually end in a **-t'** as in **chitat'** (chee-*taht'*; to read), **govorit'** (guh-vah-*reet'*; to speak), and **vidyet'** (*veed*-yet'; to see).

Some Russian verbs (which are usually irregular) take the infinitive endings **-ti** as in **idti** (ee-*tee*; to walk) and **-ch'** as in **moch'** (mohch'; to be able to). For a list of common irregular verbs, see Appendix A.

In a Russian dictionary, as in any language dictionary, verbs are always listed in their infinitive form. Why? Well, imagine a dictionary that lists all verb forms. It probably would be a dictionary the size of the Kremlin.

Living in the present tense

Russian verbs have only one present tense. Like English verbs, Russian verbs conjugate (change their form) so that they always agree in person and number with the subject of the sentence. To conjugate most Russian verbs in the present tense, you drop the infinitive ending **-t'** and replace it with one of the six endings in Table 2-11.

Table 2-11	Forming the Present Tense of Verbs	
Subject of Sentence	*Drop the Infinitive Verb Ending (-t') and Replace It With*	*Example*
ya (ya; I)	-yu	ya rabotayu (ya ruh-*boh*-tuh-yu; I work/am working)
ty (tih; you; informal singular)	-yesh'	ty rabotayesh' (tih ruh-*boh*-tuh-eesh'; You work/are working)
on/ona/ono (ohn/ah-*nah*/ah-*noh*; he/she/it)	-yet	on rabotayet (ohn ruh-*boh*-tuh-eet; He works/is working)
my (mih; we)	-yem	my rabotayem (mih ruh-*boh*-tuh-eem; We work/are working)
vy (vih; you; formal singular and plural)	-yetye	vy rabotayetye (vih ruh-*boh*-tuh-ee-tee; You work/are working)
oni (ah-*nee*; they)	-yut	oni rabotayut (ah-*nee* ruh-*boh*-tuh-yut; They work/are working)

The present tense in Russian corresponds to both the present simple and present continuous tenses in English; in other words, it denotes both the general action in the present tense (such as "I work") and the action taking place at the moment of speaking (such as "I am working").

Verbs that conjugate as **-yu, -yesh', -yet, -yem, -yetye,** and **-yut** are called first-conjugation verbs. The term in itself implies that second-conjugation verbs exist; they conjugate as **-yu, -ish', -it, -im, -itye,** and **-yat.** So how do you know whether the verb is the first or second conjugation? Easy: Dictionaries always indicate this situation. In addition, a lot of verbs conjugate — how should we

put it? — in whatever way they want to conjugate (in other words, in a completely unpredictable fashion!). How do you deal with such verbs? Always check with the dictionary; dictionaries always indicate something peculiar in verb conjugations. However, they don't list all the forms but only three of them, usually the **ya** (I), **ty** (you; informal singular), and **oni** (they) forms with the hope that you can figure out the rest of the forms.

We alert you to regular verbs that follow the second-conjugation pattern and irregular verbs with conjugation peculiarities throughout this book.

Talking about the past tense

In the following sections, we show you how to form the past tense of Russian verbs and explain the differences between imperfective and perfective verbs.

Keep it simple: Forming the past tense

To form the past tense of a Russian verb, all you need to do is drop the infinitive ending **-t'** and replace it with one of four endings in Table 2-12.

Table 2-12	Forming the Past Tense of Verbs	
If the Subject of the Sentence Is	*Drop the Infinitive Ending -t' and Replace It With*	*Example*
Masculine singular	-l	on rabotal (ohn ruh-*boh*-tuhl; He worked)
Feminine singular	-la	ona rabotala (ah-nah ruh-*boh*-tuh-luh; She worked)
Neuter singular	-lo	ono rabotalo (ah-noh ruh-*boh*-tuh-luh; It worked)
Plural	-li	oni rabotali (ah-*nee* ruh-*boh*-tuh-lee; They worked)

Perfective or imperfective? That is the question

English expresses past events either through the past simple tense (I ate yesterday) or the present perfect tense (I have eaten already). While *I ate yesterday* simply states a fact, *I have eaten already* emphasizes the result of the action. Russian verbs do something similar by using what's called *verbal aspect*. Two aspects exist in Russian: perfective and imperfective.

Up to this point, we've been withholding some very essential information from you: Every English verb in the English-Russian dictionary is represented by two Russian verbs, its imperfective equivalent and a perfective counterpart. Usually, the imperfective is listed first in the aspectual pair, like in this example:

To read — **chitat'** (chee-*taht'*)/**prochitat'** (pruh-chee-*taht'*)

In this example, **chitat'** is the imperfective infinitive, and **prochitat'** is the perfective infinitive. You form the perfective aspect by adding the prefix **pro-** to the imperfective infinitive. Don't assume, however, that you add **pro-** to every Russian imperfective verb to find its perfective aspect. It's not that simple. Sometimes the perfective aspect of a verb looks quite different from the imperfective aspect, as in the case of the verb "to look/to glance": **glyadyet'** (glee-*dyet'*) and **glyanut'** (glee-noot'). **Glyadyet'** is the imperfective infinitive and **glyanut'** is the perfective infinitive.

The formation of the perfective infinitive is as unpredictable as the rest of Russian grammar. Our advice: When you memorize a new Russian verb, memorize both its imperfective and perfective aspects.

To emphasize the fact of an action in the past or to express habitual or repeated action in the past, Russian uses the imperfective aspect form of the verb. To emphasize the result or completion of the action, Russian uses the perfective aspect of the verb. You also use the perfective aspect of a verb if you want to emphasize a single, momentary event that took place in the past, such as breaking a plate.

If you tell someone **Ya pisal ryezyumye tsyelyj dyen'** (ya pee-*sahl* ree-zyu-*meh tseh* -lihy dyen'; I was writing my resume all day), you use the past tense imperfective form of the verb **pisat'**, because your emphasis is on the fact of writing, not on the completion of the task. If you finished writing your resume, you use the past tense perfective form of the verb, because your emphasis is on the completion of the action: **Ya napisal ryesyumye.** (ya nuh-pee-*sahl* ree-zyu-*mye;* I have written my resume.)

Knowing which of the two aspects to select is important only when you speak about the past or the future (see the next section). Russian doesn't have aspects in the present tense. In other words, in describing present tense events, you can use only the imperfective form of the verb. Don't even think about using perfective form in the present tense!

Talkin' the Talk

 Viktor and Marina are former co-workers. They meet after a long absence.

Viktor:	**Privyet Marina, chto novogo? Kuda vy propali?** pree-*vyet* mah-*ree*-nuh, shtoh *noh*-vuh-vuh? koo-*dah* vih prah-*pah*-lee? Hi Marina, what's new? Where've you disappeared to?
Marina:	**Privyet, Viktor! Ya nyeskol'ko myesyatsyev otdykhala, a potom nachala rabotat' v shklolye.** Pree-*vyet, veek*-tuhr! ya *nyes*-kuhl'-kuhl' *mye*-see-tsehf uh-dih-*khah*-luh, ah pah-*tohm* nuh-chuh-*lah* rah-*boh*-tuht' f *shkoh*-lee. Hi Viktor! I relaxed for several months, and then I started to work at a school.
Viktor:	**Oj kak intyeryesno! Ya tozhye rabotal odnazhdy v shkolye. Kak vam eto nravitsya?** Ohy kahk een-tee-*ryes*-nuh! ya *toh*-zheh rah-*boh*-tuhl ahd-*nahzh*-dih f *shkoh*-lee. kahk vahm *eh*-tuh *nrah*-veet-sye? Oh, how interesting! I also worked once at a school. How do you like it?
Marina:	**Nichyego, no ya predpochitayu otdykhat'.** Nee-chee-*voh,* noh ya preet-puh-chee-*tah*-yu uh-dih-*khaht'.* Not bad, but I prefer to relax.
Viktor:	**Soglasyen, no k sozhalyeniyu nado rabotat'.** sah-*glah*-seen, noh k suh-zhah-*lye*-nee-yu *nah*-duh ruh-*boh*-tuht'. I agree, but unfortunately one has to work.

Words to Know

Chto novogo?	shtoh <u>noh</u>-vuh-vuh	What's new?
Kuda vy propali?	koo-<u>dah</u> vih prah-<u>pah</u>-lee	Where've you disappeared to?
otdykhala	uh-dih-<u>khah</u>-luh	relaxed (feminine, singular)
nyeskol'ko myesyetsev	<u>nyes</u>-kuhl'-kuh <u>mye</u>-see-tsehf	for several months
rabotat'	ruh-<u>boh</u>-tuht'	to work (imperfective)
rabotal	ruh-<u>boh</u>-tuhl	worked (masculine, singular)
odnazhdy	ahd-<u>nahzh</u>-dih	once/at one time
Kak vam nravitsya?	kahk vahm <u>eh</u>-tuh <u>nrah</u>-veet-sye	How do you like it?
Ya predpochitayu . . .	yah preet-puh-chee-<u>tah</u>-yu	I prefer to . . . (+ infinitive)
k sozhalyeniyu	k suh-zhah-<u>lye</u>-nee-yu	unfortunately

Planning for the future tense

To describe an action that will take place in the future, Russian uses the future tense. While English has many different ways to talk about the future, Russian has only two: the *future imperfective* and the *future perfective*.

You use the future imperfective when you want to emphasize the fact that something will happen or be happening in the future, but you don't necessarily want to emphasize the result or completion of an action. You use the future perfective to emphasize result or completion of an action.

To form the future imperfective, you use the future tense form of the verb **byt'** (biht'; to be) plus the imperfective infinitive. This combination translates into "will/will be." Table 2-13 shows the conjugation of the verb **byt'** in the future tense. (Find out more about this interesting verb in the next section.)

Table 2-13	Conjugation of Byt' in the Future Tense
Pronoun	*Correct Form of Byt'*
ya (I)	budu (*boo*-doo)
ty (you; informal singular)	budyesh' (*boo*-deesh')
on/ona/ono (he/she/it)	budyet (*boo*-deet)
my (we)	budyem (*boo*-deem)
vy (you; formal singular and plural)	budyetye (*boo*-dee-tee)
oni (they)	budut (*boo*-doot)

If you want to say "I will read (but not necessarily finish reading) the article," you use the **ya** (I) form of the verb **byt'** plus the imperfective infinitive **chitat'** (chee-*taht*'; to read): **Ya budu chitat' stat'yu** (ya *boo*-doo chee-*taht*' staht'-*yu*).

To form the future perfective, you simply conjugate the perfective form of the verb, as in **Ya prochitayu stat'yu syegodnya** (ya pruh-chee-*tah*-yu staht'-*yu* see-*vohd*-nye; I'll read/finish reading the article today). In other words, you use the ending **-yu** for **ya** (I) as you do in the present tense. See the previous section for more about perfective verbs.

Using the unusual verb byt' (to be)

Russian has no present tense of the verb *to be*. To say "I'm happy," you just say **Ya schastliv** (ya *sh'as*-leef; *Literally:* I happy). To say "That's John," you just say **Eto Dzhon** (*eh*-tuh dzhohn; *Literally:* That John). The being verbs *am, are,* and *is* are implicitly understood in the present tense.

To express the verb *to be* in the past tense, you need to use the proper past tense form of the verb **byt':**

- **byl** (bihl; was) if the subject is a masculine singular noun

- **byla** (bih-*lah*; was) if the subject is a feminine singular noun

- **bylo** (*bih*-luh; was) if the subject is a neuter singular noun

- **byli** (*bih*-lee; was) if the subject is a plural noun or if the subject is **vy** (vih; you; formal singular)

To express the verb *to be* in the future tense, you have to use the correct form of the verb **byt'** in the future tense. (For conjugation, refer to Table 2-13.) To say "I will be happy," you say **Ya budu schastliv** (ya *boo*-doo *sh'as*-leef), and for "I will be there," you say **Ya budu tam** (ya *boo*-doo tahm).

Providing Extra Details with Adverbs

Adverbs are words like *very, quickly,* and *beautifully.* They add information to a verb, an adjective, or even another adverb. Russian adverbs are one of the most uncomplicated parts of speech. Unlike nouns, verbs, and adjectives, adverbs never change their form. In the following sections, you discover the main categories of Russian adverbs: adverbs of manner and adverbs of time.

Describing how

You use some adverbs to describe *how* an action is performed. These adverbs are called *adverbs of manner,* and they're easy to spot because they usually end in **-o.** In fact, you can consider the ending **-o** as a kind of equivalent of the ending **-ly** in English adverbs.

Some adverbs of manner you probably hear and use a lot are **khorosho** (khuh-rah-*shoh*; well), **plokho** (*ploh*-khuh; poorly), **pravil'no** (*prah*-veel'-nuh; correctly), **nyepravil'no** (nee- *prah*-veel'-nuh; incorrectly), **bystro** (*bihs*-truh; quickly), **myedlyenno** (*myed*-lee-nuh; slowly), **lyegko** (leekh-*koh*; easily), and **prosto** (*proh*-stuh; simply).

Describing when and how often

To describe when and how often the action took place, Russian uses *time adverbs.* Like adverbs of manner, time adverbs are recognizable because they usually end in **-o** (and sometimes in **-a**).

Some of the most common time adverbs are **chasto** (*chahs*-tuh; often), **ryedko** (*ryed*-kuh; rarely), **inogda** (ee-nahg-*dah*; sometimes), **nikogda** (nee-kahg-*dah*; never), **vsyegda** (fseeg-*dah*; always), **skoro** (*skoh*-ruh; soon), **obychno** (ah-*bihch*-nuh; usually), **rano** (*rah*-nuh; early), **pozdno** (*pohz*-nuh; late), and **dolgo** (*dohl*-guh; for a long time).

Constructing Sentences Like a Pro

The whole point of learning grammar is to actually create Russian-sounding sentences. In the following sections, you discover how to do just that. You have a lot of freedom of word order when creating Russian sentences. You get tips on selecting the noun or pronoun, adjectives, and verb, and you see how to connect different parts of a sentence with conjunctions. You also find out how to form questions in Russian.

Enjoying the freedom of word order

One of the biggest differences between English and Russian is that English tends to have a fixed order of words, whereas Russian enjoys a free order of words.

In English, word order can often determine the meaning of a sentence. For example, in English you say, "The doctor operated on the patient," but you never say "The patient operated on the doctor." It just doesn't make sense.

In Russian, however, it's perfectly okay to put **patsiyenta** at the beginning of the sentence and **doktor** at the end, as in **Patsiyenta opyeriroval doktor** (puh-tsee-*yent*-uh uh-pee-*ree*-ruh-vuhl *dohk*-tuhr). It still means "The doctor operated on the patient" even though it looks like "The patient operated on the doctor." If you wanted to, you could even put **opyeriroval** first, **patsiyenta** second, and **doktor** at the end, as in **Opyeriroval patsiyenta doktor.** It still means "The doctor operated on the patient" even though it looks like "Operated on the patient the doctor."

In Russian, you can freely shift around the order of words in a sentence, because the Russian case system tells you exactly what role each word plays in the sentence. (For additional information on cases, see "Making the Russian Cases" earlier in this chapter.)

As a rule, you give new information or information you want to emphasize at the end of a Russian sentence and the least important information at the beginning of a Russian sentence.

Selecting the noun (or pronoun) and adjective

Usually, the first step in forming a sentence is deciding on which nouns and adjectives to use. If you want to say "I'm reading an interesting article," the first thing you need to decide is what role each of the nouns and pronouns plays in the sentence, so you can decide which case to put them into. In this sentence, "I" is the subject and "interesting article" is the direct object.

The subject of a sentence is always in the nominative case, and the direct object is always in the accusative case. The nominative case for the pronoun "I" is **ya,** and now we have to put **intyeryesnaya stat'ya** (een-tee-*ryes*-nuh-ye staht'-*ya*; interesting article) into the accusative case. (For details on cases, see "Making the Russian Cases" earlier in this chapter.)

Start with the feminine noun, **stat'ya.** Table 2-2 says that if a noun ends in **-ya,** then you form the accusative case by replacing **-ya** with **-yu,** so now you have **stat'yu.** And as for the adjective **intyeryesnaya,** it must agree in gender, case, and number with the noun it modifies. The dictionary form of "interesting" in Russian is **intyeryesnyj.** From Table 2-10 you know that this adjective takes the ending **-uyu** when it modifies a feminine noun in the accusative case. Presto! You now have **intyeryesnuyu.** (See "Decorating Your Speech with Adjectives" earlier in this chapter for more information.)

Choosing the verb

After you decide on the verb and tense you want to use in your sentence, you just need to make sure it agrees in number (and in gender if it's in the past tense) with the subject of the sentence. (For more, see "Adding Action with Verbs" earlier in this chapter.)

In the sentence "I'm reading an interesting article," the verb is obviously in the present tense and agrees with the singular pronoun "I." Table 2-11 in the section "Living in the present tense" earlier in this chapter says that you form the first person singular present tense verb by replacing the infinitive ending **-t'** with **-yu.** So the verb form you want is **chitayu** from the infinitive **chitat'.** The whole sentence is **Ya chitayu intyeryesnuyu stat'yu** (ya chee-*tah*-yu een-tee-*ryes*-noo-yu staht'-*yu*; I'm reading an interesting article). Congratulations! You've just created a complete Russian sentence!

Connecting with conjunctions

Sometimes you may want to connect words or phrases in a sentence with conjunctions, which are words like *and, but,* and *however.* "And" in Russian is **i** (ee), "but" is **a** (ah), and "however" is **no** (noh).

Forming questions

Forming questions in Russian is easy. You simply begin your sentence with a question word like **kto** (ktoh; who), **chto** (shtoh; what), **gdye** (gdye; where), **kogda** (kahg-*dah*; when), **pochyemu** (puh-chee-*moo*; why), or **kak** (kahk; how). And then you form your sentence as if you were making a statement.

For example, a man you know makes an exciting statement: **Ya syegodnya nye zavtrakal** (ya see-*vohd*-nye nee *zahf*-truh-kuhl; I didn't have breakfast today). Being a polite person, you need to somehow respond to this news. You may ask why your interlocutor didn't have breakfast. That'll demonstrate to him that you listened carefully to what he had to say. You ask:

> **Pochyemu ty syegodnya nye zavtrakal?** (puh-chee-*moo* tih see-*vohd*-nye nee *zahf*-truh-kuhl; Why didn't you have breakfast today?)

That's how simple it is! No auxiliary verbs, no changing the verb back to its infinitive form as you have to do in English! Asking questions is so much easier in Russian than in English, isn't it?

In Russian, you don't have to invert the subject and the verb when you're forming questions.

Counting in Russian

You're probably not going to need to know numbers beyond talking about how many siblings you have (which we explain in Chapter 4), telling time (which we talk about in Chapter 7), or counting your money (which we talk about in Chapter 14). But just in case, knowing the numbers in the following sections should help you with all other possible counting needs.

The harsh truth is that each Russian number changes its form for all six cases! But unless you plan to spend a lot of time at mathematics or accounting conferences conducted in Russian, you won't find yourself in many practical situations in which you need to know all the different forms. So we give you all the numbers you need to know only in the nominative case.

Numbers 0–9

These are the numbers you'll probably use most often when counting groceries, siblings, friends, and other people and things around the house:

- ✔ **0 nol'** (nohl')
- ✔ **1 odin** (ah-*deen*)
- ✔ **2 dva** (dvah)
- ✔ **3 tri** (tree)

- ✔ **4 chyetyrye** (chee-*tih*-ree)
- ✔ **5 pyat'** (pyat')
- ✔ **6 shyest'** (shehst')
- ✔ **7 syem'** (syem')
- ✔ **8 vosyem'** (*voh*-seem')
- ✔ **9 dyevyat'** (*dye*-veet')

But wait! You have to use a few rules when you use these numbers. The following sections give you the scoop.

The number 1 followed by a noun

If the noun you're referring to is masculine, you say **odin** followed by the noun as in **odin chyelovyek** (ah-*deen* chee-lah-*vyek*; one man). If the noun is feminine you say **odna** as in **odna dyevushka** (ahd-*nah* dye-voosh-kuh; one girl). And if the noun is neuter you say **odno** as in **odno okno** (ahd-*noh* ahk-*noh*; one window).

The number 2 followed by a noun

If you're talking about nouns that are masculine or neuter, you say **dva,** and if the noun is feminine, **dva** becomes **dvye.** After the numeral 2, you have to put the noun into the genitive case singular as in **dva chyelovyeka** (dvah chee-lah-*vye*-kuh; two men), **dva okna** (dvah ahk-*nah*; two windows), and **dvye dyevushki** (dvye *dye*-voosh-kee; two girls). For rules on forming genitive case for singular nouns, see Table 2-2 earlier in the chapter.

The numbers 3 and 4 followed by a noun

Like the numeral **dva** (dvah; two), **tri** (tree; three) and **chyetyrye** (chee-*tih*-ree; four) also require the noun used after them to be put into the genitive singular. (For rules on forming genitive case, see Table 2-2 earlier in the chapter.) Unlike **odin** and **dva,** these numbers don't change their form depending on the gender of the noun they refer to.

The numbers 5 through 9 followed by a noun

Any noun you use after the numerals 5–9 must be put into the genitive plural case, as in the phrase **pyat' dyevushyek** (pyat' *dye*-voo-shuhk; five girls) and **syem' mal'chikov** (syem' *mahl*-chee-kuhf; seven boys). (See "Changing plurals into the genitive case" earlier in this chapter.) Unlike **odin** and **dva,** these numbers don't change their form depending on the gender of the noun they are used with.

Numbers 10–19

The following are the numbers 10 through 19:

- **10 dyesyat'** (*dye*-seet')
- **11 odinnadtsat'** (ah-*dee*-nuht-tsuht')
- **12 dvyenadtsat'** (dvee-*naht*-tsuht')
- **13 trinadtsat'** (tree-*naht*-tsuht')
- **14 chyetyrnadtsat'** (chee-*tihr*-nuht-tsuht')
- **15 pyatnadtsat'** (peet-*naht*-tsuht')
- **16 shyestnadtsat'** (sheest-*naht*-tsuht')
- **17 syemnadtsat'** (seem-*naht*-tsuht')
- **18 vosyemnadtsyat'** (vuh-seem-*naht*-tsuht')
- **19 dyevyatnadtsat'** (dee-veet-*naht*-tsuht')

Starting with the numeral 11, Russian numerals up to 19 follow a recognizable pattern of adding **-nadtsat'** (*naht*-tsuht') to the numerals 1 through 9 (see the previous section). You can, however, find a few slight deviations to this rule, so watch out:

- **Dvyenadtsat'** (dvee-*naht*-tsuht'; 12) changes the **dva** (dvah; two) to a **dvye** (dve; two)
- **Chyetyrnadtsat'** (chee-*tihr*-nuht-tsuht'; 14) loses the final **e** in **chyetyrye** (chee-*tih*-ree; four)
- The numerals 15–19 all lose the final soft signs contained in 5–9 (For example, 15 is **pyatnadtsat'** and not **pyat'nadtsat'**).

Nouns following all these numerals take the genitive plural.

Numbers 20–99

To say 21, 22, 31, 32, 41, 42 . . . and so on, all you need to do is add the numerals 1 through 9 to the numeral 20, 30, 40 . . . and so on. See the following list for multiples of ten:

- **20 dvadtsat'** (*dvaht*-tsuht')
- **30 tridtsat'** (*treet*-tsuht')
- **40 sorok** (*soh*-ruhk)
- **50 pyatdyesyat'** (pee-dee-*syat*')

- 60 **shyestdyesyat'** (shees-dee-*syat'*)
- 70 **syem'dyesyat'** (*syem'*-dee-seet')
- 80 **vosyemdyesyat'** (*voh*-seem-dee-seet')
- 90 **dyevyanosto** (dee-yee-*nohs*-tuh)

Therefore, you make the numbers 21–23 like this:

- 21 **dvadtsat' odin** (*dvaht*-tsuht' ah-*deen*)
- 22 **dvadtsat' dva** (*dvaht*-tsuht' dva)
- 23 **dvadtsat' tri** (*dvaht*-tusht' tree)

When using nouns after these numerals, be sure to put the noun in the nominative after each number ending in 1 (as in 21 and 31); in the genitive singular case after each number ending in 2, 3, or 4 (as in 42, 53, and 64); and in the genitive plural case after all the others.

Numbers 100–999

You form each of the following numerals (except 200) by adding either a **sta** or a **sot** to the numerals 1–10:

- 100 **sto** (stoh)
- 200 **dvyesti** (*dvye*-stee)
- 300 **trista** (*tree*-stuh)
- 400 **chyetyryesta** (chee-*tih*-rees-tuh)
- 500 **pyat'sot** (peet'-*soht*)
- 600 **shyest'sot** (shees'-*soht*)
- 700 **syem'sot** (seem'-*soht*)
- 800 **vosyem'sot** (vuh-seem'-*soht*)
- 900 **dyevyat'sot** (dee-veet'-*soht*)

Sta (stah; 100) is actually the genitive singular form of **sto** (stoh; 100), and it makes sense that this is the form used with the "100" part of the numerals 200, 300, and 400, because 2, 3, and 4 force the noun after them into the genitive singular. It's as if the numeral 100 (**sto**) is treated like a noun when it comes after the numerals 2, 3, and 4, in 200, 300, and 400. The exception to this rule is **dvyesti** (200), in which **sto** becomes **sti** rather than **sta**. And **sot** (soht; 100) is the genitive plural form of **sto**. This fact also makes sense because the numerals 5–9 all take the genitive plural after them.

Creating composite numbers in Russian is as easy as one, two, three. Say you need to say "one hundred fifty five" in Russian. Translate "one hundred" into **sto.** "Fifty" in Russian is **pyatdyesyat.** Five is **pyat'.** There you go; the number 155 is **sto pyatdyesyat pyat'** (stoh pee-dee-*syat* pyat'). This process also applies to numbers larger than 1,000 (see the next section).

For numbers ending in 1 (such as 121, 341, and so on), the noun following them must be in the nominative case. For numbers ending in 2–4 (122, 453, 794, and so on), the noun following them must be in the genitive singular. For numbers ending in 5–9, the noun following them must be in the genitive plural.

Numbers 1,000–1,000,000

To say 1,000, you may say either just **tysyacha** (*tih*-see-chuh) or **odna tysyacha** (ahd-*nah* tih-sih-chuh; *Literally:* one thousand). Starting with 2,000, numbers in increments of 1,000 going up to 10,000, simply add **tysyachi** (*tih*-see-chee; 1,000) or **tysyach** (*tih*-seech; 1,000) to the numerals 2–9. The numbers 2,000, 3,000, and 4,000 add **tysyachi** and 5,000–9,000 add **tysyach,** as shown in the following list:

- **1,000 tysyacha** (*tih*-see-chuh)
- **2,000 dvye tysyachi** (dvye *tih*-see-chee)
- **3,000 tri tysyachi** (tree *tih*-see-chee)
- **4,000 chyetyrye tysyachi** (chee-*tih*-ree *tih*-see-chee)
- **5,000 pyat' tysyach** (pyat' *tih*-seech)

Tysyachi is the genitive singular form and **tysyach** is the genitive plural form of **tysyacha.** Notice how 2,000–4,000 require the genitive singular form and 5,000–9,000 require the genitive plural form of **tysyacha.** That's because tysyacha is treated like a noun, and nouns coming after 2, 3, and 4 must be in the genitive singular case. Nouns coming after 5–9 must be in the genitive plural.

To say 10,000, use the number **dyesyat'** (*dye*-seet'; ten) followed by the word **tysyacha** in its genitive plural form, **tysyach.** This rule also applies for numbers beyond 10,000:

- **10,000 dyesyat' tysyach** (*dye*-seet' *tih*-seech)
- **50,000 pyatdyesyat' tysyach** (pee-dee-*syat tih*-seech)
- **100,000 sto tysyach** (stoh *tih*-seech)

And one really big number is quite simple: **1,000,000 million** (mee-lee-*ohn*).

Ordinal numbers

Ordinal numbers are numbers like 1st, 2nd, and 3rd. We list the first 20 here:

- **pyervyj** (*pyer*-vihy; first)
- **vtoroj** (ftah-*rohy*; second)
- **tryetij** (*trye*-teey; third)
- **chyetvyertyj** (cheet-*vyor*-tihy; fourth)
- **pyatyj** (*pya*-tihy; fifth)
- **shyestoj** (shees-*tohy*; sixth)
- **syed'moj** (seed'-*mohy*; seventh)
- **vos'moj** (vahs'-*mohy*; eighth)
- **dyevyatyj** (dee-*vya*-tihy; ninth)
- **dyesyatyj** (dee-*sya*-tihy; tenth)
- **odinnadtsatyj** (ah-*dee*-nuht-suh-tihy; eleventh)
- **dvyennadtsatyj** (dvee-*naht*-suh-tihy; twelfth)
- **trinadtsatyj** (tree-*naht*-suh-tihy; thirteenth)
- **chyetyrnadtsatyj** (chee-*tihr*-nuht-suh-tihy; fourteenth)
- **pyatnadtsatyj** (peet-*naht*-suh-tihy; fifteenth)
- **shyestnadtsatyj** (shees-*naht*-suh-tihy; sixteenth)
- **syemnadtsatyj** (seem-*naht*-suh-tihy; seventeeth)
- **vosyem'nadtsatyj** (vuh-seem-*naht*-suh-tihy; eighteenth)
- **dyevyatnadtsatyj** (dee-veet-*naht*-suh-tihy; nineteenth)
- **dvadtsatyj** (dvuht-*sah*-tihy; twentieth)

Russian uses a principle similar to one in English with ordinal numbers higher than 20. You say the first numeral (or numerals) normally (like a cardinal number), with only the final numeral put into ordinal form:

- The 21st is **dvadtsat' pyervyj** (*dvah*-tsuht' *pyer*-vihy)
- The 46th is **sorok shyestoj** (*soh*-ruhk shees-*tohy*)
- The 65th is **shyest'dyesyat pyatyj** (shees-dee-*syat'* *pya*-tihy)
- The 177th is **sto syem'dyesyat' syed'moj** (stoh *syem'*-dee-seet' seed'-*mohy*)

In Russian, ordinal numbers behave just like adjectives, which means that they always agree in case, number, and gender with the nouns they precede. For more on this subject, see "Always consenting: Adjective-noun agreement" earlier in this chapter.

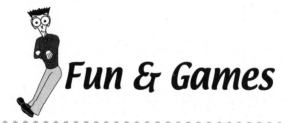

Fun & Games

What's the nominative singular form of these plural nouns? You can find the answers in Appendix C.

1. **komp'yutyery**
2. **knigi**
3. **okna**
4. **koshki**
5. **magaziny**

How many of these Russian numerals can you recognize? Check out the answers in Appendix C.

- ✔ **odin**
- ✔ **chyetyrye**
- ✔ **dvyenadtsat'**
- ✔ **dvadtsat'**
- ✔ **pyat'sot**
- ✔ **dvadtsat' tysyach trista sorok syem'**
- ✔ **shyest'sot tysyach dyevyanosto odin**

- ✔ **dva**
- ✔ **vosyem'**
- ✔ **pyatnadtsat'**
- ✔ **sto**
- ✔ **tysyacha**

Chapter 3

Zdravstvujtye! Privyet! Greetings and Introductions

In This Chapter

▶ Using informal and formal versions of "you"

▶ Knowing phrases for "hello" and "goodbye"

▶ Making sense of Russian names

▶ Introducing yourself and others

*J*ust as in English, greetings and introductions in Russian are the first steps in establishing contact with other people and making a good first impression. Greetings and introductions in Russian are a bit more formal than in English. If you greet somebody correctly in Russian, that person is impressed and probably wants to get to know you better. If, however, you botch your greeting, you may get a funny look or even offend the person you're addressing.

In this chapter, we give you details on how to make your best first impression. We cover the formal and informal versions of "you," saying "hello" and "goodbye," understanding Russian names, and introducing yourself and other folks.

To Whom Am 1 Speaking? Being Informal or Formal

When you want to say "hello" in Russian, it's important to know who you're talking to first. Unlike in English (but similar to French, German, or Spanish, for example), Russian uses two different words for the word "you" — informal **ty** (tih) and formal **vy** (vih). (In English, no matter whom you're talking to — your close friend, your boss, the President of the United States, or your dog — you use the word "you.")

Showing affection for grandparents

The distinction between **ty** and **vy** isn't only a sign of a formal or an informal situation. **Ty** also signifies affection. Although grandparents are by definition older people, their grandchildren address them with **ty**. Maybe this is because of the very special role a Russian **babushka** (*bah*-boosh-kuh; grandmother) plays in the Russian family. Traditionally, Russian mothers often leave their children with *their* mothers, or *babushkas*. *Babushkas* often live with their grownup children who already have their own families just to help them to raise the kids: They feed them, walk them, and take them to or from school — a full-time job! No wonder the grandchildren use **ty** in addressing their grandmothers.

Although a grandfather often shares these responsibilities with his wife, his role is considered significantly less important. Nonetheless, the affectionate **ty** is still used with the word **dyedushka** (*dye*-doosh-kuh; grandfather), as well.

Here's how to know when to use which form of "you":

- ✔ In Russian, you're allowed to use the informal **ty** *only* when you're speaking to your parents, grandparents, siblings, children, and close friends.

- ✔ The formal **vy** is used in more formal situations when you talk to your boss, acquaintances, older people, or people you don't know very well, and anytime you're speaking to more than one person.

If you're a young person, you can safely use **ty** when addressing people your age, such as your classmates. Don't, however, dare to use **ty** when talking to your teacher, no matter how young she is! If you use **ty** in addressing an elderly woman or your teacher, your perhaps very innocent mistake may be taken as extreme rudeness, unless people make allowances for the fact that you're not a native Russian speaker.

As a rule, you should use the formal **vy** when addressing somebody you've never met before, an official, a superior, or someone who is older than you. As you get to know somebody better, you may switch to the informal **ty**. You even have a way of asking a person whether he or she is ready to switch to **ty: Mozhno na ty?** (*Mozh*-nuh nah tih?; May I call you informal "you?") If the answer is **da!** (dah; yes), then you're free to start calling the person **ty**. If, however, the answer is **nyet!** (nyet; no), you better wait until the person feels more comfortable with you!

If you're at all unsure whether to use **vy** or **ty**, use **vy** until the person you're addressing asks you to use **ty** or addresses you with **ty**.

Comings and Goings: Saying Hello and Goodbye

Greetings and goodbyes are essential Russian phrases to know. In the following sections, we show you how to say "hello" in a variety of ways, give you a few greetings to use throughout the day, tell you how to ask and answer to "How are you," and wrap up a conversation with goodbyes.

Saying hello to different people

To greet one person with whom you're on informal **ty** (tih) terms, use the word **Zdravstvuj** (*zdrah*-stvooy; hello). To greet a person with whom you're on formal **vy** (vih) terms, use the longer word, **Zdravstvujtye** (*zdrah*-stvooy-tee; hello). (We cover **ty** and **vy** in the previous section.) Note that the first letter "v" in **Zdravstvujtye** is silent. Otherwise it would be hard even for Russians to pronounce!

Zdravstvujtye is also used to address more than one person. Use it when addressing two or more people even if they're children, members of your family, or close friends.

The informal way of saying "hello" in Russian is **privyet!** (pree-*vyet*) It's similar to the English "hi," and you should be on pretty familiar terms with a person before you use this greeting.

Greeting folks at any time of day

You have ways to greet people in Russian, other than the bulky **Zdravstvuj** or **Zdravstvujtye,** but how you use these greetings depends on what time of day it is. The most commonly used greetings are in Table 3-1.

Table 3-1	Greetings for Different Times of the Day	
Greeting	*Pronunciation*	*Meaning*
dobroye utro!	*dohb*-ruh-ee *oo*-truh	Good morning! (This is the greeting you use in the morning — until noon.)
dobryj dyen'!	*dohb*-rihy dyen'	Good afternoon! (This is the greeting you can use most of the day, except for early in the morning or late at night.)
dobryj vyechyer!	*dohb*-rihy *vye*-cheer	Good evening! (This is the greeting you would most likely use in the evening.)

Note that Russians use these expressions only as greetings but not at leave-taking. (See "Taking your leave," later in this chapter for details on good-byes.) You can also use these expressions without giving any thought to whether the person you greet should be addressed with **ty** or **vy.** No matter whom you greet, you can safely use any of these phrases.

Handling "How are you?"

The easiest and most popular way to ask "How are you?" is **Kak dyela?** (kahk dee-*lah*) You use this phrase in rather informal settings, like at parties, meeting a friend on the street, or talking on the phone.

A more formal way to ask "How are you?" is **Kak vy pozhivayetye?** (kahk vih puh-zhih-*vah*-ee-tee) You use this phrase when speaking with your boss, your professor, or somebody you've just met.

You won't offend anyone in a formal setting if you say **Kak dyela?,** but you're better off sticking to **Kak vy pozhivayete?** Russians tend to err on the side of more formality rather than less.

A word of caution. In the English-speaking world, "How are you?" is just a standard phrase often used in place of a greeting. The person asking this formulaic question doesn't expect to get the full account of how you're actually doing. But in Russia it's different. They want to know everything! When they ask you how you're doing, they are in fact genuinely interested in how you're doing and expect you to give them a more or less accurate account of the most recent events in your life.

How should you reply to **Kak dyela?** Although optimistic Americans don't hesitate to say "terrific" or "wonderful," Russians usually respond with a more reserved **Khorosho** (khuh-rah-*shoh*; good) or **Normal'no** (nahr-*mahl'*-nuh; normal or okay), or even a very neutral **Nichyego** (nee-chee-*voh*; so-so, *Literally:* nothing) or **Nyeplokho** (nee-*ploh*-khuh; not bad).

If you're truly feeling great, go ahead and answer **pryekrasno!** (pree-*krahs*-nuh; wonderful), or **vyelikolyepno!** (vee-lee-kah-*lyep*-nuh; terrific). But beware that by saying "terrific" or "wonderful," you're putting your Russian friend on guard: Russians know all too well that life is not a picnic. To a Russian, wonderful and terrific events are the exception, not the rule. To be on the safe side, just say either **Nichyego** or **Nyeplokho.**

And don't stop there! Be sure to ask the person how she's doing. You simply say **A u vas?** (ah oo vahs; and you?; formal) If you want to be less formal, you say **A u tyebya?** (ah oo tee-*bya*; and you?)

Taking your leave

The usual way to say *goodbye* in almost any situation is **Do svidaniya!** (duh svee-*dah*-nee-ye), which literally means "Till (the next) meeting." If you're on informal terms with somebody, you may also say **Poka** (pah-*kah*; 'bye or see you later).

The phrase you use while leave-taking in the evening or just before bed is **Spokojnoj Nochi** (spah-*kohy*-nuhy *noh*-chee; Good night). The phrase works both for formal and informal situations.

Talkin' the Talk

Sasha bumps into her classmate Oleg on the subway. Sasha is just about to get off.

Oleg:	**Sasha, privyet!**
	sah-shuh, pree-*vyet!*
	Sasha, hi!

Sasha: (pleasantly surprised)	**Oj, Olyeg! Privyet! Kak dyela?**
	ohy, ah-*lyek!* pree-*vyet!* kahk dee-*lah?*
	Oh, Olyeg! Hi! How are you?

Oleg:	**Nichyego. A u tyebya?**
	nee-chee-*voh.* ah oo tee-*bya?*
	Okay. And you?

Sasha:	**Nyeplokho. Oj, eto moya stantsiya. Do svidaniya, Olyeg.**
	nee-*ploh*-khuh. ohy, *eh*-tuh mah-*ya stahn*-tsih-ye. duh svee-*dah*-nee-ye, ah-*lyek.*
	Not bad. Oh, this is my station. Goodbye, Olyeg.

Oleg:	**Poka!**
	pah-*kah!*
	Bye!

Words to Know

privyet	pree-<u>vyet</u>	hi
Kak dyela?	kahk dee-<u>lah</u>	How are you?
nichyego	nee-chee-<u>voh</u>	okay
A u tyebya?	ah oo tee-<u>bya</u>	And you?
nyeplokho	nee-<u>ploh</u>-khuh	not bad
do svidaniya	duh svee-<u>dah</u>-nee-ye	goodbye
poka	pah-<u>kah</u>	'bye

Not So Simple: Deciphering Russian Names

The Russian word "name" is **imya** (*ee*-mye), but you may not hear this word when people ask about your name. That's because what they actually ask is not "What is your name?" but literally, "How do people/they call you . . . ?" — **Kak vas/tyebya zovut?** (kahk vahz/tee-*bya* zah-*voot*) Consequently, when you answer the question, you say how people in fact call you — **Myenya zovut Dzhon** (mee-*nya* zah-*voot* dzhohn; My name is John, *Literally:* They call me John).

Saying names in Russian is a bit more complicated than in English. The reason is that in introducing themselves, especially in formal situations, Russians use the *patronymic* (patronymic means father's name) right after the first name. The patronymic usually has the ending **-vich** (veech), meaning "son of," or **-ovna** (*ohv*-nuh), meaning "daughter of." For example, a man named Boris, whose father's name is Ivan, would be known as Boris Ivanovich (Ivanovich is the patronymic). A woman named Anna whose father's name is Ivan would be known as Anna Ivanovna (Ivanovna is the patronymic). A Russian almost never formally addresses a person named Mikhail as just "Mikhail" but rather as "Mikhail" plus his patronymic with the suffix **-vich** (for instance, "Mikhail Nikolayevich" or "Mikhail Borisovich").

You may say that Russians have three names. The first name is a baptismal name; the second name is his or her father's name with the ending **-vich** for men, or **-ovna** for women; and the third is the last name, or the family name.

Men's last names and women's last names have different endings. That's because Russian last names have genders. Although most Russian male last names have the ending **-ov** (of), female names take the ending **-ova** (*ohv*-nuh). Imagine that your new acquaintance, Anna Ivanovna Ivanova, is a married woman. Her husband's last name isn't **Ivanova** (ee-vuh-*noh*-vuh), but **Ivanov** (ee-vuh-*nof*).

No matter what your relation is to another person (either informal or formal), you can still address that person by his or her first name and patronymic. So if you're unsure whether you're on **ty** or **vy** terms with someone, go ahead and address the person by the first name and patronymic just to be safe. When you're clearly on friendly terms with the person, you can switch to using the first name only.

In everyday conversation Russians almost never use words like Mr., Mrs., Ms., and Miss. Russians use these kinds of titles only in extremely formal situations, such as in government proceedings or in legal contracts. In such situations you may hear somebody referred to as **Gospodin Putin** (guhs-spah-*deen* poo-teen; Mr. Putin) or **Gospozha Gorbachyova** (guhs-pah-*zhah* guhr-buh-*choh*-vuh; Mrs. Gorbachev).

Playing the Russian nickname game

By the way, what does Mr. Ivanov call his wife (whose name is Anna)? Most likely, he uses the diminutives Anya, Anechka, Anyuta, or Annushka. Russians are extremely ingenious in creating new diminutives and are constantly changing them even when addressing one and the same person. This is one of the reasons why Americans sometimes find it difficult to read Russian novels. While it seems that new characters are constantly being introduced by the author, the fact is that in many cases it's an old character with a new diminutive version of her name! For example, Ekatyerina Shchyerbatskaya, a famous character from Leo Tolstoy's *Anna Karyenina*, is sometimes affectionately called by the diminutives, Katyenka, Katiusha, and Kitty. No wonder Russian novels are so long!

Break the Ice: Making Introductions

Making a good first impression is important for the beginning of any relationship. Russians tend to be more formal than Americans in how they approach a person they've just met. In the following sections, we show you the best ways to introduce yourself to somebody you've just met. We also show you phrases to use when getting acquainted with someone, how to ask for somebody's name, and the best way to introduce your friends, colleagues, and family to new people.

Getting acquainted

In English, introducing yourself is the best way to start a conversation with somebody you don't know. Not so in Russian. When introducing themselves, Russians are a little more ceremonial. Russians like to begin with first *suggesting* to get acquainted by saying "Let's get acquainted!" They have two ways to say this, depending on whether they're on formal **vy** (vih) or informal **ty** (tih) terms with the person (see "Who Am I Speaking To? Being Informal or Formal" earlier in this chapter for info on these terms). Check out Table 3-2.

Table 3-2	Asking to Become Acquainted	
Introduction	*Pronunciation*	*Meaning*
Formal: Davajtye poznakomimsya!	duh-*vahy*-tee puhz-nuh-*koh*-meem-sye	Let's get acquainted! (addressing a person formally or two or more people)
Informal: Davaj poznakomimsya!	duh-*vahy* puhz-nuh-*koh*-meem-sye	Let's get acquainted! (addressing a person informally)

If somebody says one of these phrases to you, you should politely accept the suggestion. To respond, you can just use the first word, which makes your task much easier (see Table 3-3).

Table 3-3	Agreeing to Become Acquainted	
Response	*Pronunciation*	*Meaning*
Formal: Davajtye!	duh-*vahy*-tee	Okay (*Literally:* Let's; addressing a person formally or two or more people)
Informal: Davaj!	duh-*vahy*	Okay (*Literally:* Let's; addressing a person informally)

Asking for people's names and introducing yourself

The formal version of "What is your name?" is **Kak vas zovut?** (kahk vahz zah-*voot?*; *Literally:* What do they call you?) The informal version of "What is your name?" is **Kak tyebya zovut?** (kahk tee-*bya* zah-*voot*; *Literally:* What do they call you?)

To introduce yourself in Russian, just say **Myenya zovut** (Mee-*nya* zah-*voot*) + your name. (See "Not So Simple: Deciphering Russian Names," earlier in this chapter, for details about Russian names.)

When introducing yourself, Russian doesn't distinguish between formal and informal. You use the introduction **Menya zovut** in both formal and informal situations.

After you're introduced to someone, you may want to say, "Nice to meet you." In Russian you say **ochyen' priyatno** (oh-cheen' pree-*yat*-nuh; *Literally:* very pleasant). The person you've been introduced to may then reply **mnye tozhye** (mnye *toh*-zheh; same here). You use the phrases **ochyen' priyatno** and **mnye tozhye** in both formal and informal situations.

Introducing your friends, colleagues, and family

Everyday, common introductions are easy in Russian. When you want to introduce your friends, all you need to say is **Eto . . .** (*eh*-tuh; This is . . .) Then you simply add the name of the person (see "Not So Simple: Deciphering Russian Names" earlier in this chapter for more info about names).

To indicate that the person is an acquaintance or a colleague, you say one of two things:

- If the person is a man, you say **Eto moj znakomyj** (*eh*-tuh mohy znuh-*koh*-mihy; This is my acquaintance).

- If the person is a woman, you say **Eto moya znakomaya** (*eh*-tuh mah-*ya* znuh-*koh*-muh-ye; This is my acquaintance).

As in English, the same construction (**Eto** + the family member) applies to a broad circle of people including your family members. For example, to introduce you mother, you say **Eto moya mama** (*eh*-tuh mah-*ya mah*-muh; This is my mother); to introduce your brother, just say **Eto moj brat** (*eh*-tuh mohy braht; This is my brother). To introduce other members of your family, see Chapter 4, where we provide words indicating other family members.

Talkin' the Talk

Anna is approached by her friend, Viktor, and his acquaintance, Boris Aleksyeyevich:

Viktor:	**Oj, privyet, Anna!** ohy, pree-*vyet, ah*-nuh! Oh, hi Anna!
Anna:	**Privyet Viktor! Kak dyela?** Pree-*vyet veek*-tuhr! kahk dee-*lah*? Hi, Viktor! How are you?
Viktor:	**Nichyego. A u tyebya.** nee-chee-*voh*. ah oo tee-*bya*? Okay. And you?
Anna:	**Nyeplokho.** nee-*ploh*-khuh. Not bad.
Viktor (to Anna):	**A eto moj znakomyj, Boris Alyeksyeyevich.** ah *eh*-tuh mohy znuh-*koh*-mihy, bah-*rees uh*-leek-*sye*-ee-veech. And this is my acquaintance, Boris Alekseevich.

Chapter 3: Zdravstvujtye! Privyet! Greetings and Introductions

Anna (to Boris Aleksyeyevich):   **Zdravstvujtye! Davajtye poznakomimsya!**
zdrah-stvooy-tee! duh-*vahy*-tee puhz-nuh-*koh*-meem-sye!
Hello! Let's get acquainted!

Boris Aleksyeyevich: **Davajtye! Myenya zovut Boris.**
duh-*vahy*-tee! mee-*nya* zah-*voot* bah-*rees.*
Let's! My name is Boris.

Anna: **Ochyen' priyatno!**
oh-cheen' pree-*yat*-nuh!
Nice to meet you!

Boris Aleksyeyevich: **Mnye tozhye.**
mnye *toh*-zheh.
Nice to meet you, too. (*Literally:* same here)

Words to Know

Eto moj znakomyj	<u>eh</u>-tuh mohy znuh-<u>koh</u>-mihy	This is my acquaintance
Davajtye poznakomimsya!	duh-<u>vahy</u>-tee puhz-nuh-<u>koh</u>-meem-sye	Let's get acquainted!
Myenya zovut	mee-<u>nya</u> zah-<u>voot</u>	My name is
Ochyen' priyatno!	<u>oh</u>-cheen' pree-<u>yat</u>-nuh	Nice to meet you!
mnye tozhye	mnye <u>toh</u>-zheh	likewise

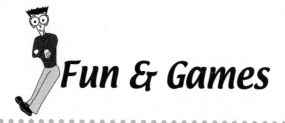

Fun & Games

Practice saying "Hello" in Russian to the following people. Should you use **Zdravstvujtye** (*Zdrah*-stvooy-tee) or **Zdravstvuj** (*Zdrah*-stvooy)? Find the correct answers in Appendix C.

1. Your close friend

2. Your boss

3. Your teacher

4. Your doctor

5. Your pet

6. A group of friends

7. Several children

Try practicing greetings by time of day. In the right column, find and say the greeting that should be used at the time of day indicated in the left column. See Appendix C for the correct answers.

3 p.m.	**Dobryj dyen'!**
11 a.m.	**Dobryj vyechyer!**
8 a.m.	**Dobroye utro!**
8 p.m.	

The dialogue between Nina and Natasha got scrambled. Take a few minutes to unscramble it and put the phrases in correct order (see Appendix C to check your answers). Nina and Natasha are both 18 years old. They study at the same school but have not met yet.

Natasha:	**Davaj!**
Nina:	**Zdravstvuj! Davaj poznakomimsya!**
Nina:	**Myenya zovut Nina. A kak tyebya zovut?**
Nina:	**Ochyen' priyatno!**
Natasha:	**Myenya zovut Natasha.**
Natasha:	**Mnye tozhye.**

Part II
Russian in Action

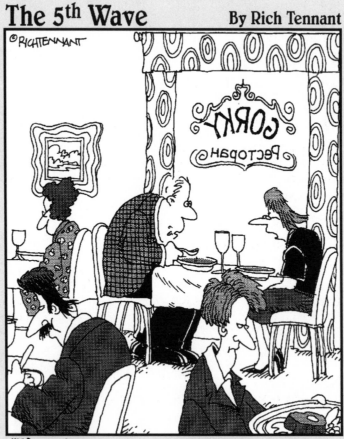

"If you're going to slurp your borscht, at least try to slurp it in Russian."

In this part . . .

Part II gives you all the Russian you need for ordinary, everyday living. You discover Russian phrases and expressions for making small talk, eating, drinking, going shopping, talking about your favorite sports and hobbies, and having fun on the town the Russian way. You also find out how to make telephone calls, send letters, and talk about the house and office in Russian.

Chapter 4

Getting to Know You: Making Small Talk

· ·

In This Chapter

▶ Breaking the ice by talking about yourself

▶ Exchanging contact information

▶ Knowing what to say when you don't understand something

· ·

The best way to start getting to know someone is through small talk. Imagine you're on a plane on your way to Russia. Chances are the person sitting next to you is Russian. So, what are you going to talk about? To break the ice you're probably going to want to talk about yourself, where you're from, your age, your job, and your family, maybe even about the weather. Just before the flight lands, you probably want to give and receive contact information.

In this chapter we show you how to do all these things in Russian and also what to say when you don't understand something. You'll be ready for your first complete conversation with a real Russian!

Russian doesn't have a translation for the phrase "small talk." That's because Russians take small talk seriously, especially when they talk to foreigners. One reason for this is that for most of its long and turbulent history, Russia was virtually cut off from the rest of the world. Chatting with foreigners has always been a way for Russians to satisfy their strong curiosity about the outside world. In other words, they really want to get to know you and everything about you and as fast as possible. Don't be shocked if their direct questions sometimes sound like KGB interrogations. They're just curious!

Let Me Tell You Something: Talking about Yourself

What do people talk about when they first meet? The topics are highly predictable: home, family, jobs, and even age. In the following sections, we deal with each of them.

The Western view of what one can ask about during the first casual conversation is quite different from the Russian view. The rules of Russian small talk are quite a bit looser and allow you to ask questions that a Western code of good manners would consider quite forward, to say the least, including such topics as money, annual income, death, illnesses, and sex, among others. For instance, a young 30-year-old man should expect to be asked why he's not yet married. And a recently married couple will probably be asked why they don't have children yet!

Stating where you're from

One of the topics that's bound to come up during your first conversations is your country of origin. Expect to hear the question, **Otkuda vy?** (aht-*koo*-duh vih; Where are you from?) To answer, you can say:

- ✔ **Ya iz Amyeriki** (ya eez uh-*mye*-ree-kee; I am from America)
- ✔ **Ya zhivu v Amyerikye** (ya zhih-*voo* v uh-*mye*-ree-kye; I live in America)

It's also common and acceptable to answer **Otkuda vy?** with a statement of nationality; for example, you can say "I am American" rather than "I live in the United States." See the next section for more about describing your nationality.

After a Russian finds out your country of origin, he may ask you where in the country you're from (such as a city or a state). You may hear questions like

---

So how much do you make?

Among the questions Russians don't hesitate to ask are **Kakaya u vas zarplata?** (kuh-*kah*-ye oo vahs/tee-*bya* zuhr-*plah*-tuh; formal), **Kakaya u tyebya zarplata?** (kuh-*kah*-ye oo tee-*bya* zuhr-*plah*-tuh; informal), and **Skol'ko vy poluchayete?** (*skoh'l*-kuh vih puh-loo-*chah*-ee-tee), which basically mean the same thing: *How much do you make?* In Russia the income one earns is usually described on a monthly basis. That's why, before answering, you may want to divide your yearly income by 12 (12 months).

✔ **V kakom shtatye vy zhivyote?** (f kuh-*kohm* shtah-tee vih zhih-*vyo*-tee; What state do you live in?)

✔ **Vy iz kakogo shtata?** (vih ees kuh-*koh*-vuh *shtah*-tuh; What state are you from?)

✔ **V kakom gorodye vy zhivyote?** (f kuh-*kohm* goh-ruh-dee vih zhih-*vyo*-tee; What city do you live in?)

✔ **Vy iz kakogo goroda?** (vih eez kuh-*koh*-vuh *goh*-ruh-duh; What city are you from?)

Later, when you're asked where in the U.S. (or England or Australia) you live, you may want to say the city or state you're from:

✔ **Ya zhivu v Siyetlye** (ya zhih-*voo* f see-*yet*-lee; I live in Seattle)

✔ **Ya iz Siyetla** (ya ees see-*yet*-luh; I am from Seattle)

Notice that when the preposition **v** is followed by a noun beginning with a consonant, it's pronounced like *f*, not *v*, and when the preposition **iz** is followed by a noun beginning with a consonant, it's pronounced *ees*, not *eez*.

When you say **Ya zhivu v . . .** (ya zhih-*voo* v; I live in . . .), use the word describing the place where you live in the prepositional case, because the preposition **v** (in) takes that case. When saying **Ya iz . . .** (ya eez; I am from . . .), use the next word in the genitive case because the preposition **iz** (eez; from) requires genitive. (For more info on cases, see Chapter 2.)

Talking about your nationality and ethnic background

Because Russia has historically been a very ethnically diverse country, Russians tend to be aware of and interested in different nationalities. From the very start of your friendship or conversation, a Russian will want to know your nationality or ethnic background. So be prepared to hear the next question: **A kto vy po-natsional'nosti?** (ah ktoh vih puh-nuh-tsee-ah-*nahl'*-nuhst-ee; And what is your nationality?)

Russian has three different words to indicate nationality. The choice of the word depends on the gender and number of the person or people whose nationality is being described. Select the phrase that describes you:

✔ **Ya amyerikanyets** (ya uh-mee-ree-*kahn*-neets; I'm an American man)

✔ **Ya amyerikanka** (ya uh-mee-ree-*kahn*-kuh; I'm an American woman)

✔ **My amyerikantsy** (mih uh-mee-ree-*kahn*-tsih; We're Americans)

You can use the phrase **My amyerikantsy** for any group of American men, women, or mixed genders.

Russian is very specific about gender. If you're a male, make sure you use the word indicating the nationality of a man, and if you're a female, use the word indicating the nationality of a woman. Imagine a man introducing himself as **Ya amyerkinanka.** Although people will understand what he's saying, they'll be quite amused, and if you're that man, you may be just a tad embarrassed.

Most Russians are highly educated people. They know that the United States, Australia, and Great Britain are ethnically diverse countries. Therefore, they also ask the question **A kto vy po-natsional'nosti?** (ah ktoh vih puh-nuh-tsee-ah-*nahl'*-nuhst-ee; And what is your nationality?) to find out your specific ethnic heritage (rather than your nationality). This situation is especially true if you don't look like a "typical American," which to a Russian means a blue-eyed, blond, tall, and athletic-looking Anglo-Saxon.

Another possibility is that your new Russian friend will attempt to guess your nationality instead of asking you outright. Most Russians are very good at recognizing foreigners in a crowd of people and sometimes are even able to guess your nationality just by looking at you. If this is the case, you may hear questions like these right off the bat:

- ✔ **Vy amyerikanyets?** (vih uh-mee-ree-*kah*-neets; Are you American? *Literally:* Are you an American man?)

- ✔ **Vy amyerikanka?** (vih uh-mee-ree-*kahn*-kuh; Are you American? *Literally:* Are you an American woman?)

- ✔ **Vy amyerikantsy?** (vih uh-mee-ree-*kahn*-tsih; Are you Americans?)

In Table 4-1 you find a list of some nationalities and specific ethnicities. Find the one that best describes your background, and note that Russian doesn't capitalize names of nationalities and ethnic backgrounds.

Table 4-1	Words Denoting Nationality and Ethnicity		
Nationality of a Man	**Nationality of a Woman**	**Nationality of People**	**Translation**
afrikanyets (uhf-ree-*kah*-neets)	afrikakanka (uhf-ree-*kahn*-kuh)	afrikantsy (uhf-ree-*kahn*-tsih)	African
amyerikanyets (uh-mee-ree-*kah*-neets)	amyerikanka (uh-mee-ree-*kahn*-kuh)	amyerikantsy (uh-mee-ree-*kahn*-tsih)	American
indyeyets (een-*dye*-eets)	indiyanka (een-dee-*ahn*-kuh)	indyejtsy (een-*dyey*-tsih)	American Indian
arab (uh-*rahp*)	arabka (uh-*rahp*-kuh)	araby (uh-*rah*-bih)	Arab(ic)

Nationality of a Man	Nationality of a Woman	Nationality of People	Translation
argyentinyets (uhr-geen-*tee*-neets)	argyentinka (uhr-geen-*teen*-kuh)	argyentintsy (uhr-geen-*teen*-tsih)	Argentinean
kitayets (kee-*tah*-eets)	kitayanka (kee-tuh-*yan*-kuh)	kitajtsy (kee-*tahy*-tsih)	Chinese
yegiptyanin (ee-geep-*tya*-neen)	yegiptyanka (ee-geep-*tyan*-kuh)	yegiptyanye (ee-geep-*tya*-nee)	Egyptian
anglichanin (uhn-glee-*chah*-neen)	anglichanka (uhn-glee-*chahn*-kuh)	anglichanye (uhn-glee-*chah*-nee)	English
frantsuz (fruhn-*tsooz)*	frantsuzhyenka (fruhn-*tsoo*-zhihn-kuh)	frantsuzy (fruhn-*tsoo*-zih)	French
nyemyets (*nye*-meets)	nyemka (*nyem*-kuh)	nyemtsy (*nyem*-tsih)	German
indus (een-*doos)*	indiyanka (een-dee-*ahn*-kuh)	indusy (een-*doo*-sih)	Indian
iranyets (ee-*rah*-neets)	iranka (ee-*rahn*-kuh)	irantsy (ee-*rahn*-tsih)	Iranian
irlandyets (eer-*lahn*-deets)	irlandka (eer-*lahn*-kuh)	irlandtsy (eer-*lahn*-tsih)	Irish
ital'yanyets (ee-tuhl-*ya*-neets)	ital'yanka (ee-tuhl-*yan*-kuh)	ital'yantsy (ee-tuhl-*yan*-tsih)	Italian
yaponyets (ee-*poh*-neets)	yaponka (ee-*pohn*-kuh)	yapontsy (ee-*pohn*-tsih)	Japanese
yevryej (eev-*ryey)*	yevryejka (eev-*ryey*-kuh)	yevryei (eev-*rye*-ee)	Jewish
myeksikanyets (meek-see-*kah*-neets)	myeksikanka (mee-ksee-*kahn*-kuh)	myeksikantsy (mee-ksee-*kahn*-tsih)	Mexican
polyak (pah-*lyak)*	pol'ka (*pohl'*-kuh)	polyaki (pah-*lya*-kee)	Polish
russkij (*roos*-keey)	russkaya (*roos*-kuh-ye)	russkiye (*roos*-kee-ye)	Russian
shotlandyets (shaht-*lahn*-deets)	shotlandka (shaht-*lahn*-kuh)	shotlandtsy (shaht-*lahn*-tsih)	Scottish
ispanyets (ees-*pah*-neets)	ispanka (ees-*pahn*-kuh)	ispnatsy (ees-*pahn*-tsih)	Spanish
turok (*too*-ruhk)	turchanka (tuhr-*chahn*-kuh)	turki (*toor*-kee)	Turkish

Most words denoting nationality of women have the ending **-ka** as in **amy-erikanka** (American woman). Many words denoting nationality of men end in **-yets** as in **kitayets** (Chinese man). Some words, however, slightly divert from this rule, such as the word **frantsuz** (frahn-*tsoos*; Frenchman). Most words denoting the nationality of people (plural) have the ending **-tsy.** Exceptions to the words you may be using a lot include the following:

- ✔ **russkij** (*roos*-keey; Russian male)

- ✔ **russkaya** (*roo*-skuh-ye; Russian female)

- ✔ **russkiye** (*roo*-skee-ye; Russians)

Other exceptions are words like **yevryei** (eev-*rye*-ee; Jewish people) and **anglichanye** (uhn-glee-*chah*-nee; English people). Unfortunately, no hard and fast rule exists for this, so you just need to memorize the words as they are.

Note the translation of the word "Indian." English uses the word "Indian" for both American and Asian Indians. Russian uses **indus** to indicate an Asian Indian man and **indyeyets** to indicate a Native American man. This difference eliminates the ambiguity of English. However, this distinction disappears in the word **indiyanka,** which denotes both an Asian Indian and an American Indian woman, but the distinction reappears when you refer to a group of Indians (either **indusy** or **indyejsty**).

Talkin' the Talk

John and Natasha are on board a flight from Frankfurt to Moscow. They've just met.

Natasha:	**Dzhohn, otkuda vy?** dzhon, aht-*koo*-duh vih? John, where are you from?
John:	**Ya amyerikanyets. A vy russkaya?** ya uh-mee-ree-*kah*-neets. ah vih *roos*-kuh-ye? I'm American. And are you Russian?
Natasha:	**Da, russkaya. Ya zhivu v Pyermi. A gdye vy zhivyotye v Amyerikye?** dah, *roos*-kuh-ye. ya zhih-*voo* f pyer-*mee*. ah gdye vih zhih-*vyo*-tee v uh-*mye*-ree-kee? Yes, I am Russian. I live in Perm. And where do you live in the U.S.?
John:	**Ya iz shtata Viskonsin. Ya zhivu i uchus' v Madisonye.** ya ees-*shtah*-tuh vees-*kohn*-seen. ya zhih-*voo* ee oo-*choos'* v *mah*-dee-sohn-ee.

I'm from the state of Wisconsin. I live and study in Madison.

Natasha: **Kak intyeryesno! Vy nye pokhozhi na amyerikantsa. Kto vy po-natsional'nosti?**
kahk een-tee-*ryes*-nuh! vih nee pah-*khoh*-zhih nuh uh-mee-ree-*kahn*-tsuh. ktoh vih puh-nuh-tsih-ah-*nahl'*-nuhs-tee?
How interesting! You don't look American. What's your nationality?

John: **Moya mama myeksikanka, a papa ital'yanyets.**
mah-*ya mah*-muh meek-see-*kahn*-kuh, uh *pah*-puh ee-tuhl-*ya*-neets.
My mother is Mexican, and my father is Italian.

Natasha: **Ponyatno.**
pah-*nyat*-nuh.
I see.

Words to Know

Otkuda vy?	aht-<u>koo</u>-duh vih	Where are you from?
Gdye vy zhivyotye?	gdye vih zhih-<u>vyo</u>-tee	Where do you live?
Ya zhivu v . . .	ya zhih-<u>voo</u> v	I live in . . .
Kto vy po natsional'nosti?	ktoh vih puh-nuhts-ee-ah-<u>nahl'</u>-nuhst-ee	What's your nationality?
Vy nye pokhozhi na . . .	vih nee pah-<u>khoh</u>-zhih nuh	You don't look like a . . .
Ya uchus' v	ya oo-<u>choos'</u> v	I study at/in
iz shtata	ees-<u>shtah</u>-tuh	from the state
Kak intyeryesno!	kahk een-tee-<u>ryes</u>-nuh	How interesting!
Ponyatno	pah-<u>nyat</u>-nuh	I see

The nationality question: A touchy subject

The question **Kto vy po natsional'nosti?** (ktoh vih puh-nuhts-ee-ah-*nahl'*-nuhst-ee; What's your nationality?) isn't just a matter of small talk for Russians. The question of one's ethnic background has been important in Russia from time immemorial. Unfortunately, Russians weren't always welcoming of foreigners. For centuries, in the big Russian Empire, non-Russians, including other Slavs such as Ukrainians, Byelorussians, and Poles were officially and unofficially considered to be inferior to the Great Russians. Great Russian nationalism, which is still very much alive today, goes back to the official policy of the Russian autocracy toward national minorities.

An example of Russian nationalism was the policy of Russification started by Catherine the Great (a German by birth) in the 18th century. Russification was an attempt to inspire a sense of Russian-ness in all peoples through a reverence for Russia's past, traditions, and culture, through the use of the Russian language, and by converting non-Christians to the Orthodox faith. Many people were forbidden to use their non-Russian language in schools and in the administration.

The results of Russification were especially evident in the policy of the authorities toward the Jews. Jews were classified as **inorodsty** (een-ah-*rohd*-tsih; non-citizens/aliens), who were non-Christian and considered second-class citizens. Joseph Stalin, who was a Georgian, used the idea of Russian supremacy as a way of establishing centralized power in the country, and he used Russian anti-Semitism as a method of inspiring feelings of Russian patriotism in all the citizens of the Soviet Union. That's why the question of one's nationality is still a touchy subject for Russians.

Telling your age

To inquire about someone's **vozrast** (*vohz*-ruhst; age) in Russian, you ask one of two questions:

> ✔ Use **Skol'ko tyebye lyet?** (*skohl'*-kuh tee-*bye* lyet; How old are you?) in a situation where you use the informal **tih** (you) address.

> ✔ Otherwise, say **Skol'ko vam lyet?** (*skohl'*-kuh vahm lyet; How old are you?) For more on formal and informal "you," see Chapter 3.

The answer to the questions **Skol'ko vam/tyebye lyet?** isn't as simple as you may think. First of all, in Russia age is seen as something that happens to you, something you can't control (and this is, after all, very true). That's why, rather than using the subject in the nominative case, Russian uses the dative form of the person whose age is being described. In Russian you say literally "To me is 23 years old."

CULTURAL WISDOM

Time flies in Russia

Attitudes toward age and aging differ in various cultures. You may notice that Russians on the whole — how should we put it? — *age earlier* than Americans. A young 26-year-old single woman is definitely "old" if not "an old maid" because marrying age in Russia begins much earlier.

Age today is an important factor in hiring decisions in Russia. A 40-year-old man may find it extremely hard to find new employment just because he is "too old." In their job announcements, employers don't hesitate to mention, for example, that they're hiring only young individuals no older than 35 to 40 years old.

As to marrying age, following the Western example, young people are starting to get married a little later today. Nonetheless, the average marrying age for Russians is in the early or mid-twenties.

The second tricky part of talking about your age is that the translation of the word "year(s)" depends on how old you are. This is how it works:

- ✔ If you're 1, 21, or 31 years old (in other words, if the numeral indicating your age is 1 or ends in 1), use the word **god** (goht; year), as in **Mnye 21 god** (mnye *dvaht*-tsuht' ah-*deen* goht; I am twenty-one years old).

- ✔ If you're 2, 3, or 4 years old (and already want to speak Russian!) or the numeral denoting your age ends in a 2, 3, or 4, use the word **goda** (*goh*-duh; years), as in **Mnye 22 goda** (mnye *dvaht*-tsuht' dvah *goh*-duh; I am twenty-two years old).

- ✔ If you're 5, 25, or 105 years old or the numeral denoting your age ends in 5, use the word **lyet,** as in **Mnye 25 lyet** (mnye *dvaht*-tsuht' pyat' lyet; I am twenty-five years old).

- ✔ If the numeral denoting your age ends in a 6, 7, 8, or 9, or if your age is 10 through 20, use the word **lyet,** as in **Mnye 27 lyet** (mney *dvaht*-tsuht' syem' lyet; I am twenty-seven years old).

Check out Chapter 2 for more about cases and numbers.

Discussing your family

Family is a big part of Russian culture, so your Russian acquaintances will certainly be curious about yours. Whether you have a small family or a large one, in this section we give all the words and phrases you need to know to talk about your family with your new Russian friends.

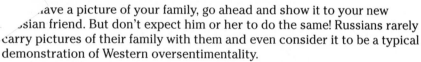

...ning with basic terms for family members

...ave a picture of your family, go ahead and show it to your new ...sian friend. But don't expect him or her to do the same! Russians rarely carry pictures of their family with them and even consider it to be a typical demonstration of Western oversentimentality.

Your best bet is to just talk about the members of your family with your new Russian friend, using the following words:

- ✔ **mat'** (maht'; mother)
- ✔ **otyets** (ah-*tyets*; father)
- ✔ **rodityeli** (rah-*dee*-tee-lee; parents)
- ✔ **syn** (sihn; son)
- ✔ **synovya** (sih-nah-*vya*; sons)
- ✔ **doch'** (dohch'; daughter)
- ✔ **dochyeri** (*doh*-chee-ree; daughters)
- ✔ **zhyena** (zhih-*nah*; wife)
- ✔ **muzh** (moosh; husband)
- ✔ **brat** (braht; brother)
- ✔ **brat'ya** (*brah*-tye; brothers)
- ✔ **syestra** (sees-*trah*; sister)
- ✔ **syostry** (*syos*-trih; sisters)
- ✔ **ryebyonok** (ree-*byo*-nuhk; child)
- ✔ **dyeti** (*dye*-tee; children)
- ✔ **babushka** (*bah*-boosh-kuh; grandmother)
- ✔ **dyedushka** (*dye*-doosh-kuh; grandfather)
- ✔ **babushka i dyedushka** (*bah*-boosh-kuh ee *dye*-doosh-kuh; grandparents; *Literally:* grandmother and grandfather)
- ✔ **vnuk** (vnook; grandson)
- ✔ **vnuki** (*vnoo*-kee; grandsons)
- ✔ **vnuchka** (*vnooch*-kuh; granddaughter)
- ✔ **vnuchki** (*vnooch*-kee; granddaughters)
- ✔ **vnuki** (*vnoo*-kee; grandchildren)
- ✔ **dyadya** (*dya*-dye; uncle)
- ✔ **tyotya** (*tyo*-tye; aunt)
- ✔ **kuzyen** (koo-*zehn*; male cousin)

- **kuzina** (koo-*zee*-nuh; female cousin)
- **plyemyannik** (plee-*mya*-neek; nephew)
- **plyemyannitsa** (plee-*mya*-nee-tsuh; niece)
- **syem'ya** (seem'-*ya*; family)

Talking about family members with the verb "to have"

When talking about your family, use phrases like "I have a brother" and "I have a big family" and "I don't have any brothers or sisters." To say these phrases you need to know how to use the verb **yest'** (yest'; to have).

Just as in English, this Russian verb expresses possession. For example, in the sentence, "My brother has a car," the phrase "my brother" indicates a possessor or owner and the word "car" indicates the thing that belongs to the owner. In Russian, the owner is expressed by the prepositional phrase **U** + a noun (or phrase) in the genitive case, followed by the verb **yest'** (have, has), and the thing that indicates what's being possessed or owned is expressed by the noun (phrase) in the nominative case. In other words, to convey the idea "My brother has a car," you have to create the Russian word combination **U** + "My brother" (genitive case) followed by the word **yest'** and then followed by the word "car" in the nominative case. The resulting Russian sentence can be literally translated into English as "At my brother there is a car": **U moyego brata yest' mashina.** (oo muh-ee-*voh brah*-tuh yest' muh-*shih*-nuh; My brother has a car.) Chapter 2 has the full scoop on cases.

Use the construction **U myenya yest'** . . . (oo mee-*nya* yest'; I have . . .) when talking about your own family:

- **U myenya yest' brat** (oo mee-*nya* yest' braht; I have a brother)
- **U myenya yest' syestra** (oo mee-*nya* yest' sees-*trah*; I have a sister)

If you want to say that you don't have a brother, a sister, a nephew, and so on, you use the construction **U myenya nyet** (oo mee-*nya* nyet) plus a noun in the genitive case:

- **U myenya nyet brata** (oo mee-*nya* nyet braht-uh; I don't have a brother)
- **U myenya nyet syestry** (oo mee-*nya* nyet sees-*trih*; I don't have a sister)

The genitive plural forms of some family members are irregular, and you need to memorize them:

- **brat'yev** (*braht'*-eef; brothers)
- **syestyor** (sees-*tyor*; sisters)
- **synovyej** (sih-nah-*vyey*; sons)
- **dochyeryej** (duh-chee-*ryey*; daughters)
- **dyetyej** (deet-*yey*; children)

Be sure to use these genitive plural forms in the construction **U myenya nyet . . .** (oo mee-*nya* nyet; I don't have . . .), as in:

- ✔ **U myenya nyet dochyeryej** (oo mee-*nya* nyet duh-chee-*ryey*; I don't have any daughters)

- ✔ **U myenya nyet synovyej** (oo mee-*nya* nyet sih-nah-*vyey*; I don't have any sons)

- ✔ **U myenya nyet dyetyej** (oo mee-*nya* nyet deet-*yey*; I don't have children)

Describing your job

Because what you do for living is crucial for a Russian's understanding of who you are, be prepared to answer the question **Kto vy po profyessii?** (ktoh vih puh-prah-*fye*-see-ee; What do you do for living? *Literally:* What's your job?) Interestingly, the very construction of this question reveals that in the Russian mentality, your profession is an expression of who you are as a person.

To answer the question about your profession, you just need the phrase **Ya** + your profession, as in **Ya yurist** (ya yoo-*reest*; I am a lawyer) or **Ya pryepodavatyel'** (ya pree-puh-duh-*vah*-teel'; I am a professor). Below is a list of the most common professions. Find the one that best fits you:

- ✔ **agyent po nyedvizhimosti** (uh-*gyent* puh need-*vee*-zhih-muhs-tee; real estate agent)

- ✔ **aktrisa** (ahk-*tree*-suh; actress)

- ✔ **aktyor** (ahk-*tyor*; male actor)

- ✔ **archityektor** (uhr-khee-*tyek*-tuhr; architect)

- ✔ **bibliotyekar'** (beeb-lee-ah-*tye*-kuhr'; librarian)

- ✔ **biznyesmyen** (beez-nehs-*myen*; businessman)

- ✔ **biznyesmyenka** (beez-nehs-*myen*-kuh; businesswoman)

- ✔ **bukhgaltyer** (bookh-*gahl*-teer; accountant)

- ✔ **domokhozyajka** (duh-muh-khah-*zyahy*-kuh; homemaker)

- ✔ **inzhyenyer** (een-zhee-*nyer*; engineer)

- ✔ **khudozhnik** (khoo-*dohzh*-neek; artist, painter)

- ✔ **muzykant** (moo-zih-*kahnt*; musician)

- ✔ **myedbrat** (meed-*braht*; male nurse)

- ✔ **myedsyestra** (meed-sees-*trah*; female nurse)

- ✔ **myenyedzhyer** (*meh*-need-zhehr; manager)

- ✔ **pisatyel'** (pee-*sah*-teel'; author, writer)

- ✔ **programmist** (pruh-gruh-*meest*; programmer)

- ✔ **pryepodavatyel'** (pree-puh-duh-*vah*-teel'; professor at the university)

- ✔ **studyent** (stoo-*dyent*; male student)

- ✔ **studyentka** (stoo-*dyent*-kuh; female student)

- ✔ **uchityel'** (oo-*chee*-teel'; male teacher)

- ✔ **uchityel'nitsa** (oo-*chee*-teel'-nee-tsuh; female teacher)

- ✔ **vospitatyel'** (vuhs-pee-*tah*-teel'; preschool teacher)

- ✔ **vrach** (vrahch; physician)

- ✔ **yurist** (yu-*reest*; attorney, lawyer)

- ✔ **zhurnalist** (zhoor-nuh-*leest*; journalist)

- ✔ **zunbnoj vrach** (zoob-*noy* vrahch; dentist)

Some professions have female versions, some are used for both men and women, and some have only male versions.

You can also specify where you work. Russian doesn't have an equivalent for the English "I work for United" or "He works for FedEx." Instead of *for*, Russian uses its equivalent of *at* — prepositions **v** or **na.** Rather than saying "I work for United," a Russian says "I work at United."

The Russian prepositions **v** and **na** (at) require that the noun denoting a place should take the prepositional case. Here are some of the most common places people work. We include the right preposition and prepositional case, so you can start telling people where you work right away. Say **Ya rabotayu . . .** (ya rah-*boh*-tuh-yu; I work . . .) plus one of these phrases:

- ✔ **doma** (*doh*-muh; from home)

- ✔ **na fabrikye** (nuh *fah*-bree-kee; at a light-industry factory)

- ✔ **na zavodye** (nuh zah-*vohd*-ee; at a heavy-industry plant)

- ✔ **v bankye** (v *bahn*-kee; at a bank)

- ✔ **v bibliotyekye** (v beeb-lee-ah-*tye*-kee; in a library)

- ✔ **v bol'nitsye** (v bahl'-*nee*-tsee; at a hospital)

- ✔ **v byuro nyedvizhimosti** (v byu-*roh* need-*vee*-zhih-muhs-tee; at a real estate agency)

- ✔ **v kommyerchyeskoj firmye** (f kah-*myer*-chees-kuhy *feer*-mee; at a business firm, company)

- ✔ **v laboratorii** (v luh-buh-ruh-*toh*-ree-ee; in a laboratory)

- ✔ **v magazinye** (v muh-guh-*zee*-nee; at a store)

✔ **v shkolye** (f *shkoh*-lee; at school)

✔ **v uchryezhdyenii** (v ooch-reezh-*dye*-nee-ee; at an office)

✔ **v univyersityetye** (v oo-nee-veer-see-*tye*-tee; at a university)

✔ **v yuridichyeskoj firmye** (v yu-ree-*dee*-chees-kuhy *feer*-mee; at a law firm)

Let's Get Together: Giving and Receiving Contact Information

Just before you're about to take your leave from a new Russian acquaintance, you probably want to exchange contact information. The easiest way to do this is just hand over your business card and say **Eto moya kartochka** (*eh*-tuh mah-*yah kahr*-tuhch-kuh; This is my card). In case you don't have a business card, you need to know these phrases:

✔ **Moj adryes . . .** (mohy *ah*-drees; My address is . . .)

✔ **Moya ulitsa . . .** (mah-*ya oo*-lee-tsuh; My street is . . .)

✔ **Moj nomyer doma . . .** (mohy *noh*-meer *doh*-muh; My house number is . . .)

✔ **Moj indyeks . . .** (mohy *een*-dehks; My zip code is . . .)

And nothing's easier than giving your phone number if you know your Russian numerals! (For more numerals, see Chapter 2.) Just say **Moj nomyer tyelyefona** (moy *noh*-mer tee-lee-*fohn*-uh; My telephone number is . . .) and the right numerals: **Moj nomer tyelyefona 555 12 34.** (moy *noh*-mer tee-lee-*fohn*-uh pyat' pyat' pyat' ah-*deen* dvah tree chee-*tih*-ree; My telephone number is 555 12 34.)

Russian telephone numbers are always written and spoken as XXX-XX-XX. For more information about telephone calls, see Chapter 9.

After you give your contact info, be sure to get your new friend's address, phone number, and e-mail address. You can use these phrases:

✔ **Kakoj u vas nomyer tyelyefona?** (kuh-*kohy* oo vahs *noh*-meer tee-lee-*foh*-nuh; What's your phone number?)

✔ **Kakoj u vas adryes?** (kuh-*kohy* oo vahs *ahd*-rees; What's your address?)

✔ **Kakoj u vas adryes po imyeilu?** (kuh-*kohy* oo vahs *ahd*-rees puh ee-*meh*-ee-loo; What's your e-mail address?)

To answer these questions, you simply say

- ✔ **Moi nomyer tyelyefona . . .** (mohy *noh*-meer tee-lee-*foh*-nuh; My telephone number is . . .)
- ✔ **Moi adryes . . .** (mohy *ahd*-rees; My address is . . .)
- ✔ **Moj adryes po imyeilu . . .** (mohy *ahd*-rees puh ee-*meh*-ee-loo; My e-mail address is . . .)

I'm Sorry! Explaining that You Don't Understand Something

When you first start conversing in Russian, there will probably be a lot you don't understand. You can signal that you don't understand something in several ways. Choose the phrase you like best, or use them all to really get the message across:

- ✔ **Izvinitye, ya nye ponyal.** (eez-vee-*nee*-tee ya nee *pohh*-nyel; Sorry, I didn't understand; masculine)
- ✔ **Izvinitye, ya nye ponyala.** (eez-vee-*nee*-tee ya nee puh-nye-*lah*; Sorry, I didn't understand; feminine)
- ✔ **Izvinitye, ya plokho ponimayu po-russki.** (eez-vee-*nee*-tee ya *ploh*-khuh puh-nee-*mah*-yu pah-*roos*-kee; Sorry, I don't understand Russian very well.)
- ✔ **Govoritye, pozhalujsta, myedlyennyeye!** (guh-vah-*ree*-tee pah-*zhahl*-stuh *myed*-lee-nee-ee; Speak more slowly, please!)
- ✔ **Kak vy skazali?** (kahk vih skuh-*zah*-lee; What did you say?)
- ✔ **Povtoritye, pozhalujsta.** (puhf-tah-*ree*-tee pah-*zhahl*-stuh; Could you please repeat that?)
- ✔ **Vy govoritye po-anglijski?** (vih guh-vah-*ree*-tee puh uhn-*gleey*-skee; Do you speak English?)

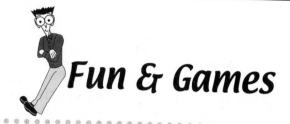

Fun & Games

Which of the two words indicates a woman? See the answers in Appendix C.

1. a. **amyerikanyets**   b. **amyerikanka**

2. a. **russkiye**   b. **russkaya**

3. a. **nyemtsy**   b. **nyemka**

4. a. **yevryejka**   b. **yevryej**

5. a. **frantsuzhyenka**   b. **frantsuz**

Which of the three words doesn't belong to the group? Check out the answers in Appendix C.

1. **plyemyannik, syestra, brat**

2. **dyeduska, babushka, otyets**

3. **mat', doch', otyets**

4. **vnuchka, babushka, vnuk**

5. **syestra, brat, otyets**

Which of the following statements just doesn't make sense? (The word **rabotayet** (ruh-*boh*-tuh-eet) means "works.") See the answers in Appendix C.

1. **Aktyor rabotayet v teatrye.**

2. **Aktrisa rabotayet v teatrye.**

3. **Profyessor rabotayet v univyersityetye.**

4. **Domokhozyajka rabotayet na fabrikye.**

5. **Inzhyenyer rabotayet na zavodye.**

Chapter 5

Making a Fuss about Food

In This Chapter

▶ Talking about food fundamentals

▶ Eating breakfast, lunch, and dinner

▶ Shopping for food

▶ Dining in restaurants and cafés

Russians are famous for their bountiful cuisine. Whether you like home-made food or prefer to go out to Russian restaurants, knowing how to talk about food is helpful. In this chapter, we dish up a hearty helping of words and phrases for expressing hunger and thirst, using eating utensils, and observing Russian food etiquette. We discuss the different meals of the day and the famous Russian farmer's market. We also discuss places to eat out, and what to say and do when you're there.

Focusing on Food Basics

Because food has always been such an important part of Russian culture, Russian has a rich variety of words and expressions related to eating and drinking. In this section, we tell you how to say you're thirsty and hungry in Russian, how to talk about the different eating utensils, and give you an overview of basic Russian table etiquette.

Eating up

When Russians are hungry they don't say "I'm hungry." Instead they say **Ya khochu yest'.** (ya khah-*choo* yest'; I'm hungry, *Literally:* I want to eat.) If you want to ask somebody if they're hungry, you say:

✔ **Ty khochyesh' yest'?** (tih *khoh*-cheesh' yest'; Are you hungry? *Literally:* Do you want to eat?; informal)

✔ **Vy khotitye yest'?** (vih khah-*tee*-tee yest'; Are you hungry? *Literally:* Do you want to eat?; formal and plural)

In addition to these expressions, you may also hear one of these phrases:

✔ **Vy golodnyj?** (vih gah-*lohd*-nihy; Are you hungry?), when speaking to a male

✔ **Vy golodnaya?** (vih gah-*lohd*-nuh-ye; Are you hungry?), when speaking to a female

✔ **Vy golodnyye?** (vih gah-*lohd*-nih-ee; Are you hungry?), when speaking to multiple people

To answer these questions, you say:

✔ **Ya golodnyj** (ya gah-*lohd*-nihy; I'm hungry), if you're male

✔ **Ya golodnaya** (ya gah-*lohd*-nuh-ye; I'm hungry), if you're female

Note that these phrases, however, have a particular flavor. In Russia **golod** (*goh*-luht; hunger) is a word that carries tragic historical connotations. So while it's perfectly acceptable to use the above expressions, you should know that they also carry this darker, secondary meaning.

Table 5-1 shows you how to conjugate the Russian verb **yest'** (yest'; to eat) for all the different pronouns. It's an irregular verb, so you just have to memorize it. (For more on regular verb conjugations, see Chapter 2.)

Table 5-1	Conjugation of Yest'	
Conjugation	*Pronunciation*	*Translation*
ya yem	ya yem	I eat or I am eating
ty yesh'	tih yesh'	You eat or You are eating (informal singular)
on/ona/ono yest	ohn/ah-*nah*/ah-*noh* yest	He/she/it eats or He/she/it is eating
my yedim	mih ee-*deem*	We eat or We are eating
vy yeditye	vih ee-*dee*-tee	You eat or You are eating (formal singular and plural)
oni yedyat	ah-*nee*-ee-*dyat*	They eat or They are eating

Drinking up

If you feel thirsty, you say **Ya khochu pit'** (ya khah-*choo* peet'; I'm thirsty, *Literally:* I want to drink). When you want to ask somebody whether they're thirsty, you say **Ty khochyesh' pit'?** (tih *khoh*-cheesh' peet'; Are you thirsty? *Literally:* Do you want to drink?; informal) or **Vy khotitye pit'?** (vih khah-*tee*-tee peet'; Are you thirsty? *Literally*: Do you want to drink?; formal)

The drinking verb **pit'** (peet'; to drink) has an unruly conjugation, as shown in Table 5-2.

Table 5-2	Conjugation of Pit'	
Conjugation	*Pronunciation*	*Translation*
ya p'yu	ya p'yu	I drink or I am drinking
ty p'yosh'	tih p'yosh'	You drink or You are drinking (informal singular)
on/ona/ono p'yot	ohn/ah-*nah*/ah-*noh* p'yot	He/she/it drinks or He/she/it is drinking
my p'yom	mih p'yom	We drink or We are drinking
vy p'yotye	vih *p'yo*-tee	You drink or You are drinking (formal singular and plural)
oni p'yut	ah-*nee* p'yut	They drink or They are drinking

Just as in English, the Russian statement **On/ona p'yot** (ohn/ah-*nah* p'yot; He/she drinks) in certain contexts can signify that the person is an alcoholic. If that's not your intention, you may want to add a direct object to the sentence to clarify your meaning.

Some common **napitki** (nuh-*peet*-kee; beverages) you may use as the direct objects are **sok** (sohk; juice), **chaj** (chahy; tea), **kofye** (*koh*-fye; coffee), **vodka** (*voht*-kuh; vodka), **pivo** (*pee*-vuh; beer), **vino** (vee-*noh*; wine), and a famous Russian **kvas** (kvahs) — a nonalcoholic beverage made of bread.

To say "I drink coffee" in Russian, you say **Ya p'yu kofye** (yah p'yu *koh*-fye). "I'm drinking vodka" is **Ya p'yu vodku** (yah p'yu *voht'*-koo). Notice that in this sentence **vodka** become **vodku,** the accusative case form of the noun, because it's the direct object of the sentence. (For more on using the accusative case with direct objects, see Chapter 2.)

Making room for the Russian tea tradition

The famous Russian tradition called **chayepitiye** (chah-ee-*pee*-tee-ye) is derived of two words — **chaj** (chahy; tea) and the noun **pitiye** (*pee*-tee-ye; drinking). Russians love tea almost like Brits do and drink it in huge quantities, usually in big glasses. In the old days, they used a **samovar** (suh-mah-*vahr*) — a special, huge tea-kettle, placed in the middle of the table. Russians usually drink tea with **sakhar** (*sah*-khuhr; sugar) and homemade berry preserves called **varayen'ye** (vah-*ryen*-ye).

Using utensils and tableware

Here's a list of the most common eating utensils and tableware:

- **blyudyechko** (*blyu*-deech-kuh; tea plate)

- **chashka** (*chahsh*-kuh; cup)

- **chaynaya lozhka** or **lozhyechka** (*chahy*-nuh-ye *lohsh*-kuh or *loh*-zhihch-kuh; teaspoon)

- **glubokaya taryelka** (gloo-*boh*-kuh-ye tuh-*ryel*-kuh; soup bowl)

- **kruzhka** (*kroosh*-kuh; mug)

- **lozhka** (*lohsh*-kuh; spoon)

- **nozh** (nohsh; knife)

- **salfyetka** (sahl-*fyet*-kuh; napkin)

- **stakan** (stuh-*kahn*; glass)

- **taryelka** (tah-*ryel*-kuh; plate)

- **vilka** (*veel*-kuh; fork)

Imagine that you're about to start eating a bowl of steaming soup but (much to your disappointment) you notice that you don't have a spoon. This is what you may want to say: **U myenya nyet lozhki.** (oo mee-*nya* nyet *lohsh*-kee; I don't have a spoon.)

After **nyet,** Russian uses the genitive case. For more on using **nyet** when expressing a lack of something, see Chapter 4. Chapter 2 has basic info on cases.

If you need to borrow a spoon from someone, you may ask that person by saying **Mozhno lozhku?** (*mohzh*-nuh *lohsh*-koo; Can I have a spoon?)

The construction **Mozhno . . .** (*mohzh*-nuh; Can/May I have . . .) + a noun is quite common in Russian. The noun takes the accusative case.

Minding basic Russian table manners

If you want to impress your Russian acquaintances, you should know basic Russian table manners. Some of the most important rules are related to using table utensils:

- ✔ Hold your fork in your left hand at all times, if you use a knife.

- ✔ Hold your fork in your right hand if you don't need a knife to cut food. When Russians eat fish, for example, they don't use a knife, and they hold the fork in the right hand.

- ✔ When eating dessert, don't use a fork; use a teaspoon instead.

Russians often find the American habit of cutting food into pieces before eating it very amusing. In Russia, only mothers do this for their young children. So when in a Russian restaurant, do as the Russians do. Never cut your food first with your knife and then put down the knife to hold your fork in the right hand. Always hold your knife in the right hand and your fork in the left hand, cutting pieces of food as necessary.

Enjoying Different Meals in Russia

Russians eat three meals a day: **zavtrak** (*zahf*-truhk; breakfast), **obyed** (ah-*byet*; dinner), and **uzhin** (*oo*-zhihn; supper). But Russian meals have quite a few peculiarities, which we tell you about in the following sections. We give you details on the amazingly flexible Russian breakfast, the hearty Russian midday meal, and the Russian dinner. Prepare your taste buds!

Russian for "to cook" is **gotovit'** (gah-*toh*-veet'). So, if cooking is one of your hobbies, you can now proudly say **Ya lyublyu gotovit'** (ya lyub-*lyu* gah-*toh*-veet'; I like/love to cook) when asked **Vy lyubitye gotovit'?** (vih *lyu*-bee-tee gah-*toh*-veet'; Do you like to cook?)

What's for breakfast? Almost anything!

The Russian breakfast is called **zavtrak** (*zahf*-truhk). What can you eat for **zav-trak?** The real question is what *can't* you eat! In contrast to American cereal, fruit, or bagels, or the British porridge, or the French croissant and jam, the Russian **zavtrak** is very flexible. Some Russian breakfast favorites include

- ✔ **butyerbrod s kolbasoj** (boo-tehr-*broht* s kuhl-buh-*sohy*; sausage sandwich)
- ✔ **butyerbrod s syrom** (boo-tehr-*broht* s *sih*-ruhm; cheese sandwich)
- ✔ **kasha** (*kah*-shuh; cooked grain served hot with milk, sugar, and butter)
- ✔ **kofye s molokom** (*koh*-fye s muh-lah-*kohm*; coffee with milk)
- ✔ **kolbasa** (kuhl-buh-*sah*; sausage)
- ✔ **kyefir** (kee-*feer*; buttermilk)
- ✔ **syelyodka s kartoshkoj** (see-*lyot*-kuh s kahr-*tohsh*-kuhy; herring with potatoes)
- ✔ **varyen'ye** (vuh-*ryen'*-ee; jam)
- ✔ **yaichnitsa** (ee-*eesh*-nee-tsuh; fried or scrambled eggs)

The management at Russian hotels in Moscow and St. Petersburg realize that such breakfast dishes as **syelyodka s kartoshkoj** may not appeal to all Western travelers, so the hotels try to accommodate their patrons' tastes. Rest assured that you can get a decent Western-style breakfast in a hotel catering to the needs of Western guests. Use the following words to order Western-style breakfast foods:

- ✔ **behkon** (*beh*-kuhn; bacon)
- ✔ **bliny** (blee-*nih*; pancakes)
- ✔ **kholodnaya kasha** (khah-*lohd*-nuh-ye *kah*-shuh; cereal)
- ✔ **kukuruznyye khlop'ya** (koo-koo-*rooz*-nih-ee *khlohp'*-ye; corn flakes)
- ✔ **moloko** (muh-lah-*koh*; milk)
- ✔ **ovsyanka** (ahf-*syan*-kuh; oatmeal)
- ✔ **sok** (sohk; juice)
- ✔ **tost** (tohst; toast)
- ✔ **yajtsa** (*yay*-tsuh; boiled eggs)

For the sake of fairness, we should mention that Russians share with Westerners their love of **bliny** (pancakes) and **yajtsa** (boiled eggs). **Bliny,** however, isn't a dish exclusive to breakfast in Russia. Also note that you use the word **yajtsa** (*yay*-tsuh; boiled eggs) only in reference to boiled eggs rather than fried or scrambled eggs, which are **yaichnitsa** (ee-*eesh*-nee-tsuh).

Let's do dinner (not lunch)

Obyed (ah-*byet*; dinner) is the main meal of the day and it's usually eaten as a midday meal between 1 p.m. and 3 p.m.

Don't make the common mistake of calling your evening meal **obyed,** because this may cause misunderstanding. **Obyed** is, in fact, your midday meal. What speakers of English call "lunch" doesn't have an equivalent in Russian.

For their midday meal, Russians enjoy a four-course meal consisting of **zakuski** (zuh-*koos*-kee; appetizers), **sup** (soop; soup), **vtoroye** (ftah-*roh*-ye; the second or main course), and **dyesyert** (dee-*syert*; dessert), also called **tryet'ye** (*trye*-t'ee; third course).

The most popular Russian **zakuski** are:

- ✔ **baklazhannaya ikra** (buh-klah-*zhah*-nuh-ye eek-*rah*; eggplant caviar)

- ✔ **kapustnyj salat** (kah-*poost*-nihy suh-*laht*; cabbage salad)

- ✔ **salat iz ogurtsov i pomidorov** (suh-*laht* iz ah-goor-*tsohf* ee puh-mee-*doh*-ruhf; salad made of tomatoes and cucumbers)

- ✔ **salat olivye** (suh-*laht* uh-lee-*v'ye*; meat salad)

- ✔ **studyen'** (*stoo*-deen'; beef in aspic)

- ✔ **syelyodka** (see-*lyot*-kuh; salt herring)

- ✔ **vinyegryet** (vee-nee-*gryet*; mixed vegetable salad made with beets, carrots, and pickle)

- ✔ **vyetchina s goroshkom** (veet-chee-*nah* s gah-*rohsh*-kuhm; ham with peas)

After **zakuski** comes the **sup.** You have many different kinds to choose from:

- ✔ **borsh'** (bohrsh'; beet root soup)

- ✔ **bul'yon** (bool'-*yon*; broth)

- ✔ **kurinyj sup** (koo-*ree*-nihy soop; chicken soup)

- ✔ **molochnyj sup** (mah-*lohch*-nihy soop; milk soup)

- ✔ **sh'i** (sh'ee; cabbage soup)

- ✔ **ukha** (oo-*khah*; fish soup)

After the **sup** comes the main course, usually called **vtoroye** (ftah-*roh*-ee; *Literally:* second course). Here are some typical Russian favorites:

- ✔ **bifshtyeks** (beef-*shtehks*; beefsteak)

- ✔ **bifstroganov** (behf-*stroh*-guh-nuhf; beef Stroganoff)

- ✔ **gamburgyer** (gahm-*boor*-geer; hamburger) Russians are still getting used to this one, but they do prefer **kotlyety** to **gamburgyery;** old habits die hard

- ✔ **golubtsy** (guh-loop-*tsih*; stuffed cabbage rolls)

- ✔ **griby** (gree-*bih*; mushrooms)

- ✔ **kotlyety** (kaht-*lye*-tih; ground meat patties)

- ✔ **kotlyety s kartoshkoj** (kaht-*lye*-tih s kuhr-*tohsh*-kuhy; meat patty with potatoes)

- ✔ **kuritsa** (*koo*-ree-tsuh; chicken)

- ✔ **makarony** (muh-kuh-*roh*-nih; pasta)

- ✔ **pitsa** (*pee*-tsuh; pizza) This one is a relative novelty in Russian cuisine.

- ✔ **pyechyen'** (*pye*-cheen'; liver)

- ✔ **ryba** (*rih*-buh; fish)

- ✔ **schnitzyel'** (*shnee*-tsehl'; schnitzel)

- ✔ **sosiski** (sah-*sees*-kee; frankfurters)

- ✔ **zharkoye** (zhuhr-*koh*-ee; any meat cooked in oven)

The main course is usually served with **kartoshka** (kuhr-*tohsh*-kuh; potatoes), **makarony** (muh-kuh-*roh*-nih; pasta), and **ris** (rees; rice), and it's always served with **khlyeb** (khlep; bread).

After the main course comes **dyesyert** (dee-*syert*; dessert), or **tryet'ye** (*trye*-t'ee; third course). This course usually consists of some kind of **tort** (tohrt; cake) or a sweet drink called **kompot** (kahm-*poht*; compote) or **kisyel'** (kee-*syel'*; drink made of fruit and starch). Another common dessert favorite is **morozhenoye** (mah-*roh*-zhih-nuh-ee; ice-cream).

For those who insist on Western-style dessert, you can find **pyechyen'ye** (pee-*chyen'*-ee; cookies), **pirog** (pee-*rohk*; pie), and **tort** (tohrt; cake).

Some typical beverages that Russians drink in the middle of the day are **sok** (sohk; juice), **chaj** (chahy; tea), **kofye** (*koh*-fye; coffee), and **voda** (vah-*dah*; water), although the latter doesn't enjoy as much popularity as it does in the U.S., for example.

A simple supper

The last meal of the day is called **uzhin** (*oo*-zhihn; supper), and it's usually eaten with the family around the kitchen or dining room table. Just as with **obyed** (dinner; see the previous section), soup and a main course are often served for **uzhin. Butyerbrody** (boo-tehr-*broh*-dih; open-sided sandwiches) may also be served, and several cups of **chaj** (chahy; tea) often conclude the evening meal. Some other Russian supper favorites include:

- ✔ **blinchiki** (*bleen*-chee-kee; crepes)
- ✔ **pyel'myeni** (peel'-*mye*-nee; Russian ravioli)
- ✔ **syrniki** (*sihr*-nee-kee; patties made of cottage cheese)
- ✔ **tvorog so smyetanoj** (*tvoh*-ruhk suh smee-*tah*-nuhy; cottage cheese with sour cream)

Russians believe that breakfast, the most important meal of the day, should be plentiful, while supper should be light. Russian folk wisdom says: "Eat your breakfast yourself, share your dinner with a friend, give your supper to your enemy." Gosh, with enemies like that, who needs friends? As for supper-time beverages, **chaj** (chahy; tea) is certainly the most popular drink. A very healthy habit is having a glass of **kyefir** (kee-*feer*; buttermilk) before going to bed. Contrary to Westerners' beliefs, Russians don't drink alcoholic drinks with supper unless it's a very special occasion.

Talkin' the Talk

Syeryozha came home early from school because he has a stomachache. His mother is concerned that it may be food poisoning.

Syeryozha's mother:	**Syeryozha, pochyemu ty tak rano prishyol iz shkoly? Chto sluchilos'?** see-*ryo*-zhuh, puh-chee-*moo* tih tahk *rah*-nuh pree-*shohl* ees *shkoh*-lih? shtoh sloo-*chee*-luhs'? Syeryozha, why did you come from school so early? What happened?
Syeryozha:	**Mama, u myenya bolit zhivot.** *mah*-muh, oo mee-*nya* bah-*leet* zhih-*voht*. Mom, I have a stomachache.
Syeryozha's mother:	**Zhivot? Chto ty syegodnya yel na zavtrak?**

zhih-*voht*? shtoh tih see-*vohd*-nye yel
nuh *zahf*-truhk?
Stomachache? What did you have for
breakfast today?

| Syeryozha: | **Ya yel kashu i pil moloko.**
ya yel *kah*-shoo ee peel muh-lah-*koh*.
I had hot cereal and drank milk. |
|---|---|

| Syeryozha's mother: | **A chto ty yel v shkolye na obyed?**
uh shtoh tih yel f *shkoh*-lee nuh
ah-*byet*?
And what did you eat for lunch at school? |
|---|---|

| Syeryozha: | **Na obyed ya yel salat, kotlyety s kar-toshkoj i pil kisyel'.**
nuh ah-*byet* ya yel suh-*laht*, kaht-*lye*-tih s kahr-*tohsh*-kuhy ee peel kee-*syel'*.
For lunch I had salad, meat patty with potatoes, and drank kissel. |
|---|---|

| Syeryozha's mother: | **A chto tih yel na pyervoye?**
uh shtoh tih yel nuh *pyer*-vuh-ee?
And what did you eat for the first course? |
|---|---|

| Syeryozha: | **Ya, nichyego nye yel. Ya nye khotyel sup.**
ya nee-chee-*voh* nee yel. ya nee khah-*tyel* soop.
I did not eat anything. I did not want to eat soup. |
|---|---|

| Syeryozha's mother: | **Syeryozha, ty dolzhyen yest' sup kazhdyj dyen'. Mozhyet byt' u tyebya bolit zhivot, potomu chto ty nye yesh' sup. Ty khochyesh yest'?**
see-*ryo*-zhuh, tih *dohl*-zhihn yest' soop *kahzh*-dihy dyen'. *moh*-zhiht biht' oo tee-bya bah-*leet* zhih-*voht,* puh-tah-*moosh*-tuh tih nee yesh' soop. tih *khoh*-cheesh yest'?
Syeryozha, you have to eat soup every day. Maybe you have a stomachache because you don't eat soup. Are you hungry? |
|---|---|

| Syeryozha: | **Nyet, ya nye khochu yest' sup. Ya khochu pit'.**
nyet, ya nee khah-*choo* yest' soop. ya khah-*choo* peet'.
No, I don't want soup. I'm thirsty. |
|---|---|

Syeryozha's mother:	**Chto ty khochyesh' pit'? Ty khochyesh' chaj?**
	shtoh tih *khoh*-cheesh' peet'? tih *khoh*-cheesh' chahy?
	What do you want to drink? Do you want tea?

Syeryozha:	**Da, khochu.**
	dah khah-*choo.*
	Yes, I do.

Syeryozha's mother:	**Khorosho, syejchas ya sdyelayu chaj.**
	khuh-rah-*shoh*, see-*chahs* ya *sdye*-luh-yu chahy.
	Okay. I'll make tea.

Words to Know

Chto sluchilos'?	shtoh sloo-<u>chee</u>-luhs'	What happened?
U myenya bolit zhivot.	oo mee-nya bah-<u>leet</u> zhih-<u>voht</u>	I have a stomachache.
Iz shkoly	ees <u>shkoh</u>-lih	From school
Chto ty yel?	shtoh tih yel	What did you eat?
Na zavtrak	nuh <u>zahf</u>-truhk	For breakfast
Na obyed	nuh ah-<u>byet</u>	For lunch
Na pyervoye	nuh <u>pyer</u>-vuh-ee	For the main course
Ya nichyego nye yel.	ya nee-chee-<u>voh</u> nee yel	I didn't eat anything.
Mozhyet byt'	<u>moh</u>-zhiht biht'	Maybe
Potomu chto	puh-tah-<u>moo</u>-shtuh	Because
Chto ty khochyesh' pit'?	shtoh tih <u>khoh</u>-cheesh' peet'?	What do you want to drink?

Going Out for Groceries

If you want to make a quick trip to the **produktovyyj magazin** (pruh-dook-*toh*-vihy muh-guh-*zeen*; grocery store) or spend a leisurely day at the Russian **rynok** (*rih*-nuhk; market), you have to know how to buy food products in Russian. In the following sections, we tell you all the different things you can buy.

Picking out produce

Buying produce at a farmer's market is very common. Russians are convinced that produce is much fresher there than in regular grocery stores. Table 5-3 has a list of some of the more popular produce items you may want to buy:

Table 5-3	Produce	
Russian	*Pronunciation*	*Translation*
yabloki	*ya*-bluh-kee	Apple
svyokla	*svyok*-luh	Beets
chyernika	cheer-*nee*-kuh	Blueberry
kapusta	kuh-*poos*-tuh	Cabbage
morkov'	mahr-*kohf'*	Carrots
vishnya	*veesh*-nye	Cherry
ogurtsy	uh-goor-*tsih*	Cucumber
balkazhany	buhk-luh-*zhah*-nih	Eggplant
chyesnok	chees-*nohk*	Garlic
vinograd	vee-nah-*grahd*	Grape
luk	look	Onion
grushi	*groo*-shih	Pears
gorokh	guh-*rohkh*	Peas
pyeryets	*pye*-reets	Pepper
ryediska	ree-*dees*-kuh	Radish
malina	muh-*lee*-nuh	Raspberry
klubnika	kloob-*nee*-kuh	Strawberry

Russian	Pronunciation	Translation
pomidory	puh-mee-*doh*-rih	Tomato
arbuz	uhr-*boos*	Watermelon

Surveying other grocery items

Chances are, most of the food items you want to buy can be found at the **rynok,** but you can also buy the food products you need at **produktovyye magaziny** (pruh-dook-*toh*-vih-ee muh-gah-*zee*-nih; grocery stores). We list some of the most common food items in Table 5-4.

Table 5-4	Common Food Items	
Russian	**Pronunciation**	**Translation**
myaso	*mya*-suh	Meat
govyadina	gah-*vya*-dee-nuh	Beef
farsh	fahrsh	Ground beef
kuritsa	*koo*-ree-tsuh	Chicken
ryba	*rih*-buh	Fish
vyetchina	veet-chee-*nah*	Ham
baranina	buh-*rah*-nee-nuh	Lamb
svinina	svee-*nee*-nuh	Pork
kolbasa	kuhl-buh-*sah*	Sausage
maslo	*mahs*-luh	Butter
kyefir	kee-*feer*	Buttermilk
syr	sihr	Cheese
yajtsa	*yahy*-tsuh	Eggs
moloko	muh-lah-*koh*	Milk
smyetana	smee-*tah*-nuh	Sour cream
jogurt	*yo*-goort	Yogurt
bubliki	*boob*-lee-kee	Bagels

(continued)

Table 5-4 (continued)

Russian	Pronunciation	Translation
khlyeb	khlyep	Bread
chyornyj khlyeb	*chyor*-nihy khlyep	Dark bread
bulka	*bool*-kuh	White bread
kofye	*koh*-fye	Coffee
sok	sohk	Juice
chaj	chahy	Tea
voda	vah-*dah*	Water
muka	moo-*kah*	Flour
majonyez	muh-ee-*nehs*	Mayonnaise
gorchitsa	gahr-*chee*-tsuh	Mustard
makarony	muh-kuh-*roh*-nih	Pasta
pyeryets	*pye*-reets	Pepper
ris	rees	Rice
sol'	sohl'	Salt
sakhar	*sah*-khuhr	Sugar
podsolnechnoye maslo	paht-*sohl*-neech-nuh-ee *mahs*-luh	Sunflower oil

Eating Out with Ease

Eating out at Russian restaurants and cafes can be a lot of fun, especially if you know Russian. In the following sections, we go over the different kinds of restaurants you can go to, how to reserve your table, the right way to order a meal, and how to pay your bill.

Deciding on a place to eat

You can find lots of different places to eat out, Russian-style, depending on your mood and budget. If you're in the mood for a night of culinary delights, with a full eight-course meal, lots of drinks, and live music, check out a fancy Russian **ryestoran** (ree-stah-*rahn*; restaurant). Be sure you have a healthy budget and are well-rested, because prices are steep and you won't be coming home 'til the wee hours of the morning!

A more affordable everyday option is a **kafye** (kuh-*feh*; café), which can serve anything from coffee and ice-cream, to pancakes, to pies. Cafés are usually privately owned and have such interesting names (often unrelated to food) that if you pass one of them on the street, you may not even recognize it as a place to eat! But if you follow that delicious smell under your nose, you may wind up at one of these delightful little places:

✔ **blinnaya** (*blee*-nuh-ye; café that serves pancakes)

✔ **chyeburyechnya** (chee-boo-*ryech*-nuh-ye; café that serves meat pies)

✔ **kafye-morozhenoye** (kuh-*feh* mah-*roh*-zhih-nuh-ee; ice-cream parlor)

✔ **pirozhkovya** (pee-rahsh-*koh*-vuh-ye; café that serves small pies)

✔ **pyel'myennya** (*peel'*-myen-nuh-ye; place that serves Russian ravioli)

✔ **pyshyechnaya** (*pih*-shihch-nuh-ye; donut shop)

✔ **stolovaya** (stah-*loh*-vuh-ye; dining room)

✔ **zakusochnaya** (zuh-*koo*-suhch-nuh-ye; snack bar)

Making reservations on the phone

After you decide which restaurant to go to, pick up the phone and make a reservation. And don't worry. The person answering the phone has probably dealt quite often with customers whose Russian isn't perfect. He or she will be happy to help you:

✔ If you're a man, say, **Ya khotyel by zakazat' stolik na syegodnya.** (ya khah-*tyel* bih zuh-kuh-*zaht'* stoh-leek nuh see-*vohd*-nye; I'd like to reserve a table for tonight.)

✔ If you're a woman, say, **Ya khotyela by zakazat' stolik na syegodnya.** (ya khah-*tye*-luh bih zuh-kuh-*zaht'* stoh-leek nuh see-*vohd*-nye; I'd like to reserve a table for tonight.)

When you say **ya khotyel(a) by,** you're using Russian subjunctive mood. It's one of the easiest things in Russian grammar. You just use the past tense of the verb + the word **by.** (For more on forming past tense, see Chapter 2.) Instead of saying the word **stol** (stohl; table), Russians like to use the diminutive form **stolik** (*stoh*-leek; *Literally:* little table) when making restaurant reservations.

If you want to reserve a table for tomorrow, just replace the phrase **na syegodnya** (nuh see-*vohd*-nye; for today) with the phrase **na zavtra** (nuh *zahf*-truh; for tomorrow). If you want to specify a day of the week, use the same preposition **na** + the day of the week in accusative case. (See Chapter 7 for the days of the week.) So if you want to make a reservation for Saturday and you're a male, you say **Ya khotyel by zakazat' stolik na subbotu.** (ya khah-*tyel* bih zuh-kuh-*zaht'* stoh-leek nuh soo-*boh*-too; I'd like to reserve a table for Saturday.)

What you'll probably hear in response is **Na skol'ko chyelovyek?** (nuh *skohl'*-kuh chee-luh-*vyek*?; For how many people?) To answer this question, decide (quickly, Russians are very impatient on the phone!) how many people are accompanying you, add yourself, and after these quick calculations say one of these phrases:

- **na dvoikh** (nuh dvah-*eekh*; for two)
- **na troikh** (nuh trah-*eekh*; for three)
- **na chyetvyerykh** (nuh cheet-vee-*rihkh*; for four)
- **na odnogo** (nuh uhd-nah-*voh*; for one person)

The person on the phone will probably want to know by what time the table should be ready for you, and he or she will ask **Na kakoye vryemya?** (nuh kah-*koh*-ee *vrye*-mye; For what time?) To answer this question, use the preposition **na** (nah; for) + the time when you're planning to arrive:

- **na syem' chasov** (nuh syem' chah-*sohf*; for 7 o'clock)
- **na vosyem' chasov** (nuh *voh*-seem' chah-*sohf*; for 8 o'clock)

(For more info on specifying the time, see Chapter 7.) Also be prepared to give your name, which you do by simply stating it.

Don't expect to be asked whether you want to sit in the smoking or non-smoking section. Too many people in Russia smoke (especially when drinking alcoholic beverages) and smokers rule. Even those people who don't generally smoke tend to smoke in restaurants.

The art of ordering a meal

After you arrive at the restaurant and are seated by **myetrdotyel'** (mehtr-dah-*tyel*; maitre d'), the **ofitsiant** (uh-fee-tsih-*ahnt*; waiter) or **ofitsiantka** (uh-fee-tsih-*ahnt*-kuh; waitress) will bring you a **myenyu** (mee-*nyu*; menu). In a nice restaurant, all the dishes in the menu are usually in English as well as Russian.

When you open the menu, you'll notice it's divided into several subsections, which is how items are usually eaten and ordered in a Russian restaurant:

- **zakuski** (zuh-*koos*-kee; appetizers)
- **supy** (soo-*pih*; soups)
- **goryachiye blyuda** (gah-*rya*-chee-ee *blyu*-duh; main dishes)
- **sladkiye blyuda** (*slaht*-kee-ee *blyu*-duh; dessert)
- **alkogol'nye napitki** (ahl-kah-*gohl'*-nih-ee nuh-*peet*-kee; alcoholic drinks)
- **bezalkogol'niye napitki** (beez-uhl-kah-*gohl'*-nih-ee nuh-*peet*-kee; nonalcoholic beverages)

When the waiter asks you **Chto vy budyetye zakazyvat'?** (shtoh vih *boo*-dee-tee zuh-*kah*-zih-vuht'; What would you like to order?), just say **Ya budu** + the name of the item you're ordering in the accusative case. (On forming the accusative, see Chapter 2.) For example, you may say something like: **Ya budu kotlyetu s kartofyelyem i salat iz pomidorov.** (ya *boo*-doo kaht-*lye*-tih s kahr-*toh*-fee-leem ee suh-*laht* ees puh-mee-*doh*-ruhf; I'll have meat patty with potatoes and tomato salad.)

The waiter may also ask you specifically **Chto vy budyetye pit'?** (shtoh vih *boo*-dee-tee peet'; What would you like to drink?) To answer, you simply say **Ya budu** (ya *boo*-doo; I will have) + the name of the drink(s) you want in the accusative case. So, if at dinner you're extremely thirsty (and aren't the designated driver), you may say **Ya budu vodku i sok i butylku vina.** (ya *boo*-doo *voht*-koo ee sohk ee boo-*tihl*-koo vee-*nah*; I'll have vodka and juice and a bottle of wine.) For details on the accusative case, see Chapter 2.

Waiters and waitresses don't take your drink orders before you start ordering meals; expect to be asked what you want to drink at the end of your order. Moreover, when the waiter asks this question, he's asking about alcoholic beverages. Water or soda with your meal isn't as common as it is in the West. As a matter of fact, many Russians believe that one shouldn't chase food with water or any other beverage because it interferes with food digestion.

When you say **Ya budu** + the food or drink item, what you're really saying is **Ya budu yest'** . . . (ya *boo*-doo yest'; I will eat . . .) or **Ya budu pit'** . . . (ya *boo*-doo peet'; I will drink . . .) The verbs **yest'** (yest'; to eat) and **pit'** (peet'; to drink) force the noun coming after them into the accusative case, because it's a direct object. When you order, you skip the verbs **yest'** and **pit',** but they're implied. (On uses of the accusative case, see Chapter 2.)

When you're done ordering, you should say **Vsyo!** (fsyo; That's it!) Otherwise, the waiter will keep standing next to you, waiting for you to order more.

Having handy phrases for the wait staff

In this section, we include some helpful phrases you may want to use when ordering or receiving a meal or drinks.

If you're a vegetarian, the best way to ask about vegetarian dishes is to say: **Kakiye u vas yest' vyegyetarianskiye blyuda?** (kuh-*kee*-ee oo vahs yest' vee-gee-tuh-ree-*ahns*-kee-ee *blyu*-duh; What vegetarian dishes do you have?) Note, however, that being a vegetarian in Russia is still seen as a very bizarre habit.

Imagine that you're a vegetarian and you're sitting in a restaurant waiting for the vegetarian dish you ordered. Instead, the waiter puts in front of you a steaming, juicy beefsteak with potatoes. What do you do? Before that waiter is gone, say **Ya eto nye zakazyval/zakazyvala!** (ya *eh*-tuh nee zuh-*kah*-zih-vuhl/zuh-*kah*-zih-vuh-luh; I did not order this!) (Use **zakazyval** if you're a man, and **zakazyvala** if you're a woman.)

If you feel like asking a waiter what dish he or she recommends or what specialties the restaurant has, be cautioned that your questions may puzzle your Russian server. Only waiters in very nice Moscow restaurants that are trying to emulate their Western counterparts are prepared to answer them. Here is the question you may want to attempt: **A chto vy ryekomyenduyetye?** (uh shtoh vih ree-kuh-meen-*doo*-ee-tee; What would you recommend?)

If you suddenly recall something you meant to include in your order or decide that you want something else, try getting the attention of your waiter (who is rushing by you) with a phrase like **Izvinitye, vy nye mogli by prinyesti vodu?** (eez-vee-*nee*-tee vih nee mahg-*lee* bih pree-nees-*tee voh*-doo; Excuse me, could you bring water?)

Other common problems you may come across can be resolved just by stating some facts about the meal that alert the waiter and make him take some counter-measures. For example, you may say:

- **Eto blyudo ochyen' kholodnoye.** (*eh*-tuh *blyu*-duh *oh*-cheen' khah-*lohd*-nuh-ye; This dish is very cold.)

- **Eto blyudo ochyen' solyonoye.** (*eh*-tuh *blyu*-duh *oh*-cheen' sah-*lyo*-nuh-ye; This dish is too salty.)

- **Eto blyudo ochyen' ostroye.** (*eh*-tuh *blyu*-duh *oh*-cheen' *ohs*-truh-ye; This dish is too spicy.)

If, on the other hand, you enjoyed your meal and service, be sure to say **Vsyo bylo ochyen' vkusno!** (vsyo *bih*-luh *oh*-cheen' *fkoos*-nuh; Everything was very tasty!) and/or **Spasibo za otlichnyj syervis!** (spuh-*see*-buh zah aht-*leech*-nihy *syer*-vees; Thank you for the excellent service!)

Receiving and paying the bill

When it comes time to ask for the bill, don't expect the waiter to bring it automatically. When the waiter is in the vicinity, try to attract his attention either by waving or smiling to him or just saying (loudly, if necessary; Russians are very direct!) **Rasschitajtye nas pozhalujsta!** (ruh-shee-*tahy*-tee nahs pah-*zhahl*-stuh; Check please!)

Asking for several separate checks isn't common in Russia. Waiters hate doing it even in Russian restaurants abroad. So ask for a check and then prepare to divide the amount by the number of eaters. If you're buying a meal for somebody or everybody at the table, announce it to the company or person you're inviting by saying: **Ya zaplachu** (ya zuh-pluh-*choo*; I will pay) or **Ya plachu** (ya pluh-*choo*; I am paying) or **Ya ugosh'yayu** (ya-oo-gah-*sh'a*-yu; *Literally:* My treat).

As in most restaurants in the world, checks aren't accepted in Russia. Before paying with a credit card, we recommend that you ask: **Vy prinimayetye kryeditnyye kartochki?** (vih pree-nee-*mah*-ee-tee kree-*deet*-nih-ee *kahr*-tuhch-kee; Do you take credit cards?)

If the waiter returns before you ask him for the bill, he may tell you how much you owe by saying **S vas . . .** (s vahs; you owe, *Literally:* from you is due . . .) If your meal costs 200 rubles 41 kopecks, the waiter will say **S vas dvyesti rublyej sorok odna kopyejka.** (s vahs *dvyes-tee*-roob-*lyey* soh-ruhk ahd-*nah* kah-*pyey*-kuh; You owe two hundred rubles and forty-one kopeks.) See Chapter 14 for more details about money.

Talkin' the Talk

Jack and his Russian fiancée, Natasha, are in a nice restaurant in downtown Moscow. They have just been seated at the table and are now ordering the meal.

Ofitsiant: (waiter)	Gotovy? Chto vy budyetye zakazyvat'? gah-*toh*-vih? shtoh vih *boo*-dee-tee zuh-*kah*-zih-vuht'? Ready? What will you be ordering?
Jack:	Na zakusku, ya budu kholodnyj yazyk s goroshkom i butyerbrod s ikroj. I shashlyk. Nuh zuh-*koos*-koo, ya *boo*-doo khah-*lohd*-nihy ee-zihk s gah-*rohsh*-kuhm ee boo-tehr-*broht* s eek-*rohy*. ee shuhsh-*lihk*. For the appetizer I will have tongue with peas and caviar sandwich. And roasted mutton.
Ofitsiant:	Chto vy budyetye pit'? shtoh vih *boo*-dee-tee peet'? What will you have to drink?
Jack:	Kakoye u vas yest' khoroshyeye vino? kuh-*koh*-ee oo vahs yest' khah-*roh*-sheh-ee vee-*noh*? What good wine do you have?
Ofitsiant:	Yest' risling, yest' khoroshyeye armyanskoye vino. yest' *rees*-leenk, yest' khah-*roh*-sheh-ee uhr-*myan*-skuh-ee vee-*noh*. We have Riesling, we have a nice Armenian wine.

Jack:	**Khorosho, prinyesitye butylku armyanskogo vina.**
	khuh-rah-*shoh*, pree-nee-*see*-tee boo-*tihl*-koo uhr-*myan*-skuh-vuh vee-*nah*.
	Okay. Bring a bottle of Armenian wine.
Ofitsiant:	**Yesh'o chto-nibud' budyetye pit'?**
	ee-*sh'yo* shtoh-nee-bood' boo-dee-tye peet'?
	What else are you going to drink?
Jack:	**I butylku minyeral'noj vody. Vsyo. Natasha, chto ty budyesh'?**
	ee boo-*tihl*-koo mee-nee-*rahl'* -nuhy vah-*dih*. fsyo. nah-*tah*-shuh, shtoh tih *boo*-deesh'?
	And a bottle of mineral water. That's it. Natasha, what will you have?
Natasha:	**Ya budu syevryugu i kotlyetu po-kiyevski.**
	ya *boo*-doo seev-*ryu*-goo ee kaht-*lye*-too puh kee-eef-skee.
	I'll have sturgeon and chicken a la Kiev.
Ofitsiant:	**Vsyo?**
	fsyo?
	That's it?
Natasha:	**Vsyo.**
	fsyo.
	That's it.
Ofitsiant:	**Vy khotitye chto-nibud' na dyesyert?**
	vih khah-*tee*-tee *shtoh*-nee-bood' nuh dee-*syert*?
	Do you want anything for dessert?
Natasha:	**Nyet, spasibo. Tol'ko kofye.**
	nyet, spa-*see*-buh. *tohl'*-kuh *koh*-fee.
	No, thank you. Only coffee.

Words to Know

Gotovy?	gah-<u>toh</u>-vih	Are you ready (to order)?
na zakusku	nuh zah-<u>koos</u>-koo	as an appetizer
Chto vy budyetye pit'?	shtoh vih <u>boo</u>-dee-tee peet'	What will you drink?
Kakoye u vas yest' khoroshyeye vino?	kuh-<u>koh</u>-ee oo vahs yest' khah-<u>roh</u>-sheh-ee vee-<u>noh</u>	What good wine do you have?
Yest' risling.	yest' <u>rees</u>-link	We have Riesling.
Chto tih budyesh'?	shtoh tih <u>boo</u>-deesh'	What will you have?
Vy khotitye chto-nibud' na dyesyert?	vih khah-<u>tee</u>-tee <u>shtoh</u>-nee-bood' nuh dee-<u>syert</u>	Do you want anything for dessert?
tol'ko	<u>tohl</u>'-kuh	only

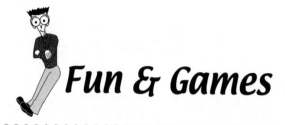

Fun & Games

Which of the following two dishes would you most likely eat for breakfast in Russia? See Appendix C for the correct answers.

1. a. **yaichnitsa** b. **ukha**

2. a. **zharkoye** b. **butyerbrod s kolbasoj**

3. a. **butyerbrod s syrom** b. **kotlyeta**

4. a. **kotlyetu s kartofyelyem** b. **kasha**

5. a. **varyen'ye** b. **kapustnyj salat**

Which of the following phrases would you probably use or hear while making a restaurant reservation? See Appendix C for the correct answers.

1. **Ya khotyel by zakazat' stolik na subbotu.**

2. **Mnye, pozhalujsta, butylku moloka.**

3. **Na dvoikh.**

4. **Skol'ko chyelovyek?**

5. **Na vosyem' chasov.**

6. **Ya khochu yest'.**

7. **Ya budu kotlyetu s kartofyelyem.**

8. **Ya khotyela by zakazat' stolik na syegodnya.**

9. **Na kakoye vryemya?**

10. **Yest' risling.**

Chapter 6

Shopping Made Easy

In This Chapter

▶ Finding out where and how to shop

▶ Looking for clothes

▶ Selecting the items you want

▶ Paying the bill

▶ Checking out great Russian souvenirs to buy

Shopping is a big part of Russian life. During the Soviet era, when getting even basic things like toothpaste was a major challenge, Russians felt deprived and developed a strong appreciation for any nice things they could buy. As a result, Russians love to hunt for nice, mostly Western-made, goods. Buying anything new, whether it's a stereo, a sofa, or a coat, is a pleasant experience and an important event. So as an American (or other Westerner) shopping in Russian stores, you should feel right at home!

In this chapter, we tell you about different kinds of stores, and show you how to call for store hours and get assistance when you're there. We also instruct you in the art of clothes-shopping, Russian-style. We show you how to get the right color and size, how to ask to try things on, and what to say when you want to compare different items. You also find out how to pay for your things in a Russian store. Plus we give you suggestions about some cool souvenirs to get while you're shopping. Now, let's go shopping!

Shop 'Til You Drop: Where and How to Buy Things the Russian Way

Stores where you can buy anything (other than food) can be divided into two categories: **univyermagi** (oo-nee-veer-*mah*-gee; department stores), most of which are located in the downtown of large cities, and smaller specialized **magaziny** (muh-guh-*zee*-nih; stores), which may specialize in anything from tableware to TVs.

In the following section, you find out about many different kinds of stores and what's sold in them. You also discover how to inquire about store hours, how to find the specific store or department you're looking for, and how to ask for assistance when you're there.

Looking at different types of stores and departments

More and more, fancy specialty stores are popping up throughout Russia and Russian neighborhoods in the U.S. Many of these stores have unique names, but many (especially in Russia) are still simply called by the name of the item they sell. This naming convention is a throwback to the Soviet era, when no concept of marketing products existed. A shoe store, for instance, may simply be called **obuv'** (*oh*-boof'; *Literally:* footwear), a toy store **igrushki** (eeg-*roosh*-kee; *Literally:* toys), and a book store **knigi** (*knee*-gee; *Literally:* books). The names of stores also may denote the name of an **otdyel** (aht-*dyel*; department) within an **univyermag** (oo-nee-veer-*mahk*; department store), where a specific item is sold.

Here's a list of some other stores and departments:

- **antikvarnyj magazin** (uhn-tee-*kvahr*-nihy muh-guh-*zeen*; antique store)
- **aptyeka** (uhp-*tye*-kuh; pharmacy)
- **byel'yo** (beel'-*yo*; intimate apparel)
- **dyetskaya odyezhda** (*dyet*-skuh-ye ah-*dyezh*-duh; children's apparel)
- **elyektrotovary** (eh-*lyek*-truh-tah-*vah*-rih; electrical goods)
- **fototovary** (*foh*-tuh-tah-*vah*-rih; photography store)
- **galantyeryeya** (guh-luhn-tee-*rye*-ye; haberdashery)
- **gazyehnyj kiosk** (guh-*zyet*-nihy kee-*ohsk*; newsstand)
- **golovnyye ubory** (guh-lahv-*nih*-ee oo-*boh*-rih; hats)
- **kantsyelyarskiye tovary** (kuhn-tsih-*lyar*-skee-ee tah-*vah*-rih; stationery products)
- **khozyajstvyennyj magazin** (khah-*zyay*-stvee-nihy muh-guh-*zeen*; household goods, hardware store)
- **komissionnyj magazin** (kuh-mee-see-*ohn*-nihy muh-guh-*zeen*; second-hand store)
- **kosmyetika** (kahs-*mye*-tee-kuh; makeup)
- **muzhskaya odyezhda** (moosh-skah-ye ah-*dyezh*-duh; men's apparel)

- **muzykal'nyye instrumyenty** (moo-zih-*kahl'*-nih-ee een-stroo-*myen*-tih; music store)

- **odyezhda** (ah-*dyezh*-duh; clothing store)

- **parfumyeriya** (puhr-fyu-*mye*-ree-ye; perfume)

- **posuda** (pah-*soo*-duh; tableware)

- **sportivnyye tovary** (spahr-*teev*-nih-ee tah-*vah*-rih; sports store)

- **suvyeniry** (soo-vee-*nee*-rih; souvenirs)

- **tkani** (*tkah*-nee; fabric)

- **tsvyety** (tsvee-*tih*; flowers)

- **vyerkhnyaya odyezhda** (*vyerkh*-nye-ye ah-*dyezh*-duh; outerwear store)

- **yuvyelirnyye tovary** (yu-vee-*leer*-nih-ee tah-*vah*-rih; jewelry store)

- **zhyenskaya odyezhda** (*zhehn*-skuh-ye ah-*dyezh*-duh; women's apparel)

Calling for store hours

The easiest way to find out whether a Russian store is open is to go there and look for a sign hanging in the door or window with one of these two words on it: **Otkryto** (aht-*krih*-tuh; Open) or **Zakryto** (zuh-*krit*-tuh; Closed). The next best way is just to call. If nobody answers, it probably means they're closed. Problem solved! But in case someone does answer, you may want to ask **Magazin otkryt?** (muh-guh-*zeen* aht-*kriht*; Is the store open?) or **Do kakogo chasa otkryt magazin?** (duh kuh-*koh*-vuh *chah*-suh aht-*kriht* muh-guh-*zeen*; 'Til what time is the store open?)

If you want to inquire whether the store is open on a particular day, you say, for example, **V voskryesyen'ye magazin otrkryt?** (v vuhs-kree-*syen'*-ee muh-guh-*zeen* aht-*kriht*; Is the store open on Sunday?) For more on talking about days of the week, see Chapter 7.

In Russian, the simplest way to say that a store (or window, door, or anything) is open or closed is by using a form of the word **otkryt** (aht-*kriht*; open) or **zakryt** (zuh-*kriht*; closed). If the noun you're referring to is masculine, just use this form. If it's feminine, add **-a** to each of these words, as in **Dvyer' otkryta.** (dvyer' aht-*krih*-tuh; The door is open.) If the noun is neuter, you add **-o**, as in **Okno zakryto.** (ahk-*noh* zuh-*krih*-tuh; The window is closed.) And if the noun is plural, you add **-y**, as in **Vsye magaziny otkryty syegodnya.** (fsye muh-guh-*zee*-nih aht-*krih*-tih see-*vohd*-nye; The stores are all open today.) (See Chapter 2 for more about the gender of nouns.)

Some other ways to ask about store hours include the following:

- ✔ **Kogda magazin zakryvayetsya?** (kahg-*dah* muh-guh-*zeen* zuh-krih-*vah*-eet-sye; When does the store close?)
- ✔ **Kogda zavtra otkryvayetsya magazin?** (kahg-*dah* zahf-truh uht-krih-*vah*-eet-sye muh-guh-*zeen*; When does the store open tomorrow?)

Otrkyvatsya (uht-krih-*vaht'*-sye; to open) and **zakryvatsya** (zuh-krih-*vaht'*-sye; to close) are called *reflexive verbs*. They don't take direct objects, because their action refers back to the subject of the sentence. So in the question **Kogda magazin zakryvayetsya?** (kahg-*dah* muh-guh-*zeen* zuh-krih-*vah*-eet-sye; When does the store close?), you're literally asking "What time does the store close itself?" That's because your emphasis is on the fact of the store's closing, and not on who's doing it. The infinitive of reflexive verbs usually end in **-sya,** and you need to add **-sya** to all the usual conjugation endings except after the **ya** (ya; I) and **vy** (vih; you; formal and plural) forms, in which case you add **-s'.**

The verb **zakryvayetsya** was formed by adding the reflexive ending **-sya** to the third person singular form, **zakryvayet** (zuh-krih-*vah*-eet; he/she/it closes), of the imperfective verb **zakryvat'** (zuh-krih-*vaht*; to close). (To refresh your memory about verb infinitives and conjugations, see Chapter 2.)

To indicate working hours in a store, Russians often use a form of the verb **rabotat'** (ruh-*boh*-tuht'; to work). When inquiring about store hours, you're likely to hear something like **Da, magazin rabotayet syegodnya do syemi.** (dah muh-guh-*zeen* ruh-*boh*-tuh-eet see-*vohd*-nye duh see-*mee*; Yes, the store is open today until 7, *Literally:* The store works today until 7.) or **Magazin nye rabotayet v voskryesyen'ye.** (muh-guh-*zeen* nee ruh-*boh*-tuh-eet v vuhs-kree-*syen'*-ee; The store isn't open on Sunday, *Literally:* The store doesn't work on Sunday.)

When you call a store or many places of business in Russia, don't expect the person on the line to introduce herself and tell you the name of the place you've called. Instead, what you most likely hear is an abrupt **Allyo!** (uh'-*lyo*; Hello!), **Slushayu!** (*sloo*-shuh-yu; *Literally*: I'm listening!), or simply **Da!** (dah; Yes!) spoken in a low, serious, or even melancholy voice. Also, try to listen very carefully to the information provided, because once the person on the other end has answered your questions, chances are she will hang up right away! See Chapter 9 for more details about speaking on the phone.

Navigating a department store

If you're in a big department store searching for that perfect souvenir, you may want to approach the **spravochnya** (sprah-*vuhch*-nuh-ye; information desk), or anybody who looks like he works there, and ask the question **Gdye**

otdyel suvyenirov? (gdye aht-*dyel* soo-vee-*nee*-ruhf; Where is the souvenir department?) or **Gdye suvyeniry?** (gdye soo-vee-*nee*-rih; Where are souvenirs?) You may also want to inquire about what floor the souvenir department is on. Just ask **Na kakom etazhye otdyel suvyernirov?** (nuh kuh-*kohm* eh-tuh-*zheh* aht-*dyel* soo-vee-*nee*-ruhf; What floor is the souvenir department on?) or simply **Na kakom etazhye suvyeniry?** (nuh kuh-*kohm* eh-tuh-*zheh* soo-vee-*nee*-rih; What floor are souvenirs on?)

Note that when you say **otdyel suvyenirov,** you're literally saying "the department of souvenirs" and you put the word for "souvenirs" in the genitive case. (For more info on case endings for nouns, see Chapter 2.)

After you ask for directions, be prepared to hear something like

- ✔ **na pyervom etazhye** (nuh *pyer*-vuhm eh-tuh-*zheh*; on the first floor)

- ✔ **na vtorom etazhye** (nuh ftah-*rohm* eh-tuh-*zheh*; on the second floor)

- ✔ **na tryetyem etazhye** (nuh *tryet'*-eem eh-tuh-*zheh*; on the third floor)

- ✔ **na etom etazhye napravo/nalyevo** (nuh *eh*-tuhm eh-tuh-*zheh* nuh-*prah*-vuh/nuh-*lye*-vah; on this floor to the right/left)

If you hear something not listed here, don't panic! Just watch the person's arm movements. Russians often like to accompany their direction-giving with big pointing gestures.

The ordinal numerals **pyervyj** (*pyer*-vihy; first), **vtoroj** (ftah-*rohy*; second), and **tryetij** (*trye'*-teey; third) act just like adjectives, which means they must agree in number, gender, and case with the nouns they modify. (For details on adjective-noun agreement, see Chapter 2.) Russian uses the prepositional case after the preposition **na** when indicating what floor something is on. To form the prepositional case of the ordinal numeral **pyervyj,** you treat the numeral as if it were an adjective and replace the masculine adjectival ending **-yj** with **-om,** as we describe in Chapter 2. And that's how you get the phrase **na pyervom etazhye** (nuh *pyer*-vuhm eh-tuh-*zheh*; on the first floor).

Asking for (or declining) assistance

When you want to ask for help in a Russian store, your first challenge is to get somebody's attention. The best way to do this is to turn to any salesperson and say **Izvinitye pozhalujsta!** (eez-vee-*nee*-tee pah-*zhahl*-stuh; Excuse me, please!) If you want a slightly softer approach, you can use the phrase **Bud'tye dobry . . .** (*bood'*-tee dahb-*ryh*; Would you be so kind as to help me, *Literally*: Would you be so kind . . .)

After you say one of these two phrases, you'll probably hear **Da, pozhalujsta?** (dah pah-*zhahl*-stuh; Yes, how can I help?) After that you can politely ask a

question, starting off with the polite phrase, **Skazhitye, pozhalujsta . . .** (skuh-*zhih*-tee pah-*zhahl*-stuh; Would you tell me please . . .) If you're still looking for souvenirs, you can politely say **Skazhitye, pozhalujsta, gdye suvyeniry?** (skuh-*zhih*-tee pah-*zhahl*-stuh gdye soo-vee-*nee*-rih; Could you please tell me where souvenirs are?)

Some other additional shopping-related phrases include the following:

- ✔ **U vas prodayotsya/prodayutsya . . . ?** (oo vahs pruh-duh-*yot*-sye/pruh-duh-*yut*-sye; Do you sell . . . ?) plus the name of the merchandise you're looking for in the nominative case.
- ✔ **U vas yest' . . . ?** (oo vahs yest'; Do you have . . . ?)
- ✔ **Gdye mozhno kupit' . . . ?** (gdye *mohzh*-nuh koo-*peet'*; Where can I buy . . . ?) plus the thing(s) you want to buy in the accusative case.
- ✔ **Pokazhitye, pozhalujsta etot/eto/etu/eti . . .** (puh-kuh-*zhih*-tee pah-*zhahl*-stuh *eh*-tuht/*eh*-tuh/*eh*-too/*eh*-tee; Please show me this/that . . .) plus the item(s) you want to see in the accusative case. (For more on using the demonstrative pronoun **etot,** see "Using demonstrative pronouns" later in this chapter.)

In making your requests or asking questions, try to avoid phrases such as "I am looking for . . ." or "I would like to see . . ." When translated into Russian, these phrases include the first-person pronoun **ya** (I). Using them isn't culturally appropriate, because Russian tends to avoid this word in requests and in most cases requires that you make your requests impersonal.

You won't hear "May I help you?"

You seldom hear the salespeople in a Russian store say **Ya mogu vam pomoch'?** (yah mah-*goo* vahm pah-*mohch'*; May I help you?) For more than 70 years during the Soviet regime, the salesperson rather than the customer was the boss in the stores. As a matter of fact, one of the authors of this book who grew up in Russia heard the question **Ya mogu vam pomoch'?** only once in her lifetime, namely during a recent visit to a major Moscow department store in post-Soviet Russia. She attributes this occurrence to the fact that after years of living in the U.S., she looked more American than Russian, and that made the store assistant approach her with the typical American question "May I help you?",

translated of course into Russian. In most cases you don't have to bother about how you should respond to this question, but just in case you're asked, you can say **Spasibo, ya prosto smotryu.** (spuh-*see*-buh ya *prohs*-tuh smaht-*ryu*; Thanks, I'm just looking.) The good news is that nobody will ever mind your browsing if you don't even plan on buying anything. However, you should know that you'll probably be closely watched either by a **prodavyets** (pruh-duh-*vyets*; salesman), a **prodavsh'itsa** (pruh-duhv-*sh'ee*-tsuh; saleswoman), or an **okhrannik** (ah-*khrah*-neek; security guard), which almost every Russian store has today. But their main concern is not the quality of service but theft prevention!

Talkin' the Talk

 Boris needs to buy new gloves and goes to a big department store. He has a short conversation with the **rabotnik univyermaga** (ruh-*boht*-neek oo-nee-veer *mah*-guh; the employee at the information desk).

Boris:	**Skazhitye, pozhalujsta, gdye mozhno kupit' pyerchatki'?**
	skuh-*zhih*-tee, pah-*zhahl*-stuh, gdye *mohzh*-nuh koo-*peet'* peer-*chaht*-kee?
	Tell me, please, where can I buy gloves?
Rabotnik univermaga:	**V galantyerejnom otdyelye.**
	v guh-luhn-tee-*reyy*-nuhm aht-*dye*-lee.
	In the haberdashery department.
Boris:	**A gdye galantyerejnyj otdyel? Na kakom etazhye?**
	uh gdye guh-luhn-tee-*ryey*-nihy aht-*dyel*? nuh kuh-*kohm* eh-tuh-*zheh*?
	And where is the haberdashery department? On what floor?
Rabotnik univermaga:	**Galantyereya na vtorom etazhe.**
	guh-luhn-tee-*rye*-ye nuh ftah-*rohm* eh-tuh-*zheh*.
	The haberdashery is on the second floor.
Boris:	**Ponyatno. Spasibo. A gdye lyestnitsa ili lift?**
	pah-*nyat*-nuh. spuh-*see*-buh. uh gdye *lyes*-nee-tsuh ee-lee leeft?
	I see. Thank you. And where are stairs or elevator?
Rabotnik univermaga:	**Lyestnitsa napravo, a lift nalyevo.**
	lyes-nee-tsuh nuh-*prah*-vuh, uh leeft nuh-*lye*-vuh.
	The stairs are to the right and the elevator is to the left.

Words to Know

A gdye?	uh gdye	And where is . . . ?
Na kakom etahzhye?	nuh kuh-<u>kohm</u> eh-tuh-<u>zheh</u>	On what floor?
Ponyatno	pah-<u>nyat</u>-nuh	I see
lestnitsa	<u>lyes</u>-nee-tsuh	stairs
lift	leeft	elevator

You Wear It Well: Shopping for Clothes

Russian folk wisdom has it that people's first impression of you is based on the way you're dressed. That's why you're likely to see Russians well-dressed in public, even in informal situations. Clothes-shopping is a big deal to Russians and is often a full-day's affair. In the following sections, we tell you how to get the most out of your clothes-shopping by describing what you're looking for, and getting and trying on the right size.

Seeking specific items of clothing

If you're looking for outerwear (which happens to tourists who forget to plan for the weather in a foreign place!), you want to go to the store or department called **Vyerkhnyaya odyezhda** (*vyerkh*-nee-ye ah-*dyezh*-duh; outerwear). There you'll find things like a

- **kurtka** (*koort*-kuh; short coat or a warmer jacket)
- **pal'to** (puhl'-*toh*; coat)
- **plash'** (plahsh'; raincoat or trench coat)

If you need a new pair of shoes, drop in to the store or department called **Obuv'** (*oh*-boof'; footwear) and choose among

- **bosonozhki** (buh-sah-*nohsh*-kee; women's sandals)
- **botinki** (bah-*teen*-kee; laced shoes)

This or That? Deciding What You Want

One of the most exciting things about shopping for clothes (or anything, for that matter) is talking about the advantages and disadvantages of your potential purchase. In this section we give you all the words, phrases, and grammatical constructions you need to do just that. We tell you how to express likes and dislikes, how to compare items, and how to specify which item you like best of all.

Using demonstrative pronouns

When deciding which dress you want to buy, you may want to make a statement like **Eto plat'ye luchshye chyem to.** (*eh*-tuh *plaht'*-ee *looch*-sheh chehm toh; This dress is better than that one.) The words **eto** (*eh*-tuh; this) and **to** (toh; that one) are called *demonstrative pronouns*. In Russian, demonstrative pronouns function like adjectives and change their endings depending on the case, number, and gender of the nouns they modify. (See Chapter 2 for more on adjective-noun agreement.) When comparing items, you're almost always using demonstrative pronouns only in the nominative case, so here are all the forms you need to know:

- ✔ **etot** (*eh*-tuht; this or this one) for masculine nouns
- ✔ **eta** (*eh*-tuh; this or this one) for feminine nouns
- ✔ **eto** (*eh*-tuh; this or this one) for neuter nouns
- ✔ **eti** (*eh*-tee; these or these ones) for plural nouns
- ✔ **tot** (toht; that or that one) for masculine nouns
- ✔ **ta** (tah; that or that one) for feminine nouns
- ✔ **to** (toh; that or that one) for neuter nouns
- ✔ **tye** (tye; those or those ones) for plural nouns

Expressing likes and dislikes

When people go shopping, they often base their final decisions on one simple thing: You either like something or you don't! To express that you like something in Russian, you say **Mnye** (mnye; *Literally:* to me) + a form of the verb **nravitsya** (*nrah*-veet-sye; to like) + the thing(s) you like. The verb must agree in number (and gender, for past tense) with the thing(s) you like. It's a peculiar construction: What you're saying literally is "To me, something is liked." If you like a particular coat, for example, you say **Mnye nravitsya eta kurtka.** (mnye *nrah*-veet-sye *eh*-tuh *koort*-kuh; I like this coat.)

Table 6-1 has some other forms of the verb **nravitsya** you may need to use, depending on the thing(s) you're talking about and the tense you're using.

Table 6-1	Tenses of Nravit'sya
Present Tense	nravit'sya (singular), nravyatsya (plural)
Past Tense	nravilsya (masculine), narvilas' (feminine), nravilos' (neuter) naravilis' (plural)
Future Tense	budyet nravit'sya (singular) and budut nravit'sya (plural)

If you want to express that you *don't* like something, you simply add **nye** (nee; not) before **nravitsya,** as in **Mnye nye nravitsya eta kurtka.** (mnye nee *nrah*-veet-sye *eh*-tuh *koort*-kuh; I don't like this coat.)

Practice using this construction. Imagine you're in a store with your best friend whom you dragged with you to help you find a nice formal **kostyum** (kahs-t*yum*; suit) that you need for work. You like the brown suit, but your friend seems to like the blue one. These are the remarks that the two of you may exchange:

- ✔ **Mnye nravitsya korichnyevyj kostyum.** (mnye *nrah*-veet-sye kah-*reech*-nee-vihy kahs-*tyum*; I like the brown suit.)

- ✔ **Mnye nravitsya sinij kostyum.** (mnye *nrah*-veet-sye *see*-neey kahs-*tyum*; I like the blue suit.)

Contrary to your friend's advice, you buy the suit you like: the brown one. Your friend still holds to his opinion and when leaving the store he says with a deep sigh of regret: **Mnye nravilsya sinij kostyum.** (mnye *nrah*-veel-sye *see*-neey kahs-*tyum*; I liked the blue suit).

Comparing two items

To compare things, Russian uses comparative adjectives like **bol'shye** (*bohl'*-sheh; bigger), **myen'shye** (*myen'*-sheh; smaller), **luchshye** (*looch*-sheh; better) and **khuzhye** (*khoo*-zheh; worse). Just as in English, you say the name of the item + the comparative adjectives (for instance, bigger or smaller) + the word **chyem** (chyem; than) + the other item. And here's some good news: Comparative adjectives do *not* need to agree in case, number, and gender with the nouns they refer to. They use the same form for every noun!

Say you're trying on two pairs of shoes. You like the second pair better: it's more comfortable, lighter, and cheaper, too. This is what you may be thinking to yourself: **Eti tufli udobnyeye, lyegchye, i dyeshyevlye chyem tye.** (*eh*-tee *toof*-lee oo-*dohb*-nee-ee *lyekh*-chee ee dee-*shehv*-lee chyem tye; These shoes are more comfortable, lighter, and cheaper than those.)

In addition to the words we use here, some other commonly used comparative adjectives in Russian are

- **dlinnyeye** (dlee-*nye*-ee; longer)
- **dorozhye** (dah-*roh*-zheh; more expensive)
- **dyeshyevlye** (dee-*shehv*-lee; cheaper)
- **intyeryesnyeye** (een-tee-*ryes*-nee-ee; more interesting)
- **kholodnyeye** (khuh-lahd-*nye*-ee; colder)
- **korochye** (kah-*rohch*-chee; shorter)
- **krasivyeye** (kruh-*see*-vee-ee; more beautiful)
- **tolsh'ye** (*tohl*-sh'e; thicker)
- **ton'shye** (*tohn'*-sheh; thinner)
- **tyazhyelyeye** (tee-zhih-*lye*-ee; heavier)
- **tyeplyeye** (teep-*lye*-ee; warmer)

Talking about what you like most (or least)

When you look at several items (or people or things), you may like one of them most of all. To communicate this preference, you need to use the superlative form of the adjective. Just like in English, Russian simply adds the word **samyj** (*sah*-mihy; the most) before the adjective and noun you're talking about.

To express the superlative form of the adjective, put **samyj** before the neutral adjective form, not the comparative adjective form, as given in the previous section. For a list of superlative adjective forms, see Table 6-2.

Samyj is an adjective and must agree in case, number, and gender with the nouns and other adjectives it modifies. (For details on adjective-noun agreement, see Chapter 2). Table 6-2 has the forms of **samyj** you need to use.

Table 6-2	Speaking in Superlatives		
	Masculine	*Feminine*	*Neuter*
Singular	samyj (*sah*-mihy)	samaya (*sah*-muh-ye)	samoye (*sah*-muh-ye)
Plural (all genders)	samyye (*sah*-mih-ee)	samyye (*sah*-mih-ee)	samyye (*sah*-mih-ee)

If one coat is lightest of all the coats you tried on, you may want to say **Eta kurtka samaya lyogkaya.** (*eh*-tuh *koort*-kuh sah-muh-ye *lyohk*-kuh-ye; This coat is the lightest.) If you're particularly fond of one pair of earrings, you can say **Eti syer'gi samyye krasivyye.** (*eh*-tee *syer'*-gee sah-mih-ee krah-*see*-vih-ee; These earrings are the most beautiful ones.)

To communicate that something is the worst in its category, Russians today use the word **samyj plokhoj** (*sah*-mihy plah-*khohy*; worst, *Literally:* most bad) for masculine nouns, **samaya plokhaya** (*sah*-muh-ye plah-*khah*-ye) for feminine nouns, **samoye plokhoye** (*sah*-muh-ee plah-*khoh*-ee) for neuter nouns, and **samyye plokhiye** (*sah*-mih-ee plah-*khee*-ee) for plural nouns.

So if you particularly dislike one dress, you say **Eto plat'ye samoye plokhoye.** (*eh*-tuh *plaht'*-ee sah-muh-ee plah-*khoh*-ee; That dress is the worst, *Literally:* That dress is the most bad.)

You Gotta Pay to Play: Buying Items

After you decide on an item of clothing or any other piece of merchandise, you want to make sure the price is right. In the following sections, we show you how to ask how much something costs, how to indicate you'll take it, and how to find out how you should pay for it.

How much does it cost?

To ask how much something costs, you use the phrase **Skol'ko stoit . . . ?** (*skohl'*-kuh *stoh*-eet; How much does . . . cost?) + the name of the item in the nominative case, if you're buying one thing. If you're buying more than one thing, you ask **Skol'ko stoyat . . . ?** (*skohl'*-kuh *stoh*-yet; How much do . . . cost?) + the name of the items in the nominative plural. (For more on cases and forming the nominative plural of nouns, see Chapter 2.)

If you want to know the price of an umbrella, you ask **Skol'ko stoit etot zontik?** (*skohl'*-kuh *stoh*-eet *eh*-tuht *zohn*-teek; How much is this umbrella?) If you want to buy several umbrellas, you ask **Skol'ko stoyat eti zontiki?** (*skohl'*-kuh *stoh*-yet *eh*-tee *zohn*-tee-kee; How much are these umbrellas?)

The item you're considering buying may be too expensive for you, in which case you say **Eto ochyen' dorogo.** (*eh*-tuh *oh*-cheen' *doh*-ruh-guh; It's very expensive.) If, on the other hand, you're pleasantly surprised with the price, you may joyfully say **Eto dyoshyevo!** (*eh*-tuh *dyo*-shih-vuh; It's cheap!)

I'll take it!

The simplest way to express your intention to buy something is to say **Ya voz'mu eto.** (ya vahz'-*moo eh*-tuh; I'll take it.) You can also use a form of the verb **kupit'** (koo-*peet'*; to buy) and say **Ya eto kuplyu** (ya *eh*-tuh koo-*plyu*; I'll buy it.)

Kupit' is the perfective aspect of the verb and can only be used to express past or future action. (For more on aspects, see Chapter 2.) It also has an irregular conjugation pattern. See Table 6-3.

Table 6-3	Conjugation of Kupit'	
Russian	*Pronunciation*	*Translation*
ya kuplyu	ya koo-*plyu*	I'll buy
ty kupish'	tih *koo*-peesh	You'll buy (informal singular)
on/ona/ono kupit	ohn/ah-*nah*/ah-*noh* koo-peet	He/she/it will buy
my kupim	mih *koo*-peem	We'll buy
vy kupitye	vih *koo*-pee-tee	You'll buy (formal singular and plural)
oni kupyat	ah-*nee koo*-pyet	They'll buy

Say you're planning on buying the umbrella you like. You have two ways to state this fact in Russian using a form of **kupit'**: **Ya khochu kupit' zontik.** (ya khah-*choo* koo-*peet' zohn*-teek; I want to buy an umbrella.) or **Ya kuplyu zontik.** (ya koop-*lyu zohn*-teek; I will buy an umbrella.)

Where and how do I pay?

More often than not a Russian store has a **kassa** (*kah*-suh; cahier's desk) with a **kassir** (kuh-*seer*; cashier). To pay for your item, you first need to take your money to the **kassir** and get a receipt, which you then take back to the sales-person you've already dealt with. It's a bit of a pain, and that's why it's always a good idea to ask first where you're supposed to pay: **A gdye mozhno zaplatit'?** (ah gdye *mohzh*-nuh zuh-pluh-*teet'*; And where can I pay?)

When you ask **A gdye mozhno zaplatit'?**, the response may be **V kassye.** (*f kah*-see; At the cahier's desk.) or **Platitye v kassu.** (pluh-*tee*-tee f kah-soo; Pay at the cashier's desk.) If you hear one of these phrases, head for the cashier's desk if it's in view. If it's not, you can ask **A gdye kassa?** (ah gdye *kah*-suh; And where is the cashier's desk?) Hopefully they'll show you where it is, and your shopping adventure will almost be over!

If you're unsure whether the store accepts credit cards, you can ask **Vy prini-mayetye kryeditnyye kartochki?** (vih pree-nee-*mah*-ee-tee kree-*deet*-nih-ee *kahr*-tuhch-kee; Do you accept credit cards?) The answer may be **Da, prini-mayem.** (dah, pree-nee-*mah*-eem; Yes, we do.) or **Nyet, nye prinimayem, tol'ko nalichnyye.** (nyet nee pree-nee-*mah*-eem *tohl'*-kuh nah-*leech*-nih-ee; No, we don't, only cash.) See Chapter 14 for more about handling money.

Normally it's almost impossible to receive a refund in a Russian store. Our advice: Think twice before you buy anything in Russia. If you're really lucky, you may try to get a refund by saying **Ya khochu eto vyernut'.** (ya khah-*choo eh*-tuh veer-*noot'*; I want to return this.) The most common response will prob-ably be **My nye prinimayem obratno.** (mih nee pree-nee-*mah*-eem ahb-*raht*-nuh; We don't take it back.) or **My nye mozhyem vyernut' vam dyen'gi.** (mih nee *moh*-zheem veer-*noot'* vahm *dehn'*-gee; We can't do a refund, *Literally:* We can't give you back your money.) Once in a blue moon a sympathetic sales-person may agree to exchange what you bought. In this case you'll hear **Yesli khotitye, my mozhyem obmyenyat'.** (*yes*-lee khah-*tee*-tee mih *moh*-zheem ahb-mee-*nyat'*; If you want, we can exchange it.) If you hear this phrase, con-sider yourself one of the lucky few, and go for it!

Talkin' the Talk

 Zina and Nina are best friends. They call each other every day. Today Zina bought a new dress and calls Nina to share this exciting news.

Nina: **Allyo!**
         uh-*lyo!*
         Hello!

Zina: **Nina, eto ya.**
         nee-nuh, *eh*-tuh ya.
         Nina, it's me.

Nina: **Zina! Privet! Kak dela?**
         zee-nuh! pree-*vyet*! kahk dee-*lah*?
         Zina! Hi! How are you?

Zina: **Nina, ya segodnya kupila syebye plat'ye!**
         nee-nuh, ya see-*vohd*-nye koo-*pee*-luh see-*bye plaht'*-ee!
         Nina, I bought myself a dress today!

Nina: **Gdye?**
         gdye?
         Where?

Zina: **V magazinye na Sadovoj ulitsye.**
         v muh-guh-*zee*-nee nuh suh-*doh*-vuhy *oo*-lee-tseh.
         At the store on Sadovaya street.

Nina: **A za skolyko ty kupila plat'ye?**
         uh zah *skohl'*-kuh tih koo-*pee*-luh *plaht'*-ee?
         And how much did you buy the dress for?

Zina: **Dyoshyevo. Za sto pyat'dyesyat.**
         dyo-sheh-vuh. zah stoh pee-dee-*syat*.
         Cheap. For one hundred fifty rubles.

Words to Know

Ya kupila syebye . . .	ya koo-<u>pee</u>-luh see-bye	I bought myself . . .
Na . . . ulitsye	nah <u>oo</u>-lee-tseh	On . . . street
Za skol'ko ty kupila plat'ye?	zah <u>skohl'</u>-kuh tih ee-<u>voh</u> koo-<u>pee</u>-luh	How much did you buy the dress for?
Za sto pyat'dyesyat.	zah stoh pee-dee-<u>syat</u>	For one hundred fifty rubles.

Something Special: Cool Things to Buy in Russia

The best souvenir to bring home from Russia is a **palyekhskaya shkatulka** (*pah*-leekh-skuh-ye shkah-*tool*-kuh; Palekh box): a black lacquered box made from papier-mâché and decorated with paintings based on traditional Russian fairy-tale plots. The authentic boxes are manufactured only in two little Russian cities, Palekh and Khokhloma, and they're quite expensive.

Watch out for knock-offs. Don't buy a **palyekhskaya shkatulka** from street vendors, who often ask the same high price for their fake versions. Ask your guide or a hotel employee where the best place to buy these boxes is.

Another cool **suvyenir** (soo-vee-*neer*; souvenir) to bring home is the famous Russian **matryoshka** (muh-*tryosh*-kuh) doll. It's a wooden doll that, when opened at its rather wide waistline, contains at least three of its "children" hiding inside of each other, each one smaller than the next. **Matryoshki** (muh-*tryosh*-kee) come in different sizes, and the bigger the "mother," the more daughters you'll discover inside.

You may also want to bring home with you a famous Russian **myekhovaya shapka** (mee-khah-*vah*-ye *shahp*-kuh; fur hat) that Russians wear in the winter. You can buy them in either **chyornyj** (*chyohr*-nihy; black) or **korichnyevyj** (kah-*reech*-nee-vihy; brown), and the best place to buy them is in an

univyermag (oo-nee-veer-*mahk*; department store) in the **otdyel** (aht-*dyel*; department) called **golovnyye ubory** (guh-lahv-*nih*-ee oo-*boh*-rih; hats), or in any standalone store with that same name.

If you're into collecting cool memorabilia from the past, you'll definitely want to buy some **sovyetskiye voyennyye chasy** (sah-v*yet*-skee-ee vah-*yen*-nih-ee chuh-*sih*; Soviet military watches). These watches, which are now considered collectors items, usually come with many different stylish designs. They're sturdy and reliable, because they were manufactured in Soviet times specially for military personnel. You can usually buy them at any store called **suvyeniry** (soo-vee-*nee*-rih; souvenirs).

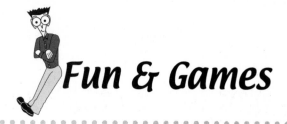

Fun & Games

At which of these stores are you likely to find the following items? See Appendix C for the correct answers.

a. **obuv'** b. **kosmyetika** c. **fototovary** d. **muzhskaya odyezhda** e. **khozya- jstvyennyj magazin** f. **kantsyelyarskiye tovary** g. **golovnyye ubory**

1. facial cream

2. suit

3. boots

4. camera

5. hat

6. soap

7. stationery

Compare the following (the correct answers are in Appendix C), using the words:

a. **bol'shye** b. **myen'shye** c. **dorozhye** d. **kholodnyeye** e. **tyazhyelyeye**

For example:

Q. **Moskva . . . chyem Pyetyerburg.** (Moscow is . . . than St. Petersburg.)

A. **Moskva bol'shye chyem Pyetyerburg.**

1. **Pyetyerburg . . . chyem Moskva.** (St. Petersburg is . . . than Moscow.)

2. **Zima v Moskvye . . . chyem v San-Frantsisko.** (Winter in Moscow is . . . than in San Francisco.)

3. **Myersyedyes . . . chyem Toyota.** (Mercedes is . . . than Toyota.)

4. **Sapogi . . . chyem tufli.** (Boots are . . . than shoes.)

Chapter 7

Going Out on the Town, Russian-Style

This chapter is all about going out on the town the Russian way. We take you to the movies, the theater, the ballet, and a museum. These places are still the most popular for Russians to go on their time off. We show you how to make plans with friends, how and where to buy tickets, how to find your seat, how to make the most of intermission, and what to say when you want to share your impressions of an event with your friends. But to make sure you're not late, we first need to tell you how to ask about and understand show times. So please be patient, or as Russians like to say, **Vsyo khorosho v svoyo vryemya** (fsyo khuh-rah-*shoh* f svah-*yo vrye*-mye; Everything in good time).

The Clock's Ticking: Telling Time

When you go out and have fun, **vryemya** (*vrye*-mye; time) is crucial. For one thing, you need to allocate time for fun in your busy schedule, or, as Russians often say, **Dyelu vryemya, potyekhye chas** (*dye*-loo *vrye*-mye pah-*tye*-khee chahs; Pleasure after business). Secondly, if you arrive late for a show or performance in Russia, they simply won't let you in! In the following sections, we help you solve these problems by telling you how to state and ask for time, and how to specify times of the day and days of the week.

> # The tortoise and the hare: Russian versus American concepts of time
>
> While Americans believe that time is money, Russians have a much different idea about time. No matter what you want to have done, everything seems to take longer in Russia. If you mail a letter to somebody, expect it to arrive at its destination in no less than a week (or even get lost on the way). If you want to pay for your dinner in a restaurant, it may take a long time for a waiter to finally show up. If you call your business partner and leave a message on her answering machine, it may take days for her to return your call. No wonder Russians are known for their patience!

Counting the hours

Just like in Europe, Russia uses the 24-hour system for each day. Instead of 3 p.m., you may hear the phrase **pyatnadtsat' chasov** (peet-*naht*-tsuht' chuh-*sohf*; fifteen o'clock, *Literally:* fifteen hours). Notice that the word for "o'clock" and "hour" is the same in Russian: **chas** (chahs). Russians use this form of time-telling for all kinds of official messages: timetables, schedules, radio and TV announcements, working hours, and so on. In everyday situations, however, most people use the first twelve numerals (as they do in the U.S.) to indicate both a.m. and p.m. hours.

If you want to indicate "a.m." when using the 12-hour system, you say **utra** (oot-*rah*; *Literally:* in the morning) after the time; you say **dnya** (dnya; *Literally:* in the day) after the time to indicate "p.m." So 5 a.m. would be **pyat' chasov utra** (pyat' chuh-*sohf* oot-*rah*), and 5 p.m. would be **pyat' chasov dnya** (pyat' chuh-*sohf* dnya). When you're using the 24-hour system, you don't have to add the words **utra** or **dnya.**

Saying "o'clock" in Russian is kind of tricky. These simple rules, however, should help you translate this word into Russian:

- ✔ If the time is one o'clock, you just use the word **chas,** as in **Syejchas chas** (see-*chahs* chahs; It's 1 o'clock). You don't even have to say **odin** (ah-*deen*; one) before the word **chas.**

- ✔ After the numeral **dvadtsat' odin** (*dvaht*-tsuht' ah-*deen*; twenty-one), use the word **chas** (chahs; o'clock), as in **Syejchas dvadtsat' odin chas** (see-*chahs dvaht*-tsuht' ah-*deen* chahs; It's 21 o'clock), or in other words, 9 p.m.

- ✔ After the numbers **dva** (dvah; two), **tri** (tree; three), **chyetyrye** (chee-*tih*-ree; four), **dvadtsat' dva** (*dvaht*-tsuht' dvah; twenty-two), **dvadtsat' tri** (*dvaht*-tsuht' tree; twenty-three), and **dvadtsat' chyetyrye** (*dvaht*-tsuht'

chee-*tih*-ree; twenty-four), use the word **chasa** (chuh-*sah,* o'clock), as in **Syejchas tri chasa** (see-*chahs* tree chuh-*sah;* It's 3 o'clock).

✔ With all other numerals indicating time, use the word **chasov** (chuh-*sohf;* o'clock), as in **Syejchas pyat chasov** (see-*chahs* pyat' chuh-*sohf;* It's 5 o'clock).

For more info about numerals, see Chapter 2.

One final tip: To say "noon" in Russian, you just say **poldyen'** (*pohl*-deen'; *Literally:* half day). When you want to say "midnight," you say **polnoch'** (*pohl*-nuhch; *Literally:* half night).

Marking the minutes

In their fast-paced lives, most people plan their days not just down to the hour but also down to the **minuta** (mee-*noo*-tuh; minute) and even the **syekunda** (see-*koon*-duh; second). In the following sections, we show you different ways to keep time by expressing minute time increments in Russian.

On the half hour

The easiest way to state the time by the half hour in Russian is to just add the words **tridtsat' minut** (*treet*-tsuht' mee-*noot;* thirty minutes) to the hour: **Syejchas dva chasa tridtsat' minut** (see-*chahs* dvah chuh-*sah treet*-tsuht' mee-*noot;* It's 2:30). In more conversational speech, it's common to drop the words **chasa** and **minut** and just say **Syejchas dva tridtsat'** (see-*chahs* dvah *treet*-tsuht'; It's 2:30).

However, you may hear other ways of talking about half hour increments, such as **Syejchas polovina pyervogo/vtorogo/tryet'yego** (see-*chahs* puh-lah-*vee*-nuh *pyer*-vuh-vuh/ftah-*roh*-vuh/*tryet'*-ee-vuh; It's half past twelve/one/two, *Literally:* It's half of one/two/three).

You may be wondering why "half past one" is **polovina vtorogo** rather than **polovina pyervogo.** That's because the word **polovina** literally means "half of," not "half past." What you're really saying is "half of" whatever the next hour is. Therefore, 1:30 in Russian is literally "half of two," or **polovina vtorogo,** and 2:30 is literally "half of three," or **polovina tryet'yego.** Remember to keep this straight, or else you're going to be an hour late for a lot of appointments!

In a phrase like **Syejchas polovina pyervogo,** the Russian word used to indicate the hour (**pyervogo**) is the genitive form of the ordinal number **pyervyj** (*pyer*-vihy; first). For more on cases and ordinal numbers, see Chapter 2.

While using **polovina** is perfectly fine in all situations, you can also replace **polovina** with the slightly more conversational word **pol** (pohl) to indicate half-hour increments, as in **Syejchas pol vtorogo** (see-*chahs* pohl ftah-*roh*-vuh; It's half past one, *Literally:* It's half of two.)

On the quarter hour

To indicate a quarter after an hour, Russian typically uses the phrase **pyat-nadtsat' minut** (peet-*naht*-tsuht' mee-*noot*; fifteen minutes). Using **pyatnad-tsat' minut** to indicate a quarter after the hour is easy. To say it's 5:15, you just say **Syejchas pyat' chasov pyatnadtsat' minut** (see-*chahs* pyat' chuh-*sohf* peet-*naht*-tsuht' mee-*noot*; Literally: It's five hours fifteen minutes). To be more conversational, you can drop **chasov** and **minut** and say **Syejchas pyat' pyatnadtsat'** (see-*chahs* pyat' peet-*naht*-tsuht'; It's 5:15).

To indicate a quarter to an hour is a little trickier. In this situation, Russian uses the word **byez** (byes; without) with **pyatnadtsati** and the hour, as in **Syejchas byez pyatnadtsati pyat'** (see-*chahs* bees peet-*naht*-tsuh-tee pyat'; It's 4:45, Literally: It's five without fifteen minutes). The pronunciation of **byez** changed in the sentence because it's followed by a word beginning with the devoiced consonant **p** (see Chapter 2 for details on devoiced consonants).

If you feel brave and want to use the word **chyetvyert'** (*chyet*-veert'; quarter) to talk about 15-minute increments, then you need to do one of the following:

- ✔ If it's a quarter past an hour, use the genitive case of the ordinal number corresponding to the next hour. For example: **Syejchas chyetvyert' syed'-mogo** (see-*chahs* chyet-veert' seed'-*moh*-vuh; It's a quarter past six, Literally: A quarter of the seventh hour has passed).

- ✔ If it's a quarter to an hour, use the phrase **byez chyetvyerti** (bees *chyet*-veer-tee), as in **Syejchas byez chyetvyerti vosyem'** (see-*chahs* bees *chyet*-veer-tee *voh*-seem'; It's a quarter to eight, Literally: It's eight minus a quarter).

Other times before or after the hour

To state times that aren't on the half or quarter hour, you can simply use the construction **Syejchas . . . chasa** (or **chasov**) + . . . **minut**, as in **Syejchas chyetyrye chasa dyesyat' minut** (see-*chahs* chee-*tih*-ree chuh-*sah dye*-seet' mee-*noot*; It's 4:10.) For more conversational speech, you can also drop the words **chasa** (or **chasov**) and **minut** and just say **Syejchas chyetyrye dyesyat'** (see-*chahs* chee-*tih*-ree *dye*-seet').

To express times right before the hour, you use the construction **Syejchas byez** plus the numbers indicating the minutes and the next hour. "It's ten to five" is **Syejchas byez dyesyati pyat** (see-*chahs* bees dee-see-*tee* pyat'; Literally: It's five minus ten minutes). In this construction, it's common to drop the words **minut** (minutes) and **chasov** (hours) after the numerals indicating the time.

When using this expression, you must always remember to put the numeral after the word **byez** into the genitive case. Here are the genitive case forms of the numerals you most often use with this expression:

- **odnoj** (ahd-*nohy*; one)
- **dvukh** (dvookh; two)
- **tryokh** (tryokh; three)
- **chyetyryokh** (chee-tih-*ryokh*; four)
- **pyati** (pee-*tee*; five)
- **dyesyati** (dee-see-*tee*; ten)
- **pyat'nadtsati** (peet-*naht*-tsuh-tee; fifteen)
- **dvadtsati** (dvaht-tsuh-*tee*; twenty)
- **dvadtsati pyati** (dvuht-tsuh-*tee* pee-*tee*; twenty-five)

Asking for the time

To ask what time it is, you say **Skol'ko syejchas vryemyeni?** (*skohl'*-kuh see-*chahs vrye*-mee-nee; What time is it?) If you ask a passerby in public, you may want to begin this question with the polite phrase **Izvinitye pozhalujsta . . .** (eez-vee-*nee*-tee pah-*zhahl*-stuh; Excuse me, please . . .) or **Skazhitye pozhalujsta . . .** (skuh-*zhih*-tee pah-*zhahl*-stuh; Could you please tell me . . .)

To ask at what time something will happen or has happened, use the phrases **Kogda** (kahg-*dah*; when) or **V kakoye vryemya . . .** (f kuh-*koh*-ee *vrye*-mye . . . ; At what time . . .)

Talkin' the Talk

John went downtown today but left his watch at home. He needs to find out what time it is and asks a very pretty **dyevushka** (*dye*-voosh-kuh; young woman) who happens to be passing by if she can tell him the time.

John: **Dyevushka, izvinitye pozhaluysta, vy nye skazhyetye skol'ko syejchas vryemyeni?**
dye-voosh-kuh eez-vee-*nee*-tee pah-*zhahl*-stuh vih nee *skah*-zhih-tee *skohl'*-kuh see-*chahs vrye*-mee-nee?
Excuse me, miss, can you tell me what time it is?

Dyevushka: **Syejchas? Syejchas byez chyetvyerti chas.**
see-*chahs*? see-*chahs* bees *chyet*-veer-tee chahs
Time? It's quarter to one.

John: **Skol'ko? Prostitye ya nye ponyal. Ya inostranyets.**
skohl'-kuh? prah-*stee*-tee ya nee *poh*-neel. ya ee-nah-*strah*-neets
What time? Sorry, I did not understand. I am a foreigner.

Dyevushka: **Syejchas byez pyatnadtsati minut chas. Vot chasy, posmotritye.**
see-*chahs* bees peet-*naht*-tsuh-tee mee-*noot* chahs.
voht chuh-*sih*, puhs-mah-*tree*-tee.
It is fifteen minutes to one. Here is my watch, take a look.

John: **A, ponyatno. Oj, ya dolzhyen byt' na vstryechye v chas tridtsat' v ryestoranye "Vostok"! Ya opazdyvayu.**
ah pah-*nyat*-nuh. ohy ya *dohl*-zhihn biht' nuh *fstrye*-chee f chahs *treet*-tsuht' v rees-tah-*rah*-nee vahs-*tohk*.
ya ah-*pahz*-dih-vuh-yu!
Oh, I see. Oh, I have to meet somebody at the restaurant "Vostok" at 1:30. I am running late.

Dyevushka: **Oj, eto ryadom. U vas vstryecha v polovinye vtorogo? Tuda idti pyatnadtsat' minut. Vy tam budyetye v chas.**
ohy *eh*-tuh *rya*-duhm. oo vahs *fstrye*-chuh f puh-lah-*vee*-nee ftah-*roh*-vuh? too-*dah* eet-*tee* peet-*naht*-tsuht' mee-*noot*. vih tahm *boo*-dee-tee f chahs.
Oh, it's close by. Do you have a meeting at half past one? It's a 15-minute walk. You'll be there at 1.

John: **Bol'shoye vam spasibo, dyevushka.**
bahl'-*shoh*-ee vahm spuh-*see*-buh *dye*-voosh-kuh.
Thank you so much, miss.

Words to Know

Vy nye skazhyetye?	vih nee <u>skah</u>-zhih-tee	Can you tell me?
Prostitye ya nye ponyal.	prah-<u>stee</u>-tee ya nee <u>poh</u>-neel	Sorry, I did not understand.
inostranyets	ee-nah-<u>strah</u>-neets	foreigner
Vot chasy.	voht chuh-<u>sih</u>	Here is (my) watch.
Posmotritye.	puh-smah-<u>tree</u>-tee	Take a look.
Ya dolzhyen byt' na vstryechye.	ya <u>dohl</u>-zhihn biht' nuh <u>fstrye</u>-chee	I have to be at a meeting/to meet somebody.
Ya opazdyvayu.	Ya ah-<u>pahz</u>-dih-vuh-yoo	I'm running late.
Tuda idti . . . minut.	too-<u>dah</u> eet-<u>tee</u> . . . mee-<u>noot</u>	It's a . . . minute walk.
Vy tam budyetye v	vih tahm <u>boo</u>-dee-tee v	You'll be there at

Knowing the times of the day

People all over the world seem to agree on three main time periods: **utro** (*oo-*truh; morning), **dyen'** (dyen'; afternoon), and **vyechyer** (*vye-*cheer; evening). **Noch'** (nohch; night) is the time when most people sleep. To state that something happens within these time periods, use these phrases:

- **utrom** (*oo-*truhm; in the morning)
- **dnyom** (dnyom; in the afternoon)
- **vyechyerom** (*vye-*chee-ruhm; in the evening)
- **noch'yu** (*nohch-*yu; late at night or early in the morning)

While English uses the prepositional phrase "in + time of the day" to indicate times of the day, in Russian you put the words **utro, dyen', vyechyer,** and **noch'** in instrumental case. (For more on instrumental case, see Chapter 2.) Also note that the word **dyen'** drops the letter **ye** in the process and becomes

dnyom rather than **denyom.** Nouns sometimes have this habit of "losing" letters in the process of declining for cases in Russian.

Distinguishing the days of the week

To indicate days of the week, use these Russian words:

- ✔ **ponyedyel'nik** (puh-nee-*dyel'*-neek; Monday)
- ✔ **vtornik** (*ftohr*-neek; Tuesday)
- ✔ **sryeda** (sree-*dah*; Wednesday)
- ✔ **chyetvyerg** (cheet-*vyerk*; Thursday)
- ✔ **pyatnitsa** (*pyat*-nee-tsuh; Friday)
- ✔ **subbota** (soo-*boh*-tuh; Saturday)
- ✔ **voskryesyen'ye** (vuhs-kree-*syen'*-ee; Sunday)

If somebody asks you what day of the week it is, he says: **Kakoj syegodnya dyen'?** (kuh-*kohy* see-*vohd*-nye dyen'; What day is it today?) To answer this question, you say **Syegodnya** plus the day of the week. For example: **Syegodnya ponyedyel'nik** (see-*vohd*-nye puh-nee-*dyel'*-neek; It's Monday today). It's that simple!

Note that while in English the words indicating days of the week are written with capital letters, in Russian they aren't.

To say that something happens, happened, or will happen on a certain day, you need to add the preposition **v,** and you put the word denoting the day of the week into the accusative case. (For more on cases, see Chapter 2.)

As a result, the phrases you use are the following:

- ✔ **v ponyedyel'nik** (f puh-nee-*dyel'*-neek; on Monday)
- ✔ **vo vtornik** (vah *ftohr*-neek; on Tuesday)
- ✔ **v sryedu** (f *srye*-doo; on Wednesday)
- ✔ **v chyetvyerg** (f cheet-*vyerk*; on Thursday)
- ✔ **v pyatnitsu** (f *pyat*-nee-tsuh; on Friday)
- ✔ **v subbotu** (f soo-*boh*-too; on Saturday)
- ✔ **v voskryesyen'ye** (v vuhs-kree-*syen'*-ee; on Sunday)

You may wonder why some of the days change in the accusative case, while others don't. The explanation is simple: Masculine nouns denoting inanimate objects don't change their form in accusative case and retain their nominative (dictionary) form. You may also wonder why the word **vtornik** is used with the preposition **vo** rather than **v** as other days of the week do. Well, mostly for phonetic reasons: It's very hard (even for Russians!) to pronounce **v** with the word that also begins with the sound **v.** The sounds get glued to each other in the process of speaking and it's hard to understand whether the person speaking is saying "on Tuesday" or just "Tuesday." You use **vo,** however, only if the stress of the following word falls on the first syllable. That's why we can use **v** rather than **vo** when we say **v voskryesyen'ye** (on Sunday).

Other phrases related to the days of the week include

- ✔ **dyen'** (dyen'; day)
- ✔ **syegodnya** (see-*vohd*-nye; today)
- ✔ **syegodnya utrom** (see-*vohd*-nye *oo*-truhm; this morning)
- ✔ **syegodnya vyechyerom** (see-*vohd*-nye *vye*-chee-ruhm; this evening)
- ✔ **nyedyelya** (nee-*dye*-lya; week)

Talking about time relative to the present

Just as in English, Russian has lots of phrases to talk about a certain time in the past or future that relates to the present moment. Some time-related words that you may hear or say often in Russian are

- ✔ **syejchas** (see-*chahs*; now)
- ✔ **skoro** (*skoh*-ruh; soon)
- ✔ **pozdno** (*pohz*-nuh; late)
- ✔ **pozzhye** (*poh*-zheh; later)
- ✔ **rano** (*rah*-nuh; early)
- ✔ **ran'shye** (*rahn'*-sheh; earlier)
- ✔ **vchyera** (vchee-*rah*; yesterday)
- ✔ **pozavchyera** (puh-zuhf-chee-*rah*; the day before yesterday)
- ✔ **zavtra** (*zahf*-truh; tomorrow)
- ✔ **poslyezavtra** (*poh*-slee-*zahf*-truh; the day after tomorrow)

If you want to express that something will happen in a week, a month, or a year, you use **chyeryez** plus the accusative form of either **nyedyelya** (nee-*dye*-lya; week), **myesyats** (*mye*-seets; month), or **god** (goht; year):

- ✔ **chyeryez nyedyelyu** (*cheh*-reez nee-*dye*-lyu; in a week)
- ✔ **chyeryez myesyats** (*cheh*-reez *mye*-seets; in a month)
- ✔ **chyeryez god** (*cheh*-reez goht; in a year)

To say that something happened last week, month, or year, you say

- ✔ **na proshloj nyedyele** (nuh *prohsh*-luhy nee-*dye*-lee; last week)
- ✔ **v proshlom myesyatsye** (v *prohsh*-luhm *mye*-see-tseh; last month)
- ✔ **v proshlom godu** (v *prohsh*-luhm gah-*doo*; last year)

Together Wherever We Go: Making Plans to Go Out

It's always more fun to go out on the town with friends. In the following sections, we give you all the words and expressions you need to invite your friends out with you, and we tell you how to accept or decline invitations you receive. We also tell you how to find out what time an event starts.

Do you want to go with me?

Here are common phrases people use to invite you to do things with them:

- ✔ **Pojdyom v . . .** (pahy-*dyom* v; Let's go to the . . .; informal)
- ✔ **Pojdyomtye v . . .** (pahy-*dyom*-tee v; Let's go to the . . .; formal or plural)
- ✔ **Davaj pojdyom v . . .** (duh-*vahy* pahy-*dyom* v; Let's go to the . . .; informal)
- ✔ **Davajtye pojdyom v . . .** (duh-*vahy*-tee pahy-*dyom* v; Let's go to the . . .; formal or plural)
- ✔ **Ty khochyesh' pojti v . . .** (tih *khoh*-cheesh' pahy-*tee* v; Do you want to go to the . . .; informal)
- ✔ **Vy khotitye pojti v . . .** (vih khah-*tee*-tee pahy-*tee* v; Do you want to go to the . . .; formal or plural)

To express "Do you want to . . . ," you say either **Vy khotitye . . .** (vih khah-*tee*-tee; Do you want to . . .; formal) or **Ty khochyesh' . . .** (tih *khoh*-cheesh; Do you want to . . .; informal) plus a verb infinitive. For example, the informal version of "Do you want to watch a movie?" is **Ty khochyesh' smotryet' film'?**

(tih _khoh_-cheesh smah-_tret'_ feel'm). The formal version of "Do you want to play soccer?" is **Vy khotitye igrat' v futbol?** (vih khah-_tee_-tee ee-_graht_ v foot-_bohl_). For more on infinitives, see Chapter 2.

Don't forget to use the formal form of you (**vy**) when inviting somebody you don't know too well to do something. For more info, see Chapter 3.

Davaj/davajtye is not only an invitation formula but also a very useful construction in almost any social situation. You can use it to suggest doing something: **Davajtye zakroyem okno** (duh-_vahy_-tee zuhk-_roh_-eem ahk-_noh_; Let's close the window). It's also an easy way to agree to do something with a good deal of enthusiasm: **Davaj pojdyom v kino! — Davaj!** (dah-_vahy_ pahy-_dyom_ v kee-_noh_ — dah-_vahy_; Let's go to the movies — Sure, let's do it!) Some young Russians even use it as an informal "good-bye": **Nu, davaj!** (noo dah-_vahy_; Take care, see you later!)

To let everybody around know that you want to go somewhere tonight, you may say **Ya khochu pojti v . . . syegodnya vyechyerom** (ya khah-_choo_ pahy-tee f . . . see-_vohd_-nye _vye_-chee-ruhm; I want to go to . . . tonight).

To make plans to go somewhere on a certain day of the week, you can use either **Davaj/davajtye pojdyom . . .** or **Ya khochu pojti v . . .** + one of the expressions denoting days of the week, which we cover earlier in this chapter. For example, "I want to go to the movies on Thursday" would be **Ya khochu pojti v kino v chyetvyerg** (ya khah-_choo_ pahj-tee f kee-_noh_ f cheet-_vyerk_).

After you ask someone to make plans with you (or after someone asks you), the big question is whether to decline or accept. We cover both options in the following sections.

Declining an invitation

Russians don't easily take **nyet** for an answer! So if you need to decline an invitation, we recommend softening your response with one of the following:

- **K sozhalyeniyu, ya nye mogu** (k suh-zhuh-_lye_-nee-yu ya nee mah-_goo_; Unfortunately, I can't)

- **Ochyen' zhal', no ya v etot dyen' zanyat** (_oh_-cheen' zhahl' noh ya v eh-tuht dyen' _zah_-neet; I am very sorry, but I am busy that day)

- **Mozhyet byt', v drugoj dyen'?** (_moh_-zhiht biht' v droo-_gohy_ dyen'; Maybe on a different day?)

- **Mozhyet, luchshye pojdyom v kafye?** (_moh_-zhiht _looch_-shih pahy-_dyohm_ f kah-_feh_; Maybe we could go to a coffee shop instead?)

Accepting an invitation

Here are some ways to spice up your **da:**

- ✔ **Spasibo, s udovol'stviyem!** (spah-*see*-buh s oo-dah-*vohl'*-stvee-eem; Thank you, I would be happy to!)

- ✔ **Bol'shoye spasibo, ya obyazatyel'no pridu.** (bahl'-*shoh*-ee spuh-*see*-buh, ya ah-bee-*zah*-teel'-nuh pree-*doo*; Thank you very much, I'll come by all means.)

- ✔ **Spasibo, a kogda? Vo skol'ko?** (spah-*see*-buh ah kahg-*dah*? vah *skohl'*-kuh?; Thank you, and when? What time?)

What time does it start?

If you want to know when an event (such as a movie or a performance) begins, this is how you ask: **Kogda nachinayetsya . . . ?** (kahg-*dah* nuh-chee-*nah*-eet-sye; When does . . . start?) The event you're asking about goes into the nominative case. (Check out Chapter 2 for more about cases.) For example, "When does the film start?" would be **Kogda nachinayetsya fil'm?** (kahg-*dah* nuh-chee-*nah*-eet-sye feel'm)

When talking about event start times, the verb "to start/to begin" is indispensable. Here's how you translate it into Russian:

- ✔ If the verb "to start/to begin" has an object, translate it into Russian as **nachinat',** as in **My nachinayem fil'm** (mih nuh-chee-*nah*-eem feel'm; We are beginning the show). The object must go into the accusative case.

- ✔ If the verb "to start/to begin" doesn't have an object, translate it as **nachinat'sya,** as in **Fil'm nachinayetsya v chyetyrye tridtsat'** (feel'm nuh-chee-*nah*-eet-sye v chee-*tih*-ree *treet*-tsuht'; The show begins at 4:30).

The verb **nachinat'sya** is called a *reflexive verb.* Reflexive verbs end in **-sya** or **-s'** and don't take direct objects because their action refers back to the subject of the sentence. In the phrase **Fil'm nachinayetsya v . . . ,** what you're really saying is "The movie starts itself up at . . ." Other common reflexive verbs are **otrkyvatsya** (uht-krih-*vaht*-sye; to open) and **zakryvatsya** (zuh-krih-*vaht'*-sye; to close). See Chapter 6 for more about reflexive verbs.

On the Big Screen: Going to the Movies

Going to see a **fil'm** (feel'm; movie) in Russia may be kind of challenging because most Russian movies are — you guessed it! — in Russian. Unless you just want to enjoy the music of the language or pick up some phrases and

words here and there, your best bet is to rent Russian movies with subtitles or find a **kino** (kee-*noh*; theater) that features movies with subtitles. If, however, you want to check out a real Russian film, in the following sections we show you different types of movies, how to buy a ticket, and how to find your seat at the movie theater.

Whereas English just uses the word "theater" for a movie theater, Russian is more exact in expressing the difference between a movie theater and a play, opera, or ballet theater. The word **kino** (kee-*noh*) or the more formal **kinotyeatr** (kee-nuh-tee-*ahtr*) are the only words you can use to denote "movie theater" in Russian.

Picking a particular type of movie

Check out the following list for the names of different film genres in Russian:

- **dyetyektiv** (deh-tehk-*teef*; detective film)
- **ekranizatsiya khudozhyestvyennoj lityeratury** (eh-kruh-nee-*zah*-tsih-ye khoo-*doh*-zhihs-tvee-nuhy lee-tee-ruh-*too*-rih; screen version of a book)
- **fil'm uzhasov** (feel'm *oo*-zhuh-suhf; horror film)
- **komyediya** (kah-*mye*-dee-ye; comedy)
- **mul'tfil'm** (mool't-*feel'm*; cartoon)
- **myuzikl** (*m'yu*-zeekl; musical)
- **nauhcnaya fantastika** (nuh-*ooch*-nuh-ye fuhn-*tahs*-tee-kuh; science fiction)
- **priklyuchyenchyeskij fil'm** (pree-klyu-*chyen*-chees-keey feel'm; adventure film)
- **trillyer** (*tree*-lyer; thriller)
- **vyestyern** (*vehs*-tehrn; western)

What genres do Russains prefer? It's hard to generalize. We should mention one thing, though: Russians don't seem to like happy endings as much as most Americans do, and they tend to prefer harsh reality to beautiful dreams in their movies.

Buying tickets

If you decide to go to the movies, you need a **bilyet** (bee-*lyet*; ticket). The ticket office is generally somewhere near the entrance to the movie theater. Most likely it has a sign that says **Kassa** (*kah*-suh; ticket office) or **Kassa kinotyeatra** (*kah*-suh kee-nuh-tee-*aht*-ruh; *Literally:* ticket office of the movie theater).

To ask for a ticket, customers often use a kind of a stenographic language. **Kassiry** (kuh-*see*-rih; cashiers) are generally impatient people, and you may have a line behind you. So try to make your request for a ticket as brief as you can. If you want to go to the 2:30 p.m. show, you say one of these phrases:

- ✔ **Odin na chyetyrnadtsat' tridtsat'** (ah-*deen* nah chee-*tihr*-nuh-tsuht' *treet*-tsuht'; One for 2:30)

- ✔ **Dva na chyetyrnadtsat' tridtsat'** (dvah nah chee-*tihr*-nuh-tsuht' *treet*-tsuht'; Two for 2:30)

Because probably only one movie will be showing at that time, the **kassir** (kuh-*seer*; cashier) will know which movie you want to see. But if two movies happen to be showing at the same time, or if you want to make sure that you get tickets to the right movie, you can simply add the phrase **na** (nah; to) plus the title of the movie to your request.

Choosing a place to sit and watch

In Russia, when you buy a ticket to the movie, you're assigned a specific seat, so the **kassir** (kuh-*seer*; cashier) may ask you where exactly you want to sit. You may hear **Gdye vy khotitye sidyet'?** (gdye vih khah-*tee*-tee see-*dyet*'; Where do you want to sit?) or **Kakoj ryad?** (kuh-*kohy* ryat; Which row?)

The best answer is **V syeryedinye** (f see-ree-*dee*-nee; in the middle). If you're far-sighted, you may want to say **Podal'shye** (pah-*dahl'*-sheh; further away from the screen). But if you want to sit closer, you say **Poblizhye** (pah-*blee*-zheh; closer to the screen). You may also specify a row by saying **pyervyj ryad** (*pyer*-viy ryat; first row) or **vtoroj ryad** (vtah-*roy* ryat; second row). See Chapter 2 for more about ordinal numbers.

When you finally get your ticket, you must be able to read and understand what it says. Look for the words **ryad** (ryat; row) and **myesto** (*myes*-tuh; seat). For example, you may see **Ryad: 5, Myesto: 14.** That's where you're expected to sit!

In the following sections, we cover two handy verbs to know at the movies: the verbs "to sit" and "to watch."

The verb "to sit"

The verb **sidyet'** (see-*dyet*'; to sit) has a very peculiar conjugation; the **d** changes to **zh** in the first person singular. Because you'll use this verb a lot, it's a good idea to have the full conjugation. Check out Table 7-1.

Table 7-1	Conjugation of Sidyet'	
Conjugation	*Pronunciation*	*Translation*
ya sizhu	ya see-*zhoo*	I sit or I am sitting
ty sidish'	tih see-*deesh*	You sit or You are sitting (informal singular)
on/ona/ono sidit	ohn/ah-*nah*/ah-*noh* see-*deet*	He/she/it sits or He/she/it is sitting
my sidim	mih see-*deem*	We sit or We are sitting
vy siditye	vih see-*dee*-tee	You sit or You are sitting (formal singular and plural)
oni sidyat	ah-*nee* see-*dyat*	They sit or They are sitting

The verb "to watch"

The verb **smotryet'** (smah-*tret'*; to watch) is another useful word when you go to the movies. Table 7-2 shows how you conjugate it in the present tense.

Table 7-2	Conjugation of Smotryet'	
Conjugation	*Pronunciation*	*Translation*
ya smotryu	ya smah-*tryu*	I watch or I am watching
ty smotrish'	tih *smoht*-reesh	You watch or You are watching (informal singular)
on/ona/ono smotrit	ohn/ah-*nah*/ah-*noh* *smoht*-reet	He/she/it watches or He/she/it is watching
my smotrim	mih *smoht*-reem	We watch or We are watching
vy smotritye	vih *smoht*-ree-tee	You watch or You are watching (formal singular and plural)
oni smotryat	ah-*nee* *smoht*-ryet	They watch or They are watching

It's Classic: Taking in the Russian Ballet and Theater

If a Russian ballet company happens to be in your area, don't miss it! And if you're in Russia, don't even think of leaving without seeing at least one performance either in Moscow's Bol'shoy Theater or St. Petersburg's Mariinski Theater. No ballet in the world can compare with the Russian **balyet** (buh-*lyet*; ballet) in its grand, powerful style, lavish decor, impeccable technique, and its proud preservation of the classical tradition.

The Russian **teatr** (tee-*ahtr*; theater) is just as famous and impressive as the ballet, but most theater performances are in Russian, so you may not understand a lot until you work on your Russian for a while. Still, if you want to see great acting and test your Russian knowledge, by all means check out the theater, too!

In the following sections, we show how to get your tickets and what to do during the intermission.

Handy tips for ordering tickets

The technique of buying a ticket to the ballet or theater is basically the same as it is for the movie theater. Each performance hall has a **kassa** (*kah*-suh; ticket office) and a **kassir** (kuh-*seer*; cashier). You may hear **Gdye vy khotitye sidyet'?** (gdye vih khah-*tee*-tee see-*dyet'*; Where do you want to sit?) or **Kakoj ryad?** (kah-*kohy* ryat; Which row?) See the sections "Buying tickets" and "Choosing a place to sit and watch" earlier in this chapter.

Your answer to this question is a little bit different than in a movie theater. If you prefer a centrally located seat, you say **V partyerye** (f puhr-*teh*-ree; In the orchestra seats). But a Russian ballet hall is more complicated than a movie theater, and it has many other seating options you may want to consider, depending on your budget and taste:

- ✔ **lozha** (*loh*-zhuh; box seat)
- ✔ **byenuar** (bee-noo-*ahr*; lower boxes)
- ✔ **byel'etazh** (behl'-eh-*tahsh*; tier above **byenuar**)
- ✔ **yarus** (*ya*-roos; tier above **bel'ehtazh**)
- ✔ **galyeryeya** (guh-lee-*rye*-ye; the last balcony)
- ✔ **balkon** (buhl-*kohn*; balcony)

You can try your luck at ordering tickets over the phone too. If you're lucky enough to have somebody pick up the phone when you call the ticket office, and you're a male, you say **Ya khotyel by zakazat' bilyet na . . .** (ya khah-*tyel* bih zuh-kuh-*zaht'* bee-*lyet* nah; I would like to order a ticket for . . .) + the name of the performance. If you're a female, you say **Ya khotyela by zakazat' bilyet na . . .** (ya khah-*tye*-luh bih zuh-kuh-*zaht'* bee-*lyet* nah; I would like to order a ticket for . . .) + the name of the performance.

Next, you most likely hear **Na kakoye chislo?** (nah kah-*koh*-ee chees-*loh*; For what date?) Your response should begin with **na** (nah; for) followed by the date you want to attend the performance, such as **Na pyatoye maya** (nuh *pya*-tuh-ye *mah*-ye; For May 5). You can also say things like **na syegodnya** (nah see-*vohd*-nye; for today) or **na zavtra** (nuh *zahf*-truh; for tomorrow). And if you want to buy a ticket for a specific day of the week, you say **na** plus the day of the week in the accusative case. For example, "for Friday" is **na pyatnitsu** (nuh *pyat*-nee-tsoo; for Friday).

When you indicate a date, use the ordinal number and the name of the month in the genitive case. For more information on ordinal numerals, see Chapter 2. For information on months, see Chapter 11.

Things to do during the intermission

During the **antrakt** (uhn-*trahkt*; intermission), we recommend that you take a walk around the **koridor** (kuh-ree-*dohr*; hall) and look at the pictures of the past and current **aktyory** (uhk-*tyo*-rih; actors), **aktrisy** (uhk-*tree*-sih; actresses), **baleriny** (buh-lee-*ree*-nih; ballerinas), and **rezhissyory** (ree-zhih-*syo*-rih; theater directors) that are usually displayed. Another thing you may want to do is grab a bite to eat at the **bufyet** (boo-*fyet*; buffet), which is designed to make you feel that coming to the theater is a very special occasion. Typical buffet delicacies are **butyerbrody s ikroj** (boo-tehr-broht s eek-*rohy*; caviar sandwiches), **butyerbrody s kopchyonoj ryboj** (boo-tehr-broht s kuhp-*chyo*-nuhy *rih*-buhy; smoked fish sandwiches), **pirozhnyye** (pee-*rohzh*-nih-ee; pastries), **shokolad** (shuh-kah-*laht*; chocolate), and **shampanskoye** (shuhm-*pahn*-skuh-ee; champagne).

Spectators aren't allowed to wear overcoats, raincoats, or hats in the seating area. Theater-goers are expected to leave street clothing in the **gardyerob** (guhr-dee-*rohp*; cloakroom). Marching into a seating area with your coat or hat on may anger the theater attendants, who won't hesitate to express it to you quite loudly in public.

Enjoying (or just plain surviving) the Philharmonic

Are you a classical music lover? If so, then the Russian Philharmonic may be just what you're looking for. But if not, then we recommend you try to avoid the Philharmonic, even if tickets are free. If you're not used to classical music or if you can tolerate it only in limited amounts of time, going to the Philharmonic may be a very trying experience. For one thing, you have to sit almost motionless for over two hours, staring at the **orkyestr** (ahr-*kyestr*; the orchestra) or **ispol-nityel'** (ees-pahl-*nee*-teel'; performer/soloist).

Secondly, you're not allowed to talk with your friend sitting next to you, eat candy, chew gum, or produce any sound that may disturb your fellow music lovers.

When you're at the Philharmonic, you're expected to do one thing and one thing only: **slushat' muzyku!** (*sloo*-shuht' *moo*-zih-koo; to listen to the music!) Whether you actually hear the music is up to you!

Culture Club: Visiting a Museum

Russians are a nation of museum-goers. Visiting a **myzyej** (moo-*zyey*; museum) is seen as a "culture" trip. This view explains why Russian parents consider their first duty to be taking their kids to all kinds of museums on a weekend. Apart from the fact that Russian cities and even villages usually have a lot of museums, whenever Russians go abroad they immediately start looking for museums they can go to. A trip anywhere in the world should certainly contain a number of museums.

In almost every city you're likely to find the following museums to satisfy your hunger for culture:

- ✔ **Muzyej istorii goroda** (moo-*zyey* ees-*toh*-ree-ee *goh*-ruh-duh; museum of the town history)

- ✔ **Muzyej istorii kraya** (moo-*zyey* ees-*toh*-ree-ee *krah*-ye; regional history museum)

- ✔ **Istorichyeskij muzyej** (ee-stah-*ree*-chees-keey moo-*zyey*; historical museum)

- ✔ **Kartinnaya galyeryeya** (kuhr-*tee*-nuh-ye guh-lee-*rye*-ye; art gallery)

- ✔ **Etnografichyeskij muzyej** (eht-nuh-gruh-*fee*-chees-keey moo-*zyey*; ethnographic museum)

Also, you may want to visit any of the large number of Russian museums dedicated to famous and not so famous Russian **pisatyeli** (pee-*sah*-tye-lee; writers), **poety** (pah-*eh*-tih; poets), **aktyory** (uhk-*tyo*-rih; actors) and **aktrisy**

(uhk-*tree*-sih; actresses), **khudozhniki** (khoo-*dohzh*-nee-kee; artists), **uchyonyye** (oo-*choh*-nih-ee; scientists), and **politiki** (pah-*lee*-tee-kee; politicians). For example, in St. Petersburg alone, you find the A.S. Pushkin museum, F.M. Dostoyevsky museum, A.A. Akhmatova museum, and many, many more — almost enough for every weekend of the year.

In addition to the previously listed museums, you should also know that a lot of former tsar residences were converted into museums by the special decree of the new Soviet government after the October revolution of 1917. At that time, one of the main purposes of this action was to show the working people of Russia the revolting luxury the former Russian rulers lived in by exploiting their people. A lot of these museums are in St. Petersburg and its vicinity. Four of the most popular are **Zimnyj Dvoryets** (*zeem*-neey dvah-*ryets*; Winter Palace), **Lyetnij Dvoryets Pyetra Vyelikogo** (*lyet*-neey dvah-*ryets* peet-*trah* vee-*lee*-kuh-vuh; Summer Palace of Peter the Great), **Yekatirininskij Dvoryets** (yee-kuh-tee-*ree*-neens-skeey dvah-*ryets*; Catherine's Palace), and **Pavlovskij Dvoryets** (*pahv*-luhf-skeey dvah-*ryets*; Paul's Palace).

Some other words and expressions you may need in a museum are

- **ekskursiya** (ehks-*koor*-see-ye; tour)
- **ekskursovod** (ehks-koor-sah-*voht*; guide)
- **ekskursant** (ehks-koor-*sahnt*; member of a tour group)
- **putyevodityel'** (poo-tee-vah-*dee*-teel'; guidebook)
- **zal** (zahl; exhibition hall)
- **eksponat** (ehks-pah-*naht*; exhibit)
- **vystavka** (*vihs*-tuhf-kuh; exhibition)
- **ekspozitsiya** (ehks-pah-*zee*-tsih-ye; display)
- **iskusstvo** (ees-*koos*-tvuh; arts)
- **kartina** (kuhr-*tee*-nuh; painting)
- **skul'ptura** (skool'-*ptoo*-ruh; sculpture or piece of sculpture)
- **Muzyyej otkryvayetsya v . . .** (moo-*zyey* uht-krih-*vah*-eet-sye v; The museum opens at . . .)
- **Muzyyej zakryvayetsya v . . .** (moo-*zyey* zuh-krih-*vah*-eet-sye v; The museum closes at . . .)
- **Skol'ko stoyat vkhodnyye bilyety?** (*skohl'*-kuh *stoh*-eet fkhahd-*nih*-ee bee-*lye*-tih; How much do admission tickets cost?)

How Was It? Talking about Entertainment

After you've been out to the ballet, theater, museum, or a movie, you probably want to share your impressions with others. The best way to share these impressions is by using a form of the verb **nravitsya** (*nrah*-veet-sye; to like). (For details on the present tense of this verb, see Chapter 6.) To say that you liked what you saw, you may want to say **Mnye ponravilsya spyektakl'/fil'm** (mnye pahn-*rah*-veel-sye speek-*tahkl'*/feel'm; I liked the performance/movie).

If you didn't like the production, just add the particle **nye** before the verb: **Mnye nye ponravilsya spyektakl'/fil'm** (mnye nee pahn-*rah*-veel-sye speek-*tahkl'*/feel'm; I did not like the performance/movie).

If you really loved a museum you visited, you say **Mnye ochen' ponravilsya muzyej** (mnye *oh*-cheen' pahn-*rah*-veel-sye moo-*zyey*; I loved the museum).

Don't use **lyubil** (lyu-*beel*; loved) in this situation. The past tense of the verb **lyubit'** (lyu-*beet'*; to love) means "I used to love," which isn't exactly what you want to say here. To read more about the verb **lyubit',** see Chapter 8.

If you want to elaborate on your opinion about the performance or museum, you may want to use words and phrases like

- ✔ **potryasayush'ye!** (puh-tree-*sah*-yu-sh'ee; amazing!)
- ✔ **khoroshii balyet/spyektakl'/kontsyert** (khah-*roh*-shihy buh-*lyet*/speek-*tahkl'*/kahn-*tsehrt*; a good ballet/performance/concert)
- ✔ **plokhoj balyet/spyektakl'/fil'm** (plah-*khohy* buh-*lyet*/speek-*tahkl'*/feel'm; a bad ballet/performance/film)
- ✔ **Eto byl ochyen' krasivyj balyet/spyektakl'/muzyej.** (*eh*-tuh bihl *oh*-cheen' krah-*see*-vihy buh-*lyet*/speek-*tahkl'*/moo-*zyey*; It was a very beautiful ballet/performance/museum.)
- ✔ **Eto byl ochyen' skuchnyj fil'm/spyektakl'/myzyej.** (*eh*-tuh bihl *oh*-cheen' *skoosh*-nihy feel'm/speek-*tahkl'*/moo-*zyey*; It was a very boring film/performance/museum.)
- ✔ **Eto byl nyeintyeryesnyj fil'm/spyektakl'/muzyej.** (*eh*-tuh bihl nee-een-tee-*ryes*-nihy feel'm/speek-*tahkl'*/ moo-*zyey*; It wasn't an interesting film/performance/museum.)

To ask a friend whether he or she liked an event, you can say **Tyebye ponravilsya spyektakl/fil'm'?** (tee-*bye* pahn-*rah*-veel-sye speek-*tahkl'*/feel'm?; Did you like the performance/movie?)

Talkin' the Talk

 Natasha and John have just attended a classical ballet at the St. Petersburg Mariinskij Theater. As they're leaving the theater, they exchange their opinions of the performance.

Natasha: **Tyebye ponravilsya spyektakl'?**
tee-*bye* pahn-*rah*-veel-sye speek-*tahkl'*?
Did you like the performance?

John: **Ochyen'. Potryasayush'ye. Ochyen' krasivyj balyet. A tyebye?**
oh-cheen'. puh-tree-*sah*-yu-sh'ee. *oh*-cheen' kruh-*see*-vihy buh-*lyet* uh tee-*bye*?
A lot. It was amazing. Very beautiful ballet. And did you like it?

Natasha: **I mnye ochyen' ponravilsya etot spyektakl'. Solistka tantsyevala ochyen' khorosho. I dyekoratsii byli pryekrasnyye.**
ee mnye *oh*-cheen' pahn-*rah*-veel-sye. sah-*leest*-kuh tuhn-tseh-*vah*-luh *oh*-cheen' khuh-rah-*shoh*. ee dee-kah-*rah*-tsih-ee *bih*-lee pree-*krahs*-nih-ee
And I liked the performance a lot. The soloist danced very well. And the décor was wonderful.

Words to Know

A tyebye?	a tee-<u>bye</u>	And did you like it?
solistka	sah-<u>leest</u>-kuh	soloist
ochyen' khorosho	<u>oh</u>-cheen' khuh-rah-<u>shoh</u>	very good/well
dyekoratsii	dee-kah-<u>raht</u>-tsee-ee	décor
pryekrasnyye	preek-<u>rahs</u>-nih-ee	wonderful

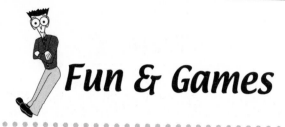

Fun & Games

Which of the following two days comes earlier during a week? Check out the correct answers in Appendix C.

1. **ponyedyel'nik, sryeda**

2. **chyetvyerg, pyatnitsa**

3. **voskryesyen'ye, vtornik**

4. **subbota, voskryesyen'ye**

Which of the two verbs — **nachinayetsya** or **nachinayet** — do you use to translate the verb "to start/to begin" in the following sentences? Check out the correct answers in Appendix C.

1. Peter begins his working day at 5 a.m.

2. The show begins at 7 p.m.

3. Dinner begins at 6 p.m.

4. The boss always begins the meeting on time.

Which of the following phrases would you probably use to express that you liked the show or performance you attended? Find the correct answers in Appendix C.

1. **Mnye ponravilsya spyektakl'.**

2. **Potryasayush'ye!**

3. **Ochyen' skuchnyj fil'm.**

4. **Nyeintyeryesnyj fil'm.**

5. **Ochyen' krasivyj balyet.**

Chapter 8

Enjoying Yourself: Recreation and Sports

. . . .

In This Chapter

▶ Discussing your hobbies

▶ Reading everything from detectives to Dostoevsky

▶ Enjoying nature

▶ Collecting things, working with your hands, and playing sports

. . . .

*T*he art of conversation isn't a forgotten skill among Russians. They love trading stories, relating their experiences, and exchanging opinions. And what's a better conversation starter than asking people about things they like to do? Go ahead and tell your new acquaintances about your sports obsession, your reading habits, or your almost complete collection of Star Wars action figures. In this chapter, we show you how to talk about your hobbies. You also discover some activities that Russians especially enjoy, and find out what to say when you're participating in them.

Shootin' the Breeze about Hobbies

Before getting to the nitty-gritty of your **khobbi** (*khoh*-bee; hobby or hobbies — the word is used for both singular and plural forms), you probably want to test the water so that you don't exhaust your vocabulary of Russian exclamations discussing Tchaikovsky with someone who prefers boxing. In the following sections, you find out how to talk about your recent experiences, your plans for the weekend, and your general likes and dislikes.

What did you do last night?

The easiest way to ask this question is

- ✔ **Chto ty dyelal vchyera vyechyerom?** (shtoh tih *dye*-luhl fchee-*rah vye*-chee-ruhm; What did you do last night?; informal singular)

- ✔ **Chto vy dyelali vchyera vyechyerom?** (shtoh vih *dye*-luh-lee fchee-*rah vye*-chee-ruhm; What did you do last night?; formal singular and plural)

When you're talking about the past, the form of the verb you use depends on the gender and the number of people you're addressing and the level of formality between you. (For more information, see Chapter 2.) The following are some of the forms of the verb *to do* that you want to be familiar with:

- ✔ **dyelal** (*dye*-luhl; did/was doing; male, informal singular)

- ✔ **dyelala** (*dye*-luh-luh; did/was doing; female, informal singular)

- ✔ **dyelali** (*dye*-luh-lee; did/were doing; formal singular and plural)

You can answer the question **Chto ty dyelal vchyera vyecherom?** with

- ✔ **Nichyego** (nee-chee-*voh*; nothing)

- ✔ **Ya byl doma** (ya bihl *doh*-muh; I was at home) if you're a male

- ✔ **Ya byla doma** (ya bih-*lah doh*-muh; I was at home) if you're a female

If you know that the person you're talking to was out, you can ask

- ✔ **Kuda ty vchyera khodil?** (koo-*dah* tih fchee-*rah* khah-*deel*; What did you do yesterday? *Literally:* Where did you go yesterday?; informal singular) when speaking to a male

- ✔ **Kuda ty vchyera khodila?** (koo-*dah* tih fchee-*rah* khah-*dee*-luh; What did you do yesterday? *Literally:* Where did you go yesterday?; informal singular) when speaking to a female

- ✔ **Kuda vy vchyera khodili?** (koo-*dah* vih fchee-*rah* khah-*dee*-lee; What did you do yesterday? *Literally:* Where did you go yesterday?; formal singular and plural)

To answer these questions, you can say:

- ✔ **Ya byl v . . .** (ya bihl v; I was in/at . . .) + a noun in the prepositional case if you're a male

- ✔ **Ya byla v . . .** (ya bih-*lah* v; I was in/at . . .) + a noun in the prepositional case if you're a female

✔ **Ya khodil v . . .** (ya khah-*deel* v; I went to . . .) + a noun in the accusative case if you're a male

✔ **Ya khodila v . . .** (ya khah-*deel*-luh v; I went to . . .) + a noun in the accusative case if you're a female

If you want to specify exactly when you did something (even if it wasn't yesterday or last night), you may want to use these phrases:

✔ **vchyera utrom** (fchee-*rah* *oot*-ruhm; yesterday morning)

✔ **vchyera vyechyerom** (fchee-*rah* *vye*-chee-ruhm; last night)

✔ **na proshloj nyedyelye** (nuh *proh*-shluhy nee-*dye*-lee; last week)

✔ **na vykhodnyye** (nuh vih-khahd-*nih*-ee; over the weekend)

What are you doing this weekend?

You may try to get the most out of your weeknights, but the weekend is the time for real adventure. Find out what your Russian friends do on the weekends using the following phrases:

✔ **Chto ty planiruyesh' dyelat' na vykhodnyye?** (shtoh tih plah-*nee*-roo-eesh' *dye*-luht' nuh vih-khahd-*nih*-ee; What are you doing this weekend? *Literally:* What do you plan to do this weekend?; informal singular)

✔ **Chto vy planiruyetye dyelat' na vykhodnyye?** (shtoh vih plan-*nee*-roo-ee-tee *dye*-luht' nuh vih-khahd-*nih*-ee; What are you doing this weekend? *Literally:* What do you plan to do this weekend?; formal singular and plural)

✔ **Chto ty obychno dyelayesh' na vykhodnyye?** (shtoh tih ah-*bihch*-nuh *dye*-luh-eesh' nuh vih-khahd-*nih*-ee; What do you usually do on the weekend?; informal singular)

✔ **Chto vy obychno dyelayetye na vykhodnyye?** (shtoh vih ah-*bihch*-nuh *dye*-luh-ee-tee nuh vih-khahd-*nih*-ee; What do you usually do on the weekend?; formal singular and plural)

✔ **Chto ty dyelayesh' syegodnya vyechyerom?** (shtoh tih *dye*-luh-eesh' see-*vohd*-nye *vye*-chee-ruhm; What are you doing tonight?; informal singular)

✔ **Chto vy dyelayetye syegodnya vyechyerom?** (shtoh vih *dye*-luh-ee-tee see-*vohd*-nye *vye*-chee-ruhm; What are you doing tonight?; formal singular and plural)

To answer these questions, you may say:

- ✔ **Ya planiruyu** (ya pluh-*nee*-roo-yu; I plan to . . .) + the imperfective infinitive of a verb

- ✔ **My planiruyem** (mih pluh-*nee*-roo-eem; We plan to . . .) + the imperfective infinitive of a verb

- ✔ **Ya budu** (ya *boo*-doo; I will . . .) + the imperfective infinitive of a verb

- ✔ **My budyem** (mih *boo*-deem; We will . . .) + the imperfective infinitive of a verb

- ✔ **Ya obychno** (ya ah-*bihch*-nuh; I usually . . .) + the imperfective verb in the first person singular ("I") form

- ✔ **My obychno** (mih ah-*bihch*-nuh; We usually . . .) + the imperfective verb in the first person singular ("I") form

For details about imperfective infinitives of verbs, see Chapter 2.

And if you don't have any particular plans, you may want to simply say **Ya budu doma** (ya *boo*-doo *doh*-muh; I'll be at home) or **My budyem doma** (mih *boo*-deem *doh*-muh; We'll be at home).

What do you like to do?

In conversation, you can easily switch from talking about your private life to discussing your general likes and dislikes, which Russians like to do a lot. To discover someone's likes or dislikes, you can ask one of the following:

- ✔ **Chyem ty lyubish' zanimat'sya?** (chyem tih *lyu*-beesh' zuh-nee-*maht*-sye; What do you like to do?; informal singular)

- ✔ **Chyem vy lyubitye zanimat'sya?** (chyem vih *lyu*-bee-tee zuh-nee-*maht*-sye; What do you like to do?; formal singular and plural)

- ✔ **Ty lyubish' . . . ?** (tih *lyu*-beesh'; Do you like . . . ?; informal singular) + the imperfective infinitive of a verb or a noun in the accusative case

- ✔ **Vy lyubitye . . . ?** (vih *lyu*-bee-tee; Do you like . . . ?; formal singular and plural) + the imperfective infinitive of a verb or a noun in the accusative case

For details about infinitives and cases, see Chapter 2.

You use the verb **lyubit'** (lyu-*beet*'; to love, to like) to describe your feelings toward almost anything, from **borsh'** (borsh'; borsht) to your significant other. Saying **Ya lyublyu gruppu "U2"** (ya lyu-*blyu* groo-poo yu-*too*; I like the band U2) isn't too strong, and this word is just right to express your feelings for your family members, too: **Ya lyublyu moyu malyen'kuyu syestru** (ya lyu-*blyu* mah-*yu* mah-*leen*'-koo-yu sees-*troo*; I love my little sister).

Just like in English, the activity you like is expressed by the infinitive of a verb after the verb **lyubit':** **Ya lyublyu chitat'** (ya lyu-*blyu* chee-*taht'*; I like to read). With nouns, however, the rule is different. To describe a person or object you love or like, put the noun in the accusative case: **Ya lyublyu muzyku** (ya lyu-*blyu moo*-zih-koo; I love music).

Table 8-1 shows you how to conjugate the verb **lyubit'** in the present tense.

Table 8-1	Conjugation of Lyubit'	
Conjugation	*Pronunciation*	*Translation*
ya lyublyu	yah lyu-*blyu*	I love/like
ty lyubish'	tih *lyu*-beesh'	You love/like (informal singular)
on/ona/ono lyubit'	on/ah-*nah*/ah-*noh lyu*-beet'	He/she/it loves/likes
my lyubim	mih *lyu*-beem	We love/like
vy lyubitye	vih *lyu*-bee-tee	You love/like (plural singular and formal)
oni lyubyat	ah-*nee lyu*-byet	They love/like

After Russians find out what you like to do, they're likely to come up with activities you can do together. To find out how to extend and respond to invitations, check out Chapter 7. And even if you have absolutely no interests in common, an invitation is still likely to follow: **Prikhoditye v gosti!** (pree-khah-*dee*-tee v *gohs*-tee; Come to visit!)

Reading All About It

An American who has traveled in Russia observed that on the Moscow metro, half the people are reading books, and the other half are holding beer bottles. But we don't agree with such a sharp division. Some Russians can be holding a book in one hand and a beer bottle in the other!

But, all joking aside, Russians are still reported to read more than any other nation in the world. So, get prepared to discuss your reading habits using phrases we introduce in the following sections.

Russian writers you just gotta know

A reading nation has to have some outstanding authors, and Russians certainly do. Russia is famous for the following writers:

- ✔ **Chekhov,** or **Chyekhov** (*cheh*-khuhf) in Russian, is up there with Shakespeare and Ibsen on the Olympus of world dramaturgy. His *Cherry Orchard* and *The Seagull* are some of the most heart-breaking comedies you'll ever see.

- ✔ **Dostoevsky,** or **Dostoyevskij** (duh-stah-*yehf*-skee) in Russian, is the reason 50 percent of foreigners decide to learn Russian. He was a highly intense, philosophical, 19th-century writer, whose tormented and yet strangely lovable characters search for truth while throwing unbelievably scandalous scenes in public places. "The Grand Inquisitor's Monologue" from his *Brothers*

Karamazov is probably the most frequently cited "favorite literary passage" among politicians all over the world.

- ✔ **Pushkin,** or **Pushkin** (*poosh*-keen) in Russian, is someone you can mention if you want to soften any Russian's heart. Pushkin did for Russian what Shakespeare did for English, and thankful Russians keep celebrating his birthday and putting up more and more of his statues in every town.

- ✔ **Tolstoy,** or **Tolstoj** (tahl-*stohy*) in Russian, was a subtle psychologist and connoisseur of the human soul. His characters are so vivid, you seem to know them better than you do your family members. Reading Tolstoy's *Anna Karenina* or *War and Peace* is the best-discovered equivalent of living a lifetime in 19th-century Russia.

Have you read it?

When you talk about reading, a handy verb to know is **chitat'** (chee-*taht'*; to read). This verb is a regular verb (see Chapter 2 for more information). Here are some essential phrases you need in a conversation about reading:

- ✔ **Ya chitayu . . .** (ya chee-*tah*-yu; I read/am reading . . .) + a noun in the accusative case

- ✔ **Chto ty chitayesh'?** (shtoh tih chee-*tah*-eesh'; What are you reading?; informal singular)

- ✔ **Chto vy chitayetye?** (shtoh vih chee-*tah*-ee-tee; What are you reading?; formal singular and plural)

- ✔ **Ty chital . . . ?** (tih chee-*tahl*; Have you read . . . ?; informal singular) + a noun in the accusative case when speaking to a male

- ✔ **Ty chitala . . . ?** (tih chee-*tah*-luh; Have you read . . . ?; informal singular) + a noun in the accusative case when speaking to a female

- ✔ **Vy chitali . . . ?** (vih chee-*tah*-lee; Have you read . . . ?; formal singular and plural) + a noun in the accusative case

What do you like to read?

So you're ready to talk about your favorite **kniga** (*knee*-guh; book) or **knigi** (*knee*-gee; books). Here are some words to outline your general preferences in literature, some of which may sound very familiar:

- ✔ **lityeratura** (lee-tee-ruh-*too*-ruh; literature)
- ✔ **proza** (*proh*-zuh; prose)
- ✔ **poyeziya** (pah-*eh*-zee-ye; poetry)
- ✔ **romany** (rah-*mah*-nih; novels)
- ✔ **povyesti** (*poh*-vees-tee; tales)
- ✔ **rasskazy** (ruhs-*kah*-zih; short stories)
- ✔ **p'yesy** (*p'ye*-sih; plays)
- ✔ **stikhi** (stee-*khee*; poems)

The conversation probably doesn't end with you saying **Ya lyublyu chitat' romany** (ya lyu-*blyu* chee-*taht'* rah-*mah*-nih; I like to read novels). Somebody will ask you: **A kakiye romany vy lyubitye?** (ah kuh-*kee*-ee rah-*mah*-nih vih *lyu*-bee-tee; And what kind of novels do you like?) To answer this question, you can simply say **Ya lyublyu** (ya lyu-*blyu*; I like . . .) plus one of the following genres:

- ✔ **sovryemyennaya proza** (suhv-ree-*mye*-nuh-ye *proh*-zuh; contemporary fiction)
- ✔ **dyetyektivy** (deh-tehk-*tee*-vih; mysteries)
- ✔ **trillyery** (*tree*-lee-rih; thrillers)
- ✔ **boyeviki** (buh-ee-vee-*kee*; action novels)
- ✔ **vyestyerny** (*vehs*-tehr-nih; Westerns)
- ✔ **istorichyeskaya proza** (ees-tah-*ree*-chees-kuh-ye *proh*-zuh; historical fiction)
- ✔ **fantastika** (fuhn-*tahs*-tee-kuh; science fiction)
- ✔ **lyubovnyye romany** (lyu-*bohv*-nih-ee rah-*mah*-nih; romance)
- ✔ **biografii** (bee-ahg-*rah*-fee-ee; biographies)
- ✔ **istorichyeskiye isslyedovaniya** (ees-tah-*ree*-chees-kee-ee ees-*lye*-duh-vuh-nee-ye; history, *Literally:* historical research)
- ✔ **myemuary** (meh-moo-*ah*-rih; memoirs)

Many Russian last names, like the famous Tolstoy and Dostoevsky, decline like adjectives. Even in their initial form, in the nominative case, they sound similar. When you talk about works by a specific author, you put the name of the author in the genitive case, and place it after the word **knigi** (*knee*-gee; books): **knigi Pushkina** (*knee*-gee *poosh*-kee-nuh; books by Pushkin). The genitive case conveys the meaning "belonging to someone, pertaining to someone, of someone." Examples include: **p'yesy Shyekspira** (*p'ye*-sih shehk-*spee*-ruh; Shakespeare's plays), and **rasskazy Chekhova** (ruhs-*kah*-zih *cheh*-khuh-vuh; short stories by Chekhov). For more on cases, see Chapter 2.

Now you're well-prepared to talk about literature, but what about the news, political commentary, and celebrity gossip? These phrases can help:

- **zhurnal** (zhoor-*nahl*; magazine)

- **gazyeta** (guh-*zye*-tuh; newspaper)

- **novosti** (*noh*-vuhs-tee; the news)

- **novosti v intyernyetye** (*noh*-vuhs-tee v een-tehr-*neh*-tee; news on the Internet)

- **stat'ya** (stuh-*t'ya*; article)

- **komiksy** (*koh*-meek-sih; comic books)

Talkin' the Talk

It's Claire's first time in a Russian library. A friendly **bibliotekar'** (beeb-lee-ah-*tye*-kuhr'; librarian) starts a conversation.

Bibliotekar':	**Vy lyubitye chitat'?** vih *lyu*-bee-tee chee-*taht'*? Do you like to read?
Claire:	**Da, ochyen' lyublyu. Osobyenno romany.** dah, *oh*-cheen' lyu-*blyu*. ah-*soh*-bee-nuh rah-*mah*-nih. Yes, I like it very much. Especially novels.
Bibliotekar':	**A kakie romany, istorichyeskiye ili dyetyektivy?** ah kuh-*kee*-ee rah-*mah*-nih, ees-tah-*ree*-chees-kee-ee ee-lee deh-tehk-*tee*-vih? And what kind of novels, historical or mysteries?
Claire:	**Bol'shye vsyego ya lyublyu fantastiku.** *bohl'*-sheh vsee-*voh* ya lyu-*blyu* fuhn-*tahs*-tee-koo. Most of all, I like science fiction.

Words to Know

osobyenno	ah-<u>soh</u>-bee-nuh	especially
istorichyeskiye	ees-tah-<u>ree</u>-chees-kee-ee	historical
dyetyektivy	deh-tehk-<u>tee</u>-vih	mystery
bol'she vsego	<u>bohl'</u>-sheh vsee-<u>voh</u>	most of all
fantastika	fuhn-<u>tahs</u>-tee-kah	science fiction

Where do you find reading materials?

The answer to where you can find reading material is easy: Pretty much any-where. At a Russian train station, you're likely to see more book and periodi-cal stands than hot dog vendors. They won't offer the best choices, though, unless you're looking for **dyetyektivy** (deh-tehk-*tee*-vih; mystery novels) or **boyeviki** (buh-ee-vee-*kee*; action novels). For more serious literature, you have to go to **knizhnij magazin** (*kneezh*-nihy muh-guh-*zeen*; bookstore) or **bibliotyeka** (beeb-lee-ah-*tye*-kuh; library). Both bookstores and libraries are divided into **otdyely** (aht-*dye*-lih; sections):

- ✔ **Otdyel khudozhyestvyennoj lityeratury** (aht-*dyel* khoo-*doh*-zhihs-tvee-nuhy lee-tee-ruh-*too*-rih; section of fiction)

- ✔ **Otdyel uchyebnoj lityeratury** (aht-*dyel* oo-*chyeb*-nuhy lee-tee-ruh-*too*-rih; section of educational materials)

- ✔ **Spravochnyj otdyel** (*sprah*-vuhch-nihy aht-*dyel*; reference section)

- ✔ **Otdyel audio i vidyeo matyerialov** (aht-*dyel* *ah*-oo-dee-uh ee *vee*-dee-uh muh-tee-*r'ya*-luhf; audio and video section)

Rejoicing in the Lap of Nature

Russians love nature. Every city in Russia has big parks where numerous urban dwellers take walks, enjoy picnics, and swim in suspiciously smelling ponds. Even more so, Russians like to get out of town and enjoy the nature in the wild. Luckily, the country's diverse geography offers a wide variety of

opportunities to do so. In the following sections, you discover how to make the most out of enjoying nature in Russian.

Enjoying the country house

The easiest route to nature is through the **dacha** (*dah*-chuh), which is a little country house not far from the city that most Russians have. **Poyekhat' na dachu** (pah-*ye*-khuht' nuh *dah*-choo; to go to the dacha) usually implies an overnight visit that includes barbecuing, dining in the fresh air, and, if you're lucky, **banya** (*bah*-nye) — the Russian-style sauna. Some phrases to use during your **dacha** experience include the following:

- ✔ **zharit' shashlyk** (*zhah*-reet' shuh-*shlihk*; to barbecue)
- ✔ **razvodit' kostyor** (ruhz-vah-*deet'* kahs-*tyor*; to make a campfire)
- ✔ **natopit' banyu** (nuh-tah-*peet'* bah-nyu; to prepare the sauna)
- ✔ **sad** (saht; orchard, garden)
- ✔ **ogorod** (uh-gah-*roht*; vegetable garden)
- ✔ **sobirat' ovosh'i** (suh-bee-*raht' oh*-vuh-sh'ee; to pick vegetables)
- ✔ **rabotat' v sadu** (ruh-*boh*-tuht' f suh-*doo*; to garden)

Picking foods in the forest

With their 73 percent of urban population, Russians like to go back to their roots and experience the kind of life where, instead of going to a store, you actually have to wander through the woods to find your food. Apparently, plenty of edible stuff is growing in the **lyes** (lyes; forest), and finding it is a fun activity similar to collecting points in a computer game. Just make sure to find out what you're about to eat before you put it in your mouth!

Things you may find in the forest include:

- ✔ **s'yedobniye griby** (s'ee-*dohb*-nih-ee gree-*bih*; edible mushrooms)
- ✔ **nyes'yedobniye griby** (nee-s'ee-*dohb*-nih-ee gree-*bih*; poisonous mushrooms)
- ✔ **yagody** (*ya*-guh-dih; berries)
- ✔ **dyeryevo** (*dye*-ree-vuh; tree)
- ✔ **dyeryev'ya** (dee-*ryev'*-ye; trees)
- ✔ **travy** (*trah*-vih; herbs)

To talk about collecting any or all of the foods in this section, use the verb **sobirat'** (suh-bee-*raht'*; to pick, to collect).

To describe your trip to the forest, use the expression **khodit' v lyes** (khah-*deet'* v lyes; to hike in the woods). And if your hiking trip involves a **kostyor** (kahs-*tyor*, campfire) and a **palatka** (puh-*laht*-kuh; tent), you can use the expression **idti v pokhod** (ee-*tee* f pah-*khoht*; to go camping).

Skiing in the Caucasus

The Caucasus, a picturesque mountainous region in the South of Russia, is easily accessible by train or by a flight into the city of Minvody, which actually stands for **minyeral'niye vody** (mee-nee-*rahl'*-nih-ee *voh*-dih; mineral waters). The reason for this unusual name is the numerous spas scattered around this beautiful area. Mineral water-based **sanatorii** (suh-nuh-*toh*-ree-ee; health care spas) and **doma otdykha** (dah-*mah oht*-dih-khuh; resorts) promise a cure for almost any health problem.

The best places to ski in the Caucasus (called **Kavkaz** in Russian) include **Dombaj** (dahm-*bahy*) and **Priyel'brus'ye** (pree-ehl'-*broo*-s'ee). The word **Priel'brus'ye** actually means "next to El'brus," with **El'brus** (ehl'-*broos*) being the highest mountain peak in Europe (according to those who consider the Caucasus a part of Europe).

Here are some phrases to help you organize your skiing adventure:

- **gora** (gah-*rah*; mountain)
- **gory** (*goh*-rih; mountains)
- **lyzhi** (*lih*-zhih; skis)
- **snoubord** (snoh-oo-*bohrd*; snowboard)
- **katat'sya na lyzhakh** (kuh-*taht*'sye nuh *lih*-zhuhkh; to ski)
- **prokat** (prah-*kaht*; rental)
- **vzyat' na prokat** (vzyat' nuh prah-*kaht*; to rent)
- **kanatnaya doroga** (kuh-*naht*-nuh-ye dah-*roh*-guh; cable cars)
- **kanatka** (kuh-*naht*-kuh; cable cars)
- **turbaza** (toor-*bah*-zuh; tourist center)
- **kryem ot zagara** (krehm uht zuh-*gah*-ruh; sunblock)

Lying around at Lake Baikal

With its picturesque cliffs, numerous islands, and crystal clear water, **Ozyero Baikal** (*oh*-zee-ruh buhy-*kahl*; Lake Baikal) is an unforgettable vacation spot. It's a little way off the beaten path — a direct flight from Moscow to Irkutsk, the nearest big city in the Baikal area, is five and a half hours long.

If you decide to embark on this adventure, having these words at your disposal makes your experience easier:

- **byeryeg** (*bye*-reek; shore)
- **plyazh** (plyash; beach)
- **ryechnoj vokzal** (reech-*nohy* vahk-*zahl*; port)
- **katyer** (*kah*-teer; boat)
- **parom** (puh-*rohm*; ferry)
- **prichal** (pree-*chahl*; pier)
- **pristan'** (*prees*-tuhn'; loading dock)
- **ostrov** (*ohs*-truhf; island)
- **bajdarka** (buhy-*dahr*-kuh; kayak)
- **rybalka** (rih-*bahl*-kuh; fishing)
- **lovit' rybu** (lah-*veet'* rih-boo; to fish)
- **plavat'** (*plah*-vuht'; to swim)
- **komary** (kuh-muh-*rih*; mosquitoes)

Taking a cruise ship down the Volga River

If you feel like enjoying some Russian waterways, but a flight all the way to Irkutsk just doesn't find its way into your schedule, a river cruise down the Volga River is an easily arranged alternative. You can get on a **tyeplokhod** (teep-lah-*khoht*; cruise ship) in any major city in Russia, including Moscow. Now, just grab a comfortable chair, relax **na palubye** (nuh *pah*-loo-bee; on the deck), and watch centuries of Russian history go by!

The Volga River has always been in the center of Russian history. The oldest cities, churches, and monasteries are located on its banks. In Russian folk songs and fairytales, the Volga is often called **matushka** (*mah*-toosh-kuh), which is an affectionate word for *mother*.

Each Volga traveler should know these words:

- ✔ **ryeka** (ree-*kah*; river)
- ✔ **ryechnoj kruiz** (reech-*nohy* kroo-*eez*; river cruise)
- ✔ **kayuta** (kuh-*yu*-tuh; ship cabin)
- ✔ **ekskursiya** (ehks-*koor*-see-ye; excursion)
- ✔ **ekskursovod** (ehks-koor-sah-*voht*; tour guide)
- ✔ **gid** (geet; tour guide)
- ✔ **monastyr'** (muh-nuh-*stihr'*; monastery)

When talking about the Volga River, you may run into confusion: Volga is not only Russia's most famous river, but also its most popular car!

Doing Things with Your Hands

Exploring natural wonders and architectural gems is fun, but so is discovering your internal treasures. In the following sections, find out how to talk about nifty things you can do with your hands. Don't be shy; your **talant** (tuh-*lahnt*; talent) deserves to be talked about.

Being crafty

If you're one of those lucky people who can create things with your hands, don't hesitate to tell Russians about it! They'll be very impressed. The following are some words you may want to know:

- ✔ **vyazat'** (veeh-*zaht'*; to knit)
- ✔ **shit'** (shiht'; to sew)
- ✔ **risovat'** (ree-sah-*vaht'*; to draw)
- ✔ **pisat' maslom** (pee-*saht' mahs*-luhm; to paint)
- ✔ **lyepit'** (lee-*peet'*; to sculpt)
- ✔ **lyepit' iz gliny** (lee-*peet'* eez *glee*-nih; to make pottery)
- ✔ **dyelat' loskutnyye odyeyala** (*dye*-luht' lahs-*koot*-nih-ee uh-dee-*ya*-luh; to quilt)

To ask someone whether he or she can do one of these crafts, use the verb **umyet'** (oo-*myet'*; can) plus the infinitive:

- **Ty umyeyesh pisat' maslom** (tih oo-*mye*-eesh' pee-*saht'* mahs-luhm; Can you paint?; informal singular)
- **Vy umyeyetye vyazat'?** (vih oo-*mye*-ee-tee vee-*zaht'*; Can you knit?; formal singular)

To answer these kinds of questions, you can say:

- **Da, ya umyeyu** (dah ya oo-*mye*-yu; Yes, I can)
- **Nyet, ya nye umyeyu** (nyet ya nee oo-*mye*-yu; No, I can't)

Playing music

Do you like **muzyka** (*moo*-zih-kuh; music)? To talk about playing a **muzykal'nyj instrumyent** (moo-zih-*kahl'*-nihy een-stroo-*myent*; musical instrument), use the verb **igrat'** (eeg-*raht'*; to play) + the preposition **na** (nah) and the name of the instrument in the prepositional case (for prepositional case endings, see Chapter 2).

Use the preposition **na** when you're talking about playing a musical instrument. Unlike in English, missing a preposition in the sentence **Ya igrayu na gitarye** (ya eeg-*rah*-yu nuh gee-*tah*-ree; I play the guitar) makes it meaningless in Russian.

You can ask the following questions:

- **Ty umyeyesh' igrat' na . . . ?** (tih oo-*mye*-eesh' eeg-*raht'* nah; Can you play . . . ?; informal) + the name of the instrument in the prepositional case
- **Vy umyeyetye igrat' na . . . ?** (vih oo-*mye*-ee-tee eeg-*raht'* nah; Can you play . . . ?; formal and plural) + the name of the instrument in the prepositional case

Some musical instruments you may want to mention include the following:

- **pianino** (pee-uh-*nee*-nuh; piano)
- **skripka** (*skreep*-kuh; violin)
- **flyejta** (*flyey*-tuh; flute)
- **klarnyet** (kluhr-*nyet*; clarinet)
- **baraban** (buh-ruh-*bahn*; drum)
- **gitara** (gee-*tah*-ruh; guitar)

> ✔ **saksofon** (suhk-sah-*fohn*; saxophone)
>
> ✔ **trombon** (trahm-*bohn*; trombone)
>
> ✔ **truba** (troo-*bah*; tuba)

Collecting Cool Stuff

If you're a proud collection owner, read through this section to find out how to talk about your hobby. These words get you started:

> ✔ **kollyektsiya** (kah-*lyek*-tsih-ye; collection)
>
> ✔ **kollyektsionyer** (kuh-leek-tsih-ah-*nyer*; collector)
>
> ✔ **marki** (*mahr*-kee; stamps)
>
> ✔ **monyeti** (mah-*nye*-tih; coins)
>
> ✔ **antikvariat** (uhn-tee-kvuh-ree-*aht*; antiques)

You can use two verbs to describe collecting something. One of them is recognizable, but rather cumbersome: **kollyektsionirovat'** (kuh-leek-tsih-ah-*nee*-ruh-vuht'; to collect). Another is more Russian and a little shorter: **sobirat'** (suh-bee-*raht'*; to collect). Here are some examples of something a collector may say:

> ✔ **Ya sobirayu marki** (ya suh-bee-*rah*-yu *mahr*-kee; I collect stamps)
>
> ✔ **A chto vy kollyektsioniruyetue?** (ah shtoh vih kuh-leek-tsih-ah-*nee*-roo-ee-tee; And what do you collect?)

Scoring with Sports

Whatever your relationship with sport is, this section equips you with the necessary tools to talk about it. To talk about playing sports, use the verb **zanimat'sya** (zuh-nee-*maht'*-sye; to engage in/to play a sport). The name of the sport after this verb should be in the instrumental case (see Chapter 2 for case details). The word for "sports" is **sport** (spohrt); it's always singular.

Zanimat'sya is a reflexive verb. That means that at the end of it, you have a little **-sya** particle that remains there no matter how you conjugate the verb. This **-sya** particle is what remained of **syebya** (see-*bya*; oneself). The use of this particle directs the action onto the speaker. Thus, **zanimat'sya** means "to engage oneself." The same verb without the **-sya** particle, **zanimat'**, means "to engage somebody else." Reflexive verbs aren't very numerous in Russian; we warn you whenever we come across them.

To conjugate the verb **zanimat'sya,** think of it as consisting of two parts: the verb **zanimat'** and **-sya.** Conjugate the verb **zanimat'** as a regular verb. Then add the particle **-sya** to the end of each conjugated form, such as **zanimayesh'sya** (zuh-nee-*mah*-eesh'-sye; you engage in). If a conjugated form of the verb ends in a vowel, then **-sya** becomes **-s',** such as in **zanimayus'** (zuh-nee-*mah*-yus'; I engage in). For more on the conjugation patterns of regular verbs, see Chapter 2.

You can ask somebody **Ty zanimayesh'sya sportom?** (tih zuh-nee-*mah*-eesh-sye *spohr*-tuhm; Do you play sports? *Literally:* Do you engage in sports?) You can answer this question by saying one of two phrases:

- **Da, ya zanimayus'** . . . (dah ya zuh-nee-*mah*-yus'; Yes, I play . . .) + the name of the sport in the instrumental case

- **Nyet, ya ne zanimayus' sportom** (nyet ya nee zuh-nee-*mah*-yus' *spohr*-tuhm; No, I don't play sports)

If you're talking about a team sport that can also be called an **igra** (eeg-*rah*; game), you can use the expression **igrat' v** (eeg-*raht'* v . . .; to play) + the name of the sport in the accusative case. For instance: **Ty igrayesh' v futbol?** (tih eeg-*rah*-eesh' f foot-*bohl*; Do you play soccer?)

Here's a list of sports you may want to talk about:

- **baskyetbol** (buhs-keet-*bohl*; basketball)

- **byejsbol** (beeys-*bohl*; baseball)

- **futbol** (foot-*bohl*; soccer)

- **vollyejbol** (vuh-leey-*bohl*; volleyball)

- **tyennis** (*teh*-nees; tennis)

- **gol'f** (gohl'f; golf)

To talk about watching a game, you can use the verb **smotryet** (smaht-*ryet'*; to watch). For more information on this verb, see Chapter 7.

Talkin' the Talk

Tom and Boris met at a party. Boris immediately starts talking about his favorite pastime, sports.

Boris:	**Ty zanimayesh'sya sportom?**
	tih zuh-nee-*mah*-eesh'-sye spohr-*tuhm*?
	Do you play sports?

Tom:	**Da, ya zanimayus' tyennisom. A ty?** dah, ya zuh-nee-*mah*-yus' *teh*-nee-suhm. uh tih? Yes, I play tennis. What about you?
Boris:	**A ya igrayu v futbol. Ty lyubish' futbol?** uh ya eeg-*rah*-yu f foot-*bohl*. tih *lyu*-beesh' foot-*bohl*? I play soccer. Do you like soccer?
Tom:	**Nye znayu. Ya nikogda nye vidyel igru.** nee *znah*-yu. ya nee-kahg-*dah* nee *vee*-deel eeg-*roo*. I don't know. I've never seen the game.
Boris:	**Pravda? Togda davaj pojdyom na match "Spartak"–"Dinamo."** *prahv*-duh? tahg-*dah* duh-*vahy* pahy-*dyom* nuh mahch spahr-*tahk* dee-*nah*-muh. Really? Let's go then to see a match between "Spartak" and "Dinamo."
Tom:	**Davaj! A kogda?** duh-*vahy*! uh kahg-*dah*? Yes, let's do it. And when?

Words to Know

Nye znayu.	nee <u>znah</u>-yoo	I don't know.
Ya nikogda nye vidyel igru.	ya nee-kahg-<u>dah</u> nee <u>vee</u>-deel eeg-<u>roo</u>	I've never seen the game.
Pravda?	<u>prahv</u>-duh	Really?
Togda davaj pojdyom na match.	tahg-<u>dah</u> duh-<u>vahy</u> pahy-<u>dyom</u> nuh mahch	Let's go then to see a match.

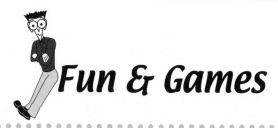

Fun & Games

- -

Match the questions in the left column with the most likely answers on the right. The correct answers are in Appendix C.

1. **Chto vy dyelayetye syegodnya vyechyerom?**

a. **Nyet, ya lyublyu tyennis.**

2. **Chto vi kollyektsionyruyetye?**

b. **Ya budu doma.**

3. **Vy igrayetye na pianino?**

c. **Ya sobirayu marki.**

4. **Vy lyubitye futbol?**

d. **Nyet, na skripkye.**

Where are you most likely to see all these things? For each group, choose an answer from the list below. The correct answers are in Appendix C.

1. **Knigi, zhurnaly, gazyety, otdyel audio i vidyeo matyerialov**

2. **Lyzhi, snoubordy, kanatka, gory**

3. **Katyer, ostrov, parom, baidarka**

a. **Ozyero Baikal**   b. **Kavkaz**   c. **knizhnij magazin**

What do they like to do? Look at this list of famous people and choose their favorite activities from the list on the right.

Vanessa Mae . . .

lyubit pisat' maslom

Renoir . . .

lyubit igrat' na gitarye

Michelangelo . . .

lyubit pisat' romany

Tolstoy . . .

lyubit igrat' na skripkye

Santana . . .

lyubit lyepit'

- -

Chapter 9

Talking on the Phone and Sending Mail

*T*elephones have become an indispensable part of our busy lives. Thanks to modern technology, we can now talk on the phone almost anywhere. In this chapter, you discover the words and expressions you need when using a telephone. You find out basic phone vocabulary, such as different parts of the phone, and we provide you with the tips on how to start, conduct, and conclude your telephone conversations. We also tell you the basics of sending letters, e-mails, and faxes.

Ringing Up Telephone Basics

Before you find out how to make a call, knowing a little bit about the phone itself is helpful. In the following sections, we give you some basic vocabulary related to phones and describe the different types of phones and phone calls.

Brushing up on phone vocabulary

You need to know a number of important words associated with the use of the **tyelyefon** (tee-lee-*fohn*; telephone). When somebody wants to talk to you, he or she may want to **zvonit'** (zvah-*neet'*; to call) you. The caller needs to **nabirat'** (nuh-bee-*raht'*; to dial) your **nomyer tyelyefona** (*noh*-meer tee-lee-*foh*-nuh; telephone number), and when the call goes through, you hear a **zvonok** (zvah-*nohk*, ring).

The main part of the telephone is the **trubka** (*troop*-kuh; receiver). On your landline, the **trubka** rests on the **tyelyefonnyj apparat** (tee-lee-*fohn*-nihy uh-puh-*raht*; the body of the phone).

You can do a lot of different things with the **trubka.** You can **podnimat' trubku** (puhd-nee-*maht' troop*-koo; to pick up the receiver), **vyeshat' trubku** (*vye*-shuht' *troop*-koo; to hang up the receiver), or **klast' trubku** (klahst' *troop*-koo; to put down the receiver). Other words related to phones include

- ✔ **knopka** (*knohp*-kuh; button)
- ✔ **gudok** (goo-*dohk*; beep, tone)
- ✔ **dolgij gudok** (*dohl*-geey goo-*dohk*; dial tone, *Literally:* long tone)
- ✔ **korotkiye gudki** (kah-*roht*-kee-ee goot-*kee*; busy signal, *Literally:* short tones)
- ✔ **kod goroda** (koht *goh*-ruh-duh; area code)
- ✔ **tyelyefonnaya kniga** (tee-lee-*fohn*-nuh-ye *knee*-guh; telephone book)

You also need to be able to give other people your phone number and to understand the phone numbers dictated to you. Usually, Russians give phone numbers in chunks. For instance, if your phone number is 123-45-67, you say it as **sto dvadtsat' tri, sorok pyat', shyestdyesyat' syem'** (stoh *dvaht*-tsuht' tree, *soh*-ruhk pyat', shees-dee-*syat'* syem; one hundred twenty-three, forty-five, sixty-seven).

Distinguishing different types of phones

Recent advances in technology have brought many different types of phones. In addition to the standard landline, or **tyelyefon,** most people today in Russia have **sotovye tyelyefony** (*soh*-tuh-vih-ee tee-lee-*foh*-nih; cellular phones), which are also called **mobil'nye tyelyefony** (mah-*beel'*-nih-ee tee-lee-*foh*-nih; mobile phones), **trubki** (*troop*-kee; *Literally:* receivers), or **mobil'niki** (mah-*beel'*-nee-kee; mobile phones). The singular forms of these words are **sotovyj tyelyefon** (*soh*-tuh-vihy tee-lee-*fohn*; cellular phone), **mobil'nyj tyelyefon** (mah-*beel'*-nihy tee-lee-*fohn*; mobile phone), **trubka** (*troop*-kuh; mobile phone, *Literally:* receiver) and **mobil'nik** (mah-*beel'*-neek; mobile phone).

Other specific types of phones include

- ✔ **diskovyj tyelyefon** (*dees*-kuh-vihy tee-lee-*fohn*; rotary phone)
- ✔ **knopochnyj tyelyefon** (*knoh*-puhch-nihy tee-lee-*fohn*; touch-tone phone)
- ✔ **byesprovodnoj tyelyefon** (bees-pruh-vahd-*nohy* tee-lee-*fohn*; cordless phone)

If you're not at home and you don't have a cell phone with you, look for what Russians call a **tyelyefonnaya budka** (tee-lee-*fohn*-nuh-ye *boot*-kuh; telephone booth), which is not always an easy task. Have you noticed that with the arrival of cellular phones, telephone booths have become an almost extinct species? Well, telephone booths were a dying species in Russia even before cell phones, mostly because the booth phones usually didn't work!

Our recommendation: When in Russia, try to have a reliable cell phone with you at all times. You have to remember, though, that the cell phone you use at home may not work in Russia unless you purchase a special card to insert into it that enables you to use it abroad. Another way to solve the problem is to just get a new cell phone in Russia.

Knowing different kinds of phone calls

If you call somebody in your calling area, you make a **myestnyj zvonok** (*myest*-nihy zvah-*nohk*; local call), and you aren't charged. If the person or institution you call is in a different city, you make a **myezdugorodnyj zvonok** (myezh-doo-gah-*rohd*-nihy zvah-*nohk*; long-distance call, *Literally:* intercity). If you want to call back home from Russia, you make a **myezhdunarodnyj zvonok** (myezh-doo-nuh-*rohd*-nihy zvah-*nohk*; international call).

Russia has no collect or operator-assisted calls. So when you're in Russia and you want to make a call, be sure to have a Russian-speaking friend around!

Dialing It In and Making the Call

When you want to make a phone call, you can't translate your desire into reality without first dialing the number of the person or institution you're calling. In order to **nabirat' nomyer** (nuh-bee-*raht' noh*-meer; to dial the number), use a **tsifyerblat** (tsih-feer-*blaht*; dial-plate), which, in many Russian homes, is still rotary rather than a push button. To help you handle this task, we provide you with the conjugation of the verb **nabirat'** in the present tense in Table 9-1.

Table 9-1	Conjugation of Nabirat'	
Conjugation	*Pronunciation*	*Translation*
ya nabirayu	ya nuh-bee-*rah*-yu	I dial or I am dialing
ty nabirayesh'	tih nuh-bee-*rah*-eesh'	You dial or You are dialing (informal singular)

(continued)

Table 9-1 *(continued)*

Conjugation	Pronunciation	Translation
on/ona nabirayet	ohn/ah-*nah* nuh-bee-*rah*-eet	He/she dials or He/she is dialing
my nabirayem	mih nuh-bee-*rah*-eem	We dial or We are dialing
vy nabirayetye	vih nuh-bee-*rah*-ee-tee	You dial or You are dialing (formal singular and plural)
oni nabirayut	ah-*nee* nuh-bee-*rah*-yut	They dial or They are dialing

Russian makes a grammatical distinction between calling a person, calling an institution, and calling a different city or a country. The following rules apply (see Chapter 2 for more details about cases):

✔ If you're calling a person, use the dative case, as in **Ya khochu zvonit' Natashye** (ya khah-*choo* zvah-*neet'* nuh-*tah*-shih; I want to call Natasha).

✔ If you're calling an institution, after the verb, use the preposition **v** or **na** + the accusative case to indicate the institution you're calling, as in **zvonit' na rabotu** (zvah-*neet'* nuh ruh-*boh*-too; to call work) or **zvonit' v magazin** (zvah-*neet'* v muh-guh-*zeen*; to call a store).

✔ If you're calling a foreign country or another city, after the verb, use **v** + the accusative form of the city or country you're calling, as in **zvonit' v Amyeriku** (zvah-*neet'* v uh-*mye*-ree-koo; to call the U.S.).

Unfortunately, **zvonit'** is nothing but an infinitive, and you can't do much with infinitives if you intend to engage in serious conversation about telephone matters. So we thought it would be a good idea to provide you with the present tense of this important verb in Table 9-2.

Table 9-2   Conjugation of Zvonit'

Conjugation	Pronunciation	Translation
ya zvonyu	ya zvah-*nyu*	I call or I am calling
ty zvonish'	tih zvah-*neesh*	You call or You are calling (informal singular)
on/ona zvonit	ohn/ah-*nah* zvah-*neet*	He/she calls or He/she is calling
my zvonim	mih zvah-*neem*	We call or We are calling

Conjugation	Pronunciation	Translation
vy zvonitye	vih zvah-*nee*-tee	You call or You are calling (formal singular and plural)
oni zvonyat	ah-*nee* zvah-*nyat*	They call or They are calling

Now, imagine that you head to the phone and pick up the receiver. If you hear **dolgiye gudki** (*dohl*-gee-ee goot-*kee*; long zoom), it means that the phone is **svobodyen** (svah-*boh*-deen; not busy), and you need to be patient until somebody answers the phone. While you're waiting for somebody to answer, you may think to yourself, **Nikto nye podkhodit k tyelyefonu** (neek-*toh* nee paht-*khoh*-deet k tee-lee-*foh*-noo; Nobody is picking up the phone).

After waiting for a couple of minutes (depending on the amount of patience you have), you may say **Nikto nye podoshol k tyelyefonu** (neek-*toh* nee puh-dah-*shohl* k tee-lee-*foh*-noo; Nobody answered the phone).

If the person you're calling is already talking on the phone with somebody else, you hear **korotkiye gudki** (kah-*roht*-kee-ee goot-*kee*; busy signal, *Literally:* short tones). This signal means the phone is busy, and you need to **povyesit' trubku** (pah-*vye*-seet' *troop*-koo; to hang up) and **pyeryezvonit'** (pee-ree-zvah-*neet'*; to call back). See the next section for details on what to do when you reach the person you want to speak to.

Arming Yourself with Basic Telephone Etiquette

Every culture has its own telephone etiquette, and Russia is no exception. In the following sections, you discover how to ask for the person you want to speak to, what you may hear in response, and how to leave a message with a person or an answering machine.

Saving time by not introducing yourself

When you make a phone call in Russia, you may get the impression that the person who answers is an extremely impatient individual who can't afford the luxury of wasting time answering the phone. That's why the person's **Alyo!** (uh-*lyo*; Hello!) — a standard way to answer the phone — may sound abrupt, unfriendly, or even angry. Don't waste time introducing yourself (even if it's a business call). Hurry up and tell the person your business right away. You may also hear just **Da** (dah; Yes) or **Slushayu** (*sloo*-shuh-yu; I'm listening).

Asking for the person you want to speak to

In English, you often say something like "Is John there?" Not so in Russian. In fact, a Russian may not even understand what you mean by that question. Instead, get to your request right away, using the phrase **Mozhno . . .** (*mohzh*-nuh; May I speak to . . .) + the name of the person you want to talk to. If you want to talk to a woman named **Natalya Ivanovna,** you say **Mozhno Natalyu Ivanovnu?** (*mohzh*-nuh nuh-*tahl'*-yu ee-*vah*-nuhv-noo; Can I talk to Natalya Ivanovna?)

Note that you have to use the name of the person you want to talk to in the accusative case. That's because what you're saying is an abbreviated **Mozhno pozvat' k tyelyefonu Natalyu Ivanovnu** (*mohzh*-nuh pahz-*vaht'* k tee-lee-*foh*-noo nuh-*tahl'*-yu ee-*vah*-nuhv-noo; Can you call to the phone Natalya Ivanovna?), and the verb **pozvat'** (pahz-*vaht'*; to call) requires that the noun after it is used in the accusative case. (For more on the accusative case, see Chapter 2.) You can make this phrase more polite by adding the phrase **Bud'tye dobry** (*bood'*-tee dahb-*rih*; Will you be so kind) at the beginning.

Anticipating different responses

Here are some of the more common things you may hear in response after you ask for the person you want to speak to:

- ✔ If you call somebody at home and he or she is not at home, you most likely hear **Yego/yeyo nyet doma** (ee-*voh*/ee-*yo* nyet *doh*-muh; He/she is not at home).

- ✔ If the person you call *is* at home but he or she is not the one who answered the phone, you hear **Syejchas** (see-*chahs*; Hold on) or **Syejchas pozovu** (see-*chahs* puh-zah-*voo*; Hold on, I'll get him/her).

- ✔ When the person you want finally answers the phone (or if he or she actually picked up the phone when you called), he or she will say **Alyo** (uh-*lyo*; Hello) or **Slushayu** (*sloo*-shuh-yu; Speaking) or simply **Da** (dah; Yes).

- ✔ You probably have the wrong number if you hear **Kogo?** (kah-*voh*; Whom?) If the person knows you called the wrong number, you most likely hear **Vy nye tuda popali** (vih nee too-*dah* pah-*pah*-lee; You dialed the wrong number).

  You can also check to make sure you dialed the right number by saying something like **Eto pyat'sot dyevyanosto vosyem' sorok pyat' dvadtsat odin?** (*eh*-tuh peet-*soht* dee-vee-*nohs*-tuh *voh*-seem' *soh*-ruhk pyat' *dvaht*-tsuht' ah-*deen*; Is this five nine eight four five two one? *Literally:* Is this five hundred ninety-eight forty-five twenty-one?) If you dialed another number, you may hear **Nyet, vy nyepravil'no nabirayete** (nyet vih nee-*prah*-veel'-nuh nuh-bee-*rah*-ee-tee; No, you've dialed the wrong number).

Talkin' the Talk

 Jack met Boris at a party. Boris gave Jack his phone number. It's Sunday night and Jack decides to call his new friend. **Zhensh'ina** (*zhehn*-sh'ee-nuh; a woman) answers the phone and it looks like Jack dialed the wrong number.

Zhensh'ina: **Alyo!**
uh-*lyo*!
Hello!

Jack: **Mohzno Borisa?**
mohzh-nuh bah-*ree*-suh?
Can I talk to Boris?

Zhensh'ina: **Kogo?**
kah-*voh*?
Who?

Jack: **Borisa.**
bah-*ree*-suh.
Boris.

Zhensh'ina: **Zdyes' takikh nyet.**
zdyes' tuh-*keekh* nyet.
Literally: There are no such people here.

Jack: **Izvinitye, ya nye ponyal. Chto vy skazali?**
eez-vee-*nee*-tee ya nee *poh*-neel. shtoh vih skuh-*zah*-lee?
Sorry, I did not understand. What did you say?

Zhensh'ina: **Molodoj chyelovyek, ya skazala chto zdyes' takikh nyet! Vy nye tuda popali.**
muh-lah-*dohy* chee-lah-*vyek*, ya skuh-*zah*-luh shtoh zdyes' tuh-*keekh* nyet! vih nee too-*dah* puh-*pah*-lee.
Young man, I said there is no Boris here. You dialed the wrong number.

Jack: **Nye tuda popal?**
nee too-*dah* pah-*pahl*?
I got the wrong number?

Zhensh'ina: **Molodoj chyelovyek, kakoj tyelyefon vy nabirayete? Kakoj nomyer tyelyefona vy nabirayetye?**
muh-lah-*dohy* chee-lah-*vyek*, kuh-*kohy* tee-lee-*fohn* vih nuh-bee-*rah*-ee-tee? kuh-*kohy* *noh*-meer tee-lee-*foh*-nuh vih nuh-bee-*rah*-ee-tee?

Young man, what telephone are you dialing? What phone number are you dialing?

Jack: **Ya nabirayu dvyesti sorok vosyem' dvyenadtsat' dyevyanosto tri.**
ya nuh-bee-*rah*-yu *dvyes*-tee *soh*-ruhk *voh*-seem' dvee-*naht*-tsuht' dee-vee-*nohs*-tuh tree.
I am dialing 248-12-93.

Zhensh'ina: **A eto dvyesti sorok vosyem' dvyenadtsat' dyevyanosto dva.**
uh *eh*-tuh *dvyes*-tee *soh*-ruhk *voh*-seem' dvee-*naht*-tsuht' dee-vee-*nohs*-tuh dvah.
And this is 248-12-92.

Jack: **Oy, izvinitye!**
ohy eez-vee-*nee*-tee!
Oh, sorry.

Zhensh'ina: **Nichyego.**
nee-chee-*voh*.
That's okay.

Words to Know

Zdyes' takikh nyet.	zdyes' tuh-<u>keekh</u> nyet	There's nobody by that name here.
Izvinitye.	eez-vee-<u>nee</u>-tee	Sorry.
Ya nye ponyal.	ya nee <u>poh</u>-neel	I didn't understand.
Chto vy skazali?	shtoh vih skuh-<u>zah</u>-lee	What did you say?
Nye tuda popal?	nee too-<u>dah</u> pah-<u>pahl</u>	I got the wrong number?
Kakoj tyelyefon vy nabirayetye?	kuh-<u>kohy</u> tee-lee-<u>fohn</u> vih nuh-bee-<u>rah</u>-ee-tee	What telephone are you dialing?
Kakoj nomyer tyelyefona vy nabirayete?	kuh-<u>kohy</u> <u>noh</u>-meer tee-lee-<u>foh</u>-nuh vih nuh-bee-<u>rah</u>-ee-tee	What number are you dialing?

Leaving a message with a person

If you call somebody and the person isn't available, you probably hear one of these phrases:

- **A kto yego sprashivayet?** (uh ktoh ee-*voh* sprah-shih-vuh-eet; And who is asking for him?)

- **A kto yeyo sprashivayet?** (uh ktoh ee-*yo* sprah-shih-vuh-eet; And who is asking for her?)

- **A chto yemu pyeryedat'?** (uh shtoh ee-*moo* pee-ree-*daht'*; Can I take a message?) if the person you're leaving a message for is a man

- **A chto yej pyeryedat'?** (uh shtoh yey pee-ree-*daht'*; Can I take a message?) if the person you're leaving a message for is a woman

When asked who is calling, say: **Eto zvonit** + your name (*eh*-tuh zvah-*neet*; This is . . . calling). Then you may simply want to give your phone number and say **Spasibo** (spuh-*see*-buh; thank you).

To ask to leave a message, begin your request with **A vy nye mozhyetye yemu/yey pyeryedat'?** (uh vih nee-*moh*-zhih-tee ee-*moo*/yey pee-ree-*daht'*; Can I leave a message for him/her?)

No matter what your message is, it should begin with the phrase **Pyeryedajte pozhalujsta . . .** (pee-ree-*dahy*-tee pah-*zhahl*-stuh; Please tell him/her . . .) Most likely, you want to say

- **Pyeryedajte pozhalujsta chto zvonil** + your name (pee-ree-*dahy*-tee pah-*zhahl*-stuh shtoh zvah-*neel*; Please tell him/her that . . . called) if you are a man

- **Pyeryedajte pozhalujsta chto zvonila** + your name (pee-ree-*dahy*-tee pah-*zhahl*-stuh shtoh zyah-*nee*-luh; Please tell him/her that . . . called) if you are a woman

Talkin' the Talk

Kira and Vyera are school friends. Kira calls Vyera to suggest going to the movies together. Vyera's mother, Olga Nikolayevna, answers the phone.

Olga Nikolayevna:	**Alyo!** uh-*lyo*! Hello!
Kira:	**Mozhno Vyeru?** *mohzh*-nuh *vye*-roo? Can I talk to Vyera?

Olga Nikolayevna:	**Vyery nyet doma. A kto yeyo sprashiv-ayet? Eto yeyo mama.** *vye*-rih nyet *doh*-muh. uh ktoh ee-*yo* sprah-shih-vuh-eet? *eh*-tuh ee-*yo mah*-muh. Vyera is not at home. And who is it? This is her mother speaking.
Kira:	**Eto yeyo podruga Kira. Zdravstvujtye! Vy nye znayete gdye ona?** *eh*-tuh ee-*yo* pahd-*roo*-guh *kee*-ruh. *zdrahs*-tvooy-tee! vih nee *znah*-ee-tee gdye ah-*nah*? It's her friend Kira. Hello! Do you happen to know where she is?
Olga Nikolayevna:	**A, Kira? Kira, a Vyera poshla v bassyejn.** ah *kee*-ruh? *kee*-ruh, uh *vye*-ruh pahsh-*lah* v buh-*seh*-een. Oh, Kira? Kira, Vyera went to the swimming pool.
Kira:	**V bassyejn? Kogda ona budyet doma?** v buh-*seh*-een? kahg-*dah* ah-*nah boo*-deet *doh*-muh? To the swimming pool? When will she be home?
Olga Nikolayevna:	**Ona dolzhna vyernut'sya cheryez polchasa. Mozhyet byt' chto-nibud' pyeryedat'?** ah-*nah* dahl-*zhnah* veer-*noot*'-sye chee-rees puhl-chuh-*sah*. *moh*-zhit biht' *shtoh*-nee-boot' pee-ree-*daht*'? She should be back in half an hour. Would you like to leave a message?
Kira:	**Nyet, spasibo. Ya pyeryezvonyu.** nyet spuh-*see*-buh. ya pee-reez-vah-*nyu*. No, thanks. I will call her back.
Olga Nikolayevna:	**Nu, khorosho. Ya yej skazhu chto ty zvonila.** noo khuh-rah-*shoh*. ya *yey* skuh-*zhoo* shtoh tih zvah-*nee*-luh. Okay. I will tell her that you called.
Kira:	**Spasibo.** spuh-*see*-buh. Thanks.

Words to Know

Vy nye znayetye gdye ona?	vih nee <u>znah</u>-ee-tee gdye ah-<u>nah</u>	Do you happen to know where she is?
Kogda ona budyet doma?	kahg-<u>dah</u> ah-<u>nah</u> <u>boo</u>-deet <u>doh</u>-muh	When will she be home?
Ona dolzhna vyernut'sya	ah-<u>nah</u> dahl-<u>zhnah</u> veer-<u>noot'</u>-sye	She should be back . . .
Mozhyet byt' chto-nibud' pyeryedat'?	<u>moh</u>-zhit biht' <u>shtoh</u>-nee-boot' pee-ree-<u>daht'</u>	Would you like to leave a message?
Ya pyeryezvonyu.	ya pee-reez-vah-<u>nyu</u>	I'll call back.
Ya yej skazhu, chto ty zvonila.	ya yey skuh-<u>zhoo</u> shtoh tih zvah-<u>nee</u>-luh	I will tell her that you called.

Talking to an answering machine

Avtootvyetchiki (uhf-tuh-aht-*vyet*-chee-kee; answering machines) are still relatively rare in Russian homes. But just in case you get an **avtootvyetchik** (answering machine), the first thing you'll probably hear is **Zdravstvujtye, nas nyet doma. Ostav'tye, pozhalujsta soobsh'yeniye poslye gudka.** (*zdrah*-stvooy-tee, nahs nyet *doh*-muh. ahs-*tahf*-tee, pah-*zhahl*-stuh suh-ahp-*sh'ye*-nee-ee *pohs*-lee goot-*kah*; Hello, we're not home. Please leave your message after the beep.)

On a cell phone answering machine, you're likely to hear a slightly different message than on a regular answering machine: **Abonyent nye dostupyen. Ostav'tye soobsh'yeniye poslye signala.** (uh-bah-*nyent* nee dahs-*too*-peen ahs-*tahf*-tee suh-ahp-*sh'ye*-nee-ee *pohs*-lee seeg-*nah*-luh; The person you are calling is not available. Leave a message after the beep.)

When leaving a message, you can say something along these lines: **Zdravstvujtye. Eto** + your name. **Pozvonitye mnye pozhalujsta. Moj nomyer tyelyefona** + your phone number (*zdrah*-stvooy-tee. *eh*-tuh . . . puhz-vah-*nee*-tee mnye pah-*zhal*-stuh. moy *noh*-meer tee-lee-*foh*-nuh . . . ; Hello! This is . . . Call me please. My phone number is . . .)

Sending a Letter, a Fax, or an E-mail

Strange as it may seem today in the age of e-mail and cell phones, people still sometimes write and send **pis'ma** (*pees'*-muh; letters).

The imperfective verb **posylat'** (puh-sih-*laht'*; to send) and its perfective counterpart **poslat'** (pahs-*laht'*) have different patterns of conjugation. While **posylat'** is a nice regular verb and **poslat'** has nothing special about it in the past tense, it has a peculiar pattern of conjugation in the future tense, shown in Table 9-3. You may need to know it so you can promise your new Russian friends that you'll send them letters, e-mail, and faxes. (Check out Chapter 2 for more about verbs in general, including imperfective and perfective verbs.)

Table 9-3	Conjugation of Poslat' in the Future Tense	
Conjugation	*Pronunciation*	*Translation*
ya poshlyu	ya pahsh-*lyu*	I will send
ty poshlyosh'	tih pahsh-*lyosh'*	You will send (informal singular)
on/ona poshlyot	ohn/ah-nah pahsh-*lyot*	He/she will send
my poshlyom	mih pahsh-*lyom*	We will send
vy poshlyotye	vih pah-*shlyo*-tee	You will send (formal singular and plural)
oni poshlyut	ah-*nee* pahsh-*lyut*	They will send

Just as in English, when sending written correspondence in Russian, it's customary to address the person you're writing to with the word "dear":

✔ **dorogoj** (duh-rah-*gohy*; dear; masculine) + the person's name

✔ **dorogaya** (duh-rah-*gah*-ye; dear; feminine) + the person's name

✔ **dorogiye** (duh-rah-*gee*-ee; dear; plural) + the people's names

In more formal situations, you should also include the date in upper left-hand corner. (For more info on dates, see Chapter 11.)

The close of your letter may include the standard **vash** (vahsh; yours; formal) or **tvoj** (tvohy; yours; informal) plus your name. Or you use one of the following phrases, depending on your intention and relationship with the recipient:

✔ **s uvazheniyem** (s oo-vuh-*zheh*-nee-eem; respectfully)

✔ **s lyubov'yu** (s lyu-*bohv'*-yu; with love)

✔ **tseluyu** (tsih-*loo*-yu; love, *Literally:* I kiss you)

When you talk about **imyeil** (ee-*meh*-eel; e-mail) and **faks** (fahks; fax), use the same verb pair of **posylat'** and **poslat'** (to send) as you do when you talk about letters. For example, suppose you want to promise your friend that you'll send him an e-mail; you simply say **Ya poshlyu tyebye imejl** (ya pahsh-*lyu* tee-*bye* ee-*meh*-eel; I'll e-mail you). If you promise to send him a fax, you say **Ya poshlyu tyebye faks** (ya pahsh-*lyu* tee-*bye* fahks; I'll send you a fax). You also use the same verb pair when you attach documents to your e-mail. **Prikryeplyeniye** (pree-kree-*plye*-nee-ee) is the Russian (and very clumsy-sounding) equivalent for the English word "attachment."

If you want to ask somebody what his or her e-mail address is, just say **Kakoj u vas imyeil?** (kuh-*kohy* oo vahs ee-*meh*-eel; What is your e-mail address? *Literally:* What is your e-mail?) But before you ask this question, you may want to make sure that this person has an e-mail account by asking **U vas yest' imyeil?** (oo vas yest' ee-*meh*-eel; *Literally:* Do you have e-mail?)

Other words and expressions associated with correspondence include

- ✔ **pis'mo** (pees'-*moh*; letter)
- ✔ **pochtovyj yash'ik** (pahch-*toh*-vihy *ya*-sh'eek; mailbox)
- ✔ **pochta** (*pohch*-tuh; post office)
- ✔ **nomyer faksa** (*noh*-meer *fahk*-suh; fax number)
- ✔ **prochitat' imyejly** (pruh-chee-*taht'* ee-*mehy*-lih; to check your e-mail, *Literally:* to read e-mails)

All the words in this section are helpful when you're at the office; for more details about working at an office, see Chapter 10.

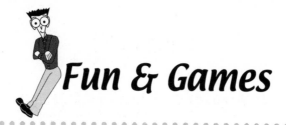

Fun & Games

Which of the following words and expressions indicate types of phones? Find the answers in Appendix C.

1. **mobil'nik**

2. **knopochnyj tyelyefon**

3. **prikryeplyeniye**

4. **pis'mo**

5. **trubka**

Put the following telephone dialogue in the right order (the right answers are in Appendix C):

a. **Mariny nyet doma. A kto yeyo sprashivayet?**

b. **Khorosho.**

c. **Eto Pyetya. Pyeryedajtye pozhalujsta chto zvonil Pyetya.**

d. **Mozhno Marinu?**

Match the Russian equivalents on the left for the English phrases on the right. See Appendix C for the correct answers.

1. **Mozhno Lyenu?**	a. Can I take a message?
2. **Yeyo nyet doma.**	b. Can I talk to Lena?
3. **Vy nye tuda popali.**	c. She's not at home.
4. **A chto yej pyeryedat'?**	d. Wrong number!

Chapter 10

Around the House and at the Office

As a Russian proverb says, **v gostyakh khorosho, a doma luchshye** (v gahs-*tyakh* khuh-rah-*shoh*, ah *doh*-muh *looch*-shih; East or West, home is best. *Literally:* It's good to be a guest, but it's better to be home). In this chapter, we show you how to set up a home in Russian, from getting exactly what you want from your real estate agent to decorating your new place. And so you can afford to set up your Russian home just the way you want it, we also tell you how to find and hold a job, all in Russian.

Hunting for an Apartment or a House

Finding an apartment or a house is stressful enough in English. Are you looking for a good view or a central location? What's more important: a big kitchen or hardwood floors? And how squeaky are those hardwood floors? Equip yourself with phrases introduced in the following sections, and good luck in your hunt for a home!

Talking about an apartment

A Russian **kvartira** (kvuhr-*tee*-ruh; apartment) is generally smaller than the apartments you may be used to. For example, **odnokomnatnaya** (uhd-nah-*kohm*-nuht-nuh-ye) **kvartira** literally means one-room apartment. You may be tempted to think of it as a one-bedroom apartment, but watch out! While the

one-bedroom apartment that you're thinking of has a living room and, possibly, a dining room, **odnokomnatnaya kvartira** doesn't. It has, literally, one room, and a kitchen (which is usually used as a dining room, no matter how tiny it is). So, a more accurate equivalent for a Russian **odnokomnatnaya kvartira** is "a studio apartment."

The most common type of an apartment for rent is the **odnokomnatnaya kvartira.** If you like to live large, you may want to look at a **dvukhkomnatnaya kvartira** (dvookh-*kohm*-nuht-nuh-ye kvuhr-*tee*-ruh; two-room apartment) or even a **tryokhkomnatnaya kvartira** (tryokh-*kohm*-nuht-nuh-ye kvuhr-*tee*-ruh; three-room apartment). Some other phrases you use and hear when talking about an apartment are:

- ✔ **snyat' kvartiru** (snyat' kvuhr-*tee*-roo; to rent an apartment)

- ✔ **sdat' kvartiru** (zdaht' kvuhr-*tee*-roo; to rent out an apartment)

- ✔ **kvartira s myebyel'yu** (kvuhr-*tee*-ruh s *mye*-bee-l'yu; furnished apartment)

- ✔ **kvartira na pyervom etazhye** (kvuhr-*tee*-ruh nuh *pyer*-vuhm eh-tuh-*zheh*; a first-floor apartment)

- ✔ **kvartira na vtorom etazhye** (kvuhr-*tee*-ruh nuh ftah-*rohm* eh-tuh-*zheh*; a second-floor apartment)

Although Russians do use the word **ryenta** (*ryen*-tuh; rent), it isn't usually used to talk about private apartments. To inquire about the price of an apartment, ask about **oplata za kvartiru** (ahp-*lah*-tuh zuh kvuhr-*tee*-roo; payment for the apartment) or **stoimost' prozhivaniya v myesyats** (*stoh*-ee-muhst' pruh-zhih-*vah*-nee-ye v *mye*-seets; cost of living per month). When you make your payments, use the expression **platit' za kvartiru** (pluh-*teet'* zuh kvuhr-*tee*-roo; pay for the apartment).

In big cities like Moscow and St. Petersburg, you can probably find an apartment on the Internet. In other places, you may have to resort to good old newspaper ads. Look for the section **Ob'yavleniya** (ahb'-eev-*lye*-nee-ye; classified). You have several ways to say "apartments for rent" in Russian. Any of the following is likely to pop up in the newspaper you're looking at:

- ✔ **kvartiry v nayom** (kvuhr-*tee*-rih v nuh-*yom*; apartments to rent)

- ✔ **aryenda kvartir** (uh-*ryen*-duh kvuhr-*teer*; rent of apartments)

- ✔ **sdayu** (sduh-*yu*; *Literally:* I am renting out)

- ✔ **snyat' zhil'yo** (snyat' zhihl'-*yo*; *Literally:* to rent a place)

The ads you find are probably saturated with abbreviations such as **kmn** for **komnata** (*kohm*-nuh-tuh; room) and **m.** for **metro**, or **stantsiya myetro** (*stahn*-tsih-ye meet-*roh*; subway station). Because the metro is such a prominent means of getting around, Russians use names of metro stations to describe location. Thus, if the ad says **m. "Tverskaya,"** the apartment is located next to metro station **"Tverskaya"** — downtown Moscow!

CULTURAL WISDOM

In close quarters: Communal living

Although scarce in number, **kommunalki** (kuh-moo-*nahl*-kee; communal apartments) still exist in some Russian cities. **Kommunalki** came into being during the Soviet revolution, when huge and luxurious aristocratic apartments were expropriated by the Soviet government and divided among three to ten poor families. The new aristocracy purchased some of those apartments, which regained their luxurious status, but others are still populated by way too many unrelated people. So, unless you're ready to live in an improvised commune, make sure to ask your real estate agent: **A eto ne kommunalka?** (uh *eh*-tuh nee kuh-moo-*nahl*-kuh; Is this a communal apartment?)

Your ad may also say **nye agenstvo** (nee uh-*gyehn*-stvuh; not an agency). What it means is that the ad was posted by the landlord himself, which allows him to cut the cost of a rental agency fee.

Discussing a house

The rules for finding a house are pretty much the same as those for finding an apartment. You can check out newspaper ads about selling **nyedvizhimost'** (need-*vee*-zhih-muhst'; real estate) or talk to an **agyent po prodazhye nyedvizhimosti** (uh-*gyent* puh prah-*dah*-zhih need-*vee*-zhih-muhs-tee; real estate agent).

If you want to rent a **dom** (dohm; house) in a big city, you're likely to find **dom v prigorodye** (dohm f *pree*-guh-ruh-dee; house in the suburbs). Even if you don't have a car, it's not usually a problem: Russia has a good system of **elyektrichki** (eh-leek-*treech*-kee; suburban trains), which take you virtually anywhere. Find out about transportation options, though, before making your decision.

Asking the right questions

REMEMBER

Some questions you definitely want to ask your **agyent po s'yomu zhil'ya** (uh-*gyent* pah s'*yo*-moo zhih-*l'ya*; real estate agent) or **khozyain/khozyajka** (khah-*zya*-een/khah-*zyay*-kuh; landlord/landlady):

- ✔ **Mnye nuzhno platit' dyeposit?** (mnye *noozh*-nuh plah-*teet'* dee-pah-*zeet*; Do I need to pay the deposit?)

- ✔ **Kto platit za uslugi (elyektrichyestvo, gaz, voda)?** [ktoh *plah*-teet zuh oos-*loo*-gee (eh-leek-*tree*-chees-tvuh, gahs, vah-*dah*); Who pays for utilities (electricity, gas, water)?]

- ✔ **Kakaya oplata v myesyats?** (kuh-*kah*-ye ahp-*lah*-tuh v *mye*-seets; What are the monthly payments?)

- ✔ **Vy khotitye, chtoby ya platil rublyami ili dollarami?** (vih khah-*tee*-tee *shtoh*-bih ya pluh-*teel* roob-*lya*-mee *ee*-lee *doh*-luh-ruh-mee; Do you want me to pay in rubles or in dollars?)

- ✔ **Eto spokojnyj rayon?** (*eh*-tuh spah-*kohy*-nihy ruh-*yon*; Is it a safe neighborhood?)

- ✔ **Kto zanimayetsya pochinkoj nyeispravnostyej?** (ktoh zuh-nee-*mah*-ee-tsye pah-*cheen*-kuhy nee-ees-*prahv*-nuhs-teey; Who performs the maintenance? *Literally:* Who performs the repairs of things that are out of order?)

Don't rush to exchange your money to pay the rent! Some landlords may prefer that you pay in dollars.

The main things to find out about a house specifically are the following:

- ✔ **Eto dom v gorodye ili v prigorodye?** (*eh*-tuh dohm v *goh*-ruh-dee *ee*-lee f *pree*-guh-ruh-dee; Is the house in the city or in the suburbs?)

- ✔ **Kakoj vid transporta tuda khodit?** (kuh-*kohy* veet *trahn*-spuhr-tuh too-dah khoh-deet; Which public transportation runs there?)

- ✔ **Skol'ko v domye etazhyej?** (*skohl'*-kuh v *doh*-mee eh-tuh-*zhehy*; How many floors does the house have?)

- ✔ **Kakoye v domye otoplyeniye?** (kuh-*koh*-ee v *doh*-mee uh-tah-*plye*-nee-ee; How is the house heated?)

- ✔ **V domye yest' garazh?** (v *doh*-mee yest' guh-*rahsh*; Is there a garage in the house?)

Sealing the deal

When you find a place to rent that strikes your fancy, you're ready to **podpisat' kontrakt** (puhd-pee-*saht'* kahn-*trahkt*; sign the lease). In your **kontrakt na aryendu zhil'ya** (kahn-*trahkt* nuh uh-*ryen*-doo zhihl'-*ya*; lease), look for the following key points:

- ✔ **srok** (srohk; duration of the lease)

- ✔ **oplata/plata** (ah-*plah*-tuh/*plah*-tuh; rent)

- ✔ **podpis'** (*poht*-pees'; signature)

Talkin' the Talk

 Josh is looking for an apartment in Moscow. He's at a rental agency, talking to an **agyent** (uh-*gyent*; a real estate agent).

Josh: **Ya khochu snyat' kvartiru. Odnokomnatnuyu, nye ochyen' doroguyu, v tsyentrye.**
ya khah-*choo* snyat' kvuhr-*tee*-roo. uhd-nah-*kohm*-nuht-noo-yu, nee *oh*-cheen' duh-rah-*goo*-yu, f *tsehn*-tree.
I want to rent an apartment. A studio, not too expensive, in the downtown area.

Agyent: **My mozhyem vam pryedlozhit' elitnuyu kvartiru v domye okolo Moskvy-ryeki. Pyatyj etazh, balkon. Vid na Kryeml'.**
mih *moh*-zhihm vahm preed-lah-*zhiht'* eh-*leet*-noo-yu kvuhr-*tee*-roo v *doh*-mee *oh*-kuh-luh mahsk-*vih* ree-kee. *pya*-tihy eh-*tahsh*, buhl-*kohn*. veet nuh kryeml'.
We can offer you an elite apartment next to Moscow River. The fifth floor, a balcony. A view of the Kremlin.

Josh: **A kakaya aryendnaya plata?**
ah kuh-*kah*-ye uh-*ryend*-nuh-ye *plah*-tuh?
And what is the rent?

Agyent: **2,000 dollarov v myesyats.**
dvye *tih*-see-chee *doh*-luh-ruhf v *mye*-seets.
$2,000 a month.

Josh: **Nyet, eto slishkom dorogo.**
nyet, *eh*-tuh *sleesh*-kuhm *doh*-ruh-guh.
No, that's too expensive.

Words to Know

v tsyentrye	f _tsehn_-tree	in the downtown area
My mozhyem vam pryedlozhit'	mih _moh_-zhihm vahm preed-lah-_zhiht'_	We can offer you
balkon	buhl-_kohn_	balcony
vid na	veet nuh	a view of
aryendnaya plata	uh-_ryend_-nuh-ye _plah_-tuh	rent
slishkom dorogo	_sleesh_-kuhm _doh_-ruh-guh	too expensive

Settling into Your New Digs

Congratulations on moving into your new home! In the following sections, you discover how to talk about your home and the things you have there.

Knowing the names of different rooms

Russians don't usually have as many rooms as Americans do. And the rooms they have are often reversible: a **divan-krovat'** (dee-_vahn_ krah-_vaht'_; sofa bed) can turn a cozy **gostinnaya** (gahs-_tee_-nuh-ye; living room) into a **spal'nya** (_spahl'_-nye; bedroom). In the morning, the same room can magically turn into a **stolovaya** (stah-_loh_-vuh-ye; dining room) when the hosts bring in their **skladnoj stol** (skluhd-_nohy_ stohl; folding table)!

Here are some names for rooms to navigate you through a Russian apartment:

- **kukhnya** (_kookh_-nye; kitchen)
- **prikhozhaya** (pree-_khoh_-zhuh-ye; hall)
- **koridor** (kuh-ree-_dohr_; corridor)
- **dyetskaya** (_dyet_-skuh-ye; children's room)
- **kabinyet** (kuh-bee-_nyet_; study)

The English word "bathroom" corresponds to two different notions in Russian: **vannaya** (*vahn*-nuh-ye) and **tualyet** (too-uh-*lyet*). **Vannaya** is the place where **vanna** (*vahn*-nuh; bathtub), **dush** (doosh; shower), and **rakovina** (*rah*-kuh-vee-nuh; sink) are. The **tualyet** is usually a separate room next to the **vannaya.**

One of the most important phrases in any language is this one: **Gdye tualyet?** (gdye too-uh-*lyet*; Where is the bathroom?)

Most Russian room names, such as **gostinnaya** and **stolovaya,** don't decline like nouns. Instead, they decline like feminine adjectives. The explanation to this mystery is easy: **stolovaya** is what remained in modern Russian of **stolovaya komnata** (dining room), where the word **stolovaya** was, in fact, an adjective, describing the feminine noun **komnata** (room). For more info on adjective declension, see Chapter 2.

Buying furniture

The easiest place to find **myebyel'** (*mye*-beel'; furniture) is **myebyel'nij magazin** (*mye*-beel'-nihy muh-guh-*zeen*; furniture store). Here are some Russian words for various pieces of furniture:

- **divan** (dee-*vahn*; sofa)
- **dukhovka** (doo-*khohf*-kuh; oven)
- **kholodil'nik** (khuh-lah-*deel'*-neek; refrigerator)
- **knizhnaya polka** (*kneezh*-nuh-ye *pohl*-kuh; bookshelf)
- **kovyor** (kah-*vyor*; carpet/rug)
- **krovat'** (krah-*vaht*; bed)
- **kryeslo** (*kryes*-luh; armchair)
- **kukhonnyj stol** (*koo*-khuh-nihy stohl; kitchen table)
- **lampa** (*lahm*-puh; lamp)
- **magnitofon** (muhg-nee-tah-*fohn*; stereo)
- **mikrovolnovka** (meek-ruh-vahl-*nohf*-kuh; microwave)
- **pis'myennyj stol** (*pees'*-mee-nihy stohl; desk/writing table)
- **plita** (plee-*tah*; stove)
- **posudomoyechnaya mashina** (pah-*soo*-dah-*moh*-eech-nuh-ye muh-*shih*-nuh; dishwasher)
- **shkaf** (shkahf; cupboard/closet/wardrobe)
- **stiral'naya mashina** (stee-*rahl'*-nuh-ye muh-*shih*-nuh; washing machine)
- **stol** (stohl; table)

- **stul** (stool; chair)
- **sushilka** (soo-*shihl*-kuh; dryer)
- **zhurnal'nyj stolik** (zhoor-*nahl'*-nihy *stoh*-leek; coffee table)
- **zyerkalo** (*zyer*-kuh-luh; mirror)

Talkin' the Talk

Matt is at a furniture store in Moscow. The **prodavets** (pruh-duh-*vyets*; shop assistant) is helping him choose furniture for his new apartment.

Matt: **Izvinitye, pohzalujsta. Gdye tut u vas krovati?**
eez-vee-*nee*-tee, pah-*zhahl*-stuh. gdye toot oo vahs krah-*vah*-tee?
Excuse me, where are the beds?

Prodavets: **Krovati vot zdyes'. Vot otlichnij divan-krovat', on na rasprodazhye, nyedorogo.**
krah-*vah*-tee voht zdyes'. voht aht-*leech*-nihy dee-*vahn* krah-*vaht'*, ohn nuh ruhs-prah-*dah*-zhih, nee-*doh*-ruh-guh.
Beds are over here. Here's a great sofa bed, it's on sale, it's inexpensive.

Matt: **Nyet, spasibo, ya ish'u obyknovyennuyu krovat'.**
nyet, spuh-*see*-buh, ya ee-*sh'oo* uh-bihk-nah-*vye*-noo-yu krah-*vaht'*.
No, thanks, I am looking for a regular bed.

Prodavets: **Odnospal'nuyu ili dvuspal'nuyu?**
ahd-nahs-*pahl'*-noo-yu ee-lee dvoo-*spahl'*-noo-yu?
Twin or queen size?

Matt: **Ya yesh'yo nye ryeshil. U myenya v kvartirye nye ochyen' mnogo myesta.**
ya ee-*sh'oh* nee ree-*shihl*. oo mee-*nya* f kvahr-*tee*-ree nee *oh*-cheen' *mnoh*-guh *myes*-tuh.
I haven't decided yet. I don't have that much space in my apartment.

Words to Know

Gdye tut u vas krovati?	gdye toot oo vahs krah-_vah_-tee	Where are the beds?
na rasprodazhye	nuh ruhs-prah-_dah_-zhih	on sale
Nyedorogo.	nee-_doh_-ruh-guh	It's inexpensive.
Ya yesh'yo nye reshil.	ya ee-_sh'oh_ nee ree-_shihl_	I haven't decided yet.
U myenya v kvartirye nye ochyen' mnogo myesta.	oo mee-_nya_ f kvuhr-_tee_-ree nee _oh_-cheen' _mnoh_-guh _myes_-tuh	I don't have that much space in my apartment.

Searching for a Job

A great Russian proverb, one may claim, summarizes Russians' attitude to work: **Rabota — nye volk, v lyes nye ubyezhit.** (ruh-_boh_-tuh nee vohlk, v lyes nee oo-bee-_zhiht_; Work isn't a wolf, it won't run away from you into the forest.) This proverb represents the same kind of thinking that inspired Mark Twain to give a new meaning to the famous words of wisdom: "Do not put off until tomorrow what can be put off till day after tomorrow just as well." But whatever Russians claim in their proverbs, the professional market in some Russian cities is thriving. In the following sections, you discover all you need to know about finding a job in Russian.

Discovering where to look

Looking for a job in Russia isn't much different than job-searching elsewhere in the world. Your options are:

- Going to a **kadrovoye agyenstvo** (_kahd_-ruh-vuh-ee uh-_gyens_-tvuh; recruiting agency)
- Posting your **ryezyumye** (ree-zyu-_meh_; resume) on a **sajt po poisku raboty** (sahjt pah _poh_-ees-koo ruh-_boh_-tih; job finder Web site)

✔ Looking for **ob'yavlyeniye** (uhb-yeev-*lye*-nee-ee; announcement/ad) in a newspaper or a magazine

✔ Harassing your friends

If you decide to go with option two, http://www.job-promo.xvx.ru/katalog.htm can help you. It's a Web site maintained by **Rossijskaya sluzhba zanyatosti** (rah-*seey*-skuh-ye *sloozh*-buh *zah*-nee-tuhs-tee; Russian federal placement service) that offers a thorough online catalog of Web sites devoted to finding a job in Russia.

The most popular newspapers that offer employment information are **"Rabota dlya vas"** (ruh-*boh*-tuh dlya vahs; Jobs for You), **"Rabota i zarplata"** (ruh-*boh*-tuh ee zuhr-*plah*-tuh; Jobs and Wages), and **"Elitnyj pyersonal"** (eh-*leet*-nihy peer-sah-*nahl*; Elite Personnel).

Some phrases to look for when you're scanning the ads:

✔ **vakansiya** (vuh-*kahn*-see-ye; vacancy)

✔ **opyt raboty** (*oh*-piht ruh-*boh*-tih; experience in the field)

✔ **ryekommyendatsii** (ree-kuh-meen-*dah*-tsih-ee; recommendations)

✔ **zarplata** (zuhr-*plah*-tuh; wage)

✔ **strakhovka** (struh-*khohf*-kuh; insurance)

✔ **otpusk** (*oht*-poosk; vacation time)

Contacting employers

When you identify a **rabotodatyel'** (ruh-*boh*-tuh-*dah*-teel'; employer) that you're interested in, you want to **poslat' ryezyumye** (pahs-*laht'* ree-zyu-*meh*; to send a resume). You have several ways to do it; to find out which way is preferred by your employer, you can ask: **Mnye prislat' ryezyumye . . . ?** (mnye pahs-*laht'* ree-zyu-*meh*; Should I send my resume . . . ?)

✔ . . . **imejlom?** (ee-*mehy*-luhm; by e-mail)

✔ . . . **faksom?** (*fahk*-suhm; by fax)

✔ . . . **pochtoj?** (*pohch*-tuhy; by mail)

A Russian resume, unlike an American one, includes your gender, birth date, and **syemyejnoye polozhyeniye** (see-*myey*-nuh-ee puh-lah-*zheh*-nee-ee; marital status). Some employers may even ask you to include your picture!

The next step is **intyerv'yu** (een-tehr-*v'yu*; interview). If you want to bring some supporting documents to the interview, but aren't sure which, you may want to ask **Kakiye dokumyenty mnye prinyesti na intyerv'yu?** (kuh-*kee*-ee

duh-koo-*myen*-tih mnye pree-nees-*tee* nuh een-tehr-*v'yu*; Which documents should I bring to the interview?) The answers can include

- **diplom** (deep-*lohm*; diploma)
- **razryeshyeniye na rabotu** (ruhz-ree-*sheh*-nee-ee nuh ruh-*boh*-too; work authorization)
- **ryekommyendatsiya** (ree-kuh-meen-*dah*-tsih-ye; reference)

Clarifying job responsibilities

To find out about your **obyazannosti** (ah-*bya*-zuh-nuhs-tee; job responsibili-ties), you need to ask questions. A good place to start is **Chto vkhodit v moi obyazannosti?** (shtoh f *khoh*-deet v mah-*ee* ah-*bya*-zuh-nuhs-tee; What do my job responsibilities include?) The variety of professional skills is endless, but these words are likely to be useful:

- **pyechatat'** (pee-*chah*-tuht'; to type)
- **rabotat' s komp'yutyerom** (ruh-*boh*-tuht' s kahm-p'*yoo*-teh-ruhm; to work with a computer)
- **pyeryevodit'** (pee-ree-vah-*deet'*; to translate)

Talkin' the Talk

Ann just finished an interview at a high school in Vladimir, where she applied for a teaching position. The **diryektor** (dee-*ryek*-tuhr; princi-pal) is congratulating Ann and explaining her job responsibilities.

Diryektor:	**Pozdravlyayu vas! Vy nam podkhoditye.** puhz-druhv-*lya*-yu vahs! vih nahm paht-*khoh*-dee-tee. Congratulations! You will be a good fit.
Ann:	**Spasibo. U myenya yest' vopros. Skol'ko urokov ya budu pryepodavat'?** spuh-*see*-buh. oo mee-*nya* yest' vahp-*rohs*. skohl'-kuh oo-*roh*-kuhf ya *boo*-doo pree-puh-duh-*vaht'*? Thank you. I have a question. How many classes will I teach?
Diryektor:	**Tri uroka kazhdyj dyen'.** tree oo-*roh*-kuh *kahzh*-dihy dyen'. Three classes every day.

Ann:	Kogda ya mogu nachat'?
	kahg-*dah* ya mah-*goo* nuh-*chaht'*?
	When can I start?

Diryektor:	Vy mozhyetye nachat' zavtra. Zarplata — tri tysyachi rublyej v myesyats.
	vih *moh*-zhih-tee nuh-*chaht'* zahf-truh. zuhr-*plah*-tuh tree *tih*-see-chee roob-*lyey* v *mye*-seets.
	You can start tomorrow. Your wage is 3,000 a month.

Words to Know

Vy nam podkhoditye.	vih nahm paht-<u>khoh</u>-dee-tee	You will be a good fit.
U myenya yest' vopros.	oo mee-<u>nya</u> yest' vahp-<u>rohs</u>	I have a question.
kazhdyj dyen'	<u>kahzh</u>-dihy dyen'	every day
Kogda ya mogu nachat'?	Kahg-<u>dah</u> ya mah-<u>goo</u> nuh-<u>chaht</u>	When can I start?
Vy mozhyetye nachat' zavtra.	vih <u>moh</u>-zhih-tee nuh-<u>chaht'</u> <u>zahf</u>-truh	You can start tomorrow.

Succeeding in the Workplace

When in Rome, do as the Romans do. Or, as the Russians say, **V chuzhoj monastyr' so svoim ustavom nye khodyat.** (f choo-*zhohy* muh-nuh-*stihr'* suh svah-*eem* oos-*tah*-vuhm nee *khoh*-dyet; Don't go to someone else's monastery with your own regulations.) The workplace may be pretty different when you're working in a foreign country, or even at home for a foreign company. The following sections equip you with the necessary phrases to thrive in a Russian workspace.

Making your way around the office

It's one thing to make it into an office, and quite another to survive there. All those special rooms and gadgets can make anyone go dizzy, even if you don't

need to refer to them in a foreign language. In the following sections, we tell you how to navigate your way around the office with maximum ease.

Surveying supplies

When you're **v ofisye** (v *oh*-fees-ee; at the office), English speakers definitely have a huge advantage: Out of the zillion little things inhabiting the office, a good portion have highly recognizable English-borrowed names. Even if you knew no Russian whatsoever, wouldn't you suspect something if you heard the phrase: **Mnye nuzhyen kartridzh dlya printyera** (mnye *noo*-zheen *kahr*-treedzh dlya *preen*-tee-ruh; I need a cartridge for my printer)? Here's a list of common office supplies to know:

- **komp'yutyer** (kahm-*p'yu*-tehr; computer)
- **noutbuk** (nuh-oot-*book*; laptop)
- **fax** (fahks; fax)
- **ksyeroks** (*ksye*-ruhks; copy machine)
- **skanyer** (*skah*-nehr; scanner)
- **modyem** (mah-*dehm*; modem)
- **monitor** (muh-nee-*tohr*; monitor)
- **tyelyefon** (tee-lee-*fohn*; telephone)
- **ruchka** (*rooch*-kuh; pen)
- **karandash** (kuh-ruhn-*dahsh*; pencil)
- **styorka** (*styor*-kuh; eraser)
- **tyetrad'** (teet-*raht'*; notebook)
- **papka** (*pahp*-kuh; file)
- **bumaga** (boo-*mah*-guh; paper)
- **zamazka** (zuh-*mahs*-kuh; liquid corrector)
- **skryepki** (*skryep*-kee; paper clips)
- **klyejkaya lyenta** (*klyey*-kuh-ye *lyen*-tuh; tape)
- **styeplyer** (*stehp*-leer; stapler)

Check out Chapter 9 for general information on making phone calls and sending faxes and e-mails.

Navigating rooms

You may want to know the names for other important work functions, such as **stolovaya** (stah-*loh*-vuh-ye; cafeteria), **komnata otdykha** (*kohm*-nuh-tuh *oht*-dih-khuh; lounge), and **kurilka** (koo-*reel*-kuh), a room designated for smoking, where you see the most of your colleagues.

Financial matters can be settled in the **buhkgaltyeriya** (boo-guhl-*tye*-ree-ye; accounts office). The room you want to avoid is the **kabinyet nachal'nika** (kuh-bee-*nyet* nuh-*chahl'*-nee-kuh; boss's office).

Your actual work is usually done in a **kabinyet** (kuh-bee-*nyet*; office room) and a **konfyeryentszal** (kuhn-fee-*ryents*-zahl; meeting room).

Communicating in the workplace

The thing about the workplace is that you're never alone. You often need to talk to a **kollyega** (kah-*lye*-guh; coworker), your **nachal'nik** (nuh-*chahl'*-neek; boss), and a **kliyent** (klee-*yent*; client). In the following sections, find out what to say in the workplace and how to say it in Russian.

Making an appointment

Here are the standard phrases used to **naznachit' vstryechu** (nuh-*znah*-cheet' *fstrye*-choo; make an appointment):

- **Davajtye vstryetimsya v dyevyat' chasov utra.** (duh-*vahy*-tee *fstrye*-teem-sye v *dye*-veet' chuh-*sohf* oo-*trah*; Let's meet at 9 a.m.)

- **Ya budu vas zhdat' v tri chasa dnya.** (ya *boo*-doo vahs zhdaht' f tree chuh-*sah* dnya; I'll be waiting for you at 3 p.m.)

If you're arranging for a phone call, you can say:

- **Ya budu zhdat' vashyego zvonka v dyesyat' chasov utra.** (ya *boo*-doo zhdaht' *vah*-shih-vuh zvahn-*kah* v *dye*-seet' chuh-*sohf* oo-*trah*; I'll be waiting for your phone call at 10 a.m.)

- **Ya vam pozvonyu v dva chasa dnya.** (ya vahm puh-zvah-*nyu* v dvah chuh-*sah* dnya; I'll call you at 2 p.m.)

For details on telling time, see Chapter 7.

Sticking to workplace etiquette

Russian business etiquette is not as strict as that of some other cultures. Just garnish your speech generously with **pozhalujsta** (pah-*zhahl*-stuh; please) and **spasibo** (spuh-*see*-buh; thank you), and you'll already sound more formal than an average Russian in the workplace.

The main thing you notice about Russian **dyelovoj etikyet** (dee-lah-*vohy* eh-tee-*kyet*; workplace etiquette) is that it's less formal than what you may be used to. Engaging in humorous exchanges that fall far from political correctness is considered normal, and your coworkers are likely to throw plenty of improvised parties at the office. Bosses and clients, however, are excluded from these friendly interactions unless they decide to set the playful tone themselves.

Always use the formal **vy** (vih; you; formal singular and plural) whenever you communicate with anyone in the workplace. If your coworkers and, especially, your boss, want to switch to less formal terms, they'll tell you so. Wait for the initiative to come from them.

To avoid uncomfortable situations, always use the first name plus patronymic form to address your colleagues. If they want you to switch to the Western first-name manner, they'll tell you: **Myenya mozhno zvat' prosto Sasha.** (mee-*nya mohzh*-nuh zvaht' *proh*-stuh *sah*-shuh; You can call me simply Sasha.) For more information on Russian names, see Chapter 3.

Here are some general polite phrases to use in the workplace:

- ✔ **Ya mogu vam chyem-nibud' pomoch'?** (ya mah-*goo* vahm *chehm*-nee-boot' pah-*mohch*; Can I help you with anything?)
- ✔ **Bol'shoye spasibo, vy mnye ochyen' pomogli.** (bahl'-*shoh*-ee spuh-*see*-buh vih mnye *oh*-cheen' puh-mahg-*lee*; Thank you very much, you helped me a lot.)

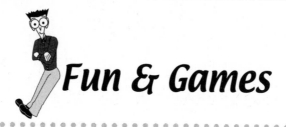

Fun & Games

Match the rooms from the list on the left with the most appropriate furniture from the list on the right. See Appendix C for the answers.

1. **Stolovaya**   a. **Krovat'**

2. **Spal'nya**   b. **Kryeslo**

3. **Gostinnaya**   c. **Stol**

In which of the following sections of the Classified ads do you NOT find information about apartments for rent? Check out Appendix C for the answer.

1. **Sdayu**

2. **Aryenda kvartir**

3. **Rabota**

4. **Kvartiry v nayom**

5. **Snyat' zhil'yo**

Part III
Russian on the Go

The 5th Wave   By Rich Tennant

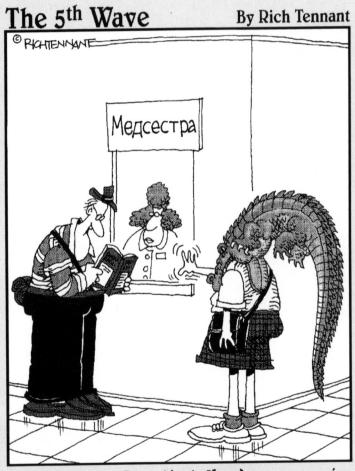

" Honey, please! Be patient! How's anyone going
to know what's wrong unless I find the
Russian word for 'alligator'?"

In this part . . .

If you're the kind of person who's constantly on the go, then Part III is for you. In this part, you find the phrases you need for booking and taking trips; getting around the city and the world on planes, trains, and more; and making the most of your hotel experience. You also discover how to talk about money, how to ask for directions, and the best way to handle emergencies in Russian. By the time you're done with Part III, you're armed with all the Russian you need to travel nearly anywhere on Earth, and maybe even a little further!

Chapter 11

Planning a Trip

- -

- -

Do you like to **putyeshyestvovat'** (poo-tee-*shehs*-tvuh-vuht'; to travel)? If so, then this chapter is for you! In this chapter, you discover how to express when and where you want to travel, how to speak to a travel agent, and how to secure a passport and a visa. We also provide you with some useful phrases and give you packing tips for a **putyeshyestviye** (poo-tee-*shehs*-tvee-ee; trip) to Russia. And now, as Russians often say: **Poyekhali!** (pah-*ye*-khuh-lee; Let's go!/start!/move!)

When Can We Go? Choosing the Date for Your Trip

The excitement of travel sets in the minute you begin to think about it. The first thing we always do when planning a trip is decide on the dates when we want to leave and come back. In the following sections, you find out the names of months and seasons, and we show you how to state the year and specific dates for travel. (See Chapter 7 for details about times of the day and the days of the week.)

Recognizing the names of the months

To help you to decide when to take a trip, here's a list of the **myesyatsy** (*mye*-see-tsih; months). Note that each **myesyats** (*mye*-seets; month) in Russian has a name that sounds very similar to its English counterpart.

- **yanvar'**(een-*vahr'*; January)
- **fyevral'** (feev-*rahl'*; February)
- **mart** (mahrt; March)
- **apryel'**(uhp-*ryel'*; April)
- **maj** (mahy; May)
- **iyun'**(ee-*yun'*; June)
- **iyul'** (ee-*yul'*; July)
- **avgust** (*ahv*-goost; August)
- **syentyabr'** (seen-*tyabr'*; September)
- **oktyabr'** (ahk-*tyabr'*; October)
- **noyabr'** (nah-*yabr'*; November)
- **dyekabr'** (dee-*kahbr'*; December)

Note that while English capitalizes the first letter of the name of the month, Russian does not.

Say you're considering taking a trip in November or August but aren't yet sure about the date. If that's the case, you indicate the month of the trip with the phrase **v** (v; in) plus the name of the month in the prepositional case, as in **v noyabrye** (v nuh-eeb-*rye*; in November) or **v avgustye** (v *ahv*-goos-tee; in August). See Chapter 2 for details about cases.

Note that the word for November changes its original accent in the prepositional case. This change (called a "stress shift") affects all months ending on **-abr'/-yabr'**.

Talking about specific dates

When you want to say a **chislo** (chees-*loh*; date) in Russian, you need to put the ordinal number indicating the day in the form of neuter gender and the name of the month in the genitive case, as in:

- **Syegodnya pyatoye oktyabrya** (see-*vohd*-nye *pya*-tuh-ee uhk-teeb-*rya*; Today is October 5).

- **Zavtra dyesyatoye iyulya** (*zahf*-truh dee-*sya*-tuh-ee ee-*yu*-lye; Tomorrow is June 10).

- **Poslyezavtra dvadtstat' chyetvyortoye marta** (*pohs*-lee-*zahf*-truh *dvaht*-tsuht' cheet-*vyor*-tuh-ee *mahr*-tuh; The day after tomorrow is March 24).

To state that a certain event occurred, occurs, or will occur on a certain date, you (again!) have to change the case of the ordinal number indicating the day of the month. This time, the ordinal number takes the genitive case. So when making a flight reservation, you say:

> **Ya khochu vylyetyet' pyervogo syentyabrya i vyernut'sya pyatogo oktyabrya.** (ya khah-*choo vih*-lee-teet' *pyer*-vuh-vuh seen-teeb-*rya* ee veer-*noot'*-sye *pya*-tuh-vuh uhk-teeb-*rya*; I want to leave on September 1 and come back on October 5.)

If somebody asks you **Kogda vy uyezzhayetye?** (kahg-*dah* vih oo-eez-*zhah*-ee-tee; When are you leaving?) and you don't mind sharing that information, you may say **Ya uyezzhayu pyatnadtsatogo marta** (ya oo-eez-*zhah*-yu peet-*naht*-tsuh-tuh-vuh *mahr*-tuh; I'm leaving March 15). If you want the person to meet you at the airport or railway station, you may add **I vozvrash'yayus' chyetvyortogo apryelya** (ee vuhz-vruh-sh'*yah*-yus' cheet-*vyor*-tuh-vuh uhp-*rye*-lye; And I'm coming back on April 4).

For more info on ordinal numbers and the genitive case, see Chapter 2.

Saying the year

To indicate a year, you begin with the century, as in **tysyacha dyevyatsot** (*tih*-see-chuh dee-veet-*soht*; nineteen, Literally: one thousand nine hundred) for the 20th century or **dvye tysyachi** (dvye *tih*-see-chee; two thousand) for the 21st century. Then, to state the number indicating the year, use the corresponding ordinal number, as in:

- **tysyacha dyevyatsot pyat'dyesyat' vos'moj god** (*tih*-see-chuh dee-veet-*soht* pee-dee-*syat* vahs'-*mohy* goht; 1958, Literally: One thousand nine hundred fifty-eighth year)

- **dvye tysyachi syed'moj god** (dvye *tih*-see-chee seed'-*mohy* goht; 2007, Literally: Two thousand seventh year)

Note that in indicating a year, Russian, unlike English (with its reputation of being an economical language), actually uses the word **god** (goht; year). The word **god** has two plural forms: the regular **gody** (*goh*-dih; years) and the irregular **goda** (gah-*dah*; years). A very subtle stylistic difference exists between the two, so don't hesitate to use both or the one you like better.

Have you ever experienced what's often referred to as a memory block when you just don't remember what year it is now? The question to ask in this situation is **Kakoj syejchas god?** (kuh-*kohy* see-*chahs* goht; What year is it now?) If you're convinced that the current year is 2006, for example, you would say **Syejchas dvye tysyachi shyestoj god** (see-*chahs* dvye *tih*-see-chee shees-*tohy* goht; It is 2006).

More often, we use years to indicate when a certain event took, takes, or will take place. To make this statement, use preposition **v** + the year in the prepositional case + **godu** (gah-*doo*; year), as in:

- ✔ **v tysyacha dyevyatsot pyat'dyesyat vos'mom godu** (v *tih*-see-chuh dee-veet-*soht* pee-dee-*syat* vahs'-*mohm* gah-*doo*; in 1958, *Literally:* in the one thousand nine hundred fifty-eighth year)

- ✔ **v dvye tysyachi syed'mom godu** (v dvye *tih*-see-chee seed'-*mohm* gah-*doo*; in 2007, *Literally:* in the two thousand seventh year)

- ✔ **v dvye tysyachi sorok vos'mom godu** (v dvye *tih*-see-chee *soh*-ruhk vahs'-*mohm* gah-*doo*; in 2048, *Literally:* in the two thousand forty-eighth year)

To indicate the year in which an event takes place, you only have to put the last ordinal numeral describing the year into the prepositional case. For more info on ordinal numerals and forming the prepositional case, see Chapter 2.

Surveying the seasons

Although some places in the world just don't have **vryemyena goda** (vree-mee-*nah* goh-duh; seasons, *Literally:* times of the year) — take, for example, Florida or California — it's still a good idea to know how to say them in Russian. Here they are:

- ✔ **zima** (zee-*mah*; winter)
- ✔ **vyesna** (vees-*nah*; spring)
- ✔ **lyeto** (*lye*-tuh; summer)
- ✔ **osyen'** (*oh*-seen'; fall)

A popular Russian song says **V prirodye plokhoj pogodye nye byvayet** (v pree-*roh*-dee plah-*khohy* pah-*goh*-dee nee bih-*vah*-eet; Nature doesn't have bad weather). This line is another way of saying that every **vryemya goda** (*vrye*-mye goh-duh; season, *Literally:* time of the year) has its own beauty.

Where Do You Want to Go? Picking a Place for Your Trip

Have you ever asked yourself **Kuda ty khochyesh' poyekhat'?** (koo-*dah* tih *khoh*-cheesh' pah-*ye*-khuht'; Where do you want to go?) or **Kuda ya khochu poyekhat'?** (koo-*dah* ya khah-*choo* pah-*ye*-khuht'?; Where do I want to go?) In the following sections, you find out how to talk about different countries in Russian.

Checking out different countries

We assume that your travel plans are going to take you to one of the seven **kontinyenty** (kuhn-tee-*nyen*-tih; continents) in the following list. You may want to know the name of each **kontinyent** (kuhn-tee-*nyent*; continent) in Russian.

- **Yevropa** (eev-*roh*-puh; Europe)
- **Syevyernaya Amyerika** (*sye*-veer-nuh-ye uh-*mye*-ree-kuh; North America)
- **Yuzhnaya Amerika** (*yuzh*-nuh-ye uh-*mye*-ree-kuh; South America)
- **Afrika** (*ahf*-ree-kuh; Africa)
- **Aziya** (*ah*-zee-ye; Asia)
- **Avstraliya** (uhf-*strah*-lee-ye; Australia)
- **Antarktika** (uhn-*tahrk*-tee-kuh; Antarctica)

Because **Antarktika** isn't a very popular destination, we list here only the **strany** (*strah*-nih; countries) most often visited by foreigners on other continents, beginning with Europe and ending with Asia. (Australia is its own continent, and you can find it in the previous list.) Do you see a **strana** (struh-*nah*; country) that you want to visit?

- **Avstriya** (*ahf*-stree-ye; Austria)
- **Angliya** (*ahn*-glee-ye; England)
- **Frantsiya** (*frahn*-tsih-ye; France)
- **Gyermaniya** (geer-*mah*-nee-ye; Germany)
- **Gollandiya** (guh-*lahnd*-dee-ye; Holland)
- **Italiya** (ee-*tah*-lee-ye; Italy)
- **Ispaniya** (ees-*pah*-nee-ye; Spain)
- **Amyerika** (uh-*mye*-ree-kuh; the United States)
- **Kanada** (kuh-*nah*-duh; Canada)
- **Myeksika** (*myek*-see-kuh; Mexico)
- **Argyentina** (uhr-geen-*tee*-nuh; Argentina)
- **Braziliya** (bruh-*zee*-lee-ye; Brazil)
- **Yegipyet** (ee-*gee*-peet; Egypt)
- **Izrail'** (eez-*rah*-eel'; Israel)
- **Morokko** (muh-*rohk*-kuh; Morocco)
- **Turtsiya** (*toor*-tsih-ye; Turkey)
- **Kitaj** (kee-*tahy*; China)

- **Indiya** (*een*-dee-ye; India)
- **Yaponiya** (ee-*poh*-nee-ye; Japan)
- **Novaya Zyelandiya** (*noh*-vuh-ye zee-*lahn*-dee-ye; New Zealand)

Visiting Russia

If you're reading this book, you may be considering a trip to **Rossiya** (rah-*see*-ye; Russia). Great idea! You won't regret it. Where would you like to go first? We recommend that you begin with **Moskva** (mahs-*kvah*; Moscow), Russia's bustling **stolitsa** (stah-*lee*-tsuh; capital), and **Sankt-Pyetyerburg** (sahnkt-pee-teer-*boork*; St. Petersburg).

You'll find quite a few things to see in Moscow, including the following:

- **Kryeml'** (kryeml'; Kremlin, the old town and the seat of the Russian government)
- **Krasnaya plosh'ad'** (*krahs*-nuh-ye *ploh*-sh'uht'; Red Square)
- **Tryetyakovskaya galyeryeya** (tree-tee-*kohf*-skuh-ye guh-lee-*rye*-ye; Tretyakoff art gallery)
- **Pushkinskij muzyej** (*poosh*-keen-skeey moo-zyey; Pushkin art museum)
- **Kolomyenskoye** (kah-*loh*-meen-skuh-ee; the former tsars' estate)
- **Novodyevich'ye kladbish'ye** (*noh*-vah-*dye*-veech-ee *klahd*-bee-sh'ee; Novodevich'ye cemetery, the burial place of many famous Russian people)

And if you have a particular interest in staring at dead bodies, then go to **Mavzolyej** (muhv-zah-*lyey*; mausoleum). Vladimir Lenin's mummy is still there for display.

If you like Russian history, literature, and culture, then **Sankt-Pyetyerburg** is a must. Our advice: Visit St. Petersburg at the end of May and beginning of June, during the **byelyye nochi** (*bye*-lih-ee *noh*-chee; white nights). That's what Russians call the short period in early summer when it almost never gets dark in the north. **Pyetyerburg** is the city where, as **pyetyerburzhtsy** (pee-teer-*boorzh*-tsih; people born and living in St. Petersburg) say, **Kazhdyj dom muzyej** (*kahzh*-dihy dohm moo-zyey; Every building is a museum).

Here's a list of a few of the places we recommend you see in **Sankt-Pyetyerburg**:

- **Ermitazh** (ehr-mee-*tahsh*; the Hermitage museum)
- **Russkij muzyej** (*roos*-keey moo-zyey; Russian Museum)

- **Pushkin** (*poosh*-keen; the town of Pushkin) or **Tsarskoye Syelo** (*tsahr*-skuh-ee see-*loh*; the tsars' village, the former summer residence of the Russian tsars)

- **Pavlovsk** (*pahv*-luhvsk; another former residence of the Russian tsars)

- **Pyetrodvoryets** (*pyet*-truh- dvah-*ryets*; Russian Versailles founded by Peter the Great)

- **Pyetropavlovskaya kryepost'** (*peet*-rah-*pahv*-luhv-skuh-ye *krye*-puhst'; Peter and Paul's Fortress, the burial place of the Russian tsars and former political prison)

- **Isaakiyevskij sobor** (ee-suh-*ah*-kee-eef-skeey sah-*bohr*; St. Isaak's Cathedral, the world's third largest one-cupola cathedral)

- **Piskaryovskoye kladbish'ye** (pees-kuh-*ryof*-skuh-ee *klahd*-bee-sh'ee; Piskarev memorial cemetery, museum of Leningrad 900-day siege)

For those of you with a more adventurous nature, you may want to go to the Asiatic part of Russia, which is the part of Russia lying beyond **Ural'skiye Gory** (oo-*rahl'*-skee-ee *goh*-rih; Ural Mountains). How about going to **Sibir'** (see-*beer'*; Siberia)? **Sibir'** is a beautiful region, and it's not always cold there. In fact, the summers are quite hot.

How Do We Get There? Booking a Trip with a Travel Agency

After you decide where you want to go, you need to call the **byuro putyeshyestvij** (byu-*roh* poo-tee-*shehs*-tveey; travel agency) and talk to an **agyent** (uh-*gyent*; travel agent). If you're planning a trip to Russia, you may want to say the following:

- **Ya khotyel by poyekhat' v Rossiyu v maye** (ya khah-*tyel* bih pah-*ye*-khuht' v rah-*see*-yu v *mah*-ee; I would like to go to Russia in May) if you're a man

- **Ya khotyela by poyekhat' v Rossiyu v maye** (ya khah-*tye*-luh bih pah-*ye*-khuht' v rah-*see*-yu v *mah*-ee; I would like to go to Russia in May) if you're a woman.

And be sure to add: **Chto vy mozhyetye pryedlozhit'?** (shtoh vih *moh*-zhih-tee preed-lah-*zhiht'*; What can you offer? or What do you have available?)

In response, you most likely hear:

> **A kuda imyenno vy khotitye poyekhat'?** (uh koo-*dah* ee-*mee*-nuh vih khah-*tee*-tee pah-*ye*-khuht'; And where exactly would you like to travel?)

To answer this question, use the expression: **Ya khotyel/khotyela by poyekhat' v** (ya khah-*tyel*/khah-*tye*-luh bih pah-*ye*-khuht' v; I'd like to go to) + the name of the city you want to see in accusative case, as in:

> ✔ **Ya khotyel by poyekhat' v Moskvu i v Pyetyerburg** (ya khah-*tyel* bih pah-*ye*-khuht' v mahs-*kvoo* ee v pee-teer-*boork*; I would like to go to Moscow and St. Petersburg) if you're a man
>
> ✔ **Ya khotyela by poyekhat' v Moskvu i v Pyetyerburg** (ya khah-*tye*-luh bih pah-*ye*-khuht' v mahs-*kvoo* ee v pee-teer-*boork*; I would like to go to Moscow and St. Petersburg) if you're a woman

Now listen carefully as the travel agent lists available **pakyety i tury** (puh-*kye*-tih ee *too*-rih; packages and tours). If anything sounds appealing to you, your next question may be about the cost and what the package includes: **Chto eto vklyuchayet?** (shtoh *eh*-tuh fklyu-*chah*-eet; What does it include?)

With the best deal, the cost includes the following:

> ✔ **rassyelyeniye v gostinitsye** (ruhs-see-*lye*-nee-ee v gahs-*tee*-nee-tsih; hotel accommodation)
>
> ✔ **gostinitsa pyervogo/vtorogo/tryet'yego klassa** (gahs-*tee*-neet-tsuh *pyer*-vuh-vuh/ftah-*roh*-vuh/*tryet'*-ee-vuh *klah*-suh; one/two/three star hotel)
>
> ✔ **tryohk/dvukh razovoye pitaniye** (*tryokh*/*dvookh* rah-zuh-vuh-ee pee-*tah*-nee-ee; three/two meals a day)
>
> ✔ **zavtrak** (*zahf*-truhk; bed and breakfast accommodation)
>
> ✔ **ekskursya po gorodu** (ehks-*koor*-see-ye puh *goh*-ruh-doo; city tour)
>
> ✔ **poyezdki v** (pah-*yest*-kee v; trips to) + the destination in the accusative case
>
> ✔ **posyesh'yeniye muzyeyev** (pah-see-*sh'ye*-nee-ee moo-*zye*-eef; museum admission)
>
> ✔ **samolyot, tuda i obratno** (suh-mah-*lyot* too-*dah* ee ahb-*raht*-nuh; round-trip flight)
>
> ✔ **posyesh'yeniye opyery/balyeta/tsirka** (pah-see-*sh'ye*-nee-ee *oh*-pee-rih/buh-*lye*-tuh/*tsihr*-kuh; tickets to the opera/ballet/circus)

And you certainly should receive information on the number of days and nights that the cost includes. For example:

- ✔ **tri dnya, tri nochi** (tree dnya, tree *noh*-chee; three days, three nights)
- ✔ **syem' dnyej, shyest' nochyej** (syem' dnyey, shehst' nah-*chyey*; seven days, six nights)

See Chapter 2 for more about using numbers followed by nouns.

Don't Leave Home without Them: Dealing with Passports and Visas

If you're planning to go to Russia, then read this section carefully! Here you find out about the all-important documents without which you aren't allowed into (or out of!) Russia: a **pasport** (*pahs*-puhrt; passport) and a **viza** (*vee*-zuh; visa).

If you're an American citizen who has already been abroad, then you know that to travel to other countries, you need a U.S. passport. For some countries, though, this document isn't enough. To go to Russia, you also need a visa that states that the authorities of the **Rossijskaya Fyedyeratsiya** (rah-*seey*-skuh-ye fee-dee-*rah*-tsih-ye; Russian Federation) allow you to cross the Russian border and return home within the time period indicated on the visa. In other words, if you decide to arrive in Russia a day before the date indicated on your visa, the law-abiding customs officer in the Russian airport has the legal right not to let you enter the country. Likewise, if your visa states that you have to leave Russia on January 24, 2006, don't even think of leaving on February 1. You may have to pay a fine and spend a lot more time at the airport than you expected and even miss your flight while explaining to the officials why you stayed in Russia longer than your visa states.

Your passport

If you're planning to go to Russia, you need a passport. If this trip isn't your first **poyezdka za granitsu** (pah-*yezt*-kuh zuh gruh-*nee*-tsoo; trip abroad), make sure to have your passport updated. Without a valid passport, Russian authorities won't let you into the country. Period.

Your visa

Kak dostat' vizu? (kahk dahs-*taht* *vee*-zoo; How to get a visa?) is the million-dollar question for anybody wanting to travel to Russia. You have three options, depending on which of these circumstances best describes your situation:

✔ Your travel agent arranges the trip for you, and you're officially a **turist** (too-*reest*; tourist) who stays in a hotel.

✔ You're going to Russia **v komandirovku** (f kuh-muhn-dee-*rohf*-koo; on business) and have an **ofitsial'noye priglashyeniye** (uh-fee-tsih-*ahl'*-nuh-ee pree-gluh-*sheh*-nee-ee; official invitation) from an organization in Russia approved by the Russian Ministry of Internal Affairs.

✔ You have friends or relatives in Russia who are officially inviting you. These people should be extremely devoted to you and willing to state that you'll be staying with them at all times before you leave, and that they agree to feed you while you're there.

Which of the three situations gives you the easiest chance to get a visa? Certainly the first one. All you have to do is call your travel agency, and they take care of it for you. If, however, you decide on the second or third options, be sure that before going to the **Rossijskoye posol'stvo** (rah-*seey*-skuh-ee pah-*sohl'*-stvuh; the Russian Embassy) or **Konsul'stvo** (kohn-*sool'*-stvuh; Consulate), you have a stamped official letter from Russia containing the pertinent information, which we describe with the second and third options.

Here's the list of documents you need in order to **podat' zayavlyeniye na vizu** (pah-*daht'* zuh-yav-*lye*-nee-ee nuh *vee*-zoo; to apply for a visa):

✔ **pasport** (*pahs*-puhrt; passport)

✔ **dvye fotografii** (dvye fuh-tah-*grah*-fee-ee; two photos)

✔ **dyenyezhnyj ordyer na 150 ili 200 dollarov** (*dye*-neezh-nihy *ohr*-deer nuh stoh pee-dee-*syat* *ee*-lee *dvyes*-tee *doh*-luh-ruhf; money order for $150 or $200)

✔ **zayavlyenie na vizu** (zuh-yav-*lye*-nee-ee nuh *vee*-zoo; visa application)

✔ **ofitsial'noye priglashyeniye** (uh-fee-tsih-*ahl'*-nuh-ee pree-gluh-*sheh*-nee-ee; official invitation)

The mistake most people make is offering a check or a credit card in place of a money order. Please know that the employees of the Russian Embassy won't accept them, no matter how much you plead. And a final word of caution: Before you decide to apply for a visa, check with the Russian Embassy Web site at www.russianembassy.org. Regulations constantly change!

Talkin' the Talk

 Jack is going to Russia on a business trip. He goes to the Russian Consulate in San Francisco to apply for a visa. Here is his conversation with the **rabotnik konsul'stva** (ruh-*boht*-neek *kohn*-sool'-stvuh; consulate employee) in the visa department.

Jack:	**Ya yedu v Moskvu v komandirovku. Mnye nuzhna viza. Vot dokumyenty.** ya *ye*-doo v mahs-*kvoo* f kuh-muhn-dee-*rohf*-koo. mnye noozh-*nah* *vee*-zuh. voht duh-koo-*myen*-tih. I am going for a business trip to Moscow. I need a visa. Here are my documents.
Rabotnik konsul'stva:	**Tak, pasport, priglashyeniye, zayav-lyeniye, I fotografii. A gdye dyenyezhnyj ordyer?** tahk, *pahs*-puhrt, pree-gluh-*sheh*-nee-ee, zuh-eev-*lye*-nee-ee, ee fuh-tah-*grah*-fee-ee. tahk uh gdye *dye*-neezh-nihy *ohr*-deer? Okay, this is the passport, invitation, application, and pictures. And where is the money order?
Jack:	**Dyenyezhnyj ordyer? Vot chyek na 150 dollarov.** *dye*-neezh-nihy *ohr*-deer? voht chyek nuh stoh pee-dee-*syat* *doh*-luh-ruhf. Money order? Here is a check for $150.
Rabotnik konsul'stva:	**My nye prinimayem chyeki. My prini-mayem tol'ko dyenyezhnyj ordyer.** mih nee pree-nee-*mah*-eem *chye*-kee. mih pree-nee-*mah*-eem *tohl'*-kuh *dye*-neezh-nihy *ohr*-deer. We do not accept checks. We accept only money orders.
Jack:	**Nu, ladno. Pridyotsya pridti yesh'yo raz.** noo, *lahd*-nuh. pree-*dyot*-sye preet-*tee* ee-*sh'yo* rahs. Oh, well. I will have to come again.

Words to Know

v komandirovku	f kuh-muhn-dee-_rohf_-koo	(to go) on a business trip
Mnye nuzhna viza.	mnye noozh-_nah_ _vee_-zuh	I need a visa.
Vot dokumyenty.	voht duh-koo-_myen_-tih	Here are my documents.
chyek na 150 dollarov	chyek nuh stoh pee-dee-_syat_ _doh_-luh-ruhf	check for $150
My nye prinimayem	mih nee pree-nee-_mah_-eem	We do not accept
tol'ko	_tohl_'-kuh	only
Pridyotsya pridti yesh'yo raz.	pree-_dyot_-sye preet-_tee_ ee-_sh'yo_ rahs	(I) will have to come again.

Take It with You: Packing Tips

When your trip is quickly approaching, it's time to start packing. No matter when and where you travel, you most likely take the following with you:

- **chyemodan** (chee-mah-_dahn_; suitcase)
- **sumka** (_soom_-kuh; bag)
- **ryukzak** (ryuk-_zahk_; backpack)
- **karta** (_kahr_-tuh; map)
- **fotooapparat** (fuh-tuh-uh-puh-_raht_; camera)
- **plyonka** (_plyon_-kuh; film)
- **vidyeo kamyera** (_vee_-dee-uh _kah_-mee-ruh; video camera)
- **mylo** (_mih_-luh; soap)
- **shampun'** (shuhm-_poon_'; shampoo)
- **dyeodorant** (deh-uh-dah-_rahnt_; deodorant)

✔ **zubnaya sh'yotka** (zoob-*nah*-ye *sh'yot*-kuh; toothbrush)

✔ **zubnaya pasta** (zoob-*nah*-ye *pahs*-tuh; toothpaste)

✔ **kosmyetika** (kahs-*mye*-tee-kuh; makeup)

If you're going to Russia during the winter months, be prepared! Here are items of clothing you want to take with you to keep warm:

✔ **shapka** (*shahp*-kuh; hat)

✔ **pal'to** (puhl'-*toh*; heavy coat or overcoat)

✔ **sharf** (shahrf; scarf)

✔ **pyerchatki** (peer-*chaht*-kee; gloves)

✔ **svityer** (*svee*-tehr; sweater)

✔ **sapogi** (suh-pah-*gee*; boots)

Chapter 6 has more info about different items of clothing that you can pack, regardless of the season when you're traveling.

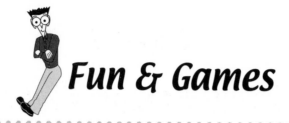

Fun & Games

Find Russian equivalents for the American-style dates given in the left column. Check out Appendix C for the correct answers.

1. **12/01/2005**   a. **pyervoye dyekabrya dvye tysyachi pyatogo goda**

2. **01/03/1999**   b. **vosyem'nadtsatoye maya tysyacha dyevyatsot shyest'dyesyat vtorogo goda**

3. **05/18/1962**   c. **dvadtsat' vtoroye syentyabrya tysyacha dyevyat'sot pyat'dyesyat shyestogo goda**

4. **09/22/1956**   d. **tryet'ye yanvarya tysyacha dyevyatsot dyevyanosto dyevyatogo goda**

Which of the following places of interest is not located in St. Petersburg? See Appendix C for the answer.

1. **Piskaryovskoye kladbish'ye**

2. **Novodyevich'ye kladbish'ye**

3. **Ermitazh**

4. **Russkij muzyej**

Chapter 12

Getting Around: Planes, Trains, and More

In This Chapter
▶ Moving along with motion verbs
▶ Making your way through the airport
▶ Exploring public transportation
▶ Traveling by train

As the Russian proverb has it, **Yazyk do Kiyeva dovyedyot** (ee-*zihk* dah *kee*-ee-vuh duh-vee-*dyot*), which translates as "Your tongue will lead you to Kiev," and basically means, "Ask questions, and you'll get anywhere." With the help of this chapter, you'll be able to ask your way into the most well-concealed corners of the Russian land via several different modes of transportation. And you'll definitely be able to make it to Kiev!

Understanding Verbs of Motion

Every language has a lot of words for things the speakers of that language know well. That's why the Eskimos have 12 different words for "snow." Russians have a lot of space to move around; maybe that's why they have so many different verbs of motion.

In English, the verb "to go" can refer to walking, flying by plane, or traveling by boat (among other options). That's not the case in Russian; in fact, for one very simple and straightforward English infinitive "to go," Russian has several equivalents. Each of these verbs has its own (and we should say, very erratic) conjugation pattern.

Your choice of verb depends on many different factors and your intended message. To mention just a few factors, the choice depends on

✔ Whether the motion is performed with a vehicle or without it

✔ Whether the motion indicates a regular habitual motion

✔ Whether the motion takes place at the moment of speaking

Why does Russian have so many words to indicate movement? Having this distinction helps make a message clearer and even saves time on unnecessary questions. For example, when you say "I want to go to the theater tonight" in English, it's not quite clear whether you're going to drive, walk, or take a train, and so the listener may have to ask for additional information, such as "How are you going to get there?" or "Will you drive?" In Russian, this information is already packed into your answer, depending on the verb that you use. Your verb choice eliminates the need to ask additional questions and may save the listener a lot of time. Neat, isn't it?

In the following sections, we explain the verbs of motion to use when you're speaking of habitual or present movement. We also show you how to talk about the exact places you're going.

Going by foot or vehicle habitually

To talk about moving around generally, you use the *multidirectional verbs* **khodit'** (khah-*deet'*; to go on foot) and **yezdit'** (*yez*-deet'; to go by vehicle). If you're talking about walking around the city or driving around the country, these two verbs are the ones to use.

You also use the multidirectional verbs **khodit'** and **yezdit'** when you talk about repeated trips there and back, such as **ya khozhu v shkolu** (ya khah-*zhoo* f shkoh-loo; I go to school) and **on yezdit na rabotu** (ohn *yez*-deet nah ruh-*boh*-too; he goes to work by vehicle).

These two verbs indicate regular habitual motion in the present tense. As an example of how to use these verbs, think of places that you go to once a week, every day, two times a month, once a year, or every weekend. Most folks, for example, have to go to work every day. In Russian you say:

✔ **Ya khozhu na rabotu kazhdyj dyen'** (ya khah-*zhoo* nuh ruh-*boh*-too *kahzh*-dihy dyen'; I go to work every day) if you go by foot

✔ **Ya yezzhu na rabotu kazhdyj dyen'** (ya *yez*-zhoo nuh ruh-*boh*–too *kahzh*-dihy dyen'; I go to work every day) if you go by vehicle

The verb **khodit'** is conjugated in Table 12-1.

Table 12-1	Conjugation of Khodit'	
Conjugation	*Pronunciation*	*Translation*
ya khozhu	ya khah-*zhoo*	I go on foot
ty khodish'	tih *khoh*-deesh'	You go on foot (informal singular)
on/ona/ono khodit	ohn/ah-*nah*/ah-*noh* khoh-deet	He/she/it goes on foot
my khodim	mih *khoh*-deem	We go on foot
vy khoditye	vih *khoh*-dee-tee	You go on foot (formal singular and plural)
oni khodyat	ah-*nee khoh*-dyet	They go on foot

When you talk about walking, you also can use the expression **khodit' pyeshkom** (khah-*deet'* peesh-*kohm;* to go by foot, to walk). This expression sounds redundant, but that's the way it's used in Russian.

The verb **yezdit'** is conjugated in Table 12-2.

Table 12-2	Conjugation of Yezdit'	
Conjugation	*Pronunciation*	*Translation*
ya yezzhu	ya *yez*-zhoo	I go by vehicle
ty yezdish'	tih *yez*-deesh'	You go by vehicle (informal singular)
on/ona/ono yezdit	ohn/ah-*nah*/ah-*noh* yez-deet	He/she/it goes by vehicle
my yezdim	mih *yez*-deem	We go by vehicle
vy yezdite	vih *yez*-dee-tee	You pl. go by vehicle (formal singular and plural)
oni yezdyat	ah-*nee yez*-dyet	They go by vehicle

You also can specify the vehicle you're using with one of these phrases:

- ✔ **yezdit' na taksi** (*yez*-deet' nah tuhk-*see;* to go by taxi)
- ✔ **yezdit' na marshrutkye** (*yez*-deet' nah muhr-*shroot*-kee; to go by minivan)
- ✔ **yezdit' na avtobusye** (*yez*-deet' nah uhf-*toh*-boo-see; to go by bus)
- ✔ **yezdit' na myetro** (*yez*-deet' nah mee-*troh*; to go by metro)

✔ **yezdit' na poyezdye** (*yez*-deet' nah *poh*-yeez-dee; to go by train)

✔ **yezdit' na mashinye** (*yez*-deet' nah muh-*shih*-nee; to go by car)

Going by foot or vehicle at the present time

In Russian, your word choice depends on whether you're moving around generally (such as driving around the city or walking around your house) or purposefully moving in a specific direction or to a specific place. To talk about moving around generally, you use the *multidirectional verbs* **khodit'** and **yezdit',** which we discuss in the previous section.

You use different verbs (called *unidirectional verbs*) to specify that you're moving in a specific direction or to a specific place. You also use these verbs to indicate motion performed at the present moment.

For walking, use the verb **idti** (ee-*tee*; to go in one direction by foot), such as in the phrase **Ya idu na rabotu** (ya ee-*doo* nuh ruh-*boh*-too; I am walking to work). Here's the conjugation of **idti:**

✔ **Ya idu** (yah ee-*doo*; I am going)

✔ **Ty idyosh'** (tih ee-*dyohsh'*; You are going; informal singular)

✔ **On/on/ono idyot** (ohn/ah-*nah*/ah-*noh* ee-*dyot*; He/she/it is going)

✔ **My idyom** (mih ee-*dyom*; We are going)

✔ **Vy idyotye** (vih ee-*dyo*-tee; You are going; formal singular and plural)

✔ **Oni idut** (ah-*nee* ee-*doot*; They are going)

For moving by a vehicle, use the unidirectional verb **yekhat'** (*ye*-khaht'; to go in one direction by a vehicle):

✔ **Ya yedu** (ya *ye*-doo; I am going)

✔ **Ty yedyesh'** (tih *ye*-deesh'; You are going; informal singular)

✔ **On/ona/ono yedyet** (ohn/ah-*nah*/ah-*noh* *ye*-deet; He/she/it is going)

✔ **My yedyem** (mih *ye*-deem; We are going)

✔ **Vy yedyetye** (vih *ye*-dee-tee; You are going; formal singular and plural)

✔ **Oni yedut** (ah-*nee* *ye*-doot; They are going)

Explaining where you're going

To tell where you're going specifically, use the prepositions **v** (v; to) or **na** (nah; to) + the accusative case of the place you're going. See Chapter 15 for details on these particular prepositions:

- ✔ **Ya idu v tyeatr** (ya ee-*doo* f tee-*ahtr*; I am going to the theater)
- ✔ **Ona idyot na kontsyert** (ah-*nah* ee-*dyot* nuh kahn-*tsehrt*; She is going to the concert)

For walking or driving around a place, use the preposition **po** (pah; around) + the dative case (for more information on cases, see Chapter 2):

- ✔ **Ona khodit po Moskvye** (ah-*nah* khoh-deet puh mahsk-*vye*; She walks around Moscow)
- ✔ **My yezdim po tsyentru goroda** (mih *yez*-deem pah *tsehnt*-roo *goh*-ruh-duh; We drive around downtown)

Now the good news! As long as you're moving within the city, you don't need to make a distinction between going by vehicle and walking. Even if you change three modes of public transportation on the way to the library, you're still perfectly fine saying **ya idu v bibliotyeku** (ya ee-*doo* v beeb-lee-ah-*tye*-koo; I'm going to the library). This distinction has remained in the language since the times when cities were small enough so that it was possible to walk everywhere. If you're going out of town, however, it's obvious that you need to use transportation, unless you're prepared to walk for months.

Remember to use **yezdit'** or **yekhat'** (to go by vehicle) when you talk about going to other cities! Otherwise, if you say **ya idu v Moskvu** (ya ee-*doo* v mahsk-*voo*), you make it sound like you're embarking on an enduring walking pilgrimage to Moscow, which is probably not your intention.

Sometimes Russians drop pronouns in sentences when using verbs of motion; it's more conversational. For example, instead of **Kuda ty idyosh'?** (koo-*dah* tih ee-*dyosh'*; Where are you going?) you may hear simply **Kuda idyosh'?** (koo-*dah* ee-*dyosh'*; Where are you going?) And instead of saying **Ya idu v tyeatr** (ya ee-*doo* f tee-*ahtr*; I'm going to the theater), you may simply say **Idu v tyeatr** (ee-*doo* f tee-*ahtr*; I'm going to the theater).

Talkin' the Talk

Sarah got a new job in Moscow. On the way to work, she meets her Russian friend Kolya.

Sarah: **Privyet! Kuda idyosh'?**
pree-*vyet*! koo-*dah* ee-*dyosh*'?
Hi! Where are (you) going?

Kolya: **Na rabotu. Ya khozhu na rabotu pyeshkom kazhdyj dyen'.**
nuh ruh-*boh*-too. ya khah-*zhoo* nuh ruh-*boh*-too peesh-*kohm kahzh*-dihy dyen'.
I'm going to work. I walk to work every day.

Sarah: **A ya yezzhu na myetro. Kolya, u tyebya yest' plany na vyechyer? Davaj pojdyom v kino.**
ah ya *ye*-zhoo nuh mee-*troh*. koh-lye, oo tee-*bya* yest' *plah*-nih nuh *vye*-cheer? duh-*vahy* pahy-*dyom* v kee-*noh*.
And I go by metro. Kolya, do you have plans for tonight? Let's go to the movies.

Kolya: **Syegodnya nye mogu. Idu s rodityelyami v tyeatr.**
see-*vohd*-nye nee mah-*goo*. ee-*doo* s rah-*dee*-tee-lee-mee f tee-*ahtr*.
Tonight, I can't. I'm going to the theater with my parents.

Words to Know

U tyebya yest' plany na vyechyer?	oo tee-<u>bya</u> yest' <u>plah</u>-nih nuh <u>vye</u>-cheer	Do you have plans for tonight?
Syegodnya nye mogu.	see-<u>vohd</u>-nye nee mah-<u>goo</u>	Tonight, I can't.
s rodityelyami	s rah-<u>dee</u>-tee-lee-mee	with my parents

Navigating the Airport

Chances are, if you visit Russia, you enter by **samolyot** (suh-mah-*lyot*; plane). If not, you probably fly somewhere within the country during your visit — those 6.6 million square miles of land make air travel especially appealing. Whether you're leaving Moscow for a 20-minute flight to St. Petersburg or a 9-hour flight to Vladivostok, the vocabulary you find in the following sections helps you plan and enjoy your trip by air.

Using the verb "to fly"

You use a special verb of motion when you talk about flying: **lyetyet'** (lee-*tyet'*; to fly). You can't use the verb **yekhat'** (covered in "Going by foot or vehicle at the present time" earlier in this chapter) when you talk about traveling by plane, unless the plane is wheeling around the airport without actually leaving the ground. If the plane actually takes off, you have to use the verb **lyetyet'**, conjugated in Table 12-3.

Table 12-3	Conjugation of Lyetyet'	
Conjugation	*Pronunciation*	*Translation*
ya lyechu	ya lee-*choo*	I fly or I am flying
ty lyetish'	tih lee-*teesh'*	You fly or You are flying (informal singular)
on/ona/ono lyetit	ohn/ah-*nah*/ah-*noh* lee-*teet*	He/she/it flies or He/she/it is flying
my lyetim	mih lee-*teem*	We fly or We are flying
vy lyetitye	vih lee-*tee*-tee	You fly or You are flying (formal singular and plural)
oni lyetyat	ah-*nee* lee-*tyat*	They fly or They are flying

Checking in and boarding your flight

After you arrive at the **aeroport** (ah-eh-rah-*pohrt*; airport), you need to choose between the areas called **zal prilyota** (zahl pree-*lyo*-tuh; arrivals) and **zal vylyeta** (zahl *vih*-lee-tuh; departures). To inquire about the status of your flight, look at the **informatsionnoye tablo** (een-fuhr-muh-tsih-*oh*-nuh-ye tahb-*loh*; departures and arrivals display). Arrivals are called **pribytiye** (pree-*bih*-tee-ee) and departures are called **otpravlyeniye** (uht-pruhv-*lye*-nee-ee).

When you come for **ryegistratsiya** (ree-geest-*rah*-tsih-ye; check-in), you need to have your **bilyet** (bee-*lyet*; ticket) and your **pasport** (*pahs*-puhrt; passport). It also helps to know your **nomyer ryejsa** (*noh*-meer *ryey*-suh; flight number). Here are some questions you may hear as you check in:

- ✔ **Vy budyetye sdavat' bagazh?** (vih *boo*-dee-tee zdah-*vaht'* buh-*gahsh*; Are you checking any luggage?)

- ✔ **Vy ostavlyali vash bagazh byez prismotra?** (vih ahs-tahv-*lya*-lee vahsh buh-*gahsh* byes pree-*smoh*-truh; Have you left your luggage unattended?)

Be prepared to **projti provyerku** (prahy-*tee* prah-*vyer*-koo; to go through check-in) and then **sluzhba byezopasnosti** (*sloozh*-buh bee-zah-*pahs*-nuhs-tee; security check), where you probably have to pass through a **myetal-loiskatyel'** (mee-*tah*-luh-ees-*kah*-teel'; metal detector). If you forget your gate number, you can ask **Kakoj u myenya nomyer vykhoda?** (kuh-*kohy* oo mee-*nya noh*-meer *vih*-khuh-duh; What's my gate number?) At the gate, you may ask the **styuard** (styu-*ahrt*; male flight attendant) or **styuardyessa** (styu-uhr-*dye*-suh; female flight attendant): **Eto ryejs v . . . ?** (*eh*-tuh ryeys v; Is this the flight to . . . ?)

Have your **posadochnyj talon** (pah-*sah*-duhch-nihy tuh-*lohn*; boarding pass) ready; **posadka** (pah-*saht*-kuh; boarding) is about to begin. Don't forget your **ruchnoj bagazh** (rooch-*nohy* buh-*gahsh*; carry-on). And find out whether your seat is a **myesto u okna** (*myes*-tuh oo ahk-*nah*; window seat), **myesto u prokhoda** (*myes*-tuh oo prah-*khoh*-duh; aisle seat), or a **myesto v syeryedinye** (*myes*-tuh f see-ree-*dee*-nee; middle seat). When you're **na bortu** (nuh bahr-*too*; on board), you meet your **pilot** (pee-*loht*; pilot) and **ekipazh** (eh-kee-*pahsh*; crew).

Handling passport control and customs

If you're taking an international flight, shortly before arrival you're handed **tamozhyennaya dyeklaratsiya** (tuh-*moh*-zhih-nuh-ye deek-luh-*rah*-tsih-ye; customs declaration). Fill it out on the plane to save yourself some time in the chaos of the airport. If you notice a bored-looking Russian in the seat next to you, feel free to ask him or her for assistance: **Pomogitye mnye, pozhalujsta, zapolnit' tamozhyennuyu dyeklaratsiyu?** (puh-mah-*gee*-tee mnye pah-*zhahl*-stuh zuh-*pohl*-neet' tuh-*moh*-zhih-noo-yu deek-luh-*rah*-tsih-yu; Would you please help me to fill out the customs declaration?)

After leaving the plane and walking through a corridor maze, you see a crowded hall with **pasportnyj kontrol'** (*pahs*-puhrt-nihy kahnt-*rohl'*; passport control). To save yourself some frustration, make sure you get into the right line: One line is for **grazhdanye Rossii** (*grahzh*-duh-nee rah-*see*-ee; Russian citizens), and one is for **inostranniye grazhdanye** (ee-nahs-*trah*-nih-ee *grahzh*-duh-nee; foreign citizens).

At passport control, you show your **pasport** (*pahs*-puhrt; passport) and **viza** (*vee*-zah; visa); see Chapter 11 for more about these documents. A **pogranich-nik** (puhg-ruh-*neech*-neek; border official) asks you **Tsyel' priyezda?** (tsehl' pree-*yez*-duh; The purpose of your visit?) You may answer:

- ✔ **turizm** (too-*reezm*; tourism)
- ✔ **rabota** (ruh-*boh*-tuh; work)
- ✔ **uchyoba** (oo-*choh*-buh; studies)
- ✔ **chastnyj vizit** (*chahs*-nihy vee-*zeet*; private visit)

After you're done with passport control, it's time to pick up your **bagazh.** To find the baggage claim, just follow the signs saying **Bagazh** (buh-*gahsh*; luggage). This word means both "luggage" and "baggage claim." The next step is going through **tamozhyennyj dosmotr** (tuh-*moh*-zhih-nihy dahs-*mohtr*; customs). The best way to go is **zyelyonyj koridor** (zee-*lyo*-nihy kuh-ree-*dohr*; nothing to declare passage way, *Literally:* green corridor). Otherwise, you have to deal with **tamozhyenniki** (tuh-*moh*-zhih-nee-kee; customs officers) and answer the question **Chto dyeklariruyete?** (shtoh deek-luh-*ree*-roo-ee-tee; What would you like to declare?)

To answer, say **Ya dyeklariruyu . . .** (ya deek-luh-*ree*-roo-yu; I'm declaring . . .) + the word for what you are declaring in the accusative case (see Chapter 2 for case details). The following items usually need to be declared:

- ✔ **alkogol'** (uhl-kah-*gohl'*; alcohol)
- ✔ **dragotsyennosti** (druh-gah-*tseh*-nuhs-tee; jewelry)
- ✔ **proizvyedyeniya iskusstva** (pruh-eez-vee-*dye*-nee-ye ees-*koost*-vuh; works of art)

Talkin' the Talk

Tony just arrived in Moscow by plane. He's going through passport control at the airport.

Tony:	**Dobryj dyen'. Vot moj pasport.**
	dohb-rihy dyen'. voht mohy *pahs*-puhrt.
	Good afternoon. Here's my passport.

Tamozhennik: **(customs officer)**	**Khorosho. A gdye viza?**
	khuh-rah-*shoh*. ah gdye *vee*-zuh?
	Great. And where is your visa?

Tony:	**Vot ona.**
	voht ah-*nah*.
	Here it is.

Tamozhennik:	Aga, vizhu. Tsyel' priyezda?
	ah-*gah*, *vee*-zhoo. tsehl' pree-*yez*-duh?
	All right, I see. The purpose of your visit?
Tony:	Turizm.
	too-*reezm*.
	Tourism.

Words to Know

Vot moj pasport.	voht mohy <u>pahs</u>-pahrt	Here's my passport.
A gdye viza?	ah gdye <u>vee</u>-zuh	And where is your visa?
Vot ona.	voht ah-<u>nah</u>	Here it is.

Leaving the airport

The moment you step out of customs, you're attacked by an aggressive mob of cab drivers. They speak numerous foreign languages and offer ungodly fares to go to the city. Ignore them and move toward the **vykhod** (*vih*-khuht; exit), where the more timid (and usually more honest) cab drivers reside. You may try to negotiate your fare (see "Taking a taxi" later in this chapter).

If you're up for an adventure and don't mind dragging your luggage around through the crowds, you also can leave the airport via public transportation. A **marshrutka** (muhr-*shroot*-kuh; minivan) is usually a fast way to make it to the city (see "Using minivans" later in this chapter for details). Some airports, such as the one in Moscow, have **elyektrichki** (eh-leek-*treech*-kee; trains) running to the city. The **avtobus** (uhf-*toh*-boos; bus) isn't a very good way to leave the airport; they're slow and far between.

Before you leave the airport, you see **obmyen valyut** (ahb-*myen* vuh-*lyut*; currency exchange). Normally, you don't need to change your currency at the airport; the exchange rate isn't very good, and any cab driver eagerly accepts U.S. dollars. Just make sure you have a variety of small bills; they aren't too good at providing change. Watch out for the way your bills look, too: Old, torn, or worn bills won't be accepted, especially outside of the cities. See Chapter 14 for additional money matters.

Conquering Public Transportation

Russians hop around their humongous cities with butterfly ease, changing two to three means of public transportation during a one-way trip to work. And so can you. Being a public transportation guru isn't necessary. You just need to know where to look for the information and how to ask the right questions, which you discover in the following sections.

Taking a taxi

The easiest way to get around unfamiliar cities and to have your share of good conversation with interesting personalities is, of course, a cab ride. Russian **taksi** (tuhk-*see*; cabs) don't always look like cabs. While the official ones are decorated with a checkers-like design or have **TAKSI** in large print on their sides, you also see plenty of regular-looking cars that stop when you raise your arm to hail a cab. Those cars are neither cabs in disguise nor necessarily serial killers; they're just regular citizens trying to make an extra $10 on the way to work. Most Russians feel safe riding with them; if you don't, then you're better off calling the **sluzhba taksi** (*sloozh*-buh tuhk-*see*; cab service). When you call the **sluzhba taksi,** they ask:

- ✔ **vash adryes** (vahsh *ahd*-rees; your address)
- ✔ **Kuda yedyetye?** (koo-*dah* ye-dee-tee; Where are you going?)

You use **kuda** (koo-*dah*; where to) rather than **gdye** (gdye; where) when you're asking about movement *toward* a destination. You can think of **kuda** as meaning "where to?" and **gdye** as simply "where?" Likewise, you use **tuda** (too-*dah*; to there) instead of **tam** (tahm; there) when you want to emphasize movement *toward* a destination. Simply stated: With verbs of motion, you usually use **kuda** rather than **gdye** and **tuda** rather than **tam.**

You can ask for your fare while you're ordering your cab: **Skol'ko eto budyet stoit'?** (*skohl'*-kuh *eh*-tuh *boo*-deet *stoh*-eet'; How much would that be?) This fare is usually non-negotiable. If you hail a cab in the street, however, you have plenty of room for negotiating.

Open your conversation with the question **Skol'ko voz'myotye do Bol'shogo?** (*skohl'*-kuh vahz'-*myo*-tee duh bahl'-*shoh*-vuh; How much will you charge me to go to the Bolshoy?) After the driver offers his fare, such as **sto rublyej** (stoh roob-*lyey*; 100 rubles), offer half the sum: **Davajtye za pyatdyesyat'!** (dah-*vahy*-tee zuh pee-dee-*syat*; what about 50? *Literally:* Let's do it for 50!) If the driver says **nyet,** add a little to your price: **Togda davajtye za syem'dyesyat!** (tahg-*dah* duh-*vahy*-tee zuh *syem'*-dee-seet; What about 70 then? *Literally:* Let's do it for 70!) Sooner or later, you find the common ground. (For more on numbers, see Chapter 2.)

You don't need to **davat' chayevye** (duh-*vaht'* chuh-ee-*vih*-ee; to give a tip) to cab drivers in Russia.

Using minivans

The transport of choice in today's Russia is the **marshrutka** (muhr-*shroot*-kuh), a minivan with a set route. **Marshrutki** (muhr-*shroot*-kee; minivans) are usually fast and often go to any destination. They stop only where passengers need to get off, so make sure you tell the driver something like **Ostanovitye, pozhalujsta, u vokzala?** (uh-stuh-nah-*vee*-tee pah-*zhahl*-stuh oo vahk-*zah*-luh; Would you please stop at the railway station?)

Marshrutki have different routes, marked by numbers. You can recognize a **marshrutka** by a piece of paper with its number in the front window. To board a **marshrutka,** you need to go to a place where it stops. These places aren't usually marked, so you need to ask a local **Gdye ostanavlivayutsya marshrutki?** (gdye uhs-tuh-*nahv*-lee-vuh-yut-sye muhr-*shroot*-kee; Where do the minivans stop?) **Marshrutki** have a set fare usually written on a piece of paper above the driver's head, and you need cash to pay for **marshrutki.**

Catching buses, trolley buses, and trams

The first difficulty with all this variety of Russian public transportation is that in English, all these things are called "buses." Here's a short comprehensive guide on how to tell one item from another:

- **avtobus** (uhf-*toh*-boos) — a bus as you know it
- **trollyejbus** (trah-*lye*-boos) — a bus connected to electric wires above
- **tramvaj** (truhm-*vahy*) — a bus connected to electric wires and running on rails

If you find yourself on something moving on rails and not connected to electric wires above, it's a train, and it's probably taking you to a different city! See "Embarking on a Railway Adventure" later in this chapter for more.

Now that you can identify the modes of transportation, you're half set. Catch the **avtobus, trollyejbus,** or **tramvaj** at the **avtobusnaya ostanovka** (uhf-*toh*-boos-nuh-ye uhs-tuh-*nohf*-kuh; bus stop), **trollyejbusnaya ostanovka** (trah-*lye*-boos-nuh-ye uhs-tuh-*nohf*-kuh; trolleybus stop), and **tramvajnaya ostanovka** (truhm-*vahy*-nuh-ye uhs-tuh-*nohf*-kuh; tram stop), respectively. You see a sign with **A** for **avtobus** and **T** for **trollyejbus** or **tramvaj.** You may also see a **raspisaniye** (ruhs-pee-*sah*-nee-ye; schedule) and a **karta marshruta** (*kahr*-tuh muhr-*shroo*-tuh; route map).

Unless you're into orienteering, the best way to find your route is to ask the locals. They're usually extremely friendly and happy to provide you with more information than you want to have. Just ask these questions:

- **Kak mnye doyekhat' do Krasnoj Plosh'adi?** (kahk mnye dah-*ye*-khuht' dah *krahs*-nuhy *ploh*-sh'ee-dee; How can I get to the Red Square?)

- **Etot avtobus idyot do Ermitazha?** (*eh*-tuht uhf-*toh*-boos ee-*dyot* duh ehr-mee-*tah*-zhuh; Will this bus take me to the Hermitage?)

- **Gdye mozhno kupit' bilyety?** (gdye *mohzh*-nuh koo-*peet'* bee-*lye*-tih; Where can I buy tickets?)

Ways to pay for a bus ride vary. In some cities, you need to buy **bilyety** (bee-*lye*-tih; tickets) ahead of time in **kioski** (kee-*ohs*-kee; ticket kiosks). In others, you pay directly to the **vodityel'** (vah-*dee*-teel'; driver) or **konduktor** (kahn-*dook*-tuhr; bus conductor) when you board the bus.

Hopping onto the subway

During Soviet times, all Russian cities were divided into those that have a **myetro** (mee-*troh*; subway) and those that don't. Life in cities with the **myetro** was considered a step better than in those without. Having a **myetro** was a sign of living in a big city. Nowadays, all cities in Russia are divided into two categories: Moscow and non-Moscow. But the **myetro** is still a big deal.

And no wonder. The Russian **myetro** is beautiful, clean, user-friendly, and cheap. It connects the most distant parts of such humongous cities as Moscow, and it's impenetrable to traffic complications. During the day, trains come every two to three minutes. Unfortunately, it's usually closed between 1:30 a.m. and 4:30 a.m. Around 4:30 a.m., it's easy to locate a **stantsiya myetro** (*stahn*-tsee-ye meet-*roh*; subway station) on a Moscow street by a crowd of young people in clubbing clothes waiting for the **myetro** to open so they can go home.

The Moscow **myetro** has 11 lines. Each **vyetka** (*vyet*-kuh; subway line) has its own name and is marked by its own color. You can take a look at a Moscow **myetro** map at www.hotels-moscow.ru/metro.html.

To take the **myetro,** you need to buy a **kartochka** (*kahr*-tuhch-kuh; fare card) for any number of trips in the **vyestibyul' myetro** (vees-tee-*byu*-lee meet-*roh*; metro foyer) or a **proyezdnoj** (pruh-eez-*nohy*; pass).

Embarking on a Railway Adventure

Taking a **poyezd** (*poh*-eest; train) is probably one of the best adventures you can have in Russia. In the following sections, find out how to read a train schedule, how to choose the type of train that's just right for you, how to buy a ticket, and how to board the train.

Making sense of a train schedule

As you're standing in front of a giant timetable tableau **na vokzale** (nuh vahk-*zah*-lee; at a railway station), it probably seems to provide more information that you want to have. You see the following:

- **stantsiya otpravlyeniya** (*stahn*-tsih-ye uht-prahv-*lye*-nee-ye; departure station)
- **stantsiya pribytiya** (*stahn*-tsih-ye pree-*bih*-tee-ye; arrival station)
- **vryemya v puti** (*vrye*-mye f poo-*tee*; travel time)
- **nomyer poyezda** (*noh*-meer *poh*-eez-duh; train number)

The column with a bunch of unfamiliar words divided by commas is probably the list of stations where the train stops. You also see **vryemya otpravleniya** (*vrye*-mye uht-pruhv-*lye*-nee-ye; departure time) and **vryemya pribytiya** (*vrye*-mye pree-*bih*-tee-ye; arrival time).

The abbreviation **Ch** stands for **chyotnyye** (*choht*-nee-ee; even-numbered dates) and the abbreviation **Nech** stands for **nyechyotnye dni** (nee-*choht*-nee-ee dnee; odd-numbered dates), which are the days when the train runs.

Surveying types of trains and cars

The types of trains you probably want to know, in the order of increasing price and quality, are

- **elyektrichka** (eh-leek-*treech*-kuh; suburban train)
- **skorostnoj poyezd** (skuh-rahs-*nohy poh*-eest; a low-speed train)
- **skoryj poyezd** (*skoh*-rihy *poh*-eest; a faster and more expensive train)
- **firmyennyj poyezd** (*feer*-mee-nihy *poh*-eest; premium train, *Literally:* company train)

Unless you're traveling to the suburbs, the **firmyennyj poyezd** is your best choice; you'll be surprised with its speed and service. The **elyektrichka** is a good alternative to buses and taxis if you're going to the suburbs.

After you pick a train, you need to pick the right kind of **vagon** (vah-*gohn*; train car). Every train, except for the **elyektrichka,** have the following types of cars (in order of increasing cost):

- ✔ **obsh'iy vagon** (*ohb*-sh'eey vah-*gohn*) This train car consists of just benches with a bunch of people sitting around. Not recommended, unless your travel time is just a couple of hours.

- ✔ **platskart** (pluhts-*kahrt*) A no-privacy sleeping car with way too many people; not divided into compartments. Not recommended, unless you're into extreme sociological experiments.

- ✔ **kupye** (koo-*peh*) A good, affordable sleeping car with four-person compartments.

- ✔ **spal'nyj vagon** (*spahl'*-nihy vah-*gohn*) The granddaddy of them all; a two-person sleeping compartment. May be pricey.

Buying tickets

You can **kupit' bilyety** (koo-*peet'* bee-*lye*-tih; buy tickets) directly at the railway station, at a travel agency, or in a **zhyelyeznodorozhnyye kassy** (zhih-*lyez*-nuh-dah-*rohzh*-nih-ee *kah*-sih; railway ticket office), which you can find throughout the city. Remember to bring your **pasport** (*pahs*-puhrt; passport) and **nalichnyye dyen'gi** (nuh-*leech*-nih-ee *dyen'*-gee; cash); the ticket office may not accept credit cards.

You can start your dialogue with **Mnye nuzhyen bilyet v** (mnye *noo*-zheen bee-*lyet* v) + the name of the city you're heading for in the accusative case (see Chapter 2 for more about cases). The ticket salesperson probably asks you the following questions:

- ✔ **Na kakoye chislo?** (nuh kuh-*koh*-ee chees-*loh*; For what date?)

- ✔ **Vam kupye ili platskart?** (vahm koo-*peh* ee-lee pluhts-*kahrt*; Would you like a compartment car or a reserved berth?)

- ✔ **V odnu storonu ili tuda i obratno?** (v ahd-*noo* stoh-ruh-noo *ee*-lee too-dah ee ah-*braht*-nuh; One way or round trip?)

You can also tell the ticket salesperson what kind of seat you prefer: **vyerkhnyaya polka** (*vyerkh*-nee-ye *pohl*-kuh; top fold down bed) or **nizhnyaya polka** (*neezh*-nye-ye *pohl*-kuh; bottom fold down bed). On **elyektrichki** (eh-leek-*treech*-kee; suburban trains), which don't have fold down beds, seats aren't assigned.

Stocking up on essentials for your ride

After you find out what **pyeron** (pee-*rohn*; platform) your train is departing from, you can take care of important things, such as stocking up on food and reading materials. Both of these resources are readily available on the train itself; you can always buy food in the **vagon-ryestoran** (vah-*gohn* rees-tah-*rahn*; restaurant car). Numerous vendors also walk through the train offering snacks, as well as **krossvordy** (krahs-*vohr*-dih; crossword puzzles) and **anyekdoty** (ah-neek-*doh*-tih; joke collections). However, if you're a little more picky about what you read, you may want to prepare something beforehand. As for the food, excessive eating on the train is a ritual, and if you want a full train experience, you have to partake in it.

On the train, have a lot of small bills ready to pay for your **postyel'noye byel'yo** (pahs-*tyel'*-nuh-ee beel'-*yo*; bed sheets), **chaj** (chahy; tea), and the numerous snacks you buy at train stations. No ATMs are available, and ice-cream vendors don't usually accept credit cards.

Boarding the train

You find your **nomyer vagona** (*noh*-meer vah-*goh*-nuh; car number) on your **bilyet** (bee-*lyet*; ticket). When you approach your train car (it's a good idea to start moving in that direction about half an hour before the departure time), you see a friendly (or not) **provodnik** (pruh-vahd-*neek*; male train attendant) or **provodnitsa** (pruh-vahd-*nee*-tsuh; female train attendant) who wants to see your **bilyet** and **pasport.**

For traveling in Russia, always have your passport and your visa with you! You can't get on the train or the plane or check into a hotel without it. For security reasons, also make photocopies of these documents, and carry the copies in a different pocket.

When you're on the train, you check out **postyel'noye byel'yo** (pahs-*tyel'*-nuh-ee beel'-*yoh*; bed sheets) from the **provodnik,** and you're ready to go!

Discovering the joys of a train trip

Russians tend to treat a train trip like a small vacation. Even before the train takes off, they change into comfortable clothes and **tapochki** (*tah*-puhch-kee; slippers) to make it easier to get in and out of "bed." Before the train leaves the city limits, they take out plentiful snacks and start the first of the long procession of on-the-train meals. People in your compartment will definitely invite you to share their meal, so make sure you offer them something, too.

A **provodnik** (pruh-vahd-*neek*; male train attendant) or a **provodnitsa** (pruh-vahd-*nee*-tsuh; female train attendant) drops by throughout the ride offering hot tea and coffee. Take them up on the offer, at least for the joy of holding unique Russian **podstakanniki** (puhd-stuh-*kah*-nee-kee; glass holders) that can't be found anywhere except in Russian trains and rarity collections.

At the stops, people almost always get out to walk around on the platform, stretch their legs, and smoke a cigarette. It's also a good chance to buy yet more food from **babushki** (*bah*-boosh-kee; local old ladies) who sell home-made food, such as **frukty** (*frook*-tih; fruit), **morozhyenoye** (mah-*roh*-zhih-nuh-ee; ice-cream), and **pivo** (*pee*-vuh; beer) on the platform. Some phrases to use during your train ride:

- ✔ **Skol'ko stoim na etoj stantsii?** (*skohl'*-kuh stah-*eem* nuh *eh*-tuhy *stahn*-tsee-ee; How long is the stop at this station?)

- ✔ **Vy nye vozrazhayete, yesli ya otkroyu okno?** (vih nee vuhz-ruh-*zhah*-ee-tee, *yes*-lee ya aht-*kroh*-yu ahk-*noh*; Do you mind if I open the window?)

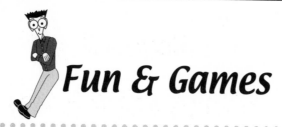

Fun & Games

Look at these sentences with motion verbs. Which of them just don't make sense? See Appendix C for the answers.

1. **Ya idu v shkolu.**

2. **Ya yedu pyeshkom.**

3. **On idyot v muzyej.**

4. **My idyom v Moskvu.**

5. **Oni yedut na mashinye.**

Which of the following will you NOT see at an airport? See Appendix C for the answer.

a. **bagazh**

b. **pasportnyj kontrol'**

c. **poyezd**

d. **zyelyonyj koridor**

Chapter 13

Staying at a Hotel

Staying in a comfortable **gostinitsa** (gahs-*tee*-nee-tsuh; hotel) while you travel is extremely important. If you have a nice and comfy hotel room, life is good and you probably love the country you're in. If, however, you stay in an old dilapidated hotel, you probably feel miserable and sorry that you ever came. To make your stay in a Russian hotel more pleasurable, in this chapter we show you how to find and book the right hotel room, what to say and do when checking in, how to resolve service problems, and how to check out and pay your bill.

Booking the Hotel That's Right for You

To ensure the hotel you're staying in doesn't disappoint you, make sure the room is what you want. In the following sections, you discover different types of hotels to choose from and find out to how to make reservations in Russian.

Distinguishing different types of hotels

Two main types of hotels exist in Russia: the more expensive, more comfortable **pyatizvyozdnyye gostinitsy** (pee-tee-*zvyozd*-nih-ee gahs-*tee*-nee-tsih; five-star hotels) and the less expensive, less comfortable **odnozvyozdnyye gostinitsy** (uhd-nah-*zvyozd*-nih-ee gahs-*tee*-nee-tsih; one-star hotels). But don't be surprised if one- or two-star hotels in Russia charge you as much as four- or even five-star hotels. Another Russian puzzle for you!

You don't just stay at a hotel, you live there

What do people do in hotels? They stay there. Although Russian does have an equivalent for this verb — **ostanavlivatysya** (uhs-tuh-*nahv*-lee-vuht'-sye; to stay), Russians like using the verb **zhit'** (zhiht'; to live) to indicate the same notion. It's very common, for example, in describing where you stayed, to say something along these lines: **My zhili v gostinitse Moskva** (mih *zhih*-lee v gahs-*tee*-nee-tsee Mahs-*kvah*; We stayed in Moscow Hotel, *Literally:* We lived in Hotel Moscow).

Russian today has two words for the English "hotel." One of them is a good old Russian word **gostinitsa** (gahs-*tee*-nee-tsuh; hotel), which literally means "a place for the guests." The other word is **otel'** (ah-*tehl'*; hotel), an offspring from the foreign word. Although from a linguistic point of view, both words are interchangeable, they're charged with slightly different meanings. Nobody in Russia uses the word **otel'** (hotel) in reference to a little old shabby hotel. In this situation, the word **gostinitsa** (hotel) is more appropriate. On the other hand, when speaking about luxurious four- or five-star hotels, Russians use both words interchangeably.

A good way to find out about hotels is to ask people who have already traveled to the city: **A gdye tam mozhno ostanovit'sya?** (uh gdye tahm *mohzh*-nuh uhs-tuh-nah-*veet'*-sye; And where can one stay there?) Don't be shy. Most people love to share this information. With a preliminary list of hotels, you can now either call your travel agent or just get more info on the Internet. (For more about dealing with travel agencies, see Chapter 11.)

Making a reservation

If you're making a reservation online, the forms that you fill out are self-explanatory. If, however, you prefer to make a reservation on the phone, you want to say: **Ya khotyel/khotyela by zabronirovat' nomyer** (ya khah-*tyel*/khah-*tye*-luh bih zuh-brah-*nee*-ruh-vuht' *noh*-meer; I would like to make a reservation for a room). Use **khotyel** if you're a man and **khotyela** if you're a woman.

When they talk about hotel rooms, Russians use the word **nomyer,** which also means "number." In a way it makes sense, because all rooms in a hotel have numbers!

You have to provide some important information when you make a hotel reservation on the phone. We steer you through the process in the following sections.

Stating how long you're going to stay

After you state that you want to make a reservation on the phone, the person you're talking to probably asks **Na kakoye chislo?** (nuh kuh-*koh*-ee chees-*loh*; For what date?)

To answer this very predictable question, use this formula: **Na** (nah; for) + the ordinal numeral indicating date in neuter + the name of the month in genitive case. For example, if you're planning to arrive on September 15, you say: **Na pyatnadtsatoye syentyabrya** (nuh peet-*naht*-tsuh-tuh-ee seen-teeb-*rya*; For September 15). (Check out details on cases in Chapter 2. For more on dates, see Chapter 11.)

You may also be asked from what date to what date you want to stay in the hotel: **S kakogo po kakoye chislo?** (s kuh-*koh*-vuh puh kuh-*koh*-ee chees-*loh*; From what date to what date?)

To answer this question, use **s** (s; from) + the genitive case of the ordinal number indicating the date + the genitive case of the word indicating the month + **po** (poh; until) +the ordinal numeral indicating the date in neuter gender (and nominative case) + name of the month in the genitive case.

If, for example, you're planning to stay in the hotel from June 21 to June 25, you say **S dvadtsat' pyervogo iyunya po dvadtsat' pyatoye iyunya** (s *dvaht*-tsuht' *pyer*-vuh-vuh ee-*yu*-nye pah *dvaht*-tsuht' *pya*-tuh-ee ee-*yu*-nye; from June 21 to June 25).

You also can simply state how many nights you're going to stay in the hotel. If you're checking in on June 21 at 3 p.m. and leaving on June 25 at 11 a.m., you'll be staying in the hotel **chyetyrye nochi** (chee-*tih*-ree *noh*-chee; four nights). For more about numbers with nouns, check out Chapter 2.

Choosing your room

When you're done talking about dates, you may hear: **Vy khotitye odnomyestnyj nomyer ili dvukhmyestnyj nomyer?** (vih khah-*tee*-tee uhd-nah-*myest*-nihy ee-lee dvookh-*myest*-nihy *noh*-meer; Do you want a single or double accommodation?)

Most rooms in hotels are either **odnomyestnyye** (uhd-nah-*myest*-nih-ee; single accommodation) or **dvukhmyestnyye** (dvookh-*myest*-nih-ee; double accommodation). If you have a third person, such as a child, you may get a **raskladushka** (ruhs-kluh-*doosh*-kuh; cot). And if you're the happy parent of two kids, you probably want to spring for an extra room.

In a Russian hotel room, you won't find king- or queen-sized beds, only **odnospal'nyye** (uhd-nah-*spahl'*-nih-ee; twins) or **dvuspal'nyye** (dvoo-*spahl'*-nih-ee; doubles).

Another very important thing you need to ask about is whether the room has a **vannaya** (*vah*-nuh-ye; bathtub), **dush** (doosh; shower) or even **tualyet** (too-uh-*lyet*; toilet). In an inexpensive hotel in a small provincial city, showers and toilets may be located **na ehtazhye** (nuh eh-tuh-*zheh*; on the floor) and not **v nomyere** (v *noh*-mee-ree; in the hotel room). To avoid such disappointments, you can ask: **V nomyere yest' vannaya, dush i tualyet?** (v *noh*-mee-ree yest' *vah*-nuh-ye doosh ee too-uh-*lyet*; Is there a bathtub, shower, and toilet in the room?) Also note that while the word **tualyet** best translates as "toilet," it really refers to the room in which a toilet is found. The actual toilet itself is called an **unitaz** (oo-nee-*tahs*).

Finding the right price

Certainly an important question to ask is **Skol'ko stoit nomyer?** (*skohl'*-kuh *stoh*-eet *noh*-meer; How much is the room?) or **Skol'ko stoyat nomyera?** (*skohl'*-kuh stoh-yet nuh-mee-*rah*; How much are the rooms?)

If the hotel you're calling has a number of vacancies, chances are the rates may be different for different rooms. If this is the case, you may hear something like: **Yest' nomyer/nomyera za syem'dyesyat yevro, za vosyem'dyesyat yevro, za sto yevro.** (yest' *noh*-meer/nuh-mee-*rah* zuh *syem'*-dee-seet *yev*-ruh, zuh *voh*-seem'-dee-seet *yev*-ruh, zuh stoh *yev*-ruh; There is a room/are rooms for 70 euros, for 80 euros, for 100 euros.)

While prices at most Russian hotels are sometimes shown in euros or dollars, you still have to pay in rubles. Why? Russian law doesn't permit most institutions to accept foreign currencies. Most Russian hotels (except for the very best five-star hotels in major cities) still don't accept credit cards. And almost no Russian hotel accepts personal checks. In general, it's a good idea to have rubles on you at all times in Russia, even before you enter the country. See Chapter 14 for more about money matters.

When you decide which room you want, say: **Ya voz'mu nomyer za vosyem'dyesyat yevro.** (ya vahz'-*moo noh*-meer zuh *voh*-seem-dee-seet *yev*-ruh; I will take a room for 80 euros.)

You may also want to inquire whether this amount includes breakfast: **Eto vklyuchayet zavtrak?** (*eh*-tuh fklyu-*chah*-eet *zahf*-truhk; Does it include breakfast?) It would be nice if it does.

Talkin' the Talk

Nancy is calling a hotel in St. Petersburg to make a reservation. She is traveling alone and is on a budget. A **rabotnik gostinitsy** (ruh-*boht*-neek gahs-*tee*-nee-tsih; hotel employee) answers the phone.

Nancy:	**Ya khotyela by zabronirovat' nomyer.** ya khah-*tye*-luh bih zuh-brah-*nee*-ruh-vuht' *noh*-meer. I would like to make a reservation for a room.
Rabotnik gostinitsy:	**Na kakoye chislo?** nuh kuh-*koh*-ee chees-*loh?* For what date?
Nancy:	**Na dvadtsatoye noyabrya.** nuh dvuht-*tsah*-tuh-ee nuh-eeb-*rya.* For November 20.
Rabotnik gostinitsy:	**Na dvadtsatoye noyabrya svobodnykh nomyerov nyet.** nuh dvuht-*tsah*-tuh-ee nuh-eeb-*rya* svah-*bohd*-nihkh nuh-mee-*rohf* nyet. There are no vacancies for November 20.
Nancy:	**A na dvadtsat' pyervoye yest' nomyera?** uh nuh *dvaht*-tsuht' *pyer*-vuh-ee yest' nuh-mee-*rah?* Are there vacancies for the 21st?
Rabotnik gostinitsy:	**Da. Odin nomyer? Na skol'ko dnyej?** dah. ah-*deen noh*-meer? nuh *skohl'*-kuh dnyey? Yes. One room? For how many days?
Nancy:	**Da, odin. Na dvye nochi. Odnomyestnyj nomyer.** dah, ah-*deen.* nuh dvye *noh*-chee. uhd-nah-*myest*-nihy *noh*-meer. Yes one. For two nights. Single accommodation.

Rabotnik gostinitsy:	**Yest' nomyer za sto yevro, za syem'dyesyat yevro.** yest' *noh*-meer zuh stoh *yev*-ruh, zuh *syem*-dee-seet *yev*-ruh. There is a room for 100 euros, and one for 70 euros.
Nancy:	**Ya voz'mu nomyer za syem'dyesyat yevro. V nomyerye yest' dush i tualyet?** ya vahz'-*moo noh*-meer zuh *syem*'-dee-seet *yev*-ruh. v *noh*-mee-ree yest' doosh ee too-uh-*lyet*? I will take the room for 70 euros. Is there a shower and toilet in the room?
Rabotnik gostinitsy:	**Da, yest'. Budyete bronirovat'?** dah, *yest'. boo*-dee-tee brah-*nee*-ruh-vuht'? Yes, there are. Will you be making a reservation?
Nancy:	**Da, budu.** Dah, *boo*-doo. Yes, I will.

Words to Know

Svobodnykh nomyerov nyet.	svah-<u>bohd</u>-nihkh nuh-mee-<u>rohf</u> nyet	There are no vacancies.
A na dvadtsat' pyervoye yest' nomyera?	uh nuh <u>dvaht</u>-suht' <u>pyer</u>-vuh-ee yest' nuh-mee-<u>rah</u>	Are there vacancies for the 21st?
na dvye nochi	nuh dvye <u>noh</u>-chee	for two nights
Budyetye bronirovat'?	<u>boo</u>-dee-tee brah-<u>nee</u>-ruh-vuht'	Will you be making reservation?
Da, budu.	Dah <u>boo</u>-doo	Yes, I will.

Checking In

Congratulations! You made it to your hotel. To make your check-in process as smooth as possible, in the following sections, we tell you what to say when checking in, how to find your room and what to expect when you get there, and how to find what you're looking for in the hotel. We also tell you about the names of important hotel employees you may want to know.

Enduring the registration process

When you arrive at your hotel, you're probably greeted (especially if you're at a nice hotel) by a **shvyejtsar** (shvyey-*tsahr*; doorman) and a **nosil'sh'ik** (nah-*seel'*-sh'ihk; porter).

Look for a sign with the word **ryegistratsiya** (ree-gee-*strah*-tsih-ye; check-in). That's where you report your arrival. Simply say **U myenya zabronirovan nomyer.** (oo mee-*nya* zuh-brah-*nee*-ruh-vuhn *noo*-meer; *Literally:* I have a room reserved.)

Expect to be asked **Kak vasha familiya?** (kahk *vah*-shuh fuh-*mee*-lee-ye; What is your last name?) Keep your passport ready — you need it for registration. To ask for your passport, the **ryegistrator** (ree-gee-*strah*-tuhr; receptionist) says: **Vash pasport** (vahsh *pahs*-puhrt; Your passport).

Beware: Your driver's license (be it Russian or foreign) isn't a valid ID in Russia. We suggest that you carry your passport with you at all times just in case.

The next step in registration is filling out the **ryegistratsionnaya kartochka** (ree-gee-struh-tsih-*oh*-nuh-ye *kahr*-tuhch-kuh; registration form). You hear **Zapolnitye, pozhalujsta, ryegistratsionnuyu kartochku.** (zuh-*pohl*-nee-tee, pah-*zhahl*-stuh, ree-gee-struh-tsih-*ohn*-noo-yu *kahr*-tuhch-koo; Fill out the registration form, please.) In most cases, this form requires you to provide the following information:

- **Imya** (*ee*-mye; first name)
- **Familiya** (fuh-*mee*-lee-ye; last name)
- **Adryes** (*ahd*-rees; address)
- **Domashnij/rabochij tyelefon** (dah-*mahsh*-neey/ruh-*boh*-cheey tee-lee-*fohn*; home/work phone number)
- **Srok pryebyvanya v gostinitsye s . . . po . . .** (srohk pree-bih-*vah*-nee-ye v gahs-*tee*-nee-tsih s . . . pah . . .; period of stay in the hotel from . . . to . . .)
- **Nomyer pasporta** (*noh*-meer *pahs*-puhr-tuh; passport number)

After you fill out all the forms and give the receptionist your passport, you receive the all-important **klyuch ot komnaty** (klyuch aht *kohm*-nuh-tih; the

key to your room) and your **kartochka gostya** (*kahr*-tuhch-kuh *gohs*-tye) or **visitka** (vee-*zeet*-kuh; hotel guest card).

Don't assume that your room number is related to the floor number. For example, if the **nomyer komnaty** (*noh*-meer *kohm*-nuh-tih; room number) is 235, it doesn't mean that the room is on the second floor; it can actually be on any floor of the hotel. Before you leave **registratsiya** (ree-gee-*strah*-tsih-ye; check-in), ask: **Na kakom etazhye moy nomyer?** (nuh kuh-*kohm* eh-tuh-*zheh* mohy *noh*-meer; On what floor is my room?)

Make sure you drop off your key with the reception desk each time you leave the hotel (and certainly pick it up when you come back). If you take your key with you, the administration of the hotel doesn't hold itself responsible for your personal belongings if anything of value left in your room mysteriously disappears.

Never leave the hotel without your **kartochka gostya** or **visitka** (hotel guest card) if you want to be let into the hotel when you come back after a long day of sightseeing. In most cases, the **visitka** (guest card) needs to be presented to the security officer that most Russian hotels are staffed with today.

Talkin' the Talk

Greg Brown has made a reservation for a hotel room in Yaroslavl' and is now checking in. Here is his conversation with the **ryegistrator** (receptionist).

Greg Brown: **U myenya zabronirovan nomyer na syegodnya.**
oo mee-*nya* zuh-brah-*nee*-ruh-vuhn *noh*-meer nuh see-*vohd*-nye.
I made a reservation for a room for today.

Ryegistrator: **Kak vasha familiya?**
kahk *vah*-shuh fuh-*mee*-lee-ye?
What is your last name?

Greg Brown: **Braun.**
brah-oon.
Brown.

Ryegistrator: **Greg Braun? Vash passport, pozhalujsta.**
grehg *brah*-oon? vahsh *pahs*-puhrt, pah-*zhahl*-stuh.
Greg Brown? Your passport, please.

Greg Brown: **Vot pozhaluysta.**
voht pah-*zhahl*-stuh.
Here it is.

Ryegistrator: **Zapolnitye, pozhalujsta, ryegistratsionnuyu kartochku.**
zuh-*pohl*-nee-tee, pah-*zhahl*-stuh, ree-gee-struh-tsih-
oh-noo-yu *kahr*-tuhch-koo.
Please fill out the registration form.

Greg Brown: **Khorosho.**
khuh-rah-*shoh.*
Okay.
(Greg fills out the form and hands it to the
receptionist.)
Vot, ya zapolnil.
voht ya zuh-*pohl*-neel.
Here, I filled it out.

Ryegistrator: **Vot vash kluch. Nomyer trista pyatnadtsat'. Vy vyp-
isyvayetyes' vos'mogo? Rasschyotnyj chas dvyenadt-
sat' chasov dnya.**
voht vahsh klyuch. *noh*-meer *trees*-tuh peet-*naht*-
tsuht'. vih vih-*pee*-sih-vuh-ee-tees' vahs'-*moh*-vuh?
ruhs-*chyot*-nihy chahs dvee-*naht*-tsuht' chuh-*sohf*
dnya.
Here is your key. You room number is 350. Are you
checking out on the 8th? Check-out time is 12 p.m.

Words to Know

na syegodnya	nuh see-<u>vohd</u>-nye	for today
Vot pozhalujsta.	voht pah-<u>zhahl</u>-stuh	Here you are.
zapolnitye	zuh-<u>pohl</u>-nee-tee	fill out
Vot, ya zapolnil.	voht ya zuh-<u>pohl</u>-neel	Here, I filled it out.
Vot vash kluch.	voht vahsh klyuch	Here is your key.
Vy vypisyvayetyes' vos'mogo?	Vih vih-<u>pee</u>-sih-vuh-ee-tees' vahs'-<u>moh</u>-vuh	You are checking out on the 8th?
rasschyotnyj chas	ruhs-<u>chyot</u>-nihy chahs	check-out time

Taking a tour of your room

What can you expect to find in your hotel room? Most likely, you see a **dvukhspal'naya krovat'** (dvookh-*spahl'*-nuh-ye krah-*vaht'*; double bed) or an **odnospal'nya krovat'**(uhd-nah-*spahl'*-nuh-ye krah-*vaht'*; twin bed) if you have a **nomyer na odnogo** (*noh*-meer nuh uhd-nah-*voh*; single room).

You also probably see a **torshyer** (tahr-*shehr*; standing lamp) or maybe a few of them, **tumbochki** (*toom*-buhch-kee; night stands), and a **pis'myennyj stol i stul** (*pees'*-mee-nihy stohl ee stool; desk and a chair). In most Russian hotel rooms, you also find a **shkaf** (shkahf; wardrobe), with **vyeshalki** (*vye*-shuhl-kee; hangers). You may (or may not) have a **tyelyefon** (tee-lee-*fohn*; telephone), a **tyelyevizor** (tee-lee-*vee*-zuhr; TV set), a **budil'nik** (boo-*deel'*-neek; alarm clock), and a **tyelyefonnyj spravochnik** (tee-lee-*foh*-nihy *sprah*-vuhch-neek; phone book containing hotel numbers). Whether you find these items in your room depends on the quality of the hotel.

If you have a bathroom in your room, you find an **unitaz** (oo-nee-*tahs*; toilet), **dush** (doosh; shower) or **vannaya** (*vah*-nuh-ye; bathtub). Check to make sure you have all the **polotyentsa** (puh-lah-*tyen*-tsuh; towels). Don't expect to see towels of various sizes in the bathroom of your hotel room. In the best case scenario, you find two kinds of towels: **vannoye polotyentsye** (*vah*-nuh-ee puh-lah-*tyen*-tseh; bath towel) and a smaller **lichnoye polotyentsye** (leech-*noh*-ee puh-lah-*tyen*-tseh; face towel).

Familiarizing yourself with the facilities

To idle away time in the hotel, you may want to explore. Here's what you may find:

- **gardyerob** (guhr-dee-*rohp*; cloak room)
- **pochta** (*pohch*-tuh; post office)
- **suvyenirnyj kiosk** (soo-vee-*neer*-nihy kee-*ohsk*; souvenir kiosk)
- **kamyera khranyeniya** (*kah*-mee-ruh khruh-*nye*-nee-ye; store room)
- **byuro obsluzhivaniya** (byu-*roh* ahp-*sloo*-zhih-vuh-nee-ye; customer service)
- **ryestoran** (rees-tah-*rahn*; restaurant)
- **bahr** (bahr; bar)

To inquire where a certain service is, go to the **byuro obsluzhivaniya** and say: **Skazhitye, pozhalujsta, gdye kamyera khranyeniya/pochta?** (skuh-*zhih*-tee pah-*zhahl*-stuh gdye *kah*-mee-ruh khruh-*nye*-nee-ee/*pohch*-tuh; Could you tell me where the store room/post office is?)

If you aren't staying in the hotel, but are just visiting somebody or having lunch in one of the hotel bars or restaurants, leaving your coat and hat in **gardyerob** (cloak room) is customary.

Meeting the staff

People who work in the earlier-mentioned facilities and other hotel services you want to know include the following:

- **administrator** (uhd-mee-nee-*strah*-tuhr; manager, person working at the front desk, or concierge)

- **gardyerobsh'ik/gardyerobsh'tsa** (guhr-dee-*rohp*-sh'eek/guhr-dee-*rohp*-sh'ee-tsuh; a person working in the cloak room)

- **nosil'sh'ik** (nah-*seel'*-sh'eek; porter)

- **shvyejtsar** (shvyey-*tsahr*; doorman)

- **gornichnaya** (*gohr*-neech-nuh-ye; maid)

Resolving Service Problems Successfully

Experienced travelers know that something always goes wrong when staying in a foreign country. In the following sections, we show you how to resolve some of the most common problems, such as reporting a broken item, asking for missing items, and requesting to change rooms.

Reporting a broken item

A very common problem is when something in your room isn't working. The key refuses to open the door, the phone is silent when you pick it up, or the shower pours only cold water on you. You need to speak to a **robotnik** (ruh-*boht*-neek; employee) in the **byuro obsluzhivaniya** (byu-*roh* ahp-*sloo*-zhih-vuh-nee-ye; customer service) to get help for these problems.

To report the problem, use the phrase **U myenya v komnatye nye rabotayet . . .** (oo mee-*nya* f *kohm*-nuh-tee nee ruh-*boh*-tuh-eet; The . . . in my room is not working) + the item that's not working. If your telephone is broken, for instance, you say **U myenya v komnatye nye rabotayet tyelyefon** (oo mee-*nya* f *kohm*-nuh-tee nee ruh-*boh*-tuh-eet tee-lee-*fohn*; The telephone in my room is not working). You put the word for the broken item into the nominative case.

Requesting missing items

The formula you need to know to report that something is missing is: **U myenya v nomyere nyet** (oo-mee-*nya* v noh-mee-ree nyet; In my room I don't have a) + the word denoting a missing thing in the genitive case. (For more information on forming the genitive case, see Chapter 2.)

Imagine that you've just taken a shower and are now reaching for the **vannoye polotyentsye** (*vah*-nuh-ee puh-lah-*tyen*-tseh; bath towel) only to discover you don't have one! Shivering from cold and dripping water from your freshly showered body, you rush to the phone to call customer service. You say: **U myenya v nomyerye nyet vannogo polotyentsa** (oo mee-*nya* v noh-mee-ree nyet *vah*-nuh-vuh puh-lah-*tyen*-tsuh; I don't have a bath towel in my room). Other things that you may request include

- **podushka** (pah-*doosh*-kuh; pillow)

- **odyeyalo** (ahd'-*ya*-luh; blanket)

- **vyeshalka** (*vye*-shuhl-kuh; hanger)

- **tualyetnaya bumaga** (too-uh-*lyet*-nuh-ye boo-*mah*-guh; toilet paper)

Asking to change rooms

To be honest, changing rooms isn't the easiest thing to do in a Russian hotel, but as they say in Russian: **Popytka nye pytka!** (pah-*piht*-kuh nee *piht*-kuh; It doesn't hurt to try!, *Literally:* An attempt is not a torture!) You should call customer service and say **Ya khotyel/khotyela by pomyenyat' nomyer** (ya khah-*tyel*/khah-*tye*-luh bih puh-mee-*nyat'* noh-meer; I would like to change my room). You say **khotyel** if you're a man and **khotyela** if you're a woman. And you need to give some convincing reasons for wanting to do so, such as:

- **V komnatye ochyen' shumno** (f *kohm*-nuh-tee *oh*-cheen' *shoom*-nuh; It is very noisy in my room).

- **V komnatye ochyen' kholodno/zharko** (f *kohm*-nuh-tee *oh*-cheen' *khoh*-luhd-nuh/*zhahr*-kuh; It is very cold/hot in my room).

- **V komnatye nyet svyeta** (f *kohm*-nuh-tee nyet *svye*-tuh; There is no light in my room).

Checking Out and Paying Your Bill

Your stay has come to an end, and now you have to pay. Or as Russians like to say: **Nastupil chas rassplaty** (nuh-stoo-*peel* chahs ruhs-*plah*-tih; It's time to pay, *Literally:* The hour of reckoning has arrived). In order to **zaplatit' za gostinitsu**

(zuh-pluh-*teet'* zuh gahs-*tee*-nee-tsoo; to pay for your hotel stay), you go to **ryegistratsiya** (ree-gee-*strah*-tsih-ye; check-in) and say **Ya vypisyvayus'. Ya khochu zaplatit'.** (ya vih-*pee*-sih-vuh-yus' ya khah-*choo* zuh-pluh-*teet'*; I am checking out. I want to pay for my stay.) Also ask **Vy prinimayetye kryedit-nyye kartochki?** (vih pree-nee-*mah*-ee-tee kree-*deet*-nih-ee *kahr*-tuhch-kee; Do you accept credit cards?) If the hotel does, inquire **Kakiye kryeditnyye kar-tochnki vy prinimayetye?** (kuh-*kee*-ee kree-*deet*-nih-ee *kahr*-tuhch-kee vih pree-nee-*mah*-ee-tee; What credit cards do you take?)

See to it that everything is correct in your receipt. It may include a **tyelyefon-nyj razgovor** (tee-lee-*foh*-nihy ruhz-gah-*vohr*; telephone call) you made from your room, or maybe **stirka** (*steer*-kuh; laundry service). If you feel that you're overcharged for some service you didn't use, point it out to the receptionist and ask politely: **A eto za chto?** (uh *eh*-tuh zah shtoh; And what is this for?) And don't forget to **poluchit' kvitantsiyu** (puh-loo-*cheet'* kvee-*tahn*-tsih-yu; to get a receipt) before you hurry out of the hotel to catch your train or plane.

As in most hotels throughout the world, the **rasschyotnyj chas** (ruhs-*chyot*-nihy chahs; check-out time) is **poldyen'** (*pohl*-deen'; noon) or **dvyenadtsat' chasov dnya** (dvee-*naht*-tsuht' chuh-*sohf* dnya; 12 p.m.). So where do you put your luggage if your plane doesn't leave until midnight? Most hotels have a **kamyera khranyeniya** (*kah*-mee-ruh khruh-*nye*-nee-ye; store room).

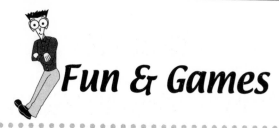

Fun & Games

Select the appropriate response for the following phrases; the answers are in Appendix C.

1. **Odnomyestnyj nomyer ili dvukhmyestnyj?**

   a. **Odnomyestnyj nomyer, pozhalujsta.**

   b. **Ya khochu zaplatit'.**

   c. **Gdye gardyerob?**

2. **Ya khotyela by zabronirovat' nomyer.**

   a. **Vy nye skazhyetye, gdye pochta?**

   b. **Na kakoye chislo?**

   c. **U myenya nye rabotayet tyelyefon.**

3. **Zdravstvujtye. U menya zabronirovan nomyer.**

   a. **Vot klyuch ot nomyera.**

   b. **U myenya v nomyere nyet polotyentsa.**

   c. **Kak vasha familiya?**

Using the information in the right-hand column, help John Evans fill out his hotel registration form in the left column. See Appendix C for the right answers.

imya _____ Evans

familiya _____ John

adryes _____ 815/555-5544

domashnij tyelyefon _____ 123 Highpoint Drive, Chicago, USA

Put these phrases from a conversation in logical order. See Appendix C for the correct answers.

a. **Moya familiya Ivanov.**

b. **U myenya zabronirovan nomyer.**

c. **Zapolnitye ryegistratsionnuyu kartochku.**

d. **Kak vasha familiya?**

Chapter 14

Money, Money, Money

*W*hat do traveling, shopping, dining, going out, and moving into a new place all have in common? They all require **dyen'gi** (*dyen'*-gee; money). This chapter takes you on a tour of the Russian monetary business. You find out about Russian currency and where to find it. You also discover phrases to use at the bank and while making payments. It pays to be prepared!

Paying Attention to Currency

In spite of ubiquitous dollar signs in fancy restaurant menus and "for rent" ads, the official Russian currency is not the U.S. dollar. In the following sections, you discover the names and denominations of Russian and international forms of money.

Rubles and kopecks

The official Russian currency is the **rubl'** (roobl'; ruble). Much like a dollar equals one hundred cents, one **rubl'** equals one hundred **kopyejki** (kah-*pyey*-kee; kopecks).

How a kopeck saved a ruble

Although Russians take pride in being extravagant with money, a Russian proverb teaches us otherwise: **Kopyejka rubl' byeryezhyot** (kah-*pyey*-kuh roobl' bee-ree-*zhoht*; A kopeck saves a ruble). Apparently, Russian folk wisdom fully agrees with the familiar "Take care of your pennies, and pounds will take care of themselves." In other words, being careful with little sums of money leads to big savings.

Kopyejki are a thing of the past now. With prices these days, nobody bothers with **kopyejki,** and they don't even appear in prices anymore.

To talk about different numbers of rubles, you need to use different cases, such as **dva rublya** (dvah roob-*lya*; two rubles) in the genitive singular, **pyat' rublyej** (pyat' roob-*lyey*; five rubles) in the genitive plural, and **dvadtsat' odin rubl'** (*dvaht*-tsuht' ah-*deen* roobl'; twenty-one rubles) in the nominative singular. For more info on numbers followed by nouns, see Chapter 2.

Before the Soviet revolution, the Russian ruble was one of the most respected currencies in Europe. Now, even Russians don't respect their currency too much. They sometimes call the ruble **dyeryevyannyj** (dee-ree-*vya*-nihy; *Literally:* wooden). Another derogatory term to refer to Russian **dyen'gi** (*dyen'*-gee; money) is **kapusta** (kuh-*poos*-tuh; *Literally:* cabbage). American dollars, on the other hand, are admirably referred to as **zyelyonyye** (zee-*lyo*-nih-ee; *Literally:* green).

Dollars, euros, and other international currencies

Although the official Russian currency is the ruble, some foreign currencies such as U.S. dollars and European euros are widely used. Although it's always better to have some rubles on you, you may be able to pay for an occasional cab ride with U.S. dollars or euros. Be careful, though: These currencies are the only two types of foreign currency that you can use in Russia. By and large, Russians aren't familiar with the way other currencies look and won't accept payment in unfamiliar-looking money. All other currencies have to be exchanged for rubles.

Here's a list of foreign currencies that you may need to exchange:

- ✔ **dollar YuS** (*doh*-luhr yu-*ehs;* U.S. dollar)
- ✔ **kanadskij dollar** (kuh-*nahts*-keey *doh*-luhr; Canadian dollar)
- ✔ **avstralijskij dollar** (uhf-struh-*leey*-skeey *doh*-luhr; Australian dollar)
- ✔ **yevro** (*yev*-ruh; euros)
- ✔ **funt styerlingov** (foont *stehr*-leen-guhf; British pound)
- ✔ **yaponskaya yena** (ee-*pohns*-kuh-ye *ye*-nuh; Japanese yen)

Changing Money

American dollars may be sufficient to take you to your hotel from the airport (at the risk of severe overpayment). After that, however, you have to jump into the "ruble zone." Big Russian cities are saturated with **punkty obmyena** (*poonk*-tih ahb-*mye*-nuh; currency exchange offices), which can also be called **obmyen valyut** (ahb-*myen* vuh-*lyut*). You can usually find a **punkt obmyena** in any hotel. The best **kurs obmyena valyut** (koors ahb-*mye*-nuh vuh-*lyut*; exchange rate), however, is offered by **banki** (*bahn*-kee; banks).

You may not get a fair exchange with street "currency exchangers." Although they may offer seductively profitable exchange rates, they offer no guarantee that what you receive in the end are, in fact, real Russian rubles. Unless you like living dangerously and Risk is your middle name, you're better off using a **bank** or **punkt obmyena.**

Some handy phrases to use when you exchange currency include

- ✔ **Ya khochu obmyenyat' dyen'gi.** (ya khah-*choo* uhb-mee-*nyat'* dyen*'*-gee; I want to exchange money.)
- ✔ **Ya khochu obmyenyat' dollary na rubli.** (ya khah-*choo* uhb-mee-*nyat'* doh-luh-rih nuh roob-*lee*; I want to exchange dollars for rubles.)
- ✔ **Kakoj kurs obmyena?** (kuh-*kohy* koors ahb-*mye*-nuh; What is the exchange rate?)
- ✔ **Nado platit' komissiyu?** (*nah*-duh pluh-*teet'* kah-*mee*-see-yu; Do I have to pay a fee?)

Most of the exchange offices require some kind of identification to allow you to exchange money; showing your passport is the safest bet.

Visiting a currency exchange office is a pretty good indicator that you have cash on you. This fact has long been known by **karmanniki** (kuhr-*mah*-nee-kee; pickpockets), who hang out by exchange office entrances and follow prospective victims after they leave the office. To avoid their unflattering attention, count your money and put it away before you step outside.

Talkin' the Talk

Jim stops by a bank to exchange dollars for rubles. He is asking the **rabotnik banka** (ruh-**boht**-neek **bahn**-kuh; bank employee) a couple of questions.

Jim:	**U vas mozhno obmyenyat' dollary na rubli?** oo vahs *mohzh*-nuh uhb-mee-*nyat' doh*-luh-rih nuh roob-*lee*? Can I exchange dollars for rubles here?
Rabotnik banka:	**Da. Kurs obmyena — odin k tridtsati.** dah. koors ahb-*mye*-nuh — ah-*deen* k tree-tsuh-*tee*. Yes. Exchange rate is one for thirty.
Jim:	**Ya khochu obmyenyat' sorok dollarov.** ya khah-*choo* uhb-mee-*nyat' soh*-ruhk *doh*-luh-ruhf. I would like to exchange forty dollars.
Rabotnik banka:	**Izvinitye, eto nyevozmozhno. Minimal'naya summa obmyena — sto dollarov.** eez-vee-*nee*-tee, *eh*-tuh nee-vahz-*mohzh*-nuh. mee-nee-*mahl'*-nuh-ye *soo*-muh ahb-*mye*-nuh — stoh *doh*-luh-ruhf. I am sorry, but that's impossible. The minimum sum for exchange is one hundred dollars.

Words to Know

U vas mozhno obmyenyat' dollary na rubli?	oo vahs <u>mohzh</u>-nuh uhb-mee-<u>nyat'</u> <u>doh</u>-luh-rih nuh roob-<u>lee</u>	Can I exchange dollars for rubles here?
odin k tridtsati	ah-<u>deen</u> k tree-tsuh-<u>tee</u>	one for thirty
Ya khochu obmyenyat' sorok dollarov.	ya khah-<u>choo</u> uhb-mee-<u>nyat'</u> <u>soh</u>-ruhk <u>doh</u>-luh-ruhf	I would like to exchange forty dollars.
Eto nyevozmozhno.	<u>eh</u>-tuh nee-vahz-<u>mohzh</u>-nuh	That's impossible.
minimal'naya summa	mee-nee-<u>mahl'</u>-nuh-ye <u>soo</u>-muh	minimum sum

Using Banks

Opening a bank account is a useful thing to do if you want to have payments deposited directly to your account, make money transfers easier, or get rid of the nerve-wracking obligation to think of your cash's safety. The following sections show you how to open and manage your bank account in Russian.

Opening an account at the bank of your choice

The first thing you need to do is decide on the type of bank you want to work with: Do you prefer a **kommyerchyeskij bank** (kah-*myer*-chees-keey bahnk; commercial bank) or **gosbank** (gohs-*bahnk*), which stands for **gosudarstvyennyj bank** (guh-soo-*dahr*-stvee-nihy bahnk; state bank)? Another way to refer to the **gosbank** is **sbyeryegatyel'naya kassa** (sbee-ree-*gah*-teel'-nuh-ye *kah*-suh); that's the phrase that you usually see on building facades. A privately owned **kommyerchyeskij bank** offers a much better **protsyent** (prah-*tsehnt*; interest rate).

In spite of a better interest rate offered by **kommyerchyeskiye banki** (kah-*myer*-chees-kee-ee *bahn*-kee; commercial banks)**, most Russians prefer to use a **gosbank.** During the numerous economic crises in Russia's recent history, **kommyerchyeskiye banki** closed and disappeared in the blink of an eye. But

if you decide to go with a **gosbank,** be prepared to face a long **ochyeryed'** (*oh*-chee-reet'; line).

Your next decision concerns the type of **schyot** (sh'oht; account) you want to open. Although **sbyeryegatyel'nyj** (sbee-ree-*gah*-teel'-nihy) literally translates as "savings," this type of **schyot** corresponds to "checking account." The accounts that involve a minimal term are called **srochnyye vklady** (*srohch*-nih-ee *fklah*-dih); they correspond to savings accounts. Also, students can open a **studyenchyeskij schyot** (stoo-*dyen*-chees-keey sh'oht; student account).

To open an account, you need to talk to a **rabotnik banka** (ruh-*boht*-neek *bahn*-kuh; bank employee). You simply say **Ya khochu otkryt' schyot** (ya khah-*choo* aht-*kriht'* sh'oht; I want to open an account). You'll need to **pokazat' pasport** (puh-kuh-*zaht'* *pahs*-puhrt; to show your passport) and to **zapolnit' zayavlyeniye** (zuh-*pohl*-neet' zuh-ee-*vlye*-nee-ee; to fill out forms). On a **zayavlyeniye,** you'll need to provide your **imya** (*ee*-mye; given name), **familiya** (fuh-*mee*-lee-ye; family name), **adryes** (*ahd*-rees; address), **nomyer pasporta** (*noh*-meer *pahs*-puhr-tuh; passport number), and the type of **schyot** (sh'oht; account) you want to open.

Talkin' the Talk

 Laura is a student at Moscow State University. She decides to open an account with a Russian bank and talks to a **rabotnik banka** (ruh-*boht*-neek *bahn*-kuh; bank employee).

Laura:	**Ya khotyela by otkryt' schyot u vas v bankye.** ya khah-*tye*-luh bih aht-*kriht'* sh'oht oo vahs v *bahn*-kee. I would like to open an account with your bank.
Rabotnik banka:	**Pozhalujsta. Posmotrityе etu broshyuru i vybyeritye, kakoj schyot vy khotitye otkryt'.** pah-*zhahl*-stuh. puh-smah-*tree*-tee *eh*-too brah-*shoo*-roo ee *vih*-bee-ree-tee, kuh-*kohy* sh'oht vih khah-*tee*-tee aht-*kriht'*. Here you go. Look at this booklet and choose the kind of account you would like to open.
Laura:	**Mnye podkhodit studyenchyeskij sbyeryegatyel'nyj schyot. Mnye na nyego budut pyeryechislyat' stipyendiyu.** mnye pahd-*khoh*-deet stoo-*dyen*-chees-keey sbee-ree-*gah*-teel'-nihy sh'oht. mnye nuh nee-*voh* *boo*-doot pee-ree-chees-*lyat'* stee-*pyen*-dee-yu.

Student savings account suits me best. I'll have my fellowship deposited into it.

Rabotnik banka: **Otlichno. Minimal'nyj vklad — dvyesti rublyej.** aht-*leech*-nuh. Mee-nee-*mahl'*-nihy fklaht — *dvyes*-tee roob-*lyey*.
Great. The minimum deposit is two hundred rubles.

Words to Know

otkryt' schyot	aht-<u>kriht'</u> sh'oht	to open an account
broshyura	brah-<u>shoo</u>-ruh	booklet
studyenchyeskij schyot	stoo-<u>dyen</u>-chees-keey sh'oht	student account
pyeryechislyat'	pee-ree-chees-<u>lyat'</u>	to deposit
minimal'nyj vklad	mee-nee-<u>mahl'</u>-nihy fklaht	minimum deposit

Making deposits and withdrawals

You have several ways to **sdyelat' vklad** (*sdye*-luht' fklaht; to deposit money) into your account:

✔ **klast' dyen'gi na schyot** (klahst' *dyen'*-gee nuh sh'oht; to deposit money directly at the bank or ATM, *Literally:* to put money into an account)

✔ **pyeryechislyat' dyen'gi na schyot** (pee-ree-chees-*lyat'* *dyen'*-gee nuh sh'oht; to deposit money into an account)

✔ **pyeryevodit' dyen'gi na schyot** (pee-ree-vah-*deet'* *dyen'*-gee nuh sh'oht; to transfer money from a different account or have it deposited by a third party, *Literally:* to transfer money to an account)

✔ **poluchat' pyeryevod** (puh-loo-*chaht'* pee-ree-*voht*; to have money wired to your account, *Literally:* to receive a transfer)

The imperfective verb **klast'** (klahst'; to put) has the perfective pair **polozhit'** (puh-lah-*zhih'*). Because the two verbs sound nothing like each other, and the frequency of their usage in conversation is so high, a good number of native speakers of Russian attempt to form the imperfective from **polozhit'** and use it in conversation. You may hear it a lot, but don't be tempted to pick it up; this form is both the most common and the most frowned upon grammatical mistake made by Russians themselves. (For more information on imperfective and perfective verbs, see Chapter 2.)

When filling out deposit slips, you're asked for the **summa vklada** (*soo*-muh *fklah*-duh; deposit amount) and **nomyer schyota** (*noh*-meer *sh'oh*-tuh; account number).

Now that you have some money in your account, you can:

- ✔ **snyat' dyen'gi so schyota** (snyat' *dyen'*-gee sah *sh'oh*-tuh; withdraw money from an account)

- ✔ **pyeryevyesti dyen'gi na drugoj schyot** (pee-ree-vees-*tee dyen'*-gee nuh droo-*gohy* sh'oht; transfer money to a different account)

- ✔ **poslat' dyenyezhnyj pyeryevod** (pahs-*laht' dyen*-neezh-nihy pee-ree-*voht*; to wire money, *Literally:* to send a money transfer)

And, finally, if you no longer need your bank account, you can just **zakryt' schyot** (zuhk-*riht'* sh'oht; to close the account).

Heading to the ATM

The fastest way to access your account is the **bankomat** (buhn-kah-*maht*; ATM). **Bankomaty** (buhn-kah-*mah*-tih; ATMs) are less ubiquitous in small cities; they're usually found in banks. Remember that you have to pay a **komissiya** (kah-*mee*-see-ye; ATM fee) each time you use a **bankomat** that belongs to a bank other than your own. The **komissiya** is usually 1.5 percent of the sum you're withdrawing, but no less than $3–$6 depending on the type of card. So, it probably makes sense to withdraw larger sums of money to avoid numerous **komissii** (kah-*mee*-see-ee; commissions) for smaller withdrawals.

Before inserting your card, make sure that the **logotip** (luh-gah-*teep*; symbol) of the card you're about to use (such as Visa or American Express) is on the **bankomat**. Otherwise, the **bankomat** may not recognize the card and may even swallow it for security purposes.

Here's your guide to the phrases you see on the **bankomat** screen:

- ✔ **vstav'tye kartu** (*fstahf'*-tee *kahr*-too; insert the card)

- ✔ **vvyeditye PIN-kod** (vee-*dee*-tee peen-*koht*; enter your PIN)

- ✔ **vvyeditye summu** (vee-*dee*-tee *soo*-moo; enter the amount)

✔ **snyat' nalichnyye** (snyat' nuh-*leech*-nih-ee; withdraw cash)

✔ **kvitantsiya** (kvee-*tahn*-tsih-ye; receipt)

✔ **zabyeritye kartu** (zuh-bee-*ree*-tee *kahr*-too; remove the card)

Spending Money

And now, on to the fun part! The best thing about money is spending it. In the following sections, discover what to do and what to say while making payments two different ways: by cash or using a credit card. You also find out where to find great bargains.

Before you run out and spend your money, you may find it helpful to know the verb **platit'** (pluh-*teet'*; to pay). Its conjugation appears in Table 14-1.

Table 14-1	Conjugation of Platit'	
Conjugation	*Pronunciation*	*Translation*
ya plachu	ya pluh-*choo*	I pay or I am paying
ty platish'	tih *plah*-teesh'	You pay or You are paying (informal singular)
on/ona/ono platit	ohn/ah-*nah*/ah-*noh* *plah*-teet	He/she/it pays or He/she/it is paying
my platim	mih *plah*-teem	We pay or We are paying
vy platitye	vih *plah*-tee-tee	You pay or You are paying (formal singular and plural)
oni platyat	ah-*nee plah*-tyet	They pay or They are paying

Finding great deals

At one time, travel in Eastern Europe was dirt cheap, which made it a perfect vacation spot for adventure-seeking college students. Well, no more; at least, not in Russia. Today, according to some polls, Moscow rates as the second most expensive city in the world. So, beware! Look out for these signs to cut down on your expenses:

✔ **rasprodazha** (ruhs-prah-*dah*-zhuh; sale)

✔ **skidka** (*skeet*-kuh; discount)

✔ **nyedorogo** (nee-*doh*-ruh-guh; inexpensive)

Another way to avoid sky-rocketing Moscow prices is to shop **na rynkye** (nuh *rihn*-kee; at the open market) rather than **v supyermarkyetye** (f soo-peer-*mahr*-kee-tee; at a supermarket), and of course, don't forget to **torgov-at'sya** (tuhr-gah-*vah*-tseh; to bargain)!

To inquire about the price of any item, ask **Skol'ko stoit . . . ?** (*skohl'*-kuh *stoh*-eet?; How much does . . . cost?) After you hear the price, you may want to specify your question to avoid the confusion:

- ✔ **Za kilogram?** (zuh kee-lahg-*rahm*; Per kilo?)
- ✔ **Za shtuku?** (zuh *shtoo*-koo; Per item?)
- ✔ **Za yash'ik?** (zuh *ya*-sh'eek; Per box?)

When you're buying several items or paying for your meal at a restaurant, a good phrase to use is **Skol'ko s myenya?** (*skohl'*-kuh s mee-*nya*; How much do I owe?)

For more information on inquiring about prices and paying for items, see Chapter 6.

Using cash

Nalichnyye (nuh-*leech*-nih-ee; cash) is still widely used in Russia. Many stores and ticket offices accept cash only, as do such places as the **rynok** (*rih*-nuhk; market) or a small **kafe** (kuh-*feh*; café). The general rule of thumb is the following: The fancier and more expensive the place is, the higher the chances that you're able to pay with a credit card (see the following section). Otherwise, prepare a stack of those rubles before you head out! To find out whether you can pay with cash, ask **U vas mozhno zaplatit' nalichnymi?** (oo vahs *mohzh*-nuh zuh-pluh-*teet'* nuh-*leech*-nih-mee; Can I pay with cash here?)

Russian rubles come both in **kupyury** (koo-*pyu*-rih; bills) and **monyety** (mah-*nye*-tih; coins). Kopecks always come in coins, but they're virtually extinct now (see "Rubles and kopecks" earlier in this chapter for more info). Here's a list of Russian bills and coins in use (so you know to be a little suspicious if you receive change in 15-ruble bills and 25-kopeck coins):

- ✔ **kupyury** (koo-*pyu*-rih; bills)
  - • **dyesyat' rublyej** (*dye*-seet' roob-*lyey*; ten rubles)
  - • **pyat'dyesyat rublyej** (pee-dee-*syat* roob-*lyey*; fifty rubles)
  - • **sto rublyej** (stoh roob-*lyey*; one hundred rubles)
  - • **pyat'sot rublyej** (peet'-*soht* roob-*lyey*; five hundred rubles)
  - • **tysyacha rublyej** (*tih*-see-chuh roob-*lyey*; one thousand rubles)

✔ **monyety** (mah-*nye*-tih; coins):

- **odna kopyejka** (ahd-*nah* kah-*pyey*-kuh; one kopeck)

- **pyat' kopyeyek** (pyat' kah-*pye*-eek; five kopecks)

- **dyesyat' kopyeyek** (*dye*-seet' kah-*pye*-eek; ten kopecks)

- **pyat'dyesyat kopyeyek** (pee-dee-*syat* kah-*pye*-eek; fifty kopecks)

- **odin rubl'** (ah-*deen* roobl'; one ruble)

- **dva rublya** (dvah roob-*lya*; two rubles)

- **pyat' rublyej** (pyat' roob-*lyey*; five rubles)

When paying **nalichnymi** (nuh-*leech*-nih-mee; with cash) in Russia, putting money into the other person's hand isn't customary. Instead, you're supposed to put the cash into a little plate usually found on the counter.

Traveler's checks may seem like a convenient way to transport money, but not in Russia. There, you may have a really hard time finding a place to exchange them. Russian doesn't even have an equivalent for "traveler's checks"; in those few places where they're recognized, they're referred to in English.

Paying with credit cards

Although **kryeditnyye kartochki** (kree-*deet*-nih-ee *kahr*-tuhch-kee; credit cards) and **bankovskiye kartochki** (*bahn*-kuhf-skee-ee *kahr*-tuhch-kee; debit cards) have long been established in cities like Moscow and St. Petersburg, in other cities your attempts to pay with a credit card may not be as welcome. When making plans to pay with a credit card, it's worth asking **U vas mozhno zaplatit' kryeditnoj kartochkoj?** (oo vahs *mohzh*-nuh zuh-pluh-*teet'* kree-*deet*-nuhy *kahr*-tuhch-kuhy; Can I pay with a credit card here?) or **Ya mogu zaplatit' kryeditnoj kartochkoj?** (ya mah-*goo* zuh-pluh-*teet'* kree-*deet*-nuhy *kahr*-tuhch-kuhy; Can I pay with a credit card?)

Some places, such as travel agencies, may charge you a fee when accepting payment by credit card. To find out where this is the case, you may want to ask **Vy vzymayetye komissionnyj sbor za oplatu kryeditnoj kartochkoj?** (vih vzih-*mah*-ee-tee kuh-mee-see-*oh*-nihy zbohr zuh ahp-*lah*-too kree-*deet*-nuhy *kahr*-tuhch-kuhy; Do you charge a fee for paying with a credit card?)

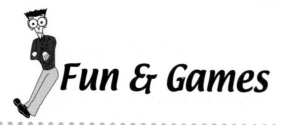

Fun & Games

Match these money-related activities in the left column with places where they are appropriate from the right column. Find the answers in Appendix C.

1. **Otkryt' schyot.**

a. **rynok**

2. **Obmyenyat' dollary.**

b. **bankomat**

3. **Vvyesti PIN-kod.**

c. **bank**

4. **Platit' nalichnymi.**

d. **obmyennyj punkt**

The following are descriptions of your interaction with a Russian bank. Put them in chronological order (see Appendix C for the answers):

a. **sdyelat' vklad**

b. **zakryt' schyot**

c. **otkryt' schyot**

Tom and Mickey go shopping. Each of them has a different means of payment on him: Tom has a credit card and Mickey has cash. Decide which of the following questions each friend is likely to ask before making his payment. (Appendix C has the answers.)

1. **Ya mogu zaplatit' kryeditnoj kartochkoj?**

2. **U vas mozhno zaplatit' nalichnymi?**

Chapter 15

Where Is Red Square?
Asking Directions

. . . .

In This Chapter

▶ Using "where" and "how"

▶ Receiving precise directions

▶ Discussing distances

. . . .

For a traveler, asking for directions (and understanding them) is an indispensable skill. In this chapter we give you the words and phrases you need when asking how to get to your destination and not get lost in the process. As exciting as it may be, being lost in a strange city can be scary and may even create panic. To avoid experiencing these unpleasant sensations, carefully read this chapter.

Asking "Where" and "How" Questions

When in doubt, just ask! In Russia, most passers-by, who at first may seem to be preoccupied with their own business, are actually very happy to help you. As a matter of fact, you may even be doing them a favor by distracting their attention from their routine duties and sometimes unhappy thoughts. In the following sections you discover how to ask for directions with two simple words: "where" and "how."

Where is it?

Russian uses two words to translate the English "where" — **gdye** (gdye; where) or **kuda** (koo-*dah*; where). But you can't use the two words interchangeably. The following is what you need to know about these words:

✔ If "where" indicates *location* rather than direction of movement and you aren't using the so-called verbs of motion (to go, to walk, to drive, and so on), use the word **gdye** (where).

✔ If "where" indicates *direction* of movement rather than location, or in other words is used in a sentence with verbs of motion (to go, to walk, to drive, and so on), use the word **kuda** (where).

When we say "verbs of motion," we mean all kinds of motion: going, walking, running, jogging, swimming, rowing, crawling, climbing, getting to . . . in other words, any verb associated with motion. For more info on verbs of motion, see Chapter 12.

Imagine you're looking for the nearest bus stop to get to a museum that's first on the list of places you want to see in a certain city. Here you are, helplessly standing on the corner of a crowded street and looking for a person with the friendliest expression to approach with your question. This young woman seems nice. Why not ask her?

Hold on! What exactly do you intend to ask her? If you're planning to ask "Where is the nearest bus stop?" think first how you're going to translate the word "where." Are you inquiring about location or destination here? Obviously, your question is about location — the location of the bus stop. Go back to the rule we just provided you. In a sentence or question asking about location, you use **gdye** (where). Now you can go ahead and ask your question:

> **Gdye blizhayshaya ostanovka avtobusa?** (gdye blee-*zhahy*-shuh-ye uhs-tuh-*nohf*-kuh uhf-*toh*-boo-suh; Where is the nearest bus stop?)

Did you notice that you don't have translate the verb "is" here and that the phrase indicating what you're looking for — the bus stop, in this case — is in the nominative case?

Look at another example. This time you're looking for a library. This is what you say in Russian:

> **Gdye bibliotyeka?** (gdye beeb-lee-ah-*tye*-kuh; Where is the library?)

Now, imagine a slightly different situation. You're at the bus station. A bus has just arrived and you want to know where it's going. The best person to ask is probably the driver himself: He should know where the bus is headed, even if today is his first day on the job. Before you ask your question, think first how you're going to begin it: with **gdye** (where) or with **kuda** (where)? Is your question "Where is the bus going?" about location or destination? Yes, you're asking a question about the destination! Go back to the earlier rules: If the main point of your question is destination, you should use the word **kuda** (where). Here's your question:

> **Kuda idyot etot avtobus?** (koo-*dah* ee-*dyot* eh-tuht uhf-*toh*-boos; Where is this bus going?)

To construct this question, you simply use **kuda,** the verb "is going" (**idyot,** in this example — see Chapter 12 for details), and the noun in the nominative case. No need to change it into another case!

How do I get there?

You're standing at the corner of a crowded street, and a young woman is passing by. You want to ask her how you can get to the **muzyyej** (moo-*zyey;* museum) you planned to see today. To ask this question, you need the verb **popast'** (pah-*pahst';* to get to). This verb, too, belongs to the category of verbs of motion (see the previous section). The phrase "How do I get to" is **Kak ya ostyuda mogu popast' v.** The following is what you want to ask:

> **Kak ya otsyuda mogu popast' v muzyej?** (kahk ya aht-*syu*-duh mah-*goo* pah-*pahst'* v moo-*zyey;* How do I get to the museum from here?)

Or you may want to make your question more impersonal by saying **Kak otsyuda mozhno popast' v** (How does one get to):

> **Kak otsyuda mozhno popast' v muzyej?** (kaht aht-*syu*-duh *mohzh*-nuh pah-*pahst'* v moo-*zyey;* How does one get to the museum from here?)

Russian uses the same prepositions, **v/na,** to express both "to (a place)" and "in/at (a place)." When you use **v/na** to indicate movement, the noun indicating the place of destination takes the accusative case. If **v/na** is used to denote location, the noun denoting location is used in prepositional case. (For more on cases, see Chapter 2.) Compare these two sentences:

> ✔ **Ya idu v bibliotyeku** (ya ee-*doo* v beeb-lee-ah-*tye*-koo; I am going to the library)
>
> ✔ **Ya v bibliotyekye** (ya v beeb-lee-ah-*tye*-kee; I am at the library)

In the first example, the noun **bibliotyeka** (beeb-lee-ah-*tye*-kuh; library) is used in the accusative case because the main message of the sentence is to indicate destination, but in the second example, the noun is in the prepositional case to denote location.

At this point you may be asking: When do you use **na** and when do you use **v?** The choice of the preposition depends on the noun it's used with. With most nouns, Russian speakers use **v.** But a number of nouns, such as those in the following list, require **na** (you just need to remember them). Note that the word after **na** in the first phrase is in the accusative case and the word after **na** in the second phrase is in the prepositional case:

> ✔ **na lyektsiyu/na lyektsii** (nuh *lyek*-tsih-yu/nuh *lyek*-tsih-ee; to a lecture/at a lecture)

- ✔ **na stadion/na stadionye** (nuh stuh-dee-*ohn*/nuh stuh-dee-*oh*-nee; to a stadium/at a stadium)

- ✔ **na stantsiyu/na stantsiye** (nuh *stahn*-tsih-yu/nuh *stahn*-tsih-ee; to a station/at a station)

- ✔ **na syeminar/na syeminarye** (nuh see-mee-*nahr*/nuh see-mee-*nah*-ree; to a seminar/at a seminar)

- ✔ **na urok/na urokye** (nuh oo-*rohk*/nuh oo-*roh*-kee; to a class/at a class)

- ✔ **na vokzal/na vokzalye** (nuh vahk-*zahl*/nuh vahk-*zah*-lee; to a railway station/at a railway station)

- ✔ **na zavod/na zavodye** (nuh zuh-*voht*/nuh zuh-*voh*-dee; to a plant/at a plant)

Understanding Specific Directions

When you're done asking for directions, it's important to understand what you're being told. In the following sections, you find out about prepositions and other words people use when talking about directions in Russian.

Recognizing prepositions

When people describe the location of something, they often use prepositions that you want to recognize in order to understand the directions given to you:

- ✔ **okolo** (*oh*-kuh-luh; near) + a noun in the genitive case

- ✔ **ryadom s** (*rya*-duhm s; next to) + a noun in the instrumental case

- ✔ **naprotiv** (nuh-*proh*-teef; opposite, across from) + a noun in the genitive case

- ✔ **za** (zah; behind, beyond) + a noun in the instrumental case

- ✔ **pozadi** (puh-zuh-*dee*; behind) + a noun in the genitive case

- ✔ **pyered** (*pye*-reet; in front of) + a noun in the instrumental case

- ✔ **myezhdu** (*myezh*-doo; between) + a noun in the instrumental case

- ✔ **vnutri** (vnoo-*tree*; inside) + a noun in the genitive case

- ✔ **snaruzhi** (snuh-*roo*-zhih; outside) + a noun in the genitive case

- ✔ **nad** (naht; above) + a noun in the instrumental case

- ✔ **pod** (poht; below) + a noun in the instrumental case

When you ask a simple question like **Gdye muzyej?** (gdye moo-*zyey*; Where is the museum?), you'll likely hear a response like:

> **Muzyej ryadom s tyeatrom, za magazinom, myezhdu aptyekoj i pochtoj, pozadi pamyatnika, naprotiv univyermaga.** (moo-*zyey rya*-duhm s tee-*aht*-ruhm, zuh muh-guh-*zee*-nuhm, *myezh*-doo uhp-*tye*-kuhy ee *pohch*-tuhy, puh-zuh-*dee pah*-meet-nee-kuh, nuh-*proh*-teef oo-nee-veer-*mah*-guh; The museum is next to the theater, beyond the store, between the pharmacy and the post office, behind the monument, opposite the department store.)

Note that each of the previously listed prepositions requires a different case for the noun or phrase following it. For more info on cases, see Chapter 2.

Do we really expect you to be able to juggle these cases? No, not at all. Your modest task for now is only to be able to understand the directions rather than provide them, unless of course you're planning on moving to Russia to become a traffic police officer.

Keeping "right" and "left" straight

When people give you directions, they also often use these words:

- **sprava ot** (*sprah*-vuh uht; to the right of) + a noun in the genitive case
- **napravo** (nuh-*prah*-vuh; to the right)
- **slyeva ot** (*slye*-vuh uht; to the left of) + a noun in the genitive case
- **nalyevo** (nuh-*lye*-vuh; to the left)
- **na lyevoj storonye** (nuh *lye*-vuhy stuh-rah-*nye;* on the left side)
- **na pravoj storonye** (nuh *prah*-vuhy stuh-rah-*nye*; on the right side)

Peter the Great's training methods

Peter the Great, the creator of the stable Russian Army, often trained the new recruits himself. The young recruits, who were often illiterate peasants, had an extremely hard time distinguishing between the two military commands — **napravo** (to the right) and **nalyevo** (to the left). To overcome this problem, the great tsar was said to have invented a new method of training new soldiers. He used the words the young peasants could distinguish very well: **syeno** (*sye*-nuh; hay) to indicate **nalyevo** (to the left), and the word **soloma** (sah-*loh*-muh; straw) to indicate **napravo** (to the right). And guess what? The method worked very well!

Here's a short exchange that may take place between you and a friendly-looking Russian woman:

You: **Izvinitye, gdye magazin?** (eez-vee-*nee*-tee gdye muh-guh-*zeen*; Excuse me, where is the store?)

The woman: **Magazin sprava ot aptyeki.** (muh-guh-*zeen sprah*-vuh uht uhp-*tye*-kee; The store is to the right of the pharmacy.)

Talkin' the Talk

Two friends, Oleg and Sergej, are talking on the phone. It's Saturday night and Oleg suggests that they go to a new restaurant tonight. He's already been there and is now explaining to Sergej where the restaurant is located.

Oleg:	**Chto ty syegodnya dyelayesh' vyechyerom?** shtoh tih see-*vohd*-nye *dye*-luh-eesh' *vye*-chee-ruhm? What are you doing this evening?
Sergej:	**Nichyego. A chto?** nee-chee-*voh*. uh shtoh? Nothing. Why?
Oleg:	**Davaj pojdyom v etot novyj ryestoran na Pyetrogradskoj storonye.** duh-*vahy puhy*-dyom v *eh*-tuht *noh*-vihy rees-tah-*rahn* nuh peet-rah-*graht*-skuhy stuh-rah-*nye*. Let's go to this new restaurant in Petrograd side (region in St. Petersburg).
Sergej:	**A, davaj. No ya tam yesh'yo nye byl. Gdye eto?** uh, duh-*vahy*. noh ya tahm ee-*sh'oh* nye bihl. *gdye eh*-tuh? Oh, okay. But I haven't been there yet. Where is it?
Oleg:	**Ty znayesh', gdye kinotyeatr Avrora?** tih *znah*-eesh', gdye kee-nuh-tee-*ahtr* uhv-*roh*-ruh? Do you know where the Aurora movie theater is?
Sergej:	**Nu?** noo? Well?
Oleg:	**Eto nyedalyeko ot Avrory, na drugoj storonye.** *eh*-tuh nee-duh-lee-*koh* uht uhv-*roh*-rih, nuh droo-*gohy* stuh-rah-*nye*. It's not far from Aurora, on the other side of the street.

Sergej:	**Eto chto, ryadom s bulochnoj?**
	eh-tuh shtoh, *rya*-duhm s *boo*-luhch-nuhy?
	Is it next to the bakery?
Oleg:	**Da, sprava ot bulochnoj i slyeva ot aptyeki.**
	dah, *sprah*-vuh aht *boo*-luhch-nuhy ee *slye*-vuh uht
	uhp-*tye*-kee.
	Yes, to the right of the bakery, to the left of the
	pharmacy.
Sergej:	**Myezhdu bulochnoj i aptyekoj?**
	myezh-doo *boo*-luhch-nuhy ee uhp-*tye*-kuhy?
	Between the bakery and the pharmacy?
Oleg:	**Da, naprotiv bara "Vostok."**
	dah, nuh-*proh*-teef *bah*-ruh vahs-*tohk.*
	Yes, opposite Vostok bar.

Words to Know

Ya tam yeshyo nye byl.	ya tahm ee-sh'oh nye bihl	I haven't been there yet.
Ty znayesh'	tih <u>znah</u>-eesh'	Do you know
Nu?	Noo?	Well? (Go on!)
Eto nyedalyeko ot	<u>eh</u>-tuh nee-duh-lee-<u>koh</u> uht	It's not far from
na drugoj storonye	nuh droo-<u>gohy</u> stuh-rah-<u>nye</u>	on the other side of the street

Making sense of commands

Usually when somebody gives you directions, they tell you where to go, not just where something is located. For this situation, we give you several common phrases that people may use when telling you where to go. These phrases also come in handy if you ever need to give somebody else directions.

The *imperative mood* is the form in which you hear and give directions. The imperative may also come in handy in other situations where you need to make a command or a polite request.

Here are some useful phrases in the imperative mood you may hear or want to use when giving directions:

- **Iditye praymo!** (ee-*dee*-tee *prya*-muh; Go straight.)

- **Iditye nazad!** (ee-*dee*-tee nuh-*zaht*; Go back.)

- **Iditye pryamo do . . . !** (ee-*dee*-tee *prya*-muh duh; Go as far as . . .) + the noun in the genitive case

- **Podojditye k . . .** (puh-duhy-*dee*-tee k; Go up to . . .) + the noun in the dative case

- **Iditye po . . .** (ee-*dee*-tee puh; Go down along . . .) + the noun in the dative case

- **Projditye mimo . . .** (prahy-*dee*-tee *mee*-muh; Pass by . . .) + the noun in the genitive case

- **Povyernitye nalyevo!** (puh-veer-*nee*-tee nuh-*lye*-vuh; Turn left or take a left turn.)

- **Povyernitye napravo!** (puh-veer-*nee*-tee nuh-*prah*-vuh; Turn right or take a right turn.)

- **Zavyernitye za ugol!** (zuh-veer-*nee*-tee *zah*-oo-guhl; Turn around the corner.)

- **Pyeryejditye ulitsu!** (pee-reey-*dee*-tee *oo*-leet-soo; Cross the street.)

- **Pyeryejditye plosh'ad'!** (pee-reey-*dee*-tee *ploh*-sh'uht'; Cross the square.)

- **Pyeryejditye chyerez dorogu!** (pee-reey-*dee*-tee *cheh*-reez dah-*roh*-goo; Cross the street/road.)

To form the imperative when you're talking to somebody with whom you're on **vy** (vih; you; formal singular and plural) terms, such as strangers, add **-tye** as we did in the previous list. When you're speaking to somebody with whom you're on **ty** (tih; you; informal singular) terms, you can remove the **-tye**. For instance, to say "turn left" to a friend, you say **Povyerni nalyevo** (puh-veer-*nee* nuh-*lye*-vuh; Turn left).

Curiously enough, Russians don't like to indicate directions with the words **vostok** (vahs-*tohk*; east), **zapad** (*zah*-puht; west), **syever** (*sye*-veer; north), and **yug** (yuk; south). They seem to avoid them when explaining how you can reach your place of destination. Phrases like "Go south," "Turn west," and "Drive south" are very rare in direction-giving.

Talkin' the Talk

 Tom is an American graduate student who came to Russia to study Russian literature. He asks a **rabotnik obsh'yezhitiya** (ruh-*boht*-neek uhp-sh'ee-*zhih*-tee-ye; dorm employee) how to get to the Dostoevsky museum.

Tom: **Skazhitye, pozhalujsta, kak mnye otsyuda popast' v muzyej Dostoyevskogo?**
skuh-*zhih*-tee, pah-*zhahl*-stuh, kahk mnye aht-*syu*-duh pah-*pahst'* v moo-*zyey* duhs-tah-*yef*-skuh-vuh?
Could you please tell me how I can get to Dostoyevsky's museum from here?

Rabotnik obsh'yezhitiya: **Muzyej Dostoyevskogo nakhoditsya na Kuznyechnom pyeryeulkye, nyeda-lyeko ot Kuznyechnogo rynka. Vy znayetye, gdye Kuznyechnyj rynok?**
moo-*zyey* duhs-tah-*yef*-skuh-vuh nuh-*khoh*-deet-sye nuh kooz-*nyech*-nuhm pee-ree-*ool*-kee, nee-duh-lee-*koh* uht kooz-*nyech*-nuh-vuh *rihn*-kuh. vih *znah*-ee-tee gdye kooz-*nyech*-nihy *rih*-nuhk?
Dostoyevsky's museum is located on Kuznyechnyj Lane, not far from Kuznyechnyj market. Do you know where Kuznyechnyj market is?

Tom: **Nyet, ya pyervyj dyen' v Pyetyerburgye.**
Nyet, ya *pyer*-vihy dyen' v pee-teer-*boor*-gee.
No, it's my first day in St. Petersburg.

Rabotnik obsh'yezhitiya: Vam nado vyjti na Nyevskij prospyekt i povyernut' napravo. Iditye pryamo po Nyevskomu prospyektu, nikuda nye svorachivaya do ulitsy Marata. Tam povyernitye opyat' napravo. Kogda dojdyotye do Kuznyechnogo pyeryeulka opyat' povyernitye napravo. Muzyej budyet na lyevoj storonye ulitsy, na uglu ulitsy Dostoyevskogo i Kuznyechnogo pyeryeulka.

vahm *nah*-duh *vihy*-tee nuh *nyef*-skeey prahs-*pyekt* ee pah-veer-*noot'* nuh-*prah*-vuh. ee-*dee*-tee *prya*-muh pah-*nyef*-skuh-moo prahs-*pyek*-too, nee-koo-*dah* nee svah-*rah*-chee-vuh-ye dah *oo*-lee-tsih muh-*rah*-tuh. tahm puh-veer-*nee*-tee ah-*pyat'* nuh-*prah*-vuh. kahg-*dah* dahy-*dyo*-tee duh kooz-*nyech*-nuh-vuh pee-ree-*ool*-kuh ah-*pyat'* puh-veer-*nee*-tee nuh-*prah*-vuh. moo-zyey *boo*-deet nuh *lye*-vuhy stuh-rah-*nye* oo-lee-tsih, nuh oog-*loo* oo-lee-tsih duhs-tah-*yef*-skuh-vuh i kooz-*nyech*-nuh-vuh pee-ree-*ool*-kuh. You need to go out to Nevsky Avenue and turn right. Go straight along Nevsky Avenue, don't turn anywhere until you reach Marat Street. Turn right again there. When you reach Kuznyechnyj Lane, turn right again. The museum is on the left-hand side, on the corner of Dostoyevsky Street and Kuznyechnyj Lane.

Tom: Tak, znachit po Nyevskomu do ulitsy Marata, napravo i opyat' napravo po Kuznyechnomu pyeryeulku?

tahk, *znah*-cheet pah *nyef*-skuh-moo dah oo-lee-tsih muh-*rah*-tuh, nuh-*prah*-vuh ee ah-*pyat'* nuh-*prah*-vuh pah kooz-*nyech*-nuh-moo pee-ree-*ool*-kuh? So, you're saying along Nevsky to Marat Street, to the right and again to the right along Kuznyechnyj Lane?

Rabotnik obsh'yezhitiya:	**Sovyershyenno vyerno.**
	suh-veer-*sheh*-nuh *vyer*-nuh.
	That's correct.

Words to Know

Kak mnye otsyuda popast' v . . .	kahk mnye aht-<u>syu</u>-duh pah-<u>pahst'</u> v	How can I get to . . . from here?
nakhoditsya	nuh-<u>khoh</u>-deet-sye	is located
vyjti na	<u>vihy</u>-tee nuh	go out to
Nikuda nye svorachivaya	nee-koo-<u>dah</u> nee svah-<u>rah</u>-chee-vuh-ye	Don't turn anywhere
Kogda dojdyotye do	kahg-<u>dah</u> dahy-<u>dyo</u>-tee duh	When you reach . . .
opyat'	ah-<u>pyat'</u>	again
na uglu	nuh oog-<u>loo</u>	on the corner

Describing Distances

Sometimes you don't want detailed information about directions. You just want to know whether someplace is near or far and how long it takes to get there. In the following sections we show you some common phrases you may use or hear when asking about distances.

Marking distances by time

Imagine you're in Moscow and you just asked a well-meaning passer-by to give you directions to Red Square. You ask a very simple question:

Skazhitye, pozhalujsta, kak mnye otsyuda popast' na Krasnuyu plosh'yad'? (skuh-*zhih*-tee pah-*zhahl*-stuh kahk mnye aht-*syoo*-duh pah-*pahst'* nuh *krahs*-noo-yu *ploh*-sh'iht; Could you tell me how I can get to Red Square from here?)

In response to your question, the sympathetic (and very talkative) Muscovite gives you an endless barrage of street names and landmarks and direction verbs to the point that you almost feel dizzy and your exhausted mind has switched off. At this point, all you want to know is whether Red Square is far away in order to decide whether you should take a taxi or some other public transportation. So with all your remaining mental energy you ask: **Eto dalyeko?** (*eh*-tuh duh-lee-*koh*; Is it far away?)

In giving directions, Russians usually like to indicate distance in terms of the time it takes to get there. Outdoorsy, younger people, may say, for example:

> **Eto nedalyeko. Minut pyatnadtsat' pyeshkom.** (*eh*-tuh nee-duh-lee-*koh*. mee-*noot* peet-*naht*-suht peesh-*kohm*; It's not far away. About fifteen minutes' walk.)

Those people who don't fancy walking that much may see the same distance differently and say:

> **Eto dalyeko. Minut pyatnadtsat' pyeshkom.** (*eh*-tuh duh-lee-*koh*. mee-*noot* peet-*naht*-suht' peesh-*kohm*; It's far. About fifteen minutes' walk.)

You may notice that in both the previous responses, the word **minut** (minutes) is placed before the numeral **pyatnadtsat'** (fifteen), and you may be wondering whether it's an error. Nope, that's not an error! Russian has a very special way of indicating approximate time, weight, distance, or even prices. Where English uses the word "about," Russian may simply use the method of reversing the order of words, as in **Minut pyatnadtsat' pyeshkom** (mee-*noot* peet-*naht*-suht' peesh-*kohm*; About fifteen minutes' walk). To be more exact, a Russian would say **Pyatnadtsat' minut pyeshkom** (peet-*naht*-suht' mee-*noot* peesh-*kohm*; Exactly fifteen minutes' walk).

A very popular way of indicating the distance in Russia is by counting the number of bus, tram, trolleybus, or subway stops to the place you're inquiring about. If you think that a fifteen-minute walk is a big deal, especially if you're tired, you may say in response:

> **Eto dovol'no dalyeko. Dvye ostanovki na tramvaye/avtobusye/trolyejbusye/myetro.** (*eh*-tuh dah-*vohl'*-nuh duh-lee-*koh*. dvye uhs-tuh-*nohf*-kee nuh truhm-*vahy*-ee/uhf-*toh*-boo-see/trah-*lyey*-boo-see/meet-*roh*; That's quite far away. Two stops by the tram/bus/trolleybus/metro.)

In addition to the well-known **taksi** (tuhk-*see*; taxi), you need to know four main kinds of transportation: **metro** (meet-*roh*; metro or subway), **avtobus** (uhf-*toh*-boos; bus), **trollyejbus** (trah-*lyey*-boos; trolleybus), and **tramvaj** (truhm-*vahy*; tram). See Chapter 12 for more details on public transportation in Russia.

Using actual measurements

Russians use the European system of measurements and define distances in terms of kilometers, meters, and centimeters. Within city limits, Russians feel more comfortable indicating distances using bus or tram stops or the time it takes one to cover the distance by walking (see the previous section); until recently, relatively few Russians had cars and most people used public transportation (which is excellent, by the way). However, when they talk about places not located within city limits, Russians usually use kilometers.

To ask a question about the distance between towns and cities, use the phrase **Skol'ko kilomyetrov ot** (*skohl'*-kuh kee-lah-*myet*-ruhf uht; How many kilometers is it from . . . ?) + the genitive case of the word denoting the name of the place + **do** (duh; to) + the genitive case of the word denoting the name of the other place. For example:

> ✔ **Skol'ko kilomyetrov ot Moskvy do Pyetyerburga?** (*skohl'*-kuh kee-lah-*myet*-ruhf uht mahs-*kvih* duh pee-teer-*boor*-guh; How many kilometers is it from Moscow to St. Petersburg?)

> ✔ **Skol'ko kilomyetrov ot Kiyeva do Moskvy?** (*skohl'*-kuh kee-luh-*myet*-ruhf uht *kee*-ee-vuh duh mahs-*kvih*; How many kilometers is it from Kiev to Moscow?)

To give a simple answer to the question, use numerals; we cover them in detail in Chapter 2. Just remember the following tips:

> ✔ After the numeral **odin** (ah-*deen*; one) or numerals ending in **odin** (one), use the word **kilomyetr** (kee-lah-*myetr*), as in **tridtsat' odin kilomyetr** (*treet*-tsuht' ah-*deen* kee-lah-*myetr*; thirty-one kilometers).

> ✔ After the numerals **dva** (dvah; two), **tri** (tree; three), **chyetyrye** (chee-*tih*-ree; four) or numerals ending in them, use the word **kilomyetra** (kee-lah-*myet*-ruh), as in **tri kilomyetra** (tree kee-lah-*myet*-ruh; three kilometers).

> ✔ After all other numerals, use the word **kilomyetrov** (kee-lah-*myet*-ruhf), as in **dvadtsat' pyat' kilomyetrov** (*dvaht*-suht' pyat' kee-lah-*myet*-ruhf; twenty-five kilometers).

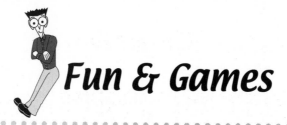

Fun & Games

Which of the two Russian words — **gdye** or **kuda** — would you use to translate the word "where" in the following sentences? See the answers in Appendix C.

1. Where are you going?

2. Where are you?

3. Where do you live?

4. Where are you driving?

5. Where did the dog go?

Select the correct translation for the following English phrases. See the correct answers in Appendix C.

1. Next to the bank

a. **ryadom s bankom**

b. **nyedalyeko ot banka**

2. Across from the bank

a. **naprotiv banka**

b. **ryadom s bankom**

3. To the right of the bank

a. **sprava ot banka**

b. **slyeva ot banka**

Which of the listed suburbs is the furthest from St. Petersburg: Pushkin, Ryepino, Zyelyenogorsk, or Ol'gino? See the answer in Appendix C.

1. **Ot Pyetyerburga do Pushkina tridtsat' kilomyetrov.**

2. **Ot Pyetyerburga do Ryepino syem'dyesyat kilomyetrov.**

3. **Ot Pyetyerburga do Zyelyenogorska shyest'dyesyat kilomyetrov.**

4. **Ot Pyetyerburga do Ol'gino pyatnadtsat' kilomyetrov.**

Chapter 16

Handling Emergencies

An emergency would be called something else if it were possible to be fully prepared for it. However, you can avoid some panic if you have a convenient reference guide that gives you just the right things to say in case an emergency interrupts your plans. In this chapter, you find out how to explain yourself in various unpleasant situations: asking for help during an emergency, getting help with a health concern, and talking to the police. Enjoy this emergency guide; we hope you never need to use it!

Finding Help in Case of Accidents and Other Emergencies

Dealing with accidents and emergencies in your native language is enough of a headache; problems seem twice as bad when you have to speak a foreign language to resolve them. But if you know how to ask for help, chances are you'll find somebody who makes resolving your problems much easier. In the following sections, you find out how to request help, call the Russian equivalent of 911, and explain your problem. And just in case — you discover the way to find somebody who speaks English!

Asking for help

The first thing you need to know is how to ask for help. If you aren't feeling well or don't know what to do during an emergency, address someone with the phrase **Izvinitye, mnye nuzhna pomosh'!** (eez-vee-*nee*-tee mnye noozh-*nah poh*-muhsh'; Excuse me, I need help!), or **Pomogitye mnye, pozhalujsta?** (puh-mah-*gee*-tee mnye pah-*zhahl*-stuh; Will you please help me?)

Make sure you explain what your problem is immediately after you ask for help so that the person you're talking to doesn't think you're a scam artist. Phrases you may want to say include the following:

- **Ya syebya plokho chuvstvuyu.** (ya see-*bya ploh*-khuh *choos*-tvoo-yu; I am not feeling well.)

- **Mnye plokho.** (mnye *ploh*-khuh; I am not feeling well.)

- **Pozvonitye v skoruyu pomosh'!** (puhz-vah-*nee*-tee v *skoh*-roo-yu *poh*-muhsh'; Call an ambulance!)

- **Pomogitye!** (puh-mah-*gee*-tee; Help!)

- **Pozovitye na pomosh'!** (puh-zah-*vee*-tee nuh *poh*-muhsh'; Call for help!)

- **Pozvonitye v militsiyu!** (puhz-vah-*nee*-tee v mee-*lee*-tsih-yu; Call the police!)

- **Dyerzhitye vora!** (deer-*zhih*-tee *voh*-ruh; Stop the thief!)

- **Pozhar!** (pah-*zhahr*; Fire!)

To get help, you can also say **Ya nye mogu . . .** (ya nee mah-*goo*; I can't . . .) + the infinitive of the verb describing what it is you can't do. For instance, try the verb **najti** (nuhy-*tee*; to find) or **otkryt'** (aht-*kriht'*; to open), and then follow with the item you can't find or open.

Calling the right number

In the United States, calling 911 is the answer to almost any emergency question, but it's not this way in Russia. There, you have three different numbers to call in cases of **pozhar** (pah-*zhahr*; fire), crime, or health problems. The numbers are easy, and any Russian knows them by heart:

- **01 — pozharnaya sluzhba** (pah-*zhahr*-nuh-ye *sloozh*-buh; fire brigade)

- **02 — militsiya** (mee-*lee*-tsih-ye; police)

- **03 — skoraya pomosh'** (*skoh*-ruh-ye *poh*-muhsh'; ambulance, *Literally:* urgent help)

Calls to 01, 02, and 03 numbers are free from any Russian pay phone.

Two other easy numbers to remember:

- ✔ **04 — sluzhba gaza** (*sloozh*-buh *gah*-zuh), the place where you call if you suspect gas leakage
- ✔ **09 — spravochnaya** (*sprah*-vuhch-nuh-ye; directory assistance)

Reporting a problem

When reporting an accident or an emergency, a good verb to use is **proiskhodit'** (pruh-ees-khah-*deet'*; to happen). To talk about something that is happening or has happened, you need only the third person singular form in the present tense — **proiskhodit** (pruh-ees-*khoh*-deet; is happening) — and the past tense forms:

- ✔ **proizoshyol** (pruh-ee-zah-*shohl*; has happened; masculine singular)
- ✔ **proizoshla** (pruh-ee-zah-*shlah*; has happened; feminine singular)
- ✔ **proizoshlo** (pruh-ee-zah-*shloh*; has happened; neuter singular)
- ✔ **proizoshli** (pruh-ee-zah-*shlee*; has happened; plural)

A common question you may be asked if you've witnessed an accident is **Chto proizoshlo?** (shtoh pruh-ee-zah-*shloh*; What happened?) You may also hear **Chto sluchilos'?** (shtoh sloo-*chee*-luhs'; What happened?) The two phrases are interchangeable.

Problems that you may have to report include:

- ✔ **avariya** (uh-*vah*-ree-ye; car accident)
- ✔ **nyeschastnyj sluchaj** (nee-*shahs*-nihy *sloo*-chuhy; accident)
- ✔ **pozhar** (pah-*zhahr*; fire)
- ✔ **ograblyeniye** (uhg-ruhb-*lye*-nee-ee; robbery)
- ✔ **otravlyeniye** (uht-ruhv-*lye*-nee-ee; poisoning)
- ✔ **infarkt** (een-*fahrkt*; heart attack)
- ✔ **ranyeniye** (ruh-*nye*-nee-ee; injury)

Check out Chapter 2 to find details about the genders of different nouns.

Talkin' the Talk

 While walking along a street in Moscow, Stacy witnesses an accident. He calls 03 and talks to the **opyerator** (uh-pee-*rah*-tuhr; operator).

Opyerator: **Skoraya pomosh'. Slushayu.**
skoh-ruh-ye *poh*-muhsh'. *sloo*-shuh-yu.
Ambulance. How can I help you? (*Literally:* I am listening.)

Stacy: **Tut proizoshla avariya. Chyelovyek popal pod mash-inu.**
toot pruh-ee-zah-*shlah* uh-*vah*-ree-ye. chee-lah-*vyek* pah-*pahl* puhd mah-*shih*-noo.
A road accident happened here. A person was hit by a car.

Opyerator: **Gdye proizoshla avariya? Adryes?**
gdye pruh-ee-zah-*shlah* uh-*vah*-ree-ye? *ahd*-rees?
Where did the accident happen? What is the address?

Stacy: **Na uglu ulitsy Tvyerskoj i Pushkinskogo bul'vara.**
nuh oog-*loo* oo-lee-tsih tveer-*skohy* ee *poosh*-keen-skuhy-vuh bool'-*vah*-ruh.
At the corner of Tverskaya Street and Pushkinskiy Avenue.

Opyerator: **V kakom sostoyanii potyerpyevshij?**
f kah-*kohm* suhs-tah-*ya*-nee-ee puh-teer-*pyef*-shihy?
What's the condition of the victim?

Stacy: **Byez soznaniya.**
byes sahz-*nah*-nee-ye.
Unconscious.

Opyerator: **Vy — rodstvyennik potyerpyevshyego?**
vih — *roht*-stvee-neek puh-teer-*pyef*-shih-vuh?
Are you a relative of the victim?

Stacy: **Nyet, ya — prosto prokhozhij, sluchajnyj svidyetyel'.**
nyet, ya — *prohs*-tuh prah-*khoh*-zhihy, sloo-*chahy*-nihy svee-*dye*-teel'.
No, I'm just a passerby, an accidental witness.

Opyerator: **Brigada vyyezzhayet.**
bree-*gah*-duh vih-eez-*zhah*-eet.
An ambulance is on its way.

Words to Know

Slushayu.	<u>sloo</u>-shuh-yu	How can I help you? (Literally: I am listening.)
Chyelovyek popal pod mashinu.	chee-lah-<u>vyek</u> pah-<u>pahl</u> puhd muh-<u>shih</u>-noo	A person was hit by a car.
Gdye proizoshla avariya?	gdye pruh-ee-zah-<u>shlah</u> uh-<u>vah</u>-ree-ye	Where did the accident happen?
V kakom sostoyanii potyerpyevshij?	f kuh-<u>kohm</u> suhs-tah-<u>ya</u>-nee-ee puh-teer-<u>pyef</u>-shihy	What is the condition of the victim?
byez soznaniya	byes sahz-<u>nah</u>-nee-ye	unconscious
v soznanii	f sahz-<u>nah</u>-nee-ee	conscious
prokhozhiy	prah-<u>khoh</u>-zhihy	passerby
svidyetyel'	svee-<u>dye</u>-teel'	witness
Brigada vyyezzhayet.	bree-<u>gah</u>-duh vih-eez-<u>zhah</u>-eet	An ambulance is on its way.

Requesting English-speaking help

In case you don't feel like practicing your Russian in the midst of an emergency, or if you just want to speed up the process, you may want to ask for English-speaking help. The question you want to use is **Zdyes' yest' kto-nibud', kto govorit po-anglijski?** (zdyes' yest' *ktoh*- nee-boot' ktoh guh-vah-*reet* puh uhng-*leey*-skee; Is there anybody here who speaks English?)

If you want to insist on finding somebody who can help you in English, say **Mnye nuzhyen kto-nibud', kto govorit po-anglijski!** (mnye *noo*-zhihn *ktoh*-nee-boot' ktoh guh-vah-*reet* puh uhng-*leey*-skee; I need somebody who speaks English!)

If you're making this request at a hospital or some other place staffed with highly educated people, you have a good chance of finding somebody who speaks English; many Russians study English in school and college.

In Moscow and St. Petersburg, you can find clinics with American and British doctors. Here are some of these clinics:

American Clinic at 31 Grokholskij Pyeryeulok, 129090 Moscow

Phones: 095-937-5757, 095-937-5774

e-mail: info@americanclinic.ru

European Medical Center at 10 2nd Spiridoniyevskij per. 5, bld. 1 Moscow

Phone: 095-933-6655

American Medical Center St. Petersburg at 10 Syerpukhovskaya St., 198013 St. Petersburg

Phone: 812-326-1730

Receiving Medical Care

If "an apple a day" doesn't work, you may need to **pojti k vrachu** (pahy-*tee* k vruh-*choo*; see a doctor). Every culture has different beliefs and procedures related to **zdorov'ye** (zdah-*rohv'*-ee; health) and **myeditsina** (mee-dee-*tsih*-nuh; medicine), and knowing what they are before visiting a doctor helps. In the following sections, you find out how to talk about medical problems in Russian, how to understand your diagnosis, and what to say and do in a pharmacy.

To make an appointment with a specific doctor at a big **poliklinika** (puh-lee-*klee*-nee-kuh; clinic), you need to go to the **ryegistratura** (ree-gees-truh-*too*-ruh; check-in desk) and say **Mnye nado zapisat'sya na priyom k . . .** (mnye *nah*-duh zuh-pee-*saht'*-sye nuh pree-*yom* k; I need to make an appointment with . . .), + the type of doctor you want to see in the dative case (for more info on case endings, see Chapter 2). At some **polikliniki** (puh-lee-*klee*-nee-kee; clinics), you may be able to make an appointment over the phone; at others, you always have to show up in person. To find out which is the case, you can call the **poliklinika** and ask: **Mozhno zapisat'sya na priyom?** (*mohzh*-nuh zuh-pee-*saht'*-sye nuh pree-*yom*; Can I make an appointment?)

For an emergency, call a **skoraya pomosh'** (*skoh*-ruh-ye *poh*-muhsh'; ambulance) by dialing 03. The ambulance will come and take the patient to the emergency room, also called **skoraya pomosh'**.

CULTURAL WISDOM

Health is more valuable than money

According to a Russian proverb, **zdorov'ye dorozhye dyenyeg** (zdah-*rohv'*-ye dah-*roh*-zhih *dye*-neek; health is more valuable than money). Believing this bit of folk wisdom was easy during the times of the Soviet Union, when medicine was free for all Soviet citizens. Nowadays, numerous **chastnyye kliniki** (*chahs*-nih-ee klee-nee-kee; private medical offices) offer a variety of **platnyye uslugi** (*plaht*-nih-ee oos-*loo*-gee; services for a fee). State-owned hospitals and medical offices are still free, but you're expected to pay for your medicine, and a monetary donation to the doctor is strongly encouraged.

Knowing your own anatomy

When you go to a doctor, you want to know how to talk about your **tyelo** (*tye*-luh; body). The following list starts with the visible parts, going from the top down:

- **golova** (guh-lah-*vah*; head)
- **shyeya** (*sheh*-ye; neck)
- **gorlo** (*gohr*-luh; throat)
- **plyecho** (plee-*choh*; shoulder)
- **grud'** (groot'; chest/breast)
- **spina** (spee-*nah*; back)
- **ruka** (roo-*kah*; arm/hand)
- **lokot'** (*loh*-kuht'; elbow)
- **zapyast'ye** (zuh-*pyast'*-ee; wrist)
- **palyets** (*pah*-leets; finger)
- **nogti** (*nohk*-tee; nails)
- **zhivot** (zhih-*voht*; stomach)
- **polovyye organy** (puh-lah-*vih*-ee *ohr*-guh-nih; genitals)
- **noga** (nah-*gah*; leg/foot)
- **kolyeno** (kah-*lye*-nuh; knee)
- **lodyzhka** (lah-*dihsh*-kuh; ankle)
- **kozha** (*koh*-zhuh; skin)

In Russian, no distinction exists between the arm and the hand; for both body parts, you use the word **ruka.** Similarly, for both leg and foot, you use the word **noga.**

Parts of your head that you may seek treatment for include the following:

- **litso** (lee-*tsoh*; face)
- **glaz** (glahs; eye)
- **ukho** (*oo*-khuh; ear)
- **nos** (nohs; nose)
- **rot** (roht; mouth)
- **zub** (zoop; tooth)
- **podborodok** (puhd-bah-*roh*-duhk; chin)
- **yazyk** (ee-*zihk*; tongue)

The internal organs you may need to talk about include these body parts:

- **syerdtsye** (*syer*-tseh; heart)
- **pyechyen'** (*pye*-chihn'; liver)
- **zhyeludok** (zhih-*loo*-duhk; stomach)
- **mozg** (mohzk; brain)
- **lyogkiye** (*lyokh*-kee-ee; lungs)
- **kost'** (kohst'; bone)
- **muskuly** (*moos*-koo-lih; muscles)
- **pochka** (*pohch*-kuh; kidney)
- **nyervy** (*nyer*-vih; nerves)

Describing your symptoms to a doctor

The first question you hear from a doctor is usually **Chto u vas bolit?** (shtoh u vahs bah-*leet*; What is hurting you?) or **Chto vas byespokoit?** (shtoh vahs bees-pah-*koh*-eet; What brought you here, *Literally:* What is bothering you?)

The best way to start describing your symptoms if you're in pain is with the verb **bolyet** (bah-*lyet'*; to hurt): **U myenya bolit . . .** (oo mee-*nya* bah-*leet*; . . . is hurting) + the name of the organ that hurts in the nominative case.

You can also point to the place where it hurts and say **U myenya bolit zdyes'** (oo mee-*nya* bah-*leet* zdyes'; It hurts me here). You may want to specify

whether it hurts **vnutri** (vnoo-*tree*; inside) or **snaruzhi** (snah-*roo*-zhih; on the outside).

To describe specific, less-painful symptoms, you say **U myenya . . .** (oo mee-*nya*; I have . . .) + one of the phrases from the following list:

- **tyempyeratura** (teem-pee-ruh-*too*-ruh; fever)
- **ponos** (pah-*nohs*; diarrhea)
- **zapor** (zuh-*pohr*; constipation)
- **toshnota** (tuhsh-nah-*tah*; nausea)
- **bolit gorlo** (bah-*leet gohr*-luh; sore throat)
- **bolit golova** (bah-*leet* guh-lah-*vah*; headache)
- **bolit zhivot** (bah-*leet* zhih-*voht*; stomachache)
- **bolit ukho** (bah-*leet oo*-khuh; earache)
- **kashyel'** (*kah*-shihl'; cough)
- **nasmork** (*nahs*-muhrk; runny nose)
- **syp'** (sihp'; rash)
- **ozhog** (ah-*zhohk*; burn)
- **bol'** (bohl'; pain)

In Russia, temperature is measured in Celsius. Normal body temperature is 36.6°C. Anything above is a **vysokaya tyempyeratura** (vih-*soh*-kuh-ye teem-pee-ruh-*too*-ruh; high fever).

Talkin' the Talk

Kate is spending her vacation in St. Petersburg. She starts to feel unwell, so she goes to see a **vrach** (vrahch; doctor).

Kate: **Doktor, ya syebya plokho chuvstvuyu.**
dohk-tuhr, ya see-*bya ploh*-khuh *choos*-tvoo-yu.
Doctor, I am not feeling well.

Vrach: **Chto vas byespokoit?**
shtoh vahs bees-pah-*koh*-eet?
What is the problem?

Kate: **U myenya bolit zhivot.**
oo mee-*nya* bah-*leet* zhih-*voht*.
My stomach is hurting.

Vrach: **Bol' ryezkaya ili noyush'aya?**
          bohl' *ryes*-kuh-ye ee-lee *noh*-yu-sh'uh-ye?
          Is the pain sharp or dull?

Kate: **Noyush'aya. I yesh'yo u myenya tyempyeratura.**
          noh-yu-sh'uh-ye. ee-*sh'oh* oo mee-*nya* teem-pee-ruh-*too*-ruh.
          It's dull. I also have a fever.

Vrach: **Toshnota ili rvota yest'?**
          tuhsh-nah-*tah* ee-lee *rvoh*-tuh yest'?
          Do you have nausea or vomiting?

Kate: **Nyet. No nyemnogo kruzhitsya golova.**
          nyet. noh nee-*mnoh*-guh *kroo*-zhiht-sye guh-lah-*vah*.
          No. But I am a little dizzy.

Vrach: **Budyem provodit osmotr. Razdyevajtyes'.**
          boo-deem pruh-vah-*deet'* ahs-*mohtr*. ruhz-dee-*vahy*-tees'.
          Let's examine you. Undress, please.

Words to Know

ryezkaya bol'	ryes-kuh-ye bohl'	sharp pain
noyush'aya bol'	noh-yu-sh'uh-ye bohl'	dull pain
yesh'yo	ee-sh'oh	also
rvota	rvoh-tuh	vomiting
No nyemnogo kruzhitsya golova.	noh neem-noh-guh kroo-zhiht-sye guh-lah-vah	But I am a little dizzy.
provodit osmotr	pruh-vah-deet' ahs-mohtr	to examine
razdyevajtyes'	ruhz-dee-vahy-tees'	undress

Announcing allergies or special conditions

Asking about allergies and special conditions isn't always a part of a Russian doctor's routine. Make sure you take the initiative and tell the doctor **U myenya allyergiya na . . .** (oo mee-*nya* uh-leer-*gee*-ye nuh; I am allergic to . . .) + the word naming the cause of the allergy in the accusative case. Common causes of allergies include:

- **pyenitsillin** (pee-nee-tsih-*leen*; penicillin)
- **oryekhi** (ah-*rye*-khee; nuts)
- **obyezbalivayush'yeye** (uh-beez-*bah*-lee-vuh-yu-sh'ee-ee; painkillers)
- **ukus pchyely** (oo-*koos* pchee-*lih*; bee stings)
- **koshki** (*kohsh*-kee; cats)
- **sobaki** (sah-*bah*-kee; dogs)
- **yajtsa** (*yahy*-tsuh; eggs)
- **pyl'tsa** (pihl'-*tsah*; pollen)
- **plyesyen'** (*plye*-seen'; mold)
- **moloko** (muh-lah-*koh*; milk)
- **mollyuski** (mah-*lyus*-kee; shellfish)
- **ryba** (*rih*-buh; fish)

If you're on some kind of medication, tell your doctor **Ya prinimayu . . .** (ya pree-nee-*mah*-yu; I am on . . ., *Literally:* I take . . .) + the name of the medication. Some other special conditions that you may need to announce to the doctor include:

- **U myenya astma.** (oo mee-*nya ahst*-muh; I have asthma.)
- **Ya yepilyeptik.** (ya ee-pee-*lyep*-teek; I have epilepsy.)
- **Ya diabyetik.** (ya dee-uh-*beh*-teek; I have diabetes.)
- **Ya byeryemyenna.** (ya bee-*rye*-mee-nuh; I am pregnant.)

Seeing a specialist

In Russia, medicine is organized differently: Each doctor specializes not on a part of the body (for example, on the foot or arm), but on a type of organ (for instance, the skin, bone, or nerves). If you go to a Russian physician and say that your foot hurts, he doesn't send you to a foot doctor, as he would in the United States. Instead, he finds out what type of problem you have and then

sends you to a **dyermatolog** (deer-muh-*toh*-luhk; dermatologist) if your problem concerns the skin of your foot; to a **khirurg** (khee-*roork*; surgeon) if you broke a bone in your foot; or to a **nyevropatolog** (neev-ruh-puh-*toh*-luhk; neuropathologist) if your problem stems from nerve connections.

Some other doctors and their areas of specialization include:

- **ukho-gorlo-nos** (*oo*-khuh *gohr*-luh nohs; *Literally:* ear-throat-nose), or **lor** (lohr) — not unpredictably, this doctor specializes in the ear-throat-nose system

- **dantist** (duhn-*teest*; dentist), also known as **zubnoj vrach** (zoob-*nohy* vrahch)

- **vyenyerolog** (vee-nee-*roh*-luhk) — specializes in venereal diseases

- **narkolog** (nahr-*koh*-luhk) — specializes in drug addictions

- **tyerapyevt** (tee-ruh-*pyeft*; internist)

- **glaznoj vrach** (gluhz-*nohy* vrahch; eye doctor)

- **ginyekolog** (gee-nee-*koh*-luhk; gynecologist)

- **ortopyed** (uhr-tah-*pyet*; orthopedist)

- **pyediatr** (pee-dee-*ahtr*; pediatrician)

- **nyevropatolog** (neev-ruh-puh-*toh*-luhk; neurologist)

- **khirurg** (khee-*roork*; surgeon)

- **psikhiatr** (psee-khee-*ahtr*; psychiatrist)

- **kardiolog** (kuhr-dee-*oh*-luhk; cardiologist)

Some employers require a **myeditsinskoye obslyedovaniye** (mee-dee-*tsihns*-kuh-ee ahbs-*lye*-duh-vuh-nee-ee; full medical examination) from their potential employees. And in Russia, going through a **myeditsinskoye obslyedovaniye** requires seeing half a dozen doctors.

Undergoing an examination and getting a diagnosis

During a medical examination, you may hear the following phrases:

- **Razdyen'tyes' do poyasa.** (ruhz-*dyen'*-tees' duh *poh*-ee-suh; Undress from your waist up.)

- **Razdyen'tyes' polnost'yu.** (ruhz-*dyen'*-tees' *pohl*-nuhst'-yu; Take off all your clothes.)

- **Zakatitye rukav.** (zuh-kuh-*tee*-tee roo-*kahf*; Please roll up your sleeve.)

✔ **Gluboko vdokhnitye.** (gloo-bah-*koh* vdahkh-*nee*-tee; Take a deep breath.)

✔ **Lozhityes'.** (lah-*zhih*-tees'; Please lie down.)

✔ **Otkrojtye rot.** (aht-*krohy*-tee roht; Open your mouth.)

✔ **Pokazhitye yazyk.** (puh-kuh-*zhih*-tee ee-*zihk*; Stick out your tongue.)

You also may have to undergo the following tests:

✔ **analiz krovi** (uh-*nah*-leez *kroh*-vee; blood test)

✔ **analiz mochi** (uh-*nah*-leez mah-*chee*; urine test)

✔ **ryengyen** (reen-*gyen*; X-ray)

✔ **yelyektrokardiogramma** (ee-*lyekt*-ruh-kuhr-dee-ahg-*rah*-muh; electrocardiogram)

✔ **sonogramma** (suh-nah-*grah*-muh; sonogram)

✔ **ul'trazvuk** (ool'-truh-*zvook*; ultrasound)

After all the turmoil of going through the **osmotr** (ahs-*mohtr*; medical examination), you're ready to hear your **diagnoz** (dee-*ahg*-nuhs; diagnosis). The doctor will probably phrase it this way: **U vas . . .** (oo vahs; you have . . .) plus the diagnosis itself. For instance, you may hear that you have one of the following:

✔ **prostuda** (prahs-*too*-duh; cold)

✔ **angina** (uhn-*gee*-nuh; sore throat)

✔ **gripp** (greep; flu)

✔ **bronkhit** (brahn-*kheet*; bronchitis)

✔ **migryen'** (mee-*gryen'*; migraine)

✔ **infyektsiya** (een-*fyek*-tsih-ye; infection)

✔ **pnyevmoniya** (pneev-mah-*nee*-ye; pneumonia)

✔ **syennaya likhoradka** (*sye*-nuh-ye lee-khah-*raht*-kuh; hay fever)

✔ **rastyazhyeniye svyazok** (ruhs-tee-*zheh*-nee-ee *svya*-zuhk; sprain)

Russian doctors aren't in the habit of explaining what they're doing, either during the examination or while prescribing you treatment. If you, on top of getting a recommendation on how to cure yourself, want to know what's actually wrong with you, you may need to ask: **A chto u myenya?** (ah shtoh oo mee-*nya*; What do I have?) or **Kakaya u myenya bolyezn'?** (kuh-*kah*-ye oo mee-*nya* bah-*lyezn'*; What kind of illness do I have?)

If the doctor recommends that you go to the hospital — **lozhit'sya v bol'nitsu** (lah-*zhiht'*-sye v bahl'-*nee*-tsoo) — you have a more serious condition. Maybe you have **appyenditsit** (ah-peen-dee-*tsiht*; appendicitis), **pyeryelom** (pee-ree-*lohm*; a broken bone), or **pish'yevoye otravlyeniye** (pee-sh'ee-*voh*-ee uht-ruhv-*lye*-nee-ee; food poisoning).

Don't panic if the doctor recommends that you go to the hospital; it doesn't necessarily mean that your condition is critical. Russians tend to go to the hospital more often and stay there longer than Americans generally do. For a comparison: A new mother with a baby stays in the hospital for two weeks in Russia, versus a stay of only 48 hours in the United States.

Your doctor can also prescribe for you to **khodit' na protsyedury** (khah-*deet'* nuh pruh-tsih-*doo*-rih; take treatment). A prescription doesn't necessarily imply that you have to stay at the hospital; you may need to come to the hospital daily, or several times a week, for a certain type of treatment. In this case, the doctor gives you a **napravlyeniye** (nuh-pruhv-*lye*-nee-ee; written treatment authorization).

Visiting a pharmacy

In most cases, a doctor will **propisat' lyekarstvo** (pruh-pee-*saht'* lee-*kahrst*-vuh; prescribe a medicine) for you. The Russian word for prescription is **ryet-syept** (ree-*tsehpt*).

The Russian word **ryetsyept** is an interpreter's false friend. To an English speaker, it sounds a lot like "receipt." Watch out, though! The Russian for "receipt" is **chyek** (chehk). **Ryetsyept,** on the other hand, means "prescription" or "recipe."

To get your **lyekarstvo,** you need to go to the **aptyeka** (uhp-*tye*-kuh; pharmacy). Unlike in the United States, a Russian pharmacy isn't usually a part of a big department store; it's a separate little store, where only medicine is sold. To get your **lyekarstvo,** you hand your **ryetsyept** to the **aptyekar'** (uhp-*tye*-kuhr'; pharmacist). Alternatively, you can say

- ✔ **Mnye nuzhyen . . .** (mnye *noo*-zhihn; I need . . .) + the masculine name of the medicine

- ✔ **Mnye nuzhna . . .** (mnye noozh-*nah*; I need . . .) + the feminine name of the medicine

- ✔ **Mnye nuzhno . . .** (mnye noozh-*noh*; I need . . .) + the neuter name of the medicine

- ✔ **Mnye nuzhny . . .** (mnye noozh-*nih*; I need . . .) + the plural name of the medicine(s)

Going herbal

Russians are big on herbal medicine, which they call **lyechyeniye travami** (lee-*chye*-nee-ye *trah*-vah-mee). Unlike in the United States, herbs are not seen as an alternative medicine; even general practitioners often prescribe something herbal. Every Russian pharmacy has a wide selection of herbs for any cause, from sleeplessness to gastritis. Pharmacists usually offer an herbal substitute or supplement for the medicine you go to buy.

Some common medicines include

- **nyejtralizuyush'yeye kislotu sryedstvo** (neey-truh-lee-*zoo*-yu-sh'ih-ee kees-lah-*too sryets*-tvuh; antacid)

- **aspirin** (uhs-pee-*reen*; aspirin)

- **kapli ot kashlya** (*kahp*-lee uht *kahsh*-lye; cough drops)

- **sirop ot kashlya** (see-*rohp* uht *kahsh*-lye; cough syrup)

- **sryedstvo dlya snizhyeniya tyempyeratury** (*sryets*-tvuh dlya snee-*zheh*-nee-ye teem-pee-ruh-*too*-rih; fever reducer)

- **bolyeutolyayush'yeye** (boh-lee-oo-tuh-*lya*-yu-sh'ee-ee; pain reliever)

- **sryedstvo ot izzhyogi** (*sryets*-tvuh uht eez-*zhoh*-gee; heartburn reliever)

You can buy many drugs that require prescriptions in the United States as over-the-counter drugs in Russia. So, to save the time you would've spent going to the doctor, you can just ask the pharmacist for **chto-nibud' ot pros-tudy** (shtoh nee-*boot'* uht prahs-*too*-dih; something for the cold).

Calling the Police When You're the Victim of a Crime

In the difficult situation of becoming a victim of crime, you need to know where to turn to for help and what to say to the people helping you. In the following sections, you find out how to talk to the police about different crimes and answer their questions.

If the crime is serious, you should try to contact your embassy before contacting the police. A person at the embassy will advise you on what to do and help you through the difficult situation.

Talking to the police

You can contact the **militsiya** (mee-*lee*-tsih-ye; police) by calling 02 (see the section "Calling the right number" earlier in this chapter) or by going directly **v otdyelyeniye militsii** (v uht-dee-*lye*-nee-ye mee-*lee*-tsih-ee; to the police station). To find the nearest police station, you can ask a passerby **Gdye blizhajshyeye otdyelyeniye militsii?** (gdye blee-*zhahy*-shih-ee uht-dee-*lye*-nee-ye mee-*lee*-tsih-ee; Where is the nearest police station?)

Here are some useful phrases you can use to describe different types of crime to the police:

- ✔ **Myenya ograbili.** (mee-*nya* ah-*grah*-bee-lee; I was robbed.)

- ✔ **Myenya obokrali.** (mee-*nya* uh-bah-*krah*-lee; I became a victim of a theft.)

- ✔ **Na myenya bylo sovyershyeno napadyeniye.** (nuh mee-*nya* *bih*-luh suh-veer-shih-*noh* nuh-puh-*dye*-nee-ee; I was attacked.)

- ✔ **Moyu kvartiru obvorovali.** (mah-*yu* kvahr-*tee*-roo uhb-vuh-rah-*vah*-lee; My apartment was broken into.)

- ✔ **Ya stal zhyertvoj moshyennichyestva.** (ya stahl *zhehr*-tvohy muh-*sheh*-nee-chihst-vuh; I became a victim of a fraud; masculine.)

- ✔ **Ya stala zhyertvoj moschyennichyestva.** (ya *stah*-lah *zhehr*-tvuhy muh-*sheh*-nee-chihst-vuh; I became a victim of a fraud; feminine.)

- ✔ **Moyu mashinu obokrali.** (mah-*yu* muh-*shih*-noo uh-bahk-*rah*-lee; My car was broken into, *Literally:* My car was robbed.)

In order to report a specific item that's stolen from you, use the phrase **U myenya ukrali . . .** (oo mee-*nya* oo-*krah*-lee; They stole . . .) + the name of the item in the accusative case. (For more info on case endings, see Chapter 2.)

Answering questions from the police

When a crime is reported, the police want to gather more information about **pryestuplyeniye** (prees-toop-*lye*-nee-ee; the crime) and **pryestupnik** (prees-*toop*-neek; the criminal).

When talking to the police and describing the incident, you may need to use the words **vor** (vohr; thief), **karmannik** (kuhr-*mah*-neek; pickpocket), or **bandit** (buhn-*deet*; gangster) to refer to the criminal.

The police may want to know the **vremya** (*vrye*-mye; time) and **myesto** (*myes*-tuh; place) of the **proisshyestviye** (pruh-ee-*shehst*-vee-ee; incident). They may ask you to describe the **vnyeshnost'** (*vnyesh*-nuhst'; appearance) of the criminal, and **kuda on skrylsya** (koo-*dah* ohn *skrihl*-sye; in what direction he escaped). They may also ask whether he was **odin** (ah-*deen*; alone) or **s soobsh'nikami** (s sah-*ohb*-sh'nee-kuh-mee; with accomplices).

If you're physically assaulted or threatened with an **oruzhiye** (ah-*roo*-zhih-ee; weapon), the police will ask **Chyem vas udarili?** (chyem vahs oo-*dah*-ree-lee; What were you hit with?) or **Chyem vam ugrozhali?** (chyem vahm oog-rah-*zhah*-lee; What were you threatened with?)

To answer the question **Chyem vas udarili,** use the noun in the instrumental case because this case expresses the means or tool with which something is done: **udarili rukoj** (oo-*dah*-ree-lee roo-*kohj*; hit with a hand) or **ugrozhali pistolyetom** (oog-rah-*zhah*-lee pees-tah-*lye*-tuhm; threatened with a gun), for example. (For details on the instrumental case, see Chapter 2.)

After answering the questions, you may need to state the same information in a **zayavlyeniye** (zuh-eev-*lye*-nee-ee; police report).

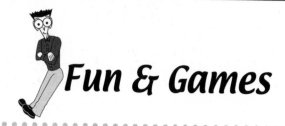

Fun & Games

Which of these places would you call in each of the following situations? Match the emergencies from the left column with the right places to call from the right column. See Appendix C for the answers.

1. **Chyelovyek popal pod mashinu**   a. **militsiya**

2. **Vas ograbili**   b. **pozharnaya sluzhba**

3. **pozhar**   c. **skoraya pomosh'**

Match these symptoms with the most probable sicknesses that cause them from the list below. Check out Appendix C for the answers.

1. **vysokaya tyempyeratura, nasmork, kashyel'**

2. **ostraya bol' v zhivotye, toshnota, rvota**

3. **bol' v gorlye**

a. **angina**   b. **prostuda**   c. **pish'yevoye otravlyeniye**

Choose the word that doesn't belong in the group. The answers are in Appendix C.

1. **moshyennichestvo, napadyeniye, gripp**

2. **aspirin, pryestupnik, aptyeka**

3. **lyekarstvo, vrach, pozhar**

Part IV
The Part of Tens

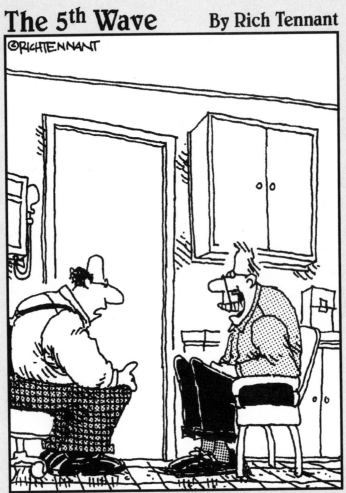

The 5th Wave   By Rich Tennant

"...and remember, no more Russian tongue twisters until you know the language better."

In this part . . .

Part IV gives you short but valuable lists of practical information on how to pick up Russian more quickly and how to start impressing native speakers with your Russian right away. To help you pick up Russian, we give you ten tried and true tips that have worked for many others, including one of the authors of this book. We also tell you ten favorite Russian expressions, which are sure to warm the heart of any Russian you say them to. We introduce you to ten Russian holidays, and we give you ten Russian phrases that are bound to win you "native speaker" points. And finally, we warn you about ten things you never want to say or do in Russia. If you follow the suggestions in this part, you're sure to win the minds and hearts of most Russians you meet!

Chapter 17

Ten Ways to Pick Up Russian Quickly

In This Chapter

▶ Engaging in activities that will advance your Russian

▶ Practicing Russian in the right places

We're not breaking any news to you by saying that the best way to learn a language is by using it. You have a much better chance of remembering **Kak dyela?** (kahk dee-*lah*; How are you?) after you say it to a Russian and actually hear **Normal'no!** (nahr-*mahl'*-nuh; Fine!) in response — just like you can read about in Chapter 3! You'll feel that your language skills are advanced, to say the least.

Coming up with new and fun ways to practice your Russian isn't always easy, though. That's why we give you some ideas in this chapter on creative ways to bring Russian into your life. Try them and feel free to come up with your own! After all, your life will contain only as much Russian as you let into it.

Check Out Russian TV, Movies, and Music

Whether you're into independent cinema or action movies, classical ballet or rock music, Russians have something to offer for any taste. Browse the foreign section of a DVD rental and the world music shelf of your local library, and you can definitely find something with which to practice your Russian. As far as movies go, be sure to get a Russian-language version with subtitles, rather than a dubbed one. And plenty of Russian-language TV channels exist in America — your cable service may even come with one!

Listen to Russian Radio Programs

You can advance your Russian without sitting down and giving it your undivided attention by listening to a Russian radio program in the car, during a walk, or while doing the dishes. Who knows how much of that new vocabulary will get stuck in your subconscious!

A variety of Russian radio stations broadcast on the Internet. For a comprehensive guide to Russian radio online, go to www.multilingualbooks.com/ online-radio-russian.html.

Read Russian Publications

Seeing a phrase in a phrase book, even if it's your favorite *Russian For Dummies,* is one thing. Seeing a phrase in a real Russian newspaper and actually recognizing it is a totally different experience.

Pick up a copy of a Russian publication, which are available in many libraries. Russian immigrant establishments, such as law offices and stores, often have local Russian-language newspapers lying around; the bonus of reading those papers is finding out what's going on locally with Russian social and cultural life. Reading such publications also is a good way to practice recognizing and "decoding" Cyrillic.

Surf the Internet

Now that the Internet exists, no one can complain about the lack of ways to practice Russian. Just remember that Russian Web sites end in ru. You may want to start your exploit from some of these Web sites:

- lenta.ru
- list.mail.ru/index.html
- menu.ru
- moskva.ru
- www.spb.ru
- www.theatre.ru/emain.html

And on blogs.mail.ru, you can read **blogi** (*bloh*-gee; blogs) in Russian, or even create your own.

Sometimes, Russian characters don't show properly on the Internet. If, instead of Cyrillic, you see a bunch of characters that look like $$##%%&&, change the encoding to Cyrillic. To do that, go to **View,** then **Encoding,** and try different Cyrillic encodings until you find the one that works.

Visit a Russian Restaurant

Most major American cities have at least one Russian restaurant. You may get more out of your visit than just a bowl of steaming **borsh'** (bohrsh') and a plate of aromatic **golubtsy** (guh-loop-*tsih;* rissoule rolled in cabbage leaves). Be ambitious, and talk to the staff exclusively in Russian. You may be pleasantly surprised by how supportive Russians can be when people try to speak their language. And who knows, your language skills may even get you a bargain! See Chapter 5 for details on visiting a restaurant.

Find a Russian Pen Pal

If you strike a personal connection with someone in a Russian chat room, you may get the chance to not only practice your Russian but also find an interesting interlocutor, and even a good friend. Some Russian **chaty** (*chah*-tih; chat rooms) to go to are chat.mail.ru, www.divan.ru, and www.games.ru/chat. You may even want to open your own Russian e-mail account to exchange messages with your new friend; good places to do so are Mail.ru and Rambler.ru.

If you want to type in Russian, but don't have a Russian keyboard, you can either put stickers with Russian letters on your regular English keyboard, or use an online Russian keyboard, such as the one at http://www.yandex.ru/keyboard_qwerty.html.

Teach English to a Russian Immigrant

Because learning is a mutual experience, teaching English to a Russian speaker may be a great way to advance your Russian. If you don't know anybody from the local Russian community, you can post an ad in a Russian store or restaurant. Writing that ad can be your first Russian exercise!

After you find a Russian establishment, you can just ask people who work there about other Russian restaurants and stores. Make sure to explain that you're looking for them to practice your language skills. Russians will be flattered by your interest in their culture and will happily share the information with you. You may even make some friends right there.

Visit a Jewish Community Center

A number of Jewish immigrants came to America throughout the 20th century and into the 21st century; many of them came from the former Soviet Union, where Russian was their native language. For many of them — especially the older generations — the Russian language is a part of their cultural heritage, and some events at a Jewish community center may be held in Russian.

You can find a Jewish community center through the Internet or in the phone book. Pay a visit there; you'll find out whether you can attend any Russian-language events. If you're willing to donate your time, offer to volunteer. Elderly immigrants may use some help from someone who speaks English, and it will be a great opportunity for you to practice your Russian.

Travel to Russia

Nothing beats traveling to the country of your interest. Whether you're going to Russia for a year of teaching English to Moscow high school students, a week of sightseeing, or a walk through the streets of St. Petersburg while your cruise ship is waiting in the port, no place makes practicing Russian easier than, well, Russia. See Chapter 11 for details on planning a trip.

Marry a Russian

If you're really set on the idea of speaking Russian like a native, you gotta do what you gotta do. Marry (or at least date) a Russian, and convince him or her to teach you the language. Of course, we're being a little tongue-in-cheek. We don't advocate that you go out and find yourself a Russian spouse just to improve your language skills. But if you do decide to date or marry a Russian, you should know that you have a great opportunity to dramatically improve your Russian. So take advantage of it! Watch out, though: Russians assimilate quickly, and you may end up spending much more time teaching English than being taught Russian. Then you'll have to resort to the secret weapon: Learning Russian from your mother-in-law!

Chapter 18

Ten Favorite Russian Expressions

In This Chapter

▶ Exploring phrases beyond their dictionary definitions

▶ Discovering the most popular Russian quotes and proverbs

*E*very culture has a way of taking familiar words and turning them into something else. The most diligent student can flip through his dictionary, and based on the literal translation, still have no idea what an expression means or why everybody is laughing. This chapter brings together ten words and expressions that Russians use a lot, and whose meanings aren't always intuitive. Recognizing these expressions in speech and using them with ease can make you sound really Russian!

Oj!

To express surprise, dismay, admiration, gratitude, or even pain — pretty much any strong feeling — Russians say **Oj!** (oy) Use **Oj!** when in English you would say "oops," "ouch," or "wow," or make a facial expression. You can confidently use **Oj!** in any of the following sentences:

✔ **Oj, kak krasivo!** (oy kahk kruh-*see*-vuh; Wow, how beautiful!)

✔ **Oj, spasibo!** (oy spuh-*see*-buh; Thank you so much!)

✔ **Oj, kto eto?** (oy ktoh *eh*-tuh; Who in the world is this?)

✔ **Oj, kak priyatno slyshat' tvoj golos!** (oy kahk pree-*yaht*-nah *slih*-shuht' tvohy *goh*-luhs; Oh, it's so nice to hear your voice!)

Russians consider **Oj!** a more feminine exclamation; men, on the other hand, are supposed to grind their teeth and keep their emotions to themselves.

Davaj

If you look up **davaj** (duh-*vahy*) in the dictionary, you find the translation "give." Russians, however, use the word in all kinds of situations. It's a popular way to suggest doing something, as in **Davaj pojdyom v kino** (duh-*vahy* pahy-*dyom* v kee-*noh*; let's go to the movies), and to answer "sure, let's do it!" (**Davaj!**) Used by itself, **davaj** means "bye, take care." (See Chapter 7 for more details.)

Pryedstav'tye Syebye

While the verb **pryedstav'tye** can mean "imagine," "picture," or even "introduce," **pryedstav'tye syebye** (preed-*stahf'*-tee see-*bye*) means "Can you believe it?" or "Imagine that!" It's a good way to begin telling a story, or to open a conversation on a subject you feel strongly about.

Poslushajtye!

Although the literal translation of **Poslushajtye!** (pahs-*loo*-shuhy-tee) is "Listen!," this translation doesn't do the expression justice. Saying "Listen!" in English sounds pushy and aggressive; in Russian, **Poslushajtye!** is a good and nice way to attract attention to your arguments. Here are some examples:

- ✔ **Poslushajtye, davajtye pojdyom na progulku!** (pahs-*loo*-shuhy-tee, duh-*vahy*-tee pahy-*dyom* nuh prah-*gool*-koo; You know what? Let's go for a walk!, *Literally:* Listen, let's go for a walk!)

- ✔ **Poslushajtye, no eto pryekrasnyj fil'm!** (pahs-*loo*-shuhy-tee, noh *eh*-tuh preek-*rahs*-nihy feel'm; But it's a wonderful movie!, *Literally:* Listen, but it's a wonderful movie!)

A less formal variant of the same expression is **Poslushaj!** (pahs-*loo*-shuhy). You can use it with someone you're on familiar terms with, someone you normally say **Ty** (tih; you; informal) to; see Chapter 2 for details on the informal "you." And if you want to be even more informal, you can use the conversational variant **Slushaj!** (*sloo*-shuhy) Just make sure the person you say it to is your good friend, and will take this informality the right way. Otherwise, stick to **Poslushaj!**

Pir Goroj

You may be at a loss to describe the grand abundance of Russian dinner parties and holiday tables. This expression, then, is useful: **pir goroj** (peer gah-*rohy*; *Literally:* feast with food piled up like a mountain). If you're hungry for more food info, check out Chapter 5.

Ya Tryebuyu Prodolzhyeniya Bankyeta

This phrase is a quote from one of the Russian's most beloved comedies, **"Ivan Vasil'yevich myenyayet profyessiyu"** (ee-*vahn* vah-*seel'*-ee-veech mee-*nya*-eet prah-*fye*-see-yu; Ivan Vasil'yevich Changes His Occupation), and is sure to make any Russian smile. Say **Ya tryebuyu prodolzhyeniya bankyeta!** (ya *trye*-boo-yu pruh-dahl-*zheh*-nee-ye buhn-*kye*-tuh; *Literally:* I insist on the continuation of the banquet!) when a party or a trip is going well, when somebody is inviting you to come over again, or when you're suggesting to do some fun activity yet another time.

"Ivan Vasil'yevich myenyayet profyessiyu" is an old Russian movie about a bland accountant, Ivan Vasil'yevich, who switches places with Tsar Ivan the Terrible with the help of a time machine invented by his neighbor. Confused, at first, to find himself in the position of Russia's 16th-century tsar (who turns out to be his identical twin), Ivan Vasil'yevich quickly takes to the tsar's lifestyle. Sitting in an ornate banquet hall of the old Kremlin, at the head of a huge table with endless delicacies, and watching a performance of his court dancers, Ivan Vasil'yevich, drunk from the rare wines and the attention of the beautiful tsarina, raises a precious goblet and exclaims, **Ya tryebuyu prodolzhyeniya bankyeta!**

Slovo — Syeryebro, A Molchaniye — Zoloto

Russians love proverbs and use them a lot. **Slovo — syeryebro, a molchaniye — zoloto** (*sloh*-vuh see-reeb-*roh* uh mahl-*chah*-nee-ee *zoh*-luh-tuh; a word is silver, but silence is gold) can be loosely translated as "Speaking is nice, but silence is supreme." This phrase is nice to say after you make a mistake speaking Russian or when you, or somebody else, says something that would be better off left unsaid.

Odna Golova Khorosho, A Dvye — Luchshye

Odna golova khorosho, a dvye — luchshye (ahd-*nah* guh-lah-*vah* khuh-rah-*shoh* ah dvye *looch*-shih; One head is good, but two heads are better) doesn't refer to science fiction mutants. Rather, it's a manifestation of the international belief that two heads are better than one. You can say this phrase when you invite somebody to do something together or when you ask for, or offer, help or advice.

Drug Poznayotsya V Byedye

Drug poznayotsya v byedye (drook puhz-nuh-*yot*-sye v bee-*dye*; A friend is tested by hardship) is the Russian equivalent of the saying, "A friend in need is a friend indeed."

Russians take friendship seriously. Their definition of a friend is not just a person you know (as in, "This is my new friend . . . what's your name again?"). Such a person would be called **znakomyj** (znuh-*koh*-mihy; acquaintance). A **drug** (drook; friend), on the other hand, is someone who cares for you. And the best way to find out whether a certain person is a friend or just an acquaintance is to see how they behave when things aren't going so great.

Staryj Drug Luchshye Novykh Dvukh

Staryj drug luchshye novykh dvukh (*stah*-rihy drook *looch*-shih *noh*-vihkh dvookh; An old friend is better than two new ones) is another speculation on the theme of friendship. An old friend (and they aren't referring to age) is better because he or she has already been tested, possibly by hardships mentioned in the previous phrase. New friends, on the other hand, are dark horses; when a bad moment strikes, they may turn out to be just acquaintances.

Chapter 19

Ten Russian Holidays to Remember

In This Chapter

▶ Finding out what holidays Russians celebrate

▶ Discovering what to expect on Russian holidays

Russians love holidays. You may say, "Who doesn't?" But there's a difference: Russians LOVE holidays — the feeling is stable and official. The government recognizes and legally acknowledges it. The difference is not only that the Russian calendar is marked by more official days off than an American one, but also that many holidays get more than one day off, because, as Russians see it, "Come on, what kind of holiday is it if you're only celebrating for a day?" Moreover, if a holiday falls on a Thursday, the government usually shifts the working schedule around so that the remaining working Friday, inconveniently stuck between the holiday and the weekend, also becomes a day off.

These arrangements, along with proximity of some important Russian holidays in time (Christmas is seven days after the New Year, Victory Day is nine days after May Day) create monstrous holiday chunks, when businesses are closed for ten consecutive days, everybody is celebrating, and attempts to get something done are not only unsuccessful but also shunned as something highly inappropriate. All this merriment is pretty enjoyable when you're included in the celebration but rather frustrating if you're trying to get some official paper. Look through this chapter to find out when you're wise to set all the business aside and celebrate.

New Year's Night

Novyj God (*noh*-vihy goht; New Year's) is celebrated on December 31 and definitely the main holiday in Russia. It's the holiday to prepare for, give the biggest **podarki** (pah-*dahr*-kee; gifts) for, and celebrate for more than a week. Think Christmas, but bigger, not religious, less family-oriented, and more party fun.

Novyj God combines traditions that Americans associate with other holidays. Russian Santa Claus, **Dyed Moroz** (dyed mah-*rohs*; Grandfather Frost) comes on New Year's night. He brings along his granddaughter **Snyegurochka** (snee-*goo*-ruch-kuh), and neither reindeer nor elves are in the picture. A Christmas tree in Russian is called a New Year's Tree — **novogodnyaya yolka** (nuh-vah-*gohd*-nee-ye *yohl*-kuh; *Literally:* New Year's pine tree).

Novogodnyaya yolka is not just a tree; it's also the name of a New Year's party for children, which is organized by all the schools, youth clubs, day care centers, and companies for their employees' children. The celebration usually consists of an interactive performance, written and staged by teachers, older students, or company enthusiasts; the traditional dance **khorovod** (khuh-rah-*voht*), when everybody holds hands and moves around the tree in circle; contests; and presents. Another surprising fact: For New Year's parties, Russians of all ages dress in costumes, just as Americans do for Halloween.

No one is supposed to stay home on New Year's night. Russians of all ages get together for New Year's parties, where they first celebrate at abundantly served tables, and then dance the night away. If the weather permits (and even if it doesn't), city authorities organize celebrations in the parks and on the main squares. You're likely to see a lot of fireworks (which you can buy on every corner), improvised **khorovody,** and people dressed up as **Dyed Moroz** riding public transportation.

Russians don't have New Year's resolutions. Instead, they make a New Year's wish, which is believed to always come true. They make it at the stroke of midnight while raising a glass of **shampanskoye** (shuhm-*pahn*-skuh-ee; champagne) — the official drink of the **Novyj God.**

If you have a chance to celebrate the **Novyj God** with Russians, do so — it's sure to be a memorable experience.

Old New Year's

Considering how much fun New Year's night is, you can understand why having just one a year isn't enough. The roots of **Staryj Novyj God** (*stah*-rihy *noh*-vihy goht; Old New Year's) go back in time to the epoch when Russia's calendar was two weeks behind the European one, thus placing New Year's day on contemporary January 14.

The celebration isn't as extensive as that of December 31 (two celebrations of that caliber would be too much even for Russians), and businesses aren't supposed to be closed on that day. Don't hope to get anything done, though; it's **Staryj Novyj God,** and no one is in the mood for work. Visit your friends, eat, and dance.

Russian Christmas

This fact may come as a surprise, but Christmas doesn't automatically mean December 25. Most Russians are Orthodox Christians, and Orthodox **Rozhdyestvo** (ruhzh-dees-*tvoh*; Christmas) is January 7. Orthodox Christianity was the first to split from the big Christian tree back in 1054. The most conspicuous features that distinguish Orthodox churches (not to go into theology) are highly ornate internal and external design, richly decorated **ikony** (ee-*koh*-nih; icons), and generous use of incense during services. On Christmas, all-night services are held in the most important Russian churches.

Those who follow the old traditions make **kutya** (koo-*t'ya*), a wheat porridge with honey, walnuts, and other ingredients, seven of them altogether; Russians believe seven to be an especially good number.

Russian Easter

Speaking of religious holidays, Russian Orthodox **Paskha** (*pahs*-khuh; Easter) doesn't coincide with Western Easter, either. **Paskha** is not only the name of the holiday, but also a special cake that Russians bake (or, more realistically, buy) for Easter. They also dye boiled **yajtsa** (*yahy*-tsuh; eggs) into cheerful colors and exchange them. On the day of Easter, instead of "Hello," Russians say to each other **Khristos voskryes!** (khrees-*tohs* vahsk-*ryes*; Christ has arisen!) The appropriate response is **Voistinu voskryes!** (vah-*ees*-tee-noo vahsk-*ryes*; He truly has!)

Women's Day

In spite of its official name, The International Day of Solidarity of Women, or, simply, **8 marta** (vahs'-*moh*-ee *mahr*-tuh; March 8), Women's Day is as far from feminism as it gets. This official day off is the day when every Russian female has a chance to "feel like a real woman." It's a mixture of Mother's Day and Valentine's Day, but more inclusive: All women, from grandmothers to neighbors to colleagues, to say nothing of mothers and sweethearts, receive flowers, gifts, and abundant compliments. This day is also the only day of the year when Russian men awkwardly cook breakfast and clean the apartment.

The Day of the Defender of the Fatherland

Dyen' zash'itnika otyechyestva (dyen' zuh-*sh'eet*-nee-kuh aht-*tye*-cheest-vuh), February 23, was initially a holiday to note men who have served or are

currently serving in the military. With time, it's become a male counterpart to Women's Day on March 8. Offices and organizations hold parties, women give presents to their male relatives and colleagues, all TV stations broadcast thematic concerts, and cities organize fireworks and open-air festivities.

Russian Mardi Gras

Maslyenitsa (*mahs*-lee-nee-tsuh) is a week of celebration right before Lent, seven weeks before Russian Easter. **Maslyenitsa** goes back to the pagan tradition of greeting the spring. The main attributes include **bliny** (blee-*nih*; pancakes), which are symbols of the sun, and open-air festivals, during which straw figures symbolizing winter are burned in bonfires.

May Day

Pyervoye Maya (*pyer*-vuh-ee *mah*-ye; May 1), started as the International Day of Solidarity of Working People, but eventually it became just another celebration of spring. On the first day of this two-day holiday, various floats, political or not, navigate down the streets of every Russian town; on the second day, everybody leaves the city for a **mayovka** (muh-*yohf*-kuh): a large-scale picnic in the lap of nature.

Victory Day

This fact is little known in the West, but the Russians took a very active part in World War II, and lost a huge number of people in it. On May 9, they celebrate **Dyen' Pobyedy** (dyen' pah-*bye*-dih; Victory Day) over Fascism with parades, fireworks, and open-air festivals.

National Unity Day

Created to replace the Day of the October Revolution (which used to be celebrated, ironically, on November 7), **Dyen' Narodnogo Yedinstva** (dyen' nuh-*rohd*-nuh-vuh ee-*deenst*-vuh; National Unity Day), celebrated on November 4, commemorates the events of 1612, when two Moscow merchants called for the unity of Russian citizens in the effort to liberate Moscow from Polish-Swedish troops. It's another occasion for parades, fireworks, and open-air festivals.

Chapter 20

Ten Phrases That Make You Sound Russian

In This Chapter
▶ Finding out what to say to really fit in with Russians
▶ Discovering traditions that help you understand Russians better

Some phrases aren't really important in a conversation. They don't really mean anything, and you can get your point across without using them. Not coincidentally, these phrases also make native speakers hit you approvingly on the back and say, "Yeah, buddy, you're one of us." A book doesn't teach you these phrases — unless the book is *Russian For Dummies*. In this chapter, you find insider's information on ten phrases that make you sound Russian.

Tol'ko Poslye Vas!

Oh, dear Old World! Russians still believe in opening doors for each other and letting others go first. If you want to be especially polite, absolutely refuse to go through a door if somebody else is aiming for it. Instead of just walking through and getting it over with, stand by the door for 15 minutes repeating **Tol'ko poslye vas!** (*tohl'*-kuh *pohs*-lee vahs; Only after you!) while your counterpart stands by the other side of the door repeating the same phrase. It may be time consuming, but it's very rewarding in the long run; you'll be recognized as a well-bred and very nice individual.

Vy Syegodnya Pryekrasno Vyglyaditye!

Speaking of being old-fashioned: Russians, for some reason, don't believe that giving compliments is considered sexual harassment. So, if you start a conversation with a Russian woman by saying **Vy syegodnya pryekrasno vyglyaditye!** (vih see-*vohd*-nye pree-*krahs*-nuh *vihg*-lee-dee-tee; You look great to

she may actually treat you nicer instead of reporting you to the authorities. It's hard to believe, but this exact phrase is considered appropriate with colleagues, shop assistants, and hotel receptionists. Just remember to stop using the phrase after you leave Russia if you want to avoid criminal charges.

If someone says **Vy syegodnya pryekrasno vyglyaditye!** to you, remember that the appropriate response isn't **spasibo** (spuh-*see*-buh; thank you); you should say **Nu, chto vy!** (noo shtoh vih; Ah, what are you talking about!) You have to show your modesty and disagree.

Zakhoditye Na Chaj!

Making a Russian friend is very easy. When you meet someone (and if you like this person enough to want to be his or her friend), don't think too hard about finding a way to create a social connection. Just say **Zakhoditye na chaj!** (zuh-khah-*dee*-tee nuh chahy; Stop by for some tea!) The person won't think you're a freak or a serial killer; he or she will most likely take your offer at face value. Keep in mind, though, that unlike "Let's do lunch," Russians take **Zakhoditye na chaj** seriously and usually accept your offer. That being said, you should actually have some tea and cookies at home, because **Zakhoditye na chaj!** implies drinking tea and conversing, unlike the American version: "Would you like to stop by my place for a drink?"

Ugosh'ajtyes'!

When you invite a new friend over for tea and whip out your strategically prepared box of cookies, a nice thing to say is **Ugosh'ajtyes!** (oo-gah-*sh'ahy*-tees'; Help yourself! *Literally:* Treat yourself!) Besides being friendly and polite, this word is just long enough to scare off foreigners. Which is, of course, a good enough reason to learn it and stand out in the crowd.

Priyatnogo Appetita!

Unless you want to strike people as a gloomy, misanthropic sociopath, don't start eating without wishing others **Priyatnogo appetita!** (pree-*yat*-nuh-vuh uh-pee-*tee*-tuh; Bon appetit!) Don't hesitate to say this phrase to people you don't know and are seeing for the first time in your life after your waiter sits them down at your table in an over-crowded restaurant.

Syadyem Na Dorozhku!

Before departing on a trip, surprise everybody by looking around thought-fully and saying **Syadyem na dorozhku!** (*sya*-deem nuh dah-*rohsh*-koo; Let's sit down before hitting the road!) Essentially a superstition, this tradition is actually useful; sitting down and staying silent for a minute before you head out the door gives you an opportunity to remember what's important. Maybe your packed lunch is still in the fridge, and your plane tickets with a sticker saying "Don't forget!" are still on your bedside table!

Sadis', V Nogakh Pravdy Nyet

Sitting down is a big deal for Russians. Which is, of course, understandable: With those vast lands, they must have had to walk a lot (especially before the invention of trains). That's why when you're sitting with somebody standing before you, or when somebody stops by and hangs out in the doorway, claim-ing to be leaving in a minute, you can say **Sadis', v nogakh pravdy nyet.** (sah-*dees'*, v nah-*gahkh prahv*-dih nyet; Sit down, there is no truth in feet.) This phrase doesn't make much sense in English. And Russians most likely don't believe that more truth exists in other parts of the body than in the feet. The phrase, however, is a nice hospitality token, and it definitely wins you some "native-speaker" points.

Ni Pukha, Ni Pyera!

Although English has its own cute little "Break a leg" phrase, nobody really uses it anymore. Russians, on the other hand, never let anyone depart on a mission — whether a lady leaves to interview for a job or guy goes to ask a girl out — without saying **Ni pukha, ni pyera!** (nee *poo*-khuh nee pee-*rah*; Good luck! *Literally:* Have neither fluff nor plume!)

The appropriate response isn't **spasibo** (spuh-*see*-buh; thank you); you should say **K chyortu!** (k *chohr*-too; To the devil!) We have no clear explana-tion for where this response came from. The **chyort** (chohrt; petty devil) part of the phrase represents a very popular character in Russian folklore. He's mentioned in a variety of expressions, such as **u chyorta na kulichkakh** (oo *chohr*-tuh nuh koo-*leech*-kukh; far away, *Literally:* at the devil's Easter cele-bration) or **chyortova dyuzhina** (*chohr*-tuh-vuh *dyu*-zhih-nuh; number 13, *Literally:* devil's dozen). The most common way **chyort** appears is in **Idi k chyortu!** (ee-*dee* k *chohr*-too; Go to the devil!) As you can tell, **K chyortu!**

sounds suspiciously close to an insult. In any other situation, **K chyortu!** would sound offensive. Responding to **Ni pukha, ni pyera!** in this manner is a precious opportunity to send the devil someone you always wanted to get rid of but were afraid to. Just be sure to smile while responding!

Tseluyu

Russians sign their letters, e-mails, and cell-phone text messages with **Tseluyu** (tsih-*loo*-yu; kisses, *Literally:* [I am] kissing [you]). You can also say **Tseluyu** at the end of a phone conversation. We don't recommend saying it in person, though: if you're face to face with someone, you may as well kiss the person instead of talking about it!

Russians are known for kissing socially. Like folks in France, Russians kiss on the cheek; unlike folks in France, Russians do it three times (because three, much like seven, is a lucky number). Social kissing is such an accepted practice in Russia that one Soviet leader caused a considerable international scandal when he whole-heartedly kissed a Western leader. Doesn't sound too scandalous? Well, being old and clumsy, the Soviet leader missed his cheek and kissed his counterpart on the mouth!

S Lyogkim Parom!

Here's a weird one: When Russians see someone who just came out of a shower, a sauna, or any place where you can, supposedly, clean yourself, they say **S lyogkim parom!** (s *lyokh*-keem *pah*-ruhm; *Literally:* Congratulations on a light steam!) This phrase is very popular, especially after it became the title of the token Russian New Year's night movie **"Ironiya sud'by, ili s lyogkim parom!"** (ee-*roh*-nee-ye sood'-*bih ee*-lee s *lyokh*-keem *pah*-ruhm; The Irony of Fate, or Congratulations on a light steam!) This romantic comedy, shown by pretty much every Russian television channel on December 31, starts in a Russian **banya** (*bah*-nye; sauna), which triggers all the adventures that follow. (See Chapter 19 for more about Russian holidays.)

You can use **S lyogkim parom!** humorously: Say it to someone who got caught in the rain or someone who spilled a drink. Yes, it sounds mean, but Russians have a dark sense of humor.

Chapter 21

Ten Things Never to Say or Do in Russia

. . . .

In This Chapter

▶ Exploring Russian social taboos

▶ Picking up some tips on proper behavior in Russia

. . . .

*E*very culture has its Do's and Don'ts. In Chapters 18 through 20, we discuss the do's. Sometimes, knowing what NOT to do is even more important if you want to fit in or at least produce a good impression. Read on to find out about ten Russian social taboos.

Don't Come to Visit Empty-Handed

If you're invited over for dinner, or just for a visit, don't come to a Russian house with empty hands. What you bring doesn't really matter — a box of chocolates, flowers, or a small toy for a child, just as long as you don't come **s pustymi rukami** (s poos-*tih*-mee roo-*kah*-mee; empty-handed). The hosts usually prepare for a visit by cooking their best dishes and buying delicacies that they normally wouldn't buy for themselves. If, after all this effort, a guest shows up without even a flower, Russians believe he doesn't care. They won't say anything, but the dinner will leave an unpleasant aftertaste.

Don't Leave Your Shoes On in Someone's Home

Russian apartments are covered in rugs. Often, they're expensive Persian rugs with intricate designs, which aren't cleaned as easily as traditional American carpeting. Besides, Russians walk a lot through dusty streets, instead of just stepping from the car directly into the home. For these reasons, and also because this tradition has gone on for centuries, Russians take

off their street shoes when they enter private residencies. The host usually offers a pair of **tapochki** (*tah*-puhch-kee; slippers); if you go to a party, women usually bring a pair of nice shoes to wear inside. And again, if you fail to take your shoes off, nobody will say anything; you're the guest, so you can do pretty much whatever you want. But sneak a peek: Are you the only person wearing your snow-covered boots at the dinner table?

Don't Joke about the Parents

Russians aren't politically correct. They casually make jokes that may cause you to cringe in your seat. No sensitive issue is spared, so you better prepare yourself. Parents, however, are the one thing that Russians just don't make jokes about, and they don't tolerate anyone else doing it either. So, go ahead and tell an **anyekdot** (uh-neek-*doht*; joke) based on ethnicity, appearance, or gender stereotypes; just steer clear of jokes about somebody's mother or father. You won't be understood.

Don't Toast with "Na Zdorov'ye!"

People who don't speak Russian usually think that they know one Russian phrase: a toast, **Na Zdorov'ye!** Little do they know that **Na Zdorov'ye!** (nuh zdah-*rohv'*-ee; for health) is what Russians say when somebody thanks them for a meal. In Polish, indeed, **Na Zdorov'ye!** or something close to it, is a traditional toast. Russians, on the other hand, like to make up something long and complex, such as, **Za druzhbu myezhdu narodami!** (zah *droozh*-boo *myezh*-doo nuh-*roh*-duh-mee; To friendship between nations!) If you want a more generic Russian toast, go with **Za Vas!** (zuh vahs; To you!)

Don't Take the Last Shirt

A Russian saying, **otdat' poslyednyuyu rubashku** (aht-*daht'* pahs-*lyed*-nyu-yu roo-*bahsh*-koo; to give away one's last shirt), makes the point that you have to be giving, no matter what the expense for yourself. In Russia, offering guests whatever they want is considered polite. Those wants don't just include food or accommodations; old-school Russians offer you whatever possessions you comment on, like a picture on the wall, a vase, or a sweater.

Now, being offered something doesn't necessarily mean you should take it. Russians aren't offering something because they want to get rid of it; they're offering because they want to do something nice for you. So, unless you feel that plundering their home is a good idea, don't just take things offered to you and leave. Refuse first, and do so a couple of times, because your hosts

will insist. And only accept the gift if you really want this special something, but then return the favor and give your hosts something nice, as well.

Don't Underdress

Russians dress up on more occasions than Americans do. Even to go for a casual walk, a Russian woman may wear high heels and a nice dress. A hardcore feminist may say women do this because they're victimized and oppressed. But Russian women themselves explain it this way, "We only live once; I want to look and feel my best." Who can blame them?

On some occasions, all foreigners, regardless of gender, run the risk of being the most underdressed person in the room. These occasions include dinner parties and trips to the theater. Going to a restaurant is also considered a festive occasion, and you don't want to show up in your jeans and T-shirt, no matter how informal you think the restaurant may be. In any case, checking on the dress code before going out somewhere is a good idea.

Don't Go Dutch

Here's where Russians differ strikingly from Western Europeans. They don't go Dutch. So, if you ask a lady out, don't expect her to pay for herself, not at a restaurant or anywhere else. You can, of course, suggest that she pay, but that usually rules out the possibility of seeing her again. She may not even have money on her. Unless they expect to run into a maniac and have to escape through the back exit, Russian women wouldn't think of bringing money when going out with a man.

And for our female readers: Even if your Russian male friend lives on a scholarship of $100 a month, he will insist on paying for everything. And if he doesn't at least insist, we recommend taking a closer look at him. Having a woman pay is a strong taboo in Russia; you may want to wonder why this man chooses to break it.

Don't Let a Woman Carry Something Heavy

This rule may make politically correct people cringe, but Russians believe that a man is physically stronger than a woman. Therefore, they believe a man who watches a woman carry something heavy without helping her is impolite.

When you see a woman (or an elderly person) carrying something heavy, offer your help with this phrase: **Razryeshitye vam pomoch'!** (ruhz-ree-*shih*-tee vahm pah-*mohch*; Let me help you!) or simply **Vam pomoch'?** (vahm pah-*mohch*; Shall I help you?) If you're offered help, you can either accept it with **Bol'shoye spasibo!** (bahl'-*shoh*-ee spuh-*see*-buh; Thank you very much!) or refuse it with **Nyet, spasibo!** (nyet spuh-*see*-buh; No, thank you!)

Don't Overlook the Elderly on Public Transportation

When Russians come to America and ride public transportation, they're very confused to see young people sitting when an elderly person is standing nearby. They don't understand that in America, an elderly person may be offended when offered a seat. Well, you don't need to worry about that in Russia. Their elderly people and pregnant women won't be offended if you offer them a seat on a bus. In fact, if you don't, the entire bus looks at you as if you're a criminal. Women, even (or should we say, especially) young ones, are also offered seats on public transportation. But that's optional. Getting up and offering a seat to an elderly person, on the other hand, is a must.

Don't Burp in Public

We hate to bring it up . . . And we're sure that this suggestion doesn't, of course, apply to our readers. But maybe you know someone you can give this piece of advice to. Know that bodily functions, such as getting rid of excess gas (yes, we're talking about burping!), are considered extremely impolite in public, even if the sound is especially long and expressive, and the author is proud of it.

Moreover, if the incident happens (we're all human), don't apologize. By apologizing, you acknowledge your authorship, and attract more attention to the fact. Meanwhile, Russians, terrified by what just happened, pretend they didn't notice, or silently blame it on the dog. Obviously, these people are in denial. But if you don't want to be remembered predominantly for this incident, steer clear of natural bodily functions in public.

Part V
Appendixes

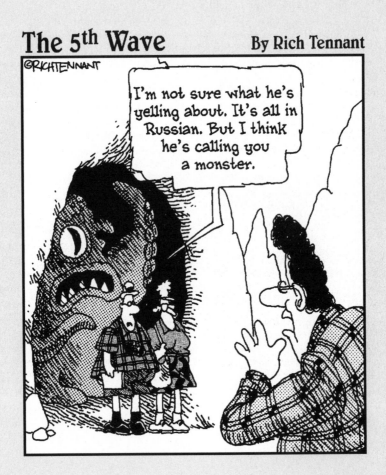

In this part . . .

The appendixes in Part V give you easy-to-use Russian reference sources. We include a sample list of commonly used regular and irregular Russian verbs with their conjugations. We provide you with a mini-dictionary with some of the words you use most often. We give you an answer key to all the Fun & Games sections that appear at the end of the chapters in this book. And finally, we list the tracks of the audio CD included with this book so you can read along and practice as you listen to real-world conversation of native Russian speakers.

Appendix A
Verb Tables

Regular Russian Verbs

Regular Verbs Ending with –at'
For example: dyelat' (to do, to make)

	Present	Past	Future
ya (I)	dyelayu	dyelal/dyelala	budu dyelat'
ty (you sing./ inform.)	dyelayesh'	dyelal/dyelala	budyesh' dyelat'
on/ona/ono (he/she/it)	dyelayet	dyelal/dyelala/ dyelalo	budyet dyelat'
my (we)	dyelayem	dyelali	budyem dyelat'
vy (you pl./form.)	dyelayetye	dyelali	budyetye dyelat'
oni (they)	dyelayut	dyelali	budut dyelat'

Regular Verbs Ending with –it'
For example: govorit' (to talk)

	Present	Past	Future
ya (I)	govoryu	govoril/govorila	budu govorit'
ty (you sing./ inform.)	govorish'	govoril/govorila	budyesh' govorit'
on/ona/ono (he/she/it)	govorit	govoril/govorila/ govorilo	budyet govorit'
my (we)	govorim	govorili	budyem govorit'
vy (you pl./form.)	govoritye	govorili	budyetye govorit'
oni (they)	govoryat	govorili	budut govorit'

Irregular Russian Verbs

byt'
to be

	Present	Past	Future
ya	None	byl/byla	budu
ty	None	byl/byla	budyesh'
on/ona/ono	None	byl/byla/bylo	budyet
my	None	byli	budyem
vy	None	byli	budyetye
oni	None	byli	budut

moch'
to be able, can

	Present	Past	Future
ya	mogu	mog/mogla	smogu
ty	mozhyesh'	mog/mogla	smozhyesh'
on/ona/ono	mozhyet	mog/mogla/moglo	smozhyet
my	mozhyem	mogli	smozhyem
vy	mozhyetye	mogli	smozhyetye
oni	mogut	mogli	smogut

zhit'
to live

	Present	Past	Future
ya	zhivu	zhil/zhila	budu zhit'
ty	zhivyosh'	zhil/zhila	budyesh' zhit'
on/ona/ono	zhivyot	zhil/zhila/zhilo	budyet zhit'
my	zhivyom	zhili	budyem zhit'
vy	zhivyotye	zhili	budyetye zhit'
oni	zhivut	zhili	budut zhit'

yest'
to eat

	Present	Past	Future
ya	yem	yel/yela	budu yest'
ty	yesh'	yel/yela	budyesh' yest'
on/ona/ono	yest	yel/yela/yelo	budyet yest'
my	yedim	yeli	budyem yest'
vy	yeditye	yeli	budyetye yest'
oni	yedyat	yeli	budut yest'

		Present	Past	Future
pit'	*ya*	p'yu	pil/pila	budu pit'
to drink	*ty*	p'yosh'	pil/pila	budyesh' pit'
	on/ona/ono	p'yot	pil/pila/pilo	budyet pit'
	my	p'yom	pili	budyem pit'
	vy	p'yotye	pili	budyetye pit'
	oni	p'yut	pili	budut pit'

		Present	Past	Future
khotyet'	*ya*	khochu	khotyel/khotyela	budu khotyet'
to want	*ty*	khochyesh'	khotyel/khotyela	budyesh' khotyet'
	on/ona/ono	khochyet	khotyel/khotyela/ khotyelo	budyet khotyet'
	my	khotim	khotyeli	budyem khotyet'
	vy	khotitye	khotyeli	budyetye khotyet'
	oni	khotyat	khotyeli	budut khotyet'

		Present	Past	Future
lyubit'	*ya*	lyublyu	lyubil/lyubila	budu lyubit'
to love, to like	*ty*	lyubish'	lyubil/lyubila	budyesh' lyubit'
	on/ona/ono	lyubit	lyubil/lyubila/ lyubilo	budyet lyubit'
	my	lyubim	lyubili	budyem lyubit'
	vy	lyubitye	lyubili	budyetye lyubit'
	oni	lyubyat	lyubili	budut lyubit'

		Present	Past	Future
platit'	*ya*	plachu	platil/platila	budu platit'
to pay	*ty*	platish'	platil/platila	budyesh' platit'
	on/ona/ono	platit	platil/platila/platilo	budyet platit'
	my	platim	platili	budyem platit'
	vy	platitye	platili	budyetye platit'
	oni	platyat	platili	budut platit'

		Present	Past	Future
vidyet'	*ya*	vizhu	vidyel/vidyela	budu vidyet'
to see	*ty*	vidish'	vidyel/vidyela	budyesh' vidyet'
	on/ona/ono	vidit	vidyel/vidyela/vidyelo	budyet vidyet'
	my	vidim	vidyeli	budyem vidyet'
	vy	viditye	vidyeli	budyetye vidyet'
	oni	vidyat	vidyeli	budut vidyet'

		Present	Past	Future
pisat'	*ya*	pishu	pisal/pisala	budu pisat'
to write	*ty*	pishyesh'	pisal/pisala	budyesh' pisat'
	on/ona/ono	pishyet	pisal/pisala/pisalo	budyet pisat'
	my	pishyem	pisali	budyem pisat'
	vy	pishyetye	pisali	budyetye pisat'
	oni	pishut	pisali	budut pisat'

Russian-English Mini-Dictionary

A

adryes (*ahd*-rees) m: address
aeroport (uh-eh-ruh-*pohrt*) m: airport
apryel' (uhp-*ryel'*) m: April
avgust (*ahv*-goost) m: August
avtobus (uhf-*toh*-boos) m: bus

B

babushka (*bah*-boosh-kuh) f: grandmother
balyet (buh-*lyet*) m: ballet
bank (bahnk) m: bank
bilyet (bee-*lyet*) m: ticket
bol'nitsa (bahl'-*nee*-tsuh) f: hospital
bol'shoj (bahl'-*shohy*): big
bolyen (*boh*-leen): ill
brat (braht) m: brother
brat'/vzyat' (braht'/vzyat'): to take
bryuki (*bryu*-kee): pants
butylka (boo-*tihl*-kuh) f: bottle
byelyj (*bye*-lihy): white
byt' (biht'): to be

C

chas (chahs) m: hour
chashka (*chahsh*-kuh) f: cup
chasy (chuh-*sih*): clock

chistyj (*chees*-tihy): clear
chitat'/prochitat' (chee-*taht'*/pruh-chee-*taht'*): to read
chto (shtoh): what
chto-to (*shtoh*-tuh): something
chyek (chyek) m: check
chyemodan (chee-mah-*dahn*) m: suitcase
chyetvyerg (cheet-*vyerk*) m: Thursday
chyornyj (*chohr*-nihy): black

D

dalyeko (duh-lee-*koh*): far
davat'/dat' (duh-*vaht'*/daht'): to give
dlinnyj (*dlee*-nihy): long
do svidaniya (duh svee-*dah*-nee-ye): goodbye
doch' (dohch') f: daughter
dolzhyen (*dohl*-zhihn): to have to
dom (dohm) m: home, house
dorogoj (duh-rah-*gohy*): dear, expensive
dostavat'/dostat' (duhs-tuh-*vaht'*/*duhs*-taht'): to get
dozhd' (dohsht') m: rain
drug (drook) m: friend
dumat' (*doo*-muht'): to think
dvoryets (dvah-*ryets*) m: palace
dvyer' (dvyer') f: door
dyedushka (*dye*-doosh-kuh) f: grandfather
dyekabr' (dee-*kahbr'*) m: December

dyelat'/sdyelat' (*dye*-luht'/*sdye*-luht'): to do, to make

dyen' (dyen') m: day

dyen'gi (*dyen'*-gee): money

dyeshyovyj (dee-*shoh*-vihy): cheap

dyesyert (dee-*syert*) m: dessert

dyevochka (*dye*-vuhch-kuh) f: girl

dzhinsy (*dzhihn*-sih): jeans

F

faks (fahks) m: fax

firma (*feer*-muh) f: firm

frukty (*frook*-tih) m: fruits

fyevral' (feev-*rahl'*) m: February

G

galstuk (*gahls*-took) m: tie

gazyeta (guh-*zye*-tuh) f: newspaper

gdye (gdye): where

glavnyj (*glahv*-nihy): main

god (goht) m: year

golova (guh-lah-*vah*) f: head

gora (gah-*rah*) f: mountain

gorod (*goh*-ruht) m: city

gost' (gohst') m: guest

gostinitsa (gahs-*tee*-nee-tsuh) f: hotel

I

idti/khodit' (eet-*tee*/khah-*deet'*): to go by foot

igrat' (eeg-*raht'*): to play

imyeil (ee-*meh*-eel) m: e-mail

imya (*ee*-mye) n: name

imyet' (ee-*myet'*): to have

indyex (*een*-dehks) m: zip code

inostrannyj (ee-nah-*strah*-nihy): foreign

intyeryes (een-tee-*ryes*) m: interest

iyul' (ee-*yul'*) m: July

iyun' (ee-*yun'*) m: June

iz (ees): from

K

kak (kahk): how

kassa (*kah*-suh) f: cash register

khlyeb (khlyep) m: bread

kholodnyj (khah-*lohd*-nihy): cold

khoroshij (khah-*roh*-shihy): good

khorosho (khuh-rah-*shoh*) m: all right, well

khotyet' (khah-*tyet'*): to want

kino (kee-*noh*) n: movie theater

klub (kloop) m: club

kniga (*knee*-guh) f: book

kofye (*koh*-fee) m: coffee

kogda (kahg-*dah*): when

kolyeno (kah-*lye*-nuh) n: knee

komnata (*kohm*-nuh-tuh) f: room

kompaniya (kahm-*pah*-nee-ye) f: company

konyets (kah-*nyets*) m: end

korichnyevyj (kah-*reech*-nee-vihy): brown

kostyum (kahs-*tyum*) m: suit

kot (koht) m: cat

kotoryj (kah-*toh*-rihy): which

krasivyj (kruh-*see*-vihy): beautiful

krasnyj (*krahs*-nihy): red

krovat' (krah-*vaht'*) f: bed

kryeditnaya kartochka (kree-*deet*-nuh-ye *kahr*-tuhch-kuh) f: credit card

kto (ktoh): who

kurtka (*koort*-kuh) f: jacket

kvartira (kvuhr-*tee*-ruh) f: apartment

L

litso (lee-*tsoh*) n: face
lozhka (*lohsh*-kuh) f: spoon
lyegko (leekh-*koh*): easy
lyekarstvo (lee-*kahrst*-vuh) n: medicine
lyetat'/lyetyet' (lee-*taht'*/lee-*tyet'*): to fly
lyeto (*lye*-tuh) n: summer
lyubit' (lyu-*beet'*): to love
lyudi (*lyu*-dee): people

M

magazin (muh-guh-*zeen*) m: shop
maj (mahy) m: May
mal'chik (*mahl'*-cheek) m: boy
malyen'kij (*mah*-leen'-keey): small
mart (mahrt) m: March
mashina (muh-*shih*-nuh) f: car
mat' (maht') f: mother
militsiya (mee-*lee*-tsih-ye) f: police
minuta (mee-*noo*-tuh) f: minute
moch'/smohch' (mohch'/smohch'): can
moj (mohy) m: my
molodoj (muh-lah-*dohy*): young
moloko (muh-lah-*koh*) n: milk
morye (*moh*-ree) n: sea
most (mohst) m: bridge
muzh (moosh) m: husband
muzhchina (moo-*sh'ee*-nuh) m: man
muzyej (moo-*zyey*) m: museum
my (mih): we
myaso (*mya*-suh) n: meat
myedsyestra (meet-sees-*trah*) f: nurse
myesto (*myes*-tuh) n: seat
myesyats (*mye*-seets) m: month
myetro (meet-*roh*) n: subway

N

nakhodit'/najti (nuh-khah-*deet'*/nahy-*tee*): to find
nalichnyye (nuh-*leech*-nih-ee): cash
nalyevo (nuh-*lye*-vuh): (to the) left
napravo (nuh-*prah*-vuh): (to the) right
nikogda (nee-kahg-*dah*): never
no (noh): but
noch' (nohch') f: night
noga (nah-*gah*) f: leg
nomyer (*noh*-meer) m: number
nos (nohs) m: nose
nosit' (nah-*seet'*): wear
novyj (*noh*-vihy): new
noyabr' (nah-*yabr'*) m: November
nozh (nohsh) m: knife
nravit'sya/ponravit'sya (nrah-veet-sye/pah-*nrah*-veet-sye): to like
nyedyelya (nee-*dye*-lye) f: week

O

obyed (ah-*byet*) m: lunch
offis (*oh*-fees) m: office
ofitsiant (uh-fee-tsih-*ahnt*) m: waiter
okno (ahk-*noh*) n: window
oktyabr' (ahk-*tyabr'*) m: October
on (ohn): he
ona (ah-*nah*): she
oni (ah-*nee*): they
ono (ah-*noh*): it
osyen' (*oh*-seen') f: fall
otdyel (aht-*dyel*) m: department
otpusk (*oht*-poosk) m: vacation
otyets (ah-*tyets*) f: father
ovosh'i (*oh*-vuh-sh'ee): vegetables

P

p'yesa (*p'ye*-suh) f: play

pal'to (puhl'-*toh*) n: coat

pasport (*pahs*-puhrt) m: passport

pis'mo (pees'-*moh*) n: letter

pit'/vypit' (peet'/*vih*-peet'): to drink

pivo (*pee*-vuh) n: beer

plash' (plahsh') m: raincoat

plat'ye (*plaht'*-ee) f: dress

platit'/zaplatit' (pluh-*teet'*/zuh-pluh-*teet'*): pay

plokhoj (plah-*khohy*): bad

pochyemu (puh-chee-*moo*): why

podarok (pah-*dah*-ruhk) m: gift

pokazyvat'/pokazat' (pah-*kah*-zih-vuht'/puh-kuh-*zaht'*): to show

pokupat'/kupit' (puh-koo-*paht'*/koo-peet'): to buy

pomogat'/pomoch' (puh-mah-*gaht'*/pah-*mohch'*): to help

ponyedyel'nik (puh-nee-*dyel'*-neek) m: Monday

povorachivat'/povyernut' (puh-vah-*rah*-chee-vuht'/puh-veer-*noot'*): to turn

poyezd (*poh*-eest) m: train

pozdno (*pohz*-nuh): late

pozhalujsta (pah-*zhahl*-stuh): please, you're welcome

pozhar (pah-*zhahr*) m: fire

prikhodit'/pridti (pree-khah-*deet'*/preet-tee): to come

prinosit'/prinyetsi (pree-nah-*seet'*/pree-nees-*tee*): to bring

privyet (pree-*vyet*): hi

problyema (prahb-*lye*-muh) f: problem

prodavat'/prodat' (pruh-duh-*vaht'*/prah-*daht'*): to sell

prodavyets (pruh-duh-*vyets*): m: sales assistant

pryedstavlyat'/pryedstavit' (preet-stuhv-*lyat'*/preet-*stah*-veet'): to introduce

putyeshyestvovat' (poo-tee-*shehst*-vuh-vuht'): to travel

pyatnitsa (*pyat*-nee-tsuh) f: Friday

R

rabota (ruh-*boh*-tuh) f: work; job

rabotat' (ruh-*boh*-tuht'): to work

rano (*rah*-nuh): early

rasprodazha (ruhs-prah-*dah*-zhuh) f: sale

rasskazyvat'/rasskazat' (ruhs-*kah*-zih-vuht'/ruhs-kuh-*zaht'*): to tell

ris (rees) m: rice

rubashka (roo-*bahsh*-kuh) f: shirt

ruka (roo-*kah*) f: arm, hand

ryba (*rih*-buh) f: fish

ryebyonok (ree-*byo*-nuhk) m: child

ryeka (ree-*kah*) f: river

ryestoran (rees-tah-*rahn*) m: restaurant

rynok (*rih*-nuhk) m: market

S

sakhar (*sah*-khuhr) m: sugar

salat (suh-*laht*) m: salad

samolyot (suh-mah-*lyot*) m: airplane

sdacha (*sdah*-chuh) f: change

shapka (*shahp*-kuh) f: hat

shkola (*shkoh*-luh) f: school

shtat (shtaht) m: state

shyeya (*sheh*-ye) f: neck

sidyet' (see-*dyet'*): to sit

sinij (*see*-neey): blue

skazat' (skuh-*zaht'*): to say

skol'ko (*skohl'*-kuh): how many, how much

skuchnyj (*skoosh*-nihy): boring

sladkij (*slaht*-keey): sweet

slishkom (*sleesh*-kuhm): too (excessively)

slovo (*sloh*-vuh) n: word

smotryet'/posmotryet' (smaht-*ryet'*/ puhs-mah-*tryet'*): to look, to watch

smyeyat'sya (smee-*yat*-sye): to laugh

snimat' (snee-*maht'*): to rent

snyeg (snyek) m: snow

sobirat'/sobrat' (sub-bee-*raht'*/sahb-*raht'*): to collect

sol' (sohl') f: salt

spasibo (spuh-*see*-buh): thank you

spat' (spaht'): to sleep

spina (spee-*nah*) f: back

sport (spohrt) m: sports

sprashivat'/sprosit' (*sprah*-shih-vuht'/sprah-*seet'*): to ask

sryeda (sree-*dah*) f: Wednesday

stakan (stuh-*kahn*) m: glass

staryj (*stah*-rihy): old

stoyat' (stah-*yat'*): to stand

strana (struh-*nah*) f: country

subbota (soo-*boh*-tuh) f: Saturday

sumka (*soom*-kuh) f: bag

suvyenir (soo-vee-*neer*) m: souvenir

syegodnya (see-*vohd*-nye): today

syejchas (see-*chahs*): now

syekryetar' (seek-ree-*tahr'*) m: secretary

syem'ya (seem'-*ya*) f: family

syentyabr' (seen-*tyabr'*) m: September

syeryj (*sye*-rihy): gray

syestra (seest-*rah*) f: sister

syevyer (*sye*-veer) n: north

syn (sihn) m: son

syr (sihr) m: cheese

T

tamozhnya (tuh-*mohzh*-nye) f: customs

taryelka (tuh-*ryel*-kuh) f: plate

tol'ko (*tohl'*-kuh): only

tozhye (*toh*-zhih): also

tsvyet (tsvyet) m: color

tsyena (tsih-*nah*) f: price

tsyerkov' (*tsehr*-kuhf') f: church

tufli (*toof*-lee): shoes

tut (toot): here

ty (tih): you (singular, informal)

tyeatr (tee-*ahtr*) m: theater

tyelyefon (tee-lee-*fohn*) m: phone

tyepyer' (tee-*pyer'*): now

tyerapyevt (teh-ruh-*pehft*) m: physician

tyoplyj (*tyop*-lihy): warm

U

uchityel' (oo-*chee*-teel') m: teacher

ukhodit'/ujti (oo-khah-*deet'*/ooy-*tee*): to leave

ulitsa (*oo*-lee-tsuh) f: street

univyersityet (oo-nee-veer-see-*tyet*) m: university

utro (*oot*-ruh) n: morning

uzhin (*oo*-zhihn) m: dinner

V

vazhnyj (*vahzh*-nihy): important

vchyera (fchee-*rah*): yesterday

vidyet' (*vee*-deet'): to see

vilka (*veel*-kuh) f: fork

vino (vee-*noh*) n: wine

viza (*vee*-zuh) f: visa

vkhod (vkhoht) m: entrance

vkhodit'/vojti (vkhah-*deet'*/vahy-*tee*):
to enter

voda (vah-*dah*) f: water

vokzal (vahk-*zahl*) m: station

volosy (*voh*-luh-sih): hair

vopros (vahp-*rohs*) m: question

voskryesyen'ye (vuhs-kree-*syen'*-ee) n:
Sunday

vostok (vahs-*tohk*) m: east

vrach (vrahch) m: doctor

vryemya (*vrye*-mye) n: time

vstryecha (*vstrye*-chuh) f: meeting

vsye (fsye): everybody

vsyo (fsyo): everything

vtornik (*ftohr*-neek) m: Tuesday

vy (vih): you (plural, formal)

vyechyer (*vye*-cheer) m: evening

vyechyerinka (vee-chee-*reen*-kuh) f:
party

vyesh' (vyesh') f: thing

vyesna (vees-*nah*) f: spring

vykhod (*vih*-khuht): exit

vysokij (vih-*soh*-keey): high, tall

Y

ya (ya): I

yanvar' (een-*vahr'*) m: January

yeda (ee-*dah*) f: food

yest' (yest'): to eat

yezdit'/yekhat' (*yez*-deet'/*ye*-khuht'):
to go by vehicle

yubka (*yup*-kuh) f: skirt

yug (yuk) m: south

yurist (yu-*reest*) m: lawyer

Z

zakanchivat'/zakonchit' (zuh-*kahn*-chee-
vuht'/zuh-*kohn*-cheet'): finish

zapad (*zah*-puht) m: west

zavtra (*zahf*-truh): tomorrow

zavtrak (*zahf*-truhk) m: breakfast

zayavlyeniye (zuh-eev-*lye*-nee-ee) n:
application

zdorov'ye (zdah-*rohv'*-ee) n: health

zdravstvujtye (*zdrah*-stvooy-tee): hello

zdyes' (zdyes'): here

zharko (*zhahr*-kuh): hot

zhdat' (zhdaht'): to wait

zhit' (zhiht'): to live

zhivot (zhih-*voht*) m: stomach

zhyena (zhih-*nah*) f: wife

zhyensh'ina (*zhehn*-sh'ee-nuh) f: woman

zhyoltyj (*zhohl*-tihy): yellow

zima (zee-*mah*) f: winter

znat' (znaht'): to know

zubnoj vrach/dantist (zoob-*nohy*
vrahch/duhn-*teest*) m: dentist

zvonit'/pozvonit' (zvah-*neet'*/puh- zvah-
neet'): to call

zyelyonyj (zee-*lyo*-nihy): green

English-Russian Mini-Dictionary

A

address: **adryes** (*ahd*-rees) m

airplane: **samolyot** (suh-mah-*lyot*) m

airport: **aeroport** (uh-eh-rah-*pohrt*) m

also: **tozhye** (*toh*-zhih)

apartment: **kvartira** (kvuhr-*tee*-ruh) f

application: **zayavlyeniye** (zuh-eev-*lye*-nee-ee) n

April: **apryel'** (uhp-*ryel'*) m

arm: **ruka** (roo-*kah*) f

ask: **sprashivat'/sprosit'** (*sprah*-shih-vuht'/sprah-*seet'*)

August: **avgust** (*ahv*-goost) m

B

back: **spina** (spee-*nah*) f

bad: **plokhoj** (plah-*khohy*)

bag: **sumka** (*soom*-kuh) f

ballet: **balyet** (buh-*lyet*) m

bank: **bank** (bahnk) m

be: **byt'** (biht')

beautiful: **krasivyj** (kruh-*see*-vihy)

bed: **krovat'** (krah-*vaht'*) f

beer: **pivo** (*pee*-vuh) n

big: **bol'shoj** (bahl'-*shohy*)

black: **chyornyj** (*chohr*-nihy)

blue: **sinij** (*see*-neey)

book: **kniga** (*knee*-guh) f

boring: **skuchnyj** (*skoosh*-nihy)

bottle: **butylka** (boo-*tihl*-kuh) f

boy: **mal'chik** (*mahl'*-cheek) m

bread: **khlyeb** (khlyep) m

breakfast: **zavtrak** (*zahf*-truhk) m

bring: **prinosit'/prinyesti** (pree-nah-*seet'*/pree-nees-*tee*)

brother: **brat'/vzyat'** (braht'/vzyat') m

brown: **korichnyevyj** (kah-*reech*-nee-vihy)

bus: **avtobus** (uhf-*toh*-boos) m

but: **no** (noh)

buy: **pokupat'/kupit'** (puh-koo-*paht'*/koo-*peet'*)

C

call: **zvonit'/pozvonit'** (zvah-*neet'*/puh-zvah-*neet'*)

can: **moch'/smoch'** (mohch'/smohch')

car: **mashina** (muh-*shih*-nuh) f

cash: **nalichnyye** (nuh-*leech*-nih-ee)

cash register: **kassa** (*kah*-suh) f

change: **sdacha** (*sdah*-chuh) f

cheap: **dyeshyovyj** (dee-*shoh*-vihy)

check: **chyek** (chyek) m

cheese: **syr** (sihr) m

child: **ryebyonok** (ree-*byo*-nuhk) m

church: **tsyerkov'** (*tsehr*-kuhf') f

city: **gorod** (*goh*-ruht) m

clock: **chasy** (chee-*sih*)

coat: **pal'to** (puhl'-*toh*) n

coffee: **kofye** (*koh*-fee) m

cold: **kholodnyj** (khah-*lohd*-nihy)

collect: **sobirat'/sobrat'** (sub-bee-*raht'*/sah-*braht'*)

come: **prikhodit'/pridti** (pree-khah-*deet'*/preet-*tee*)

company: **kompaniya** (kahm-*pah*-nee-ye) f

country: **strana** (struh-*nah*) f

credit card: **kryeditnaya kartochka** (kree-*deet*-nuh-ye *kahr*-tuhch-kuh) f

cup: **chashka** (*chahsh*-kuh) f

customs: **tamozhnya** (tuh-*mohzh*-nye) f

D

daughter: **doch'** (dohch') f

day: **dyen'** (dyen') m

dear: **dorogoj** (duh-rah-*gohy*)

December: **dyekabr'** (dee-*kahbr'*) m

dentist: **zubnoj vrach/dantist** (zoob-*nohy* vrahch/duhn-*teest*) m

department: **otdyel** (aht-*dyel*) m

dessert: **dyesyert** (dee-*syert*) m

dinner: **uzhin** (*oo*-zhihn) m

do: **dyelat'/sdyelat'** (*dye*-luht'/*sdye*-luht')

doctor: **vrach** (vrahch) m

door: **dvyer'** (dvyer') f

dress: **plat'ye** (*plaht'*-ee) n

E

early: **rano** (*rah*-nuh)

east: **vostok** (vahs-*tohk*) m

easy: **legko** (leekh-*koh*)

eat: **yest'** (yest')

e-mail: **imyeil** (ee-*meh*-eel) m

end: **konets** (kah-*nyets*) m

enter: **vkhodit'/vojti** (vkhah-*deet'*/vahy-*tee*)

entrance: **vkhod** (vkhoht) m

evening: **vyechyer** (*vye*-cheer) m

everybody: **vsye** (fsye)

everything: **vsyo** (fsyo)

exit: **vykhod** (*vih*-khuht)

expensive: **dorogoj** (duh-rah-*gohy*)

F

face: **litso** (lee-*tsoh*) n

fall: **osyen'** (*oh*-seen') f

family: **syem'ya** (seem'-*ya*) f

father: **otyets** (ah-*tyets*) m

fax: **faks** (fahks) m

February: **fevral'** (feev-*rahl'*) m

find: **nakhodit'/najti** (nuh-khah-*deet'*/nuhy-*tee*)

finish: **zakanchivat'/zakonchit'** (zuh-*kahn*-chee-vuht'/zuh-*kohn*-cheet')

fire: **pozhar** (pah-*zhahr*) m

firm: **firma** (*feer*-muh) f

fish: **ryba** (*rih*-buh) f

fly: **lyetat'/lyetyet'** (lee-*taht'*/lee-*tyet'*)

food: **yeda** (ee-*dah*) f

foreign: **inostrannyj** (ee-nahs-*trah*-nihy)

fork: **vilka** (*veel*-kuh) f

Friday: **pyatnitsa** (*pyat*-nee-tsuh) f

friend: **drug** (drook) m

from: **iz** (ees)

fruits: **frukty** (*frook*-tih) m

G

get: **dostavat'/dostat'** (duhs-tah-*vaht'*/dahs-*taht'*)

gift: **podarok** (pah-*dah*-ruhk) m

girl: **dyevochka** (*dye*-vuhch-kuh) f

give: **davat'/daht'** (duh-*vaht'*/daht')

go: **idti/yekhat'** (eet-*tee*/ye-khuht')

good: **khoroshij** (khah-*roh*-shihy)

goodbye: **do svidaniya** (duh svee-*dah*-nee-ye)

grandfather: **dyedushka** (*dye*-doosh-kuh) f

grandmother: **babushka** (*bah*-boosh-kuh) f

gray: **syeryj** (*sye*-rihy)

green: **zyelyonyj** (zee-*lyo*-nihy)

guest: **gost'** (gohst') m

H

hair: **volosy** (*voh*-luh-sih)

hand: **ruka** (roo-*kah*) f

hat: **shapka** (*shahp*-kuh) f

have: **imyet'** (ee-*myet'*)

have to: **dolzhyen** (*dohl*-zhihn)

he: **on** (ohn)

head: **golova** (guh-lah-*vah*) f

health: **zdorov'ye** (zdah-*rohv'*-ee) n

hello: **zdravstvujtye** (*zdrah*-stvooy-tee)

help: **pomogat'/pomoch'** (puh-mah-*gaht'*/pah-*mohch*)

here: **zdyes'/tut** (zdyes'/toot)

hi: **privyet** (pree-*vyet*)

high: **vysokij** (vih-*soh*-keey)

hospital: **bol'nitsa** (bahl'-*nee*-tsuh) f

hot: **zharko** (*zhahr*-kuh)

hotel: **gostinitsa** (gahs-*tee*-nee-tsuh) f

hour: **chas** (chahs) m

house: **dom** (dohm) m

how: **kak** (kahk)

how many, how much: **skol'ko** (*skohl'*-kuh)

husband: **muzh** (moosh) m

I

I: **ya** (ya)

ill: **bolyen** (*boh*-leen)

important: **vazhnyj** (*vahzh*-nihy)

introduce: **pryedstavlyat'/pryedstavit'** (preet-stuhv-*lyat'*/preet-*stah*-veet')

it: **ono** (ah-*noh*)

J

jacket: **kurtka** (*koort*-kuh) f

January: **yanvar'** (een-*vahr'*) m

jeans: **dzhinsy** (*dzhihn*-sih)

job: **rabota** (ruh-*boh*-tuh) f

July: **iyul'** (ee-*yul'*) m

June: **iyun'** (ee-*yun'*) m

K

knee: **kolyeno** (kah-*lye*-nuh) n

knife: **nozh** (nohsh) m

know: **znat'** (znaht')

L

late: **pozdno** (*pohz*-nuh)

laugh: **smyeyat'sya** (smee-*yat*-sye)

lawyer: **yurist** (yu-*reest*) m

leave: **ukhodit'/ujti** (oo-khah-*deet'*/ooy-*tee*)

leg: **noga** (nah-*gah*) f

letter: **pis'mo** (pees'-*moh*) n

like: **nravit'sya/ponravit'sya** (*nrah*-veet'-sye/pah-*nrah*-veet'-sye)

live: **zhit'** (zhiht')

long: **dlinnyj** (*dlee*-nihy)

look: **smotryet'/posmotryet'** (smaht-*ryet'*/puhs-mah-*tryet'*)

love: **lyubit'** (lyu-*beet'*)

lunch: **obyed** (ah-*byet*) m

M

main: **glavnyj** (*glahv*-nihy)

make: **dyelat'/sdyelat'**(*dye*-luht'/*sdye*-luht')

man: **muzhchina** (moo-*sh'ee*-nuh) m

March: **mart** (mahrt) m

market: **rynok** (*rih*-nuhk) m

May: **maj** (mahy) m

may: **mozhno** (*mohzh*-nuh)

meat: **myaso** (*mya*-suh) n

medicine: **lyekarstvo** (lee-*kahrst*-vuh) n

meeting: **vstryecha** (*fstrye*-chuh) f

milk: **moloko** (muh-lah-*koh*) n

minute: **minuta** (mee-*noo*-tuh) f

Monday: **ponyedyel'nik** (puh-nee-*dyel'*-neek) m

money: **dyen'gi** (*dyen'*-gee)

month: **myesyats** (*mye*-seets) m

morning: **utro** (*oot*-ruh) n

mother: **mat'** (maht') f

mountain: **gora** (gah-*rah*) f

movie theater: **kino** (kee-*noh*) n

museum: **muzyej** (moo-*zyey*) m

N

name: **imya** (*ee*-mye) n

never: **nikogda** (nee-kahg-*dah*)

new: **novyj** (*noh*-vihy)

newspaper: **gazyeta** (guh-*zye*-tuh) f

night: **noch'** (nohch') f

north: **syevyer** (*sye*-veer) n

November: **noyabr'** (nah-*yabr'*) m

now: **syejchas/tyepyer'** (see-*chahs*/tee-*pyer'*)

number: **nomyer** (*noh*-meer) m

nurse: **myedsyestra** (meet-sees-*trah*) f

O

October: **oktyabr'** (ahk-*tyabr'*) m

office: **offis** (*oh*-fees) m

old: **staryj** (*stah*-rihy)

only: **tol'ko** (*tohl'*-kuh)

P

palace: **dvoryets** (dvah-*ryets*) m

pants: **bryuki** (*bryu*-kee)

party: **vyechyerinka** (vee-chee-*reen*-kuh) f

passport: **pasport** (*pahs*-puhrt) m

pay: **platit'/zaplatit'**(pluh-*teet'*/zuh-pluh-*teet'*)

people: **lyudi** (*lyu*-dee)

phone: **tyelyefon** (tee-lee-*fohn*) m

physician: **tyerapyevt** (teh-ruh-*pehft*) m

plate: **taryelka** (tuh-*ryel*-kuh) f

please: **pozhalujsta** (pah-*zhahl*-stuh)

police: **militsiya** (mee-*lee*-tsih-ye) f

price: **tsyena** (tsih-*nah*) f

problem: **problyema** (prahb-*lye*-muh) f

Q

question: **vopros** (vahp-*rohs*) m

R

rain: **dozhd'** (dohsht') m

raincoat: **plash'** (plahsh') m

read: **chitat'/prochitat'** (chee-*taht'*/pruh-chee-*taht'*)

red: **krasnyj** (*krahs*-nihy)

rent: **snimat'/snyat'** (snee-*maht'*/*snyat'*)

restaurant: **ryestoran** (rees-tah-*rahn*) m

river: **ryeka** (ree-*kah*) f

room: **komnata** (*kohm*-nuh-tuh) f

S

salad: **salat** (suh-*laht*) m

sale: **rasprodazha** (ruhs-prah-*dah*-zhuh) f

sales assistant: **prodavyets** (pruh-duh-*vyets*) m

salt: **sol'** (sohl') f

Saturday: **subbota** (soo-*boh*-tuh) f

say: **govorit'/skazat'** (guh-vah-*reet'*/skuh-*zaht'*)

school: **shkola** (*shkoh*-luh) f

sea: **morye** (*moh*-ree) n

seat: **myesto** (*myes*-tuh) n

see: **vidyet'/uvidet'** (*vee*-deet'/oo-*vee*-deet')

sell: **prodavat'/prodat'** (pruh-duh-*vaht'*/prah-*daht'*)

September: **syentyabr'** (seen-*tyabr'*) m

she: **ona** (ah-*nah*)

shirt: **rubashka** (roo-*bahsh*-kuh) f

shoes: **tufli** (*toof*-lee)

shop: **magazin** (muh-guh-*zeen*) m

show: **pokazyvat'/pokazat'** (pah-*kah*-zih-vuht'/puh-kuh-*zaht'*)

sister: **syestra** (sees-*trah*) f

sit: **sidyet'** (see-*dyet'*)

skirt: **yubka** (*yup*-kuh) f

sleep: **spat'** (spaht')

small: **malyen'kij** (*mah*-leen'-keey)

snow: **snyeg** (snyek) m

something: **chto-to** (*shtoh*-tuh)

son: **syn** (sihn) m

south: **yug** (yuk) m

souvenir: **suvyenir** (soo-vee-*neer*) m

spoon: **lozhka** (*lohsh*-kuh) f

sports: **sport** (spohrt) m

spring: **vyesna** (vees-*nah*) f

square: **plosh'ad'** (ploh-sh'iht') f

stand: **stoyat** (stah-*yat'*)

state: **shtat** (shtaht) m

station: **vokzal** (vahg-*zahl*) m

stomach: **zhivot** (zhih-*voht*) m

street: **ulitsa** (*oo*-lee-tsuh) f

subway: **myetro** (meet-*roh*) n

sugar: **sakhar** (*sah*-khuhr) m

suit: **kostyum** (kahs-*tyum*) m

suitcase: **chyemodan** (chee-mah-*dahn*) m

summer: **lyeto** (*lye*-tuh) n

Sunday: **voskryesyen'ye** (vuhs-kree-*syen'*-ee) n

sweet: **sladkij** (*slaht*-keey)

T

take: **brat'/vzyat'** (braht'/vzyat')

tall: **vysokij** (vih-*soh*-keey)

teacher: **uchityel'** (oo-*chee*-teel') m

tell: **rasskazyvat'/rasskazat'** (ruhs-*kah*-zih-vuht'/ruhs-kuh-*zaht'*)

thank you: **spasibo** (spuh-*see*-buh)

theater: **tyeatr** (tee-*ahtr*) m

they: **oni** (ah-*nee*)

thing: **vyesh'** (vyesh') f

think: **dumat'** (*doo*-muht')

Thursday: **chyetvyerg** (cheet-*vyerk*) m

ticket: **bilyet** (bee-*lyet*) m

tie: **galstuk** (*gahls*-took) m

time: **vryemya** (*vrye*-mye) n

today: **syegodnya** (see-*vohd*-nye)

tomorrow: **zavtra** (*zahf*-truh)

too (excessively): **slishkom** (*sleesh*-kuhm)

train: **poyezd** (*poh*-eest) m

travel: **putyeshyestvovat'** (poo-tee-*shehst*-vuh-vuht')

Tuesday: **vtornik** (*ftohr*-neek) m

turn: **povorachivat'/povyernut'** (puh-vah-*rah*-chee-vuht'/puh-veer-*noot'*)

U

university: **univyersityet** (oo-nee-veer-see-*tyet*) m

V

vacation: **otpusk** (*oht*-poosk) m

vegetables: **ovosh'i** (*oh*-vuh-sh'ee)

visa: **viza** (*vee*-zuh) f

W

wait: **zhdat'** (zhdaht')

waiter: **ofitsiant** (uh-fee-tsih-*ahnt*) m

want: **khotyet'** (khah-*tyet'*)

warm: **tyoplyj** (*tyop*-lihy)

water: **voda** (vah-*dah*) f

wear: **nosit'/nyesti** (nah-*seet'*/nees-*tee*)

Wednesday: **sryeda** (sree-*dah*) f

week: **nyedyelya** (nee-*dye*-lye) f

well: **khorosho** (khuh-rah-*shoh*)

west: **zapad** (*zah*-puht) m

what: **chto** (shtoh)

when: **kogda** (kuhg-*dah*)

where: **gdye** (gdye)

white: **byelyj** (*bye*-lihy)

who: **kto** (ktoh)

why: **pochyemu** (puh-chee-*moo*)

wife: **zhyena** (zhih-*nah*) f

window: **okno** (ahk-*noh*) n

wine: **vino** (vee-*noh*) n

winter: **zima** (zee-*mah*) f

woman: **zhyensh'ina** (*zhehn*-sh'ee-nuh) f

word: **slovo** (*sloh*-vuh) n

work: **rabotat'** (ruh-*boh*-tuht')

Y

year: **god** (goht) m

yellow: **zhyoltyj** (*zhohl*-tihy)

yesterday: **vchyera** (fchee-*rah*)

you (plural, formal): **vy** (vih)

you (singular, informal): **ty** (tih)

young: **molodoj** (muh-lah-*dohy*)

you're welcome: **pozhalujsta** (pah-*zhah*-loos-tuh)

Z

zip code: **indyex** (*een*-dehks) m

Appendix C

Answer Key

• •

*T*he following are all the answers to the Fun & Games activities.

Chapter 1

Match the Russian letters with the sounds they correspond to:

1. b   2. a   3. e   4. d   5. c

Sound out the Russian words and recognize their meaning:

1. vodka   2. borsht (beet soup)   3. perestroika   4. glasnost
5. sputnik   6. tsar

Chapter 2

Find the nominative singular:

1. **komp'yutyer**   2. **kniga**   3. **okno**   4. **koshka**   5. **magazin**

How many of these Russian numerals can you recognize?

1 **odin**	2 **dva**
4 **chyetyrye**	8 **vosyem'**
12 **dvyenadtsat'**	15 **pyatnadtsat'**
20 **dvadtsat'**	100 **sto**
500 **pyat'sot**	1,000 **tysyacha**

20,347 **dvadtsat' tysyach trista sorok syem'**
600,091 **shyest'sot tysyach dyevyanosto odin**

Chapter 3

Practice saying *Hello* in Russian:

1. **Zdravstvuj!**   2. **Zdravstvujtye!**   3. **Zdravstvujtye!**
4. **Zdravstvujtye!**   5. **Zdravstvuj!**   6. **Zdravstvujtye!**
7. **Zdravstvujtye!**

Practicing greetings by the time of day:

Dobryj dyen'! (3 p.m.)   **Dobroye utro!** (11 a.m.)   **Dobroye utro!** (8 a.m.)
Dobryj vyechyer! (8 p.m.)

Unscramble the dialogue:

Nina: **Zdravstvuj! Davaj poznakomimsya!**
Natasha: **Davaj!**
Nina: **Myenya zovut Nina. A kak tyebya zovut?**
Natasha: **Myenya zovut Natasha.**
Nina: **Ochyen' priyatno!**
Natasha: **Mnye tozhye.**

Chapter 4

Which of the two words indicates a woman?

1. b. **amyerikanka**   2. b. **russkaya**   3. b. **nyemka**   4. a. **yevryejka**
5. a. **frantsuzhyenka**

Which of the three words doesn't belong to the group?

1. **plyemyannik**   2. **otyets**   3. **doch'**   4. **babushka**   5. **otyets**

Which of the following statements just doesn't make sense?

4. **Domokhozyajka rabotayet na fabrikye.**

Chapter 5

Which of the following two dishes would you most likely eat for breakfast in
Russia?

1. a. **yaichnitsa**   2. b. **butyerbrod s kolbasoj**   3. a. **butyerbrod s syrom**
4. b. **kasha**   5. a. **varyen'ye**

Which of the following phrases would you probably use or hear while making
a restaurant reservation?

1. **Ya khotyel by zakazat' stolik na subbotu.**
3. **Na dvoikh.**
4. **Skol'ko chyelovyek?**
5. **Na vosyem' chasov.**
8. **Ya khotyela by zakazat' stolik na syegodnya.**
9. **Na kakoye vryemya?**

Chapter 6

At which of these stores are you likely to find the following items?

1. b   2. d   3. a   4. c   5. g   6. e   7. f

Making comparisons:

1. b   2. d   3. c   4. e

Chapter 7

Which of the following two days comes earlier during the week?

1. **ponyedyel'nik**   2. **chyetvyerg**   3. **voskryesyen'ye**
4. **voskryesyen'ye**

Which of the two verbs — **nachinayetsya** or **nachinayet** — would you use?

1. **nachinayet**   2. **nachinayetsya**   3. **nachinayetsya**   4. **nachinayet**

Which of the following phrases would you probably use to express that you liked the show or performance you attended?

1. **Mnye ponravilsya spyektakl'.**   2. **Potryasayush'ye!**   5. **Ochyen' krasivyj balyet.**

Chapter 8

Match the phrases:

1. b   2. c   3. d   4. a

Where are you most likely to see all these things?

1. c   2. b   3. a

What do they like to do?

Vanessa Mae **lyubit igrat' na skripkye.**
Renoir **lyubit pisat' maslom.**
Michelangelo **lyubit lyepit'.**
Tolstoy **lyubit pisat' romany.**
Santana **lyubit igrat' na gitarye.**

Chapter 9

Which words and expressions indicate types of phones?

1. **mobil'nik** (mobile phone)   2. **knopochnyj tyelyefon** (touch-tone phone)
5. **trubka** (mobile phone)

The telephone dialogue in the right order:

d. **Mozhno Marinu?**
a. **Mariny nyet doma. A kto yeyo sprashivayet?**
c. **Eto Pyetya. Pyeryedajtye pozhalujsta chto zvonil Pyetya.**
b. **Khorosho.**

Match the Russian equivalents on the left for the English phrases:

1. b   2. c   3. d   4. a

Chapter 10

Match the rooms with the most appropriate furniture:

1. c   2. a   3. b

In which of the following sections of the Classifieds will you NOT find information about apartments for rent?

3. **Rabota**

Chapter 11

Find Russian equivalents for the given dates:

1. a   2. d   3. b   4. c

Which of the following places of interest is not located in St. Petersburg?

2. **Novodyevich'ye kladbish'ye**

Chapter 12

Which of these sentences don't make sense?

2. **Ya yedu pyeshkom.**
4. **My idyom v Moskvu.**

Which of the following will you NOT see at an airport?

c. **poyezd**

Chapter 13

Select the appropriate response for the following phrases:

1. a. **Odnomyestnyj nomyer, pozhalujsta.**
2. b. **Na kakoye chislo?**
3. c. **Kak vasha familiya?**

Help John Evans fill out his hotel registration form:

imya — John
familiya — Evans
adryes — 123 Highpoint Drive, Chicago, USA
domashnij tyelyefon — 815/555-5544

Unscramble the dialogue:

b. **U myenya zabronirovan nomyer.**
d. **Kak vasha familiya?**
a. **Moya familiya Ivanov.**
c. **Zapolnitye ryegistratsionnuyu kartochku.**

Chapter 14

Matching money-related activities with places where they are appropriate:

1. c   2. d   3. b   4. a

Putting descriptions of interactions with a Russian bank in chronological order:

c. **otkryt' schyot**
a. **sdyelat' vklad**
b. **zakryt' schyot**

Making payments:

1. Tom   2. Mickey

Chapter 15

Which would you use: **gdye** or **kuda**?

1. **kuda**   2. **gdye**   3. **gdye**   4. **kuda**   5. **kuda**

Select the correct translation of the English phrases:

1. a. **ryadom s bankom**
2. a. **naprotiv banka**
3. a. **sprava ot banka**

Which of the suburbs is farthest from St. Petersburg?

2. **Ryepino** — 70 kilometers away

Chapter 16

What place would you call?

1. c   2. a   3. b

Matching symptoms with the most probable sicknesses:

1. b   2. c   3. a

Picking the word that doesn't belong:

1. **gripp**   2. **pryestupnik**   3. **pozhar**

Appendix D

On the CD

Track 1: Introduction

Track 2: Pronouncing Russian letters (Chapter 1)

Track 3: Using English cognates (Chapter 1)

Track 4: Using different verb tenses (Chapter 2)

Track 5: Meeting and greeting (Chapter 3)

Track 6: Introducing people to each other (Chapter 3)

Track 7: Talking about your nationality and ethnic background (Chapter 4)

Track 8: Talking about food (Chapter 5)

Track 9: Ordering a meal (Chapter 5)

Track 10: Finding the haberdashery department (Chapter 6)

Track 11: Telling about a new dress (Chapter 6)

Track 12: Asking for the time (Chapter 7)

Track 13: Discussing a ballet performance (Chapter 7)

Track 14: Talking about books (Chapter 8)

Track 15: Discussing sports (Chapter 8)

Track 16: Getting the wrong number (Chapter 9)

Track 17: Making a phone call (Chapter 9)

Track 18: Talking about renting an apartment (Chapter 10)

Track 19: Buying furniture (Chapter 10)

Track 20: Getting a job (Chapter 10)

Track 21: Submitting documents for a visa (Chapter 11)

Track 22: Talking about moving around (Chapter 12)

Track 23: Going through passport control (Chapter 12)

Track 24: Making hotel reservations (Chapter 13)

Track 25: Checking in to a hotel (Chapter 13)

Track 26: Exchanging money (Chapter 14)

Track 27: Opening a bank account (Chapter 14)

Track 28: Giving directions to a restaurant (Chapter 15)

Track 29: Asking for directions to a museum (Chapter 15)

Track 30: Calling the ambulance (Chapter 16)

Track 31: Going to the doctor (Chapter 16)

Index

• Q •

• R •

• V •

Notes

BUSINESS, CAREERS & PERSONAL FINANCE

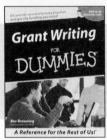

Grant Writing FOR DUMMIES

A Reference for the Rest of Us!

0-7645-5307-0

Home Buying FOR DUMMIES

A Reference for the Rest of Us!

0-7645-5331-3 *†

Also available:

- Accounting For Dummies †
  0-7645-5314-3
- Business Plans Kit For Dummies †
  0-7645-5365-8
- Cover Letters For Dummies
  0-7645-5224-4
- Frugal Living For Dummies
  0-7645-5403-4
- Leadership For Dummies
  0-7645-5176-0
- Managing For Dummies
  0-7645-1771-6

- Marketing For Dummies
  0-7645-5600-2
- Personal Finance For Dummies *
  0-7645-2590-5
- Project Management For Dummies
  0-7645-5283-X
- Resumes For Dummies †
  0-7645-5471-9
- Selling For Dummies
  0-7645-5363-1
- Small Business Kit For Dummies *†
  0-7645-5093-4

HOME & BUSINESS COMPUTER BASICS

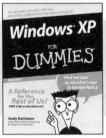

Windows XP FOR DUMMIES

A Reference for the Rest of Us!

0-7645-4074-2

Microsoft Office Excel 2003 ALL-IN-ONE DESK REFERENCE FOR DUMMIES

9 BOOKS IN 1

0-7645-3758-X

Also available:

- ACT! 6 For Dummies
  0-7645-2645-6
- iLife '04 All-in-One Desk Reference
  For Dummies
  0-7645-7347-0
- iPAQ For Dummies
  0-7645-6769-1
- Mac OS X Panther Timesaving
  Techniques For Dummies
  0-7645-5812-9
- Macs For Dummies
  0-7645-5656-8

- Microsoft Money 2004 For Dummies
  0-7645-4195-1
- Office 2003 All-in-One Desk Reference
  For Dummies
  0-7645-3883-7
- Outlook 2003 For Dummies
  0-7645-3759-8
- PCs For Dummies
  0-7645-4074-2
- TiVo For Dummies
  0-7645-6923-6
- Upgrading and Fixing PCs For Dummies
  0-7645-1665-5
- Windows XP Timesaving Techniques
  For Dummies
  0-7645-3748-2

FOOD, HOME, GARDEN, HOBBIES, MUSIC & PETS

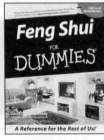

Feng Shui FOR DUMMIES

A Reference for the Rest of Us!

0-7645-5295-3

Poker FOR DUMMIES

A Reference for the Rest of Us!

0-7645-5232-5

Also available:

- Bass Guitar For Dummies
  0-7645-2487-9
- Diabetes Cookbook For Dummies
  0-7645-5230-9
- Gardening For Dummies *
  0-7645-5130-2
- Guitar For Dummies
  0-7645-5106-X
- Holiday Decorating For Dummies
  0-7645-2570-0
- Home Improvement All-in-One
  For Dummies
  0-7645-5680-0

- Knitting For Dummies
  0-7645-5395-X
- Piano For Dummies
  0-7645-5105-1
- Puppies For Dummies
  0-7645-5255-4
- Scrapbooking For Dummies
  0-7645-7208-3
- Senior Dogs For Dummies
  0-7645-5818-8
- Singing For Dummies
  0-7645-2475-5
- 30-Minute Meals For Dummies
  0-7645-2589-1

INTERNET & DIGITAL MEDIA

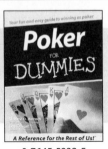

Digital Photography FOR DUMMIES

A Reference for the Rest of Us!

0-7645-1664-7

Starting an eBay Business FOR DUMMIES

A Reference for the Rest of Us!

0-7645-6924-4

Also available:

- 2005 Online Shopping Directory
  For Dummies
  0-7645-7495-7
- CD & DVD Recording For Dummies
  0-7645-5956-7
- eBay For Dummies
  0-7645-5654-1
- Fighting Spam For Dummies
  0-7645-5965-6
- Genealogy Online For Dummies
  0-7645-5964-8
- Google For Dummies
  0-7645-4420-9

- Home Recording For Musicians
  For Dummies
  0-7645-1634-5
- The Internet For Dummies
  0-7645-4173-0
- iPod & iTunes For Dummies
  0-7645-7772-7
- Preventing Identity Theft For Dummies
  0-7645-7336-5
- Pro Tools All-in-One Desk Reference
  For Dummies
  0-7645-5714-9
- Roxio Easy Media Creator For Dummies
  0-7645-7131-1

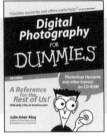

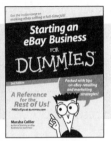

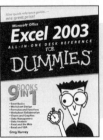

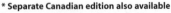

* **Separate Canadian edition also available**

† **Separate U.K. edition also available**

Available wherever books are sold. For more information or to order direct: U.S. customers visit www.dummies.com or call 1-877-762-2974.
U.K. customers visit www.wileyeurope.com or call 0800 243407. Canadian customers visit www.wiley.ca or call 1-800-567-4797.

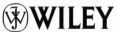 WILEY

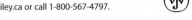

SPORTS, FITNESS, PARENTING, RELIGION & SPIRITUALITY

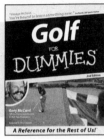

0-7645-5146-9

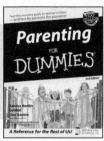

0-7645-5418-2

Also available:

- Adoption For Dummies
  0-7645-5488-3
- Basketball For Dummies
  0-7645-5248-1
- The Bible For Dummies
  0-7645-5296-1
- Buddhism For Dummies
  0-7645-5359-3
- Catholicism For Dummies
  0-7645-5391-7
- Hockey For Dummies
  0-7645-5228-7

- Judaism For Dummies
  0-7645-5299-6
- Martial Arts For Dummies
  0-7645-5358-5
- Pilates For Dummies
  0-7645-5397-6
- Religion For Dummies
  0-7645-5264-3
- Teaching Kids to Read For Dummies
  0-7645-4043-2
- Weight Training For Dummies
  0-7645-5168-X
- Yoga For Dummies
  0-7645-5117-5

TRAVEL

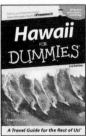

0-7645-5438-7

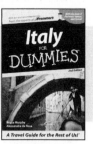

0-7645-5453-0

Also available:

- Alaska For Dummies
  0-7645-1761-9
- Arizona For Dummies
  0-7645-6938-4
- Cancún and the Yucatán For Dummies
  0-7645-2437-2
- Cruise Vacations For Dummies
  0-7645-6941-4
- Europe For Dummies
  0-7645-5456-5
- Ireland For Dummies
  0-7645-5455-7

- Las Vegas For Dummies
  0-7645-5448-4
- London For Dummies
  0-7645-4277-X
- New York City For Dummies
  0-7645-6945-7
- Paris For Dummies
  0-7645-5494-8
- RV Vacations For Dummies
  0-7645-5443-3
- Walt Disney World & Orlando For Dummies
  0-7645-6943-0

GRAPHICS, DESIGN & WEB DEVELOPMENT

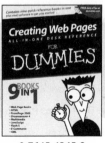

0-7645-4345-8

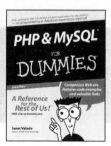

0-7645-5589-8

Also available:

- Adobe Acrobat 6 PDF For Dummies
  0-7645-3760-1
- Building a Web Site For Dummies
  0-7645-7144-3
- Dreamweaver MX 2004 For Dummies
  0-7645-4342-3
- FrontPage 2003 For Dummies
  0-7645-3882-9
- HTML 4 For Dummies
  0-7645-1995-6
- Illustrator CS For Dummies
  0-7645-4084-X

- Macromedia Flash MX 2004 For Dummies
  0-7645-4358-X
- Photoshop 7 All-in-One Desk
  Reference For Dummies
  0-7645-1667-1
- Photoshop CS Timesaving Techniques
  For Dummies
  0-7645-6782-9
- PHP 5 For Dummies
  0-7645-4166-8
- PowerPoint 2003 For Dummies
  0-7645-3908-6
- QuarkXPress 6 For Dummies
  0-7645-2593-X

NETWORKING, SECURITY, PROGRAMMING & DATABASES

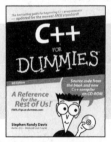

0-7645-6852-3

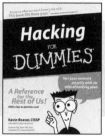

0-7645-5784-X

Also available:

- A+ Certification For Dummies
  0-7645-4187-0
- Access 2003 All-in-One Desk
  Reference For Dummies
  0-7645-3988-4
- Beginning Programming For Dummies
  0-7645-4997-9
- C For Dummies
  0-7645-7068-4
- Firewalls For Dummies
  0-7645-4048-3
- Home Networking For Dummies
  0-7645-42796

- Network Security For Dummies
  0-7645-1679-5
- Networking For Dummies
  0-7645-1677-9
- TCP/IP For Dummies
  0-7645-1760-0
- VBA For Dummies
  0-7645-3989-2
- Wireless All In-One Desk Reference
  For Dummies
  0-7645-7496-5
- Wireless Home Networking For Dummies
  0-7645-3910-8

HEALTH & SELF-HELP

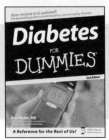
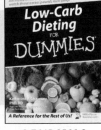

0-7645-6820-5 *†

0-7645-2566-2

Also available:

Alzheimer's For Dummies
0-7645-3899-3

Asthma For Dummies
0-7645-4233-8

Controlling Cholesterol For Dummies
0-7645-5440-9

Depression For Dummies
0-7645-3900-0

Dieting For Dummies
0-7645-4149-8

Fertility For Dummies
0-7645-2549-2

Fibromyalgia For Dummies
0-7645-5441-7

Improving Your Memory For Dummies
0-7645-5435-2

Pregnancy For Dummies †
0-7645-4483-7

Quitting Smoking For Dummies
0-7645-2629-4

Relationships For Dummies
0-7645-5384-4

Thyroid For Dummies
0-7645-5385-2

EDUCATION, HISTORY, REFERENCE & TEST PREPARATION

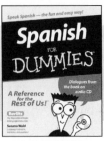
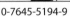
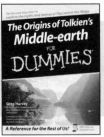

0-7645-5194-9

0-7645-4186-2

Also available:

Algebra For Dummies
0-7645-5325-9

British History For Dummies
0-7645-7021-8

Calculus For Dummies
0-7645-2498-4

English Grammar For Dummies
0-7645-5322-4

Forensics For Dummies
0-7645-5580-4

The GMAT For Dummies
0-7645-5251-1

Inglés Para Dummies
0-7645-5427-1

Italian For Dummies
0-7645-5196-5

Latin For Dummies
0-7645-5431-X

Lewis & Clark For Dummies
0-7645-2545-X

Research Papers For Dummies
0-7645-5426-3

The SAT I For Dummies
0-7645-7193-1

Science Fair Projects For Dummies
0-7645-5460-3

U.S. History For Dummies
0-7645-5249-X

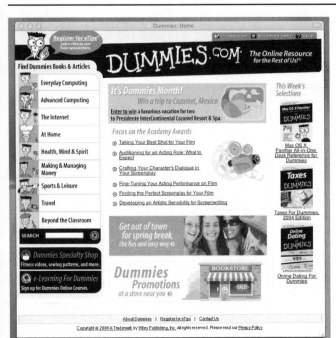

Get smart @ dummies.com®

- **Find a full list of Dummies titles**
- **Look into loads of FREE on-site articles**
- **Sign up for FREE eTips e-mailed to you weekly**
- **See what other products carry the Dummies name**
- **Shop directly from the Dummies bookstore**
- **Enter to win new prizes every month!**

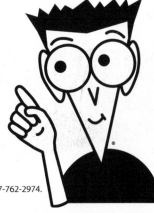

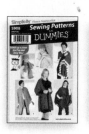
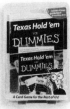
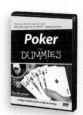
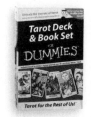
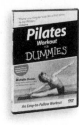
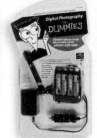
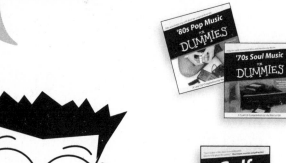
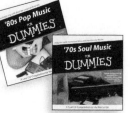
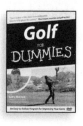
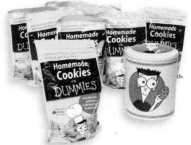
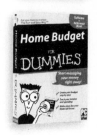
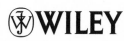

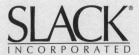

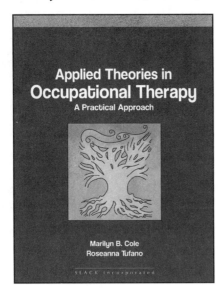